Recreational Therapy Basics, Techniques, and Interventions

Heather R. Porter, Ph.D., CTRS

Idyll Arbor's Recreational Therapy Practice Series

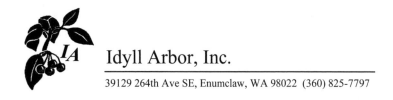

Idyll Arbor, Inc.

39129 264th Ave SE, Enumclaw, WA 98022 (360) 825-7797

Idyll Arbor's Recreational Therapy Practice Series Editor: Heather R. Porter, Ph.D., CTRS
Idyll Arbor, Inc. Editor: Thomas M. Blaschko
Cover design: Curt Pliler

To the best of our knowledge, the information and recommendations of this book reflect currently accepted practice. Nevertheless, they cannot be considered absolute and universal. Guidelines suggested by federal law are subject to change as the laws and interpretations do. Recommendations for a particular client must be considered in light of the client's needs and condition. The authors and publisher disclaim responsibility for any adverse effects resulting directly or indirectly from the suggested management practice, from any undetected errors, or from the reader's misunderstanding of the text.

ISBNs 9781882883974 paper, 9781611580570 e-book

Contents

Tables

Figures

Authors

Robert M. Beland, Ph.D.
Professor Emeritus
Department of Tourism, Recreation, and Sport
Management
University of Florida
Gainesville, FL

Genee Bower, B.S., CTRS
Therapeutic Recreation Coordinator
Oaks/Maplewood at Bethany Village
An Asbury Community
Mechanicsburg, PA

Mary Bowman, OTR/L
Occupational Therapist
Taub Training Clinic
University of Alabama at Birmingham
Birmingham, AL

Ellen Broach, Ed.D., CTRS, ATRIC
Associate Professor
Department of Health, Physical Education, and
Leisure Studies
University of South Alabama
Mobile, AL

Cynthia Carruthers, Ph.D., CTRS
Professor
Department of Educational and Clinical Studies
College of Education
University of Nevada, Las Vegas
Las Vegas, NV

Kathryn D. Elokdah, Ed.M., CTRS, ATP
Recreational Therapist
Department of Health and Human Services
National Institutes of Health
Clinical Research Center
Rehabilitation Medicine Department
Recreational Therapy Section
Bethesda, MD

Daniel D. Ferguson, Ph.D., CTRS
Professor
Department of Health, Human Performance, and
Recreation
Pittsburg State University
Pittsburg, KS

Diane Groff, Ed.D., LRT/CTRS
Associate Professor
Department of Exercise and Sport Science
Co-Founder of Get REAL and HEEL Breast
Cancer Program
University of North Carolina
Chapel Hill, NC

Elaine Hatala, Ph.D., CTRS
Assistant Professor
Department of Rehabilitation Sciences
Temple University
Philadelphia, PA

Colleen Deyell Hood, Ph.D., CTRS
Professor
Department of Recreation and Leisure Studies
Brock University
St. Catharines, ON

Susan Hutchinson, Ph.D.
Associate Professor
School of Health and Human Performance
Dalhousie University
Halifax, Nova Scotia, Canada

Glenn A. Kastrinos, M.Ed., CTRS/LRT
Assistant Professor
Department of Recreational Therapy
School of Health Sciences
Western Carolina University
Cullowhee, NC

Kari Kensinger, Ph.D., CTRS, CAS
Independent Recreational Therapy, Leisure
Behavior, and Autism Consultant
Omaha, NE

Yongho Lee, Ph.D., CTRS
Associate Professor
Department of Physical Education
Seoul National University
Seoul, Korea

Linda Levine-Madori, Ph.D., ATR-BC, CTRS, LCAT
Professor, Author, and Researcher
St. Thomas Aquinas College
Sparkill, NY
Founder and Trainer: The TTAP Method®

Donna L. Long, M.Ed., CTRS
Manager
MossRehab Clubhouse
Drucker Brain Injury Center
Philadelphia, PA

Terry Dean Long, Jr., Ph.D.
Professor
Department of Health and Human Services
Northwest Missouri State University
Maryville, MO

Neil Lundberg, Ph.D., TRS, CTRS
Associate Professor
Department of Recreation Management
Brigham Young University
Provo, UT

Alexis McKenney, Ed.D., CTRS
Associate Professor
Recreational Therapy Program
Florida International University
Miami, FL

Erin K. Moore, M.Ed., CTRS
Recreational Therapist
Belmont Behavioral Health Northeast
Philadelphia, PA

David M. Morris, Ph.D., PT
Professor
Department of Physical Therapy
University of Alabama at Birmingham
Birmingham, AL

Heather R. Porter, Ph.D., CTRS
Assistant Professor
Department of Rehabilitation Sciences
Temple University
Philadelphia, PA

Katelynn Ropars, M.S., CTRS
Recreational Therapist
Hill at Whitemarsh
Lafayette Hill, PA
and
Help-U-Bridge
West Chester, PA

Arlene A. Schmid, Ph.D., OTR
Associate Professor
Department of Occupational Therapy
Colorado State University
Fort Collins, CO

Jennifer L. Sciolla, M.S., CTRS, CCLS
Manager Child Life, Education, and Creative
Arts Therapy
The Children's Hospital of Philadelphia
Philadelphia, PA

Edward Taub, Ph.D.
University Professor
Department of Psychology
University of Alabama at Birmingham
Birmingham, AL

Marieke Van Puymbroeck, Ph.D., CTRS
Associate Professor
Department of Parks, Recreation, and Tourism
Management
Clemson University
Clemson, SC

Gena Bell Vargas, Ph.D., CTRS
Assistant Professor
Department of Rehabilitation Sciences
Temple University
Philadelphia, PA

Elizabeth H. Weybright, Ph.D., CTRS
Assistant Professor
Department of Human Development
Washington State University
Pullman, WA

J. Randal Wyble, M.S., CTRS
Assistant Professor and Therapeutic Recreation
Program Director
Therapeutic Recreation Program
College of Health Professions
Grand Valley State University
Grand Rapids, MI

Reviewers

Thanks to the individuals who graciously gave their time to review the 2006 edition and provide feedback for re-shaping this edition.

Jo Ann Coco-Ripp, Ph.D., LRT/CTRS
Associate Professor
Therapeutic Recreation Program Coordinator
School of Education and Human Performance
Winston-Salem State University
Winston-Salem, NC

Jennifer A. Piatt, Ph.D., CTRS
Assistant Professor
Department of Recreation, Park, and Tourism Studies
School of Public Health
Indiana University
Bloomington, IN

Thomas K. Skalko, Ph.D., LRT/CTRS
Professor
Recreational Therapy
College of Health and Human Performance
East Carolina University
Greenville, NC
and
Honorary Professor
College of Health Sciences
University of KwaZulu-Natal
Durban, South Africa

Research and Editing Assistants

The following individuals volunteered their time to be research and editing assistants. Their dedication to assist with recreational therapy research is highly commendable.

Rebecca Baro
Recreational Therapy Student
Temple University

Genee Bower
Recreational Therapy Student
Temple University

Joshua Cino
Recreational Therapy Student
Temple University

Morgan Ferrante
Recreational Therapy Student
Temple University

Tonya D. Fromm
Recreational Therapy Student
Temple University

Kristen Hartman
Recreational Therapy Student
Temple University

Tracy Ann Jastrzab
Recreational Therapy Student
Temple University

Lea Peterson
Recreational Therapy Student
Temple University

Erin Kate MacElroy
Recreational Therapy Student
Temple University

Yekaterina Mishin
Recreational Therapy Student
Temple University

Marianella Sanchez
Recreational Therapy Student
Temple University

Alexa Szal
Psychology Student
Temple University

Mandi Shearer
Recreational Therapy Student
Temple University

Rachel L. Thomas
Recreational Therapy Student
Temple University

Forward

In 2002, Heather R. Porter and joan burlingame embarked upon a major project — to consolidate recreational therapy practice into a handbook for students and clinicians and to explain it using the International Classification of Functioning, Disability, and Health (ICF). The project took four years and the first edition of the *Recreational Therapy Handbook of Practice: ICF-Based Diagnosis and Treatment* was published in 2006. The 770-page text was well received in the field, and earned special recognition by the Centers for Disease Control as being the first book, other than the ICF itself, to describe the ICF as a basis for healthcare practice.

Author joan burlingame moved onto other endeavors, so in 2010 I took on the task developing an updated version of the book. The first edition needed significant revision, as it was primarily based on clinical experiences. For the new edition I reached out to many content experts in the field of recreational therapy and asked them to contribute to the new evidence-based practice edition with the aim of making the text reflective of the entire profession.

As the project went forward, the publisher and I realized that there was too much information to fit into one book. We decided to create three books, one covering diagnoses (*Recreational Therapy for Specific Diagnoses and Conditions*), another describing the ICF (*Recreational Therapy and the International Classification of Functioning, Disability, and Health*), and this book (*Recreational Therapy Basics, Techniques, and Interventions*). This book offers an in-depth review of 10 recreational therapy basics and 41 techniques and interventions. In each chapter, the ICF codes have been integrated to assist therapists in identifying related codes. When we tie our practice to the set of international standards provided by the ICF, it is clear that what we do is at the cutting edge of healthcare practice. We are doing so much more than treating medical conditions. We are finding ways to restore the minds, bodies, and spirits of our clients to the best possible levels of personal, interpersonal, societal, and environmental well-being.

It is an essential resource for the education of recreational therapists, as well as a reference manual for practicing clinicians and researchers, in guiding the provision of quality evidence-based care aimed at maximizing health, function, and participation. It is with great appreciation that I thank the authors who have contributed to this set of books. Their hard work, passion, and dedication to the profession serve as an inspiration to all currently in the field and those to who will follow.

— Heather Porter

Introduction

The legitimization of a field of study and the subsequent development of best practices is based on its proven outcomes through efficacy research published in peer-reviewed journals. Evidence-based research is required to demonstrate the value of the therapy provided. In recreational therapy, we have a fair amount of case studies, survey studies, and experimental design studies without a control group. In order to strengthen our field, we need to conduct more rigorous studies, such as randomized control trials (considered the gold standard of research studies), followed by systematic reviews and meta-analyses.

This text provides techniques that have proven valuable in recreational therapy treatment and the most up-to-date efficacy research for each of them. Using this information as a starting point, we need to look at recreational therapy interventions and techniques with the goal of improving our current evidence base. As our research designs strengthen and the number of studies increases, recreational therapy stands poised to address (and show efficacy for) some of the most concerning issues in our healthcare system.

This book provides a starting point for practice and ongoing research. It is divided into two parts. Therapy Basics provides a set of background information about recreational therapy practice that is necessary for understanding how the techniques work. Techniques and Interventions describe specific treatment modalities that recreational therapists can choose from when working with clients.

In the Therapy Basics section, the book describes nine treatment considerations that are part of almost every recreational therapy intervention. While the interplay between therapist and client is evident in each of these areas, each chapter has a primary focus on either the therapist or the client. Topics the look mostly at what the recreational therapist does include Activity and Task Analysis, Body Mechanics and Ergonomics, Education and Counseling, Parameters and Precautions, Participation, and Psychoneuroimmunology. Topics that relate mostly to the client include Adjustment and Response to Disability, Consequences of Inactivity, and Stress. In addition, there is a chapter on the Theories, Models, and Concepts that provides a brief introduction to many of the models that underlie the practices of the whole healthcare team. Research, to be valuable, must be based in a sound theoretical framework.

The Techniques and Intervention section is an evidence-based review of 41 treatment techniques that are part of recreational therapy practice. As you can see from the table of contents, recreational therapy provides services to clients in all phases of healthcare. It probably has the widest range of clients of any healthcare field. An overview of each treatment is provided, along with indications, contraindications, detailed protocols and processes, outcomes, and related documentation. The connections to the International Classification of Functioning, Disability, and Health are also listed.

A variety of interventions and techniques are reviewed that relate to various health domains. Topics in the physical domain include balance training, constraint induced movement therapy, motor learning and training strategies, neuro-developmental training, transfers, walking and gait training, and wheelchair mobility. The cognitive domain techniques include cognitive retraining and rehabilitation, errorless learning, Montessori method, reality orientation, and reminiscence. The behavioral domain is covered with topics such as anger management, assertiveness training, behavior strategies and interventions, and social skills training. Psychological/emotional domain interventions include leisure-based stress coping, life review, medical play and preparation, stress management and coping, and therapeutic relationships. The sensory domain is covered in sensory interventions. Education and counseling interventions and techniques are also included, such as activity pattern development, cognitive behavioral counseling, energy conservation techniques, group psychotherapy techniques, leisure education and counseling, leisure resource awareness, sexual well-being, and values clarification. There are also activity-specific interventions. These include adaptive sports, adventure therapy, animal assisted therapy, aquatic therapy, bibliotherapy, mind-body interventions, physical activity, and therapeutic thematic arts programming. Other interventions are aimed at community participation, such as community participation, community problem solving, and disability rights education and advocacy.

Current healthcare trends are focused on low cost non-pharmacological interventions, as well as inter-ventions aimed at optimizing community participation and integration, preventing health conditions, and decreasing mortality risk while improving quality of life. One goal is to provide treatment that accomplishes these goals. Another equally important goal is to strengthen our research in these areas. This is a call to action for our profession that can be undertaken not only by recreational therapy researchers, but also by practicing clinicians. Clinicians can collect data using standardized assessment tools to answer clear research questions and partner with recreational therapy researchers to design and implement studies in the clinician's place of practice. Agencies that employ recreational therapists may also have their own research teams, as agencies are constantly striving to prove the efficacy of their work as well.

With everyone working together to find the best practices to help our clients, recreational therapy will continue to provide valuable therapy, such as that described in this book.

I. Therapy Basics

1. Activity and Task Analysis

Heather R. Porter

This chapter will look at analyzing activities for your clients and the tasks that are required to perform the activities. To understand the difference between activity analysis and task analysis, let's begin by defining the terms "activity" and "task." Activity is defined as a specific pursuit a client participates in, whereas a task is defined as a part of the activity or a specific piece of work (or play) to be done. Activities are specific pursuits such as checkers, gardening, kite flying, or weight training. Tasks are components of an activity such as setting up a checkerboard, repotting a seedling, winding up kite string, or performing one specific weight training exercise. With these concepts, it is easy to understand that activity analysis "is a procedure for breaking down and examining an activity" (Peterson and Gunn, 1984, p. 180) and task analysis is a procedure for breaking down and examining a specific task in an activity.

Activity Analysis

Conducting an activity analysis is one of the first steps in choosing activities that are appropriate to meet the specific objectives of an individual or target population. Evaluation of activity components and inherent characteristics gives the therapist information s/he needs to make appropriate clinical activity prescriptions. It is not enough to choose an activity because it is available and the client agrees to participate. The therapist should prescribe an activity that s/he knows will address particular needs of the client. This is the difference between providing activities and providing therapy.

In addition to choosing activities based on the match between inherent characteristics and client objectives, activities are chosen based on the likelihood of carryover for continued health promotion after discharge. Is the client able to afford this activity, have access to needed supplies and equipment,

have available assistance, have transportation, etc.? Peterson and Gunn (1984, p. 182) re-cap the primary benefits of activity analysis that still stand true today. Analysis provides:

- a better comprehension of the expected outcomes of participation;
- a greater understanding of the complexity of activity components, which can then be compared to the functional level of an individual or group to determine the appropriateness of the activity;
- information about whether the activity will contribute to the desired behavioral outcome when specific behavioral goals or objectives are being used;
- direction for the modification or adaptation of an activity for individuals with limitations;
- useful information for selecting an intervention, instructions, or leadership technique; and
- a rationale or explanation for the therapeutic benefits of activity involvement.

When conducting an activity analysis, therapists should use a common activity analysis form, as shown below. The analysis may need to be very detailed in identifying the key components and characteristics of the activity. Also note that the activity analysis should reflect the ICF categories (e.g., mental functions, mobility) rather than the common domain categories that many therapists are familiar with (e.g., cognitive, physical). Although the latter terms are still commonly used in practice, it is believed that with the increased use of the ICF, the use of domains will decrease and ICF categories will be the new standard.

Sample Activity Analysis Form with ICF Codes

Name of activity

_____

Type of modality

_____

Brief description of activity

_____
_____

# of participants required (min to max)

_____

Type of Play

_____

Interaction pattern
- ☐ Intra-individual (Action takes place in the mind or action involving the mind and a part of the body; requires no contact with another person or external object)
- ☐ Extra-individual (Action directed by a person toward an object; requires no contact with another person)
- ☐ Aggregate (Action directed by a person toward an object while in the company of other persons who are also directing action towards objects; action is not directed toward each other; no interaction between participants is required or necessary)
- ☐ Inter-individual (Action of a competitive nature directed by one person toward another person)
- ☐ Unilateral (Action of a competitive nature among three or more persons, one of whom is an antagonist or "it"; interaction is in simultaneous competitive relationships)
- ☐ Multilateral (Action of a competitive nature among three or more persons with no one person as an antagonist)
- ☐ Intra-group (Action of a cooperative nature by two or more persons intent upon reaching a mutual goal; action requires positive verbal or nonverbal interaction)
- ☐ Inter-group (Action of a competitive nature between two or more intra-groups)

Equipment, supplies, and tools required

_____
_____
_____
_____

Costs

_____
_____
_____

Distance between participants

_____

Facilities required

_____
_____
_____

Clothing required

_____
_____
_____

Gender identification of activity
- ☐ Primarily masculine identification
- ☐ Primarily feminine identification
- ☐ Activity is not gender specific

Type of tasks in the activity
- ☐ Single (d210 Undertaking a Single Task)
- ☐ Multiple (d220 Undertaking Multiple Tasks)

Structure of activity
- ☐ High
- ☐ Moderate
- ☐ Minimal
- ☐ Free

Noise level of activity
- ☐ High
- ☐ Moderate
- ☐ Minimal
- ☐ Quiet

Number of rules
- ☐ Many
- ☐ Moderate
- ☐ Few
- ☐ None

Complexity of rules
- ☐ Complex
- ☐ Moderate
- ☐ Simple
- ☐ NA

Leadership required
- ☐ Special activity skill expertise
- ☐ General activity skill ability
- ☐ Supervisory

☐ None needed
☐ Other

Possible adaptations to the activity, tools, equipment, supplies, positioning, environment, etc.

_____

_____

_____

_____

Precautions

_____

_____

_____

_____

Special considerations

_____

_____

_____

_____

Processing questions

_____

_____

_____

_____

_____

Preparation work to complete prior to activity

_____

_____

_____

_____

Time Factors

_____

_____

Estimated duration of entire activity
☐ Set time: _____
☐ Natural end: _____
☐ Continuous

Speed of performance
☐ Fixed
☐ Flexible

Possible delays in activity

_____

_____

_____

Inherent skills in activity

_____

_____

_____

Directionality
☐ Left/right
☐ Up/down
☐ Around
☐ Over/under
☐ Person/object
☐ Person/person
☐ Object/object

Cognitive (b1 Mental Functions, b2 Sensory Functions and Pain, d1 Learning and Applying Knowledge, and d2 General Tasks and Demands)
☐ b1140 Orientation to Time
☐ b1141 Orientation to Place
☐ b11420 Orientation to Self
☐ b11421 Orientation to Others
☐ b1400 Sustaining Attention
☐ b1401 Shifting Attention
☐ b1402 Dividing Attention
☐ b1403 Sharing Attention
☐ b1440 Short-Term Memory
☐ b1441 Long-Term Memory
☐ b1442 Retrieval of Memory
☐ b1560 Auditory Perception
☐ b1561 Visual Perception
☐ b1562 Olfactory Perception
☐ b1563 Gustatory Perception
☐ b1564 Tactile Perception
☐ b1565 Visuospatial Perception
☐ b1640 Abstraction
☐ b1641 Organization and Planning
☐ b1642 Time Management
☐ b1643 Cognitive Flexibility
☐ b1644 Insight
☐ b1645 Judgment
☐ b1646 Problem-Solving
☐ b1670 Reception of Language
☐ b1671 Expression of Language
☐ b1720 Simple Calculation
☐ b1721 Complex Calculation
☐ b260 Proprioceptive Function
☐ b2700 Sensitivity to Temperature
☐ b2701 Sensitivity to Vibration
☐ b2702 Sensitivity to Pressure
☐ d110 Watching

☐ d115 Listening
☐ d130 Copying
☐ d135 Rehearsing
☐ d163 Thinking
☐ d166 Reading
☐ d170 Writing
☐ d177 Making Decisions
☐ d240 Handling Stress and Other Psychological Demands
☐ Other:

Physical (b4 Functions of the Cardiovascular, Hematological, Immunological, and Respiratory Systems, b7 Neuromusculoskeletal and Movement-Related Functions, and d4 Mobility)
☐ b4550 General Physical Endurance
☐ b4551 Aerobic Capacity
☐ b710 Mobility of Joint Functions
☐ b730 Muscle Power Functions
☐ b740 Muscle Endurance Functions
☐ b755 Involuntary Movement Reaction Functions
☐ b760 Control of Voluntary Movement Functions
☐ d4100 Lying Down
☐ d4101 Squatting
☐ d4102 Kneeling
☐ d4103 Sitting
☐ d4104 Standing
☐ d4105 Bending
☐ d4200 Transferring Oneself While Sitting
☐ d4300 Lifting
☐ d4301 Carrying in the Hands
☐ d4302 Carrying in the Arms
☐ d4303 Carrying on Shoulders, Hip, and Back
☐ d4305 Putting Down Objects
☐ d4350 Pushing with Lower Extremities
☐ d4351 Kicking
☐ d4400 Picking Up
☐ d4401 Grasping
☐ d4402 Manipulating
☐ d4403 Releasing
☐ d4450 Pulling
☐ d4451 Pushing
☐ d4452 Reaching
☐ d4453 Turning or Twisting the Hands or Arms
☐ d4454 Throwing
☐ d4455 Catching
☐ d4500 Walking Short Distances
☐ d4501 Walking Long Distances
☐ d4502 Walking on Different Surfaces

☐ d4503 Walking around Obstacles
☐ d4550 Crawling
☐ d4551 Climbing
☐ d4552 Running
☐ d4553 Jumping
☐ d4554 Swimming
☐ d4600 Moving Around within the Home
☐ d4601 Moving Around within Buildings Other Than Home
☐ d4602 Moving Around outside the Home and Other Buildings
☐ d465 Moving Around Using Equipment
☐ d470 Using Transportation
☐ d475 Driving
☐ Other:

Communication (d3 Communication)
☐ d310 Communication with — Receiving — Spoken Messages
☐ d3150 Communicating with — Receiving — Body Gestures
☐ d3151 Communicating with — Receiving — General Signs and Symbols
☐ d3152 Communicating with — Receiving — Drawings and Photographs
☐ d320 Communicating with — Receiving — Formal Sign Language Messages
☐ d325 Communicating with — Receiving — Written Messages
☐ d330 Speaking
☐ d335 Producing Nonverbal Messages
☐ d340 Producing Messages in Formal Sign Language
☐ d345 Writing Messages
☐ d3500 Starting a Conversation
☐ d3501 Sustaining a Conversation
☐ d3502 Ending a Conversation
☐ d3503 Conversing with One Person
☐ d3504 Conversing with Many People
☐ d3550 Discussion with One Person
☐ d3551 Discussion with Many People
☐ d360 Using Communication Devices and Techniques
☐ Other:

Self-care (d5 Self-Care)
☐ d510 Washing Oneself
☐ d520 Caring for Body Parts

☐ d530 Toileting
☐ d540 Dressing
☐ d550 Eating
☐ d560 Drinking
☐ d570 Looking After One's Health
☐ Other:

Interpersonal Interactions and Relationships (d7 Interpersonal Interactions and Relationships)
☐ d7100 Respect and Warmth in Relationships
☐ d7101 Appreciation in Relationships
☐ d7102 Tolerance in Relationships
☐ d7103 Criticism in Relationships
☐ d7104 Social Cues in Relationships
☐ d7105 Physical Contact in Relationships
☐ d7200 Forming Relationships
☐ d7201 Terminating Relationships
☐ d7202 Regulating Behaviors within Interactions
☐ d7203 Interacting According to Social Rules
☐ d7204 Maintaining Social Space
☐ d730 Relating with Strangers
☐ d7400 Relating with Persons in Authority
☐ d7402 Relating with Equals
☐ Other:

Emotional and Psychological Factors (Experiences that might facilitate…)

Guilt

_____

_____

Emotional pain

_____

_____

Anger

_____

_____

Fear

_____

_____

Frustration

_____

_____

Hope and optimism

_____

_____

Creativity

_____

_____

Inner strength (drawing upon one's own or others)

_____

_____

Growth and development (continuation or in a new direction)

_____

_____

Sense of connection and belonging (within the self, with individuals/groups, with animals/nature, with higher power/spirit, with culture/history)

_____

_____

Sense of control/power (over self and things, reflected to others)

_____

_____

Sense of competence/mastery

_____

_____

Sense of freedom/autonomy

_____

_____

Sense of identity (building, expression, transforming)

_____

_____

Positive emotions of escalation (entertainment, excitement, amusement, joyfulness, happiness, playfulness)

_____

_____

Positive emotions of de-escalation (inner calmness, peace of mind, tranquility, serenity, relaxation)

_____

_____

Positive emotions of well-being (rejuvenation, satisfaction, personal fulfillment, gratification)

_____

_____

Task Analysis

Task analysis is the evaluation of a specific task in an activity. This is different from activity analysis that evaluates the activity as a whole. Task analysis lists the steps *one* person takes to complete an action or a series of related actions. Task analysis is required for any evaluation a therapist does of client ability related to activities and participation. A task analysis allows a therapist to break down a task into specific components in order to compare the client's functional abilities to each component. This assists the therapist in identifying deficits for goal and objective setting.

The field of recreational therapy has a rich history of outstanding tools that analyze activities and tasks. However, these tools go beyond what is internationally recognized as task analysis. Many of the recreational therapy methods include affective aspects of the activity, such as anger, fear, frustration, and guilt; social interaction patterns required for the activity, such as aggregate, inter-individual, and multilateral; and administrative aspects, such as leadership style required.

As the world becomes more interconnected and standards of performance span international borders, the field of recreational therapy will benefit from following international practices. This does not mean that the therapist should not consider the social or emotional impact of activity or the practical aspects of administering an activity. Each of these elements is important, but they are separate from task analysis. The overall goal of task analysis is to standardize the analysis of activities across cultures and regions. This allows the therapist practicing in a country that emphasizes "community" (the action that increases the joy of the whole is more important than the ability of the individual to experience joy) to achieve the same results as the therapist working in a country that emphasizes "individualism" (the individual has the right to excel and be personally happy even if some of the people impacted are not pleased). Task analysis typically evaluates the observable physical actions and the anticipated cognitive processing skills necessary to carry out a task.

Task analysis is a breakdown of what one individual is *required* to do to complete a task. The actions required include both physical actions and cognitive processes.

When a therapist is analyzing the actions needed to complete a task, s/he answers the question, "What are the steps that the client must go through to complete the task?" The physical and cognitive actions needed to complete a task are linear in nature, the next step logically following the one before it.

To do a task analysis, follow these steps:

1. Identify the task to be analyzed. For example, repotting a seedling.

2. Break down the task into four to ten actions. If the task selected has more than fifteen subtasks (actions), the therapist has selected too global of a task. If the action has less than four subtasks it may not be a truly independent action. In the task of repotting a seedling all the steps required to grow the seedling in the first place belong to another task or set of tasks.

3. Write down all the equipment needed to complete the task. Because the therapist will be required to "ground truth" the task analysis by performing the action as written, s/he should have all the equipment assembled: seedling, fresh soil, small hand shovel, empty pot, and filled watering can.

4. Write out the physical steps in a linear fashion, in the order that the task is completed, for repotting a plant. The easiest way to do this is for the therapist to actually write down each step while completing the task. Be sure to concentrate on a single task. If the client needs to gather his/her own equipment as part of the activity, it should be written up as a separate task.

- Scoop soil into pot until it is one inch from the top.
- With the fingers, make a hole in the soil big enough to contain the root ball of the seedling.
- Pick up the seedling.
- Place the seedling into the hole.
- Cover roots of seedling with soil.
- Gently press the soil around the seedling.
- Water seedling so soil is damp, but not soaked.
- Place pot onto a tray to catch excess water.

5. Once the therapist feels that s/he has all the required steps listed, s/he should complete the task again by taking *only* the actions that are written down.

6. Any actions that are written down on the therapist's list that are not essential to completing the task should be eliminated from the list.

7. If the therapist feels that s/he has all the required physical actions listed, then s/he should give the sequential task list to another person and see if the other person can complete the activity taking only the actions that are written down. While the other person is sequentially working through the actions for the task, the therapist should observe every movement taken to see if s/he forgot something or to note potential problems or acceptable variations.

8. At some point in the process, the therapist needs to look back at the purpose of the task, specifically at the setting in which the task will be performed, to see if there are any other requirements for completing the task successfully. In the example of repotting a seedling, the timing of removing the seedling from where it was started is important. Having the seedling exposed too long will let the seedling's roots dry out and the seedling will die. For a group it may be possible to prepare the seedlings before the activity as a separate task. If the seedlings are being repotted one at a time, "Remove the seedling from the starting soil" should be substituted for "Pick up the seedling."

9. If (or when) a client has trouble with any specific step of the actions required to complete a task, the therapist should ask if the inability to complete the step is due to (1) a physical impairment, (2) a cognitive processing impairment, (3) a social issue, (4) a cultural issue, (5) an affective (emotional) issue, (6) an environmental issue, (7) some other skill or variable that is affecting performance, or (8) a difficulty with the instructions for the step. The therapist will also want to evaluate the effectiveness and efficiency of the client's actions.

If breakdown occurs in a step and the specific problem is identified, objectives and an individually tailored treatment plan are established to restore the skill, modify the skill, or develop the skill. If success in restoring, developing, or modifying the skill is unlikely, the therapist evaluates the appropriateness of substituting one activity for another (e.g., taking a taxicab instead of a bus).

When the therapist writes up the individual steps associated with the task, there are many different formats s/he can follow. One format, an adaptation of Peabody's (2001) Task Outliner, is described below.

- The title of the task should be at the top of the page. The title of the task, because it is an action, should always start with a word that ends in "ing." For example, repotting a seedling, paying the fare on a city bus, baking corn bread.

- The second part of the form should provide a short, one sentence description of the activity to help define the scope of the task.

- A list of the equipment needed should be clearly written out.

- A description of what action or activity typically causes someone to initiate the activity should be written. Peabody calls this a "trigger." For example, the trigger for paying the fare on a city bus would be, "The client steps into the correct bus at the bus stop."

- A description of the desired outcome against which performance will be measured is written down. For example, the outcome of paying the fare on a city bus would be to pay the correct amount of bus fare at the correct time.

- Therapists often practice tasks with clients in the clinical setting before they are practiced in the setting in which they normally occur. To help clients, each therapist should use the same lead-in phrase. For example, "When you step up into the city bus, you will be expected to pay bus fare."

- The next part of the task analysis form includes the actual analysis of the specific actions required to execute the task. These steps are numbered and always start with a verb because each step is a physical or cognitive action.

- It would be appropriate to include an area for special considerations for each numbered step.

If the task has more than ten steps, the therapist should see if the task can be broken down into subtasks and then have the client chain the subtasks together to complete the full activity. For example, paying bus fare is one task, looking for and occupying an appropriate place on the bus is another task, watching or listening for the correct bus stop to depart is another task, departing from the bus (including seeing if anything is left behind on the bus seat) is another task. Once the client has overlearned one task, then the therapist and client can work on the next task associated with riding the bus. Overlearning the task is not the same thing as being able to independently complete the task. The ability to complete the task means that the client is able to do the task. However, the client may complete all the steps but do them slowly because s/he needs to think about each step. Overlearning the task means that the client is practiced enough to do the task without spending undo time or thought on the process.

Complexity of the Task

In addition to having the steps (actions) required to complete a task, the therapist will need at least two other skills: the ability to break the skill down to the right level of detail, allowing identification of specific actions that the client needs to improve, and the ability to identify other dependent and independent tasks.

Level of Detail of Tasks

The actions needed to complete a task should be written at the correct level of difficulty, using increments that match a client's ability. The therapist will need to know the level of prerequisite skills (the skills that a client has already overlearned) his/her clients are likely to have. For therapists working with clients with severe cognitive impairment, the analysis of tasks to dress for gardening outside on a brisk fall afternoon may be made up of twenty or more subtasks as the client lacks many of the prerequisite skills to complete the overall task. As an example, the client may need to learn how to put on shoes, gardening gloves, gardening apron, and coat in addition to the skills required to determine how to select the appropriate clothing. Each of these actions would have at least one task analyzed to compare performance. A client recovering from a heart attack without cognitive impairment is likely to have many more of the prerequisite skills intact, so the task analysis for this client may be very short.

Dependent versus Independent Tasks

There may be times that a client is able to demonstrate all the skills required for a specific task, such as riding the city bus, but still not be able to independently ride the bus. Tasks have dependent or independent subsets of skills. For many clients, learning the specific tasks associated with determining which bus to use, following the payment procedures for riding the bus, and knowing when to get off the bus may be challenging but doable. However, other skills (tasks) must also be integrated with the task at hand. For example, a client who is using a wheelchair for the first time not only needs to learn how to use the bus but will also need to learn mobility skills associated with riding a bus.

The following is an example of a task analysis written in Peabody's Task Outliner format.

Task: Paying Fare on a City Bus

Description: People must either pay bus fare or show a bus pass when they board public transportation. This task outline is for paying bus fare (not showing a bus pass).

Equipment needed: The off-peak fare for the city bus is $2.00 and the peak fare is $2.50. The client will need to have 10 quarters or other equivalent coin and paper money combinations to ensure adequate fair during peak hours.

Trigger: The client steps into the correct bus at the bus stop.

Desired outcome: The client pays the correct amount of fare.

Lead-in phrase: When you step up into the city bus, you will be expected to pay bus fare.

Task Analysis

1. **Walk up** to fare box located next to the bus driver.
If the client is in a wheelchair or scooter, this process may be different (d465 Moving Around Using Equipment).

2. **Read** the posted amount of fare required.
If the client has difficulty with this step, determine if the client is able to read (d166 Reading) *or has vision problems* (b210 Seeing Functions).

3. **Count** out correct change.
If the client has difficulty with this step, determine if the client is able to recognize the value of each coin or can add up coins (d860 Basic Economic Transactions).

4. **Place** correct fare in fare box.
If the client has difficulty with this step, determine where the client has problems (b7 Neuromusculoskeletal and Movement-Related Functions, s730 Structure of Upper Extremity, d440 Fine Hand Use).

5. **Watch** to make sure fare went into fare box.
If the client has difficulty with this step, determine if the client has the ability to attend to a task until completed (b160 Thought Functions, d210 Undertaking a Single Task).

6. **Take** ticket from bus driver.

Depending on the transportation system's procedures the bus rider may receive a bus ticket or a transfer pass to use on a connecting route (d210 Undertaking a Single Task).

Task analysis is the basis of most of the assessments and objectives that a therapist does as part of treatment. One of the easiest ways to determine a client's needs is to compare the client's skills against a task analysis, such as the one shown above. If the therapist has a good collection of tasks already ana-lyzed at the appropriate level for his/her clientele, then the therapist will find it easier to assess a client's functional level and to develop treatment objectives.

References

Peabody, L. (2001). *How to write policies, procedures, and task outlines: Sending clear signals in written directions*. Lacy, WA: Writing Services.

Peterson, C. & Gunn, S. (1984). *Therapeutic recreation program design: Principles and procedures* (2nd ed.). Englewood Cliffs, NJ: Prentice-Hall, Inc.

2. Adjustment and Response to Disability

Heather R. Porter

The need for psychosocial adjustment to disability is suggested when there are deficits in ICF codes b126 Temperament and Personality Functions, b130 Energy and Drive Functions, b152 Emotional Functions, d240 Handling Stress and Other Psychological Demands, d570 Looking After One's Health, d6 Domestic Life, d7 Interpersonal Interactions and Relationships, d8 Major Life Areas, and d910 Community Life. Adjustment and/or appropriate response to disability is an essential component of successful community integration and ongoing quality of life. It is an individually defined and subjective process influenced by many variables. Psychosocial adjustment is a process of emotional growth that requires the development of healthy coping mechanisms to forge a new lifestyle that optimizes assets and health. The recreational therapist helps guide a client's responses to a disability, to improve the client's ability to enjoy life and improve health.

Mary is a 32-year-old female who was in a motor vehicle accident. Fortunately, the accident did not result in brain injury. However, she did sustain a complete T-12 spinal cord injury. As she sits in a wheelchair, waiting for her next therapy appointment, she is consumed with anxiety and fear. She worries about how she is going to be able to care for her three young children (three, five, and seven), especially since she is a single mom with no other family in the area. She is also fearful of losing her independence, her career as a flight attendant, and her relationship with her boyfriend of three years.

Sally is a 34-year-old female who fell while rock climbing. She also sustained a T-12 complete spinal cord injury. Sally is a single woman with a high-power career. She is a take-control-and-fix-it type of individual who thrives on stress and deadlines. As she sits in a wheelchair, waiting for her next therapy appointment, she is thinking about all the things that

need to be done so that she can get back on track. She needs to call a contractor to have modifications made to her home, she needs to contact her employer to talk about needed changes, and she needs to set up an appointment with adaptive driving. She is overwhelmed by the multitude of tasks that she now needs to accomplish, yet she appears to be in control and organized.

Although both Mary and Sally sustained the same disability, they exhibited different initial responses to their disability. Why? Is it because of their different lifestyles, because of their different personalities, or because of their level of family responsibilities and relationships? Can one make the assumption that one will adjust better in the community than the other? The answer is no. There is no way to know how a person will react to a situation, nor can a client's initial reactions to disability predict his/her level of successful community integration. There are too many internal and external variables, such as past experiences, mental health, resource availability, coping mechanisms, belief structure, support, flexibility, and accommodation. They all interact in unpredictable ways. Therapists need to realize that each response is unique to the individual. It is not appropriate to tell a client s/he should feel a certain way. The therapist guides the client through the emotional hurdles to reach optimal emotional health.

Optimal emotional health is a primary component of the recreational therapist's job because it affects so many areas of a client's life, including the rehabilitation process. The client may have difficulty engaging in life activities, seeking out resources, or overcoming barriers. Disability may also affect the client's self-identity, life routine, leisure, relationships, self-esteem, confidence, and independence. In the rehabilitation process, a client may fail to make the most of his/her assets if depression, regression, and passivity persist. Likewise, a client who is aggressive, angry, and rigid may not be open to new ideas and techniques. In a nutshell, disability (whether temporary, permanent, chronic, or life threatening) disrupts a client's lifestyle. The ability to accommodate to disability affects the ability to be healthy.

Measuring adjustment can be a tricky process. A client can state that he is adjusting well, but his actions may not be consistent with his statement (e.g., social isolation, poor hygiene). On the other hand, a client may appear to be adjusting well to her disability (back to work, social outings with friends), yet verbally she expresses lack of identity and feelings of inadequacy. So, have these clients achieved psychosocial adjustment? The client, who is socially isolated and practices poor hygiene, may in fact be satisfied and content with his life. The client who verbalizes a lack of self-identity and adequacy may view these issues as a work-in-progress as they have been long-time issues unrelated to her current disability. Thus, psychosocial adjustment is subjective and complex. It requires attention to both actions and words, as well as how these relate to the client's belief system.

> It [is] an evolutionary, changing, and highly individualized process rather than a stable state. The problems faced by the newly disabled person are those of coping with physical and psychological loss; changes in body image, social status, and earning capacity; the anxiety and grief which often accompany these changes; and the need to learn new behaviors and make concrete plans for an uncertain future. Each individual will seek personal solutions to these problems and thus define his own adjustment to disability (Stolov & Clowers, 1981, p. 14).

Therapists who understand the factors that influence psychosocial adjustment and how a client's actions can influence those factors will be equipped to help clients along their personal journeys. Therapists must also carefully consider the words chosen when working with clients. For example, the words "adjustment," "adaptation," and "acceptance" tends to pathologize the experience of disability, conveying to the client that disability is an undesirable state (something that one has to "adjust" to, rather than "respond" to). The word "response" also lessens the

focus on disability and increases the focus on the meaning that the individual ascribes to the disability. The client decides how to "respond," rather than having to "adjust."

Premorbid Factors that Influence Psychosocial Adjustment

There are many factors that help determine how and how well a client will adjust/respond to a loss. One of the therapist's tasks is to assess factors impeding a client's adjustment/response to loss and to help develop a treatment program of emotional recovery. This section discusses some of the issues that may have already been part of the client's life before the loss.

Mental health: Depending upon the severity of the disability and how well it is being managed (e.g., with medications or the use of behavioral techniques) mental illness may affect a client's ability to adjust to disability. If a client has a history of mental illness, his/her emotional and behavioral health should be evaluated to determine a baseline. Psychotropic medications can affect a client's emotions and behavior. The team evaluates whether the client's current medications are adequate or need changing. New medications may also interact with prior medications resulting in emotional and behavioral changes leading to an impaired ability to develop functional coping skills.

Substance abuse: A client may have had a substance abuse problem prior to his/her current disability. This information is not always provided by the client or the client's family for a multitude of reasons, including embarrassment, ignorance about the impact that substance abuse has on the client's current situation, and fear of being arrested. Substance abuse can have a profound impact on a client's ability to cope with new situations. For many, substance abuse starts with soft drugs and advances to more serious drugs. The drugs are often used in the beginning for a variety of reasons including acceptance, relaxation, diminishing painful feelings, calming nerves, and increasing perceived social competence. However this initial "problem solver" often leads to dependence or abuse and an inability to develop healthy coping styles. Obtaining an addictive drug may become the primary goal of each day, impacting every other area of the person's life. The client who is in a rehabilitation facility without access to his/her substance of choice experiences withdrawal symptoms. Some of the client's unproductive behavior may be due to drugs or drug withdrawal and not the current disability. Clients with substance abuse as a secondary diagnosis should be encouraged to develop healthy coping strategies, become involved in a self-help group, or possibly receive further rehabilitation after physical rehabilitation to deal with the drug problem, including inpatient drug rehab. Individuals who have a disability, whether or not they had a history of substance abuse, are at a higher risk for substance abuse. As Trombly (1989) says,

> Reasons predisposing disabled individuals to substance abuse problems can include a family and personal history; frustration and anxieties about being disabled; experiences with unproductive, unsatisfying, and dependent roles; functional inability to release tension; attendant motor and sensory deficits that accentuate the effects of alcohol; increased isolation; a lack of a sense of the ability to control events in their lives or to reach personal goals; and rejection experiences and other stressors related to loss and life-style changes. In addition, abuse of substances provides a way of avoiding the difficult and painful work of remediation (p. 14).

Prior medical history: Prior medical history can also affect the client's ability to cope with the current disability. For example, an individual who has been living with a chronic disease, such as rheumatoid arthritis, might find it difficult to achieve a sense of control over the new disability, for example a fractured hip. The client's experience with adjusting to prior disabilities may set a tone for adjusting/responding to the current disability whether the prior strategies were healthy or not (e.g., "If I don't move around a whole lot my arthritis doesn't flare up, so I intend to do the same thing when I'm at home recovering from my hip replacement. I'm just going to stay in the house and wait until I feel better."). Education should be provided on the impact of different types of coping strategies. The therapist assists the individual in developing healthy lifestyle strategies to improve responses to disability.

Coping strategies: Everyone has different healthy and/or unhealthy coping strategies for dealing with problems. To cope some people exercise. Others talk with someone, withdraw, shop, yell, or bury themselves in work. Prior coping strategies are not always effective in dealing with new problems (e.g., used to go out for a run, but now having difficulty just walking; used to withdraw from the problems, but current problem can't be ignored). Coping strategies, even if they were effective before, may need to be changed. Learning and practicing healthy alternatives should be incorporated into the treatment plan.

Personality style: People have different types of personalities. Personality styles have been described as Type A and B, social/outgoing/extrovert, shy/quiet/introvert, just to name a few. Personality style can affect the client's ability to adjust to disability. A person who is outgoing and assertive prior to disability may find it much easier to access resources and meet needs compared to the individual who is quiet and reserved. Personality styles, although fairly consistent throughout life, can be modified. Individuals can learn assertiveness and social skills. Helping the client to understand why it is important to use a different coping strategy is an important step in the learning process. People cannot be changed, unless they want to change. Therapists are the catalysts for making change happen through education, modeling, shaping, and counseling.

Preferred patterns of life: People like to live certain ways. Some people can't envision their life outside of familiar patterns (e.g., going to work every day, going sailing, living in a cabin in the mountains). Unfortunately, there are many reasons why preferences can't be continued after a disability, including finances, accessibility, functional abilities, and level of support. Alternatives and adaptations, such as equipment, activity modification, and resources, can be explored to continue with prior life patterns, and new alternatives can be suggested. A client's ability to accommodate to changes will affect his/her ability to adjust to the loss.

Developmental life stage: Each life stage has specific developmental tasks and roles that influence the client's ability to adjust to situations. Erikson (1968) outlines eight stages of development that are divided by chronological age, however he is careful to stipulate that the developmental process is affected by life experiences and events, hindering or enhancing the developmental process. Therefore, a client's chronological age does not necessarily reflect his/her psychological, social, emotional, behavioral, cognitive, or physical functional level. In addition, current situations can affect a client's developmental performance. Regression often occurs when the client does not have enough challenges or too many new challenges. The disability may move the client to a lower developmental stage due to physiological changes, such as a traumatic brain injury, or the emotional demands of coping with the current situation when premorbid coping strategies are not effective for the current situation. In the assessment process the therapist compares the client's chronological age to the client's current functional age. Part of the assessment is to try to figure out how the client's premorbid health status, current disability, and environment interact with his/her current development stage. A client's emotional and behavior level will provide a baseline to assist the therapist in developing a plan to enhance the client's psychosocial adjustment. For example, a teenager who is currently struggling with developing his own identity and autonomy may require a different approach than a 32-year-old client who is struggling with issues related to balancing her own needs with those of loved ones.

Culture: The client's culture can affect adjustment/response to disability, especially if there are strong gender roles (man provides for family and is now unable to do so) or religious beliefs related to disability (disability is the result of being possessed). Certain cultures also place high value on being reserved and not expressing emotions, which may also affect the adjustment/response process. Language is another cultural issue to consider. Does the client understand the spoken language of the hospital? Is an interpreter needed? Does the communication reflect the client's beliefs (e.g., women do not make decisions without their husband)? If a client does not fully understand what the clinician is saying, if beliefs reflect a negative connotation of the situation, or if the culture does not value the client's new role, the adjustment process can be difficult. The therapist should not jump to the conclusion that cultural beliefs cannot be changed, nor should the therapist ignore cultural values and beliefs. An awareness of culture and the impact it may have on adjustment/response will provide the therapist with a better frame of reference for addressing adjustment/response issues.

Literacy level: The literacy level of the client can impact psychosocial adjustment/response. On average adults in the U.S. read three to five grade levels lower than years of schooling through disuse and, in order to reach 90% of people, written materials need to be at a third grade reading level (Doak, Doak, & Root, 1995). If a client has difficulty reading, s/he may not fully understand written material, resulting in an inadequate understanding of the situation. Microsoft Word contains a tool that evaluates the reading level of written material. This is usually located under "Tools: Spelling and Grammar." For non-Word documents, therapists can use the Fry Formula to determine the reading level of materials (www.readabilityformulas.com/fry-graph-readability-formula.php).

Phases of Adjustment to Disability

Adjustment to disability and the treatment required are different based on whether the disability is acquired or congenital.

Acquired Disability

Just as there are stages of grief, phases of adjustment/response to an acquired disability have also been proposed. There are generally seven phases of adjustment/response to acquired disability: (1) shock/initial impact, (2) defensive retreat/denial, (3) depression/mourning, (4) personal questioning, (5) anger, (6) growth and integration, and (7) transcendence (Smart, 2001; Falvo, 2013; Stolov & Clowers, 1981). Despite the responses being in somewhat of a logical sequence, people do not always progress in this manner. Clients may skip stages, exhibit multiple phases at one time, such as depression and personal questioning, and go backwards. For example a new personal stressor may cause a person to go back to defensive retreat. In addition, therapists must realize that not everyone is able to reach the growth/integration and transcendence phases. The time people stay at certain phases is also variable, as are the catalysts that effectively move someone to the next phase.

Shock, initial impact: Shock occurs at diagnosis or when there is a drastic change in functioning. The client's thinking is often disorganized, and s/he feels numb (unable to think or feel), overwhelmed, and confused (unable to absorb what is happening). This is the person's natural reaction to such events to prevent "emotional flooding." In order to keep emotional homeostasis, the mind shuts down to protect itself from the emotional stress. In therapy, the client may ask questions that don't appear to make sense, be unable to recall information taught, appear to be not paying attention, ask the same questions over and over again, and/or tell you that s/he feels overwhelmed and confused. In response, the therapist should provide small doses of information, be concise and clear while avoiding medical jargon, provide print materials at the appropriate literacy level, ask the person to bring someone with him/her to therapy sessions, be patient, reassure the client that s/he will not be abandoned, and convey that you and the client are a team that will work though this together.

Defensive retreat/denial: At this phase the client may deny the presence of disability (e.g., "I'm fine. I'm just tired, that's all.") or minimize the effect of the disability. The client may try to live in his/her "pre-disability world" (e.g., "I don't have to change my plans. I'll be walking again soon."). Families might also be in denial (e.g., "When will he be able to walk out of here?"). This type of behavior can be a protective response to "emotional flooding" which allows the person to gradually assimilate both the permanence and full implications of the disability and/or a defensive mechanism to preserve self-identity. In therapy, the client may refuse to accept information about the disability, insist that there has been a mistake, seek out other service providers for second opinions, and exhibit a lack of motivation to learn or understand how to live with a disability. Therapists should provide information in small doses at a time to allow the person to assimilate the information at a more controlled, self-determined rate. If the client feels overwhelmed with information, the material is less likely to be accepted. Failure on the part of the therapist to recognize and accommodate to an individual's tolerance level for distressing information may also impact therapy participation and resultant outcomes. Therapists should provide print materials at the appropriate literacy level, make themselves available for questions, and consider the use of experiential learning in an emotionally safe environment to increase insight.

Depression/mourning: In the previous phase of denial the person focuses on the past only and doesn't want to consider the future. This is different from depression, which sets in when the person recognizes the present situation and is saddened about the future outlook. In this phase the person struggles with questions about an uncertain future and an uncertain identity. It can also be difficult to cope with something when the inescapable disability is always "with" the person. The person may turn to unhealthy coping mechanisms, such as drugs or alcohol, and may express suicidal ideation. Broadly speaking, depression is a response to feeling a lack of hope and inability to meet goals that are meaningful to the person. In therapy, the client may verbalize suicidal thoughts or feelings of sadness, emptiness, and worthlessness; be tearful; have diminished interest or pleasure in almost all activities; have significant weight loss or gain; have problems with sleep, either insomnia or hypersomnia; exhibit psychomotor retardation (slowing down) or agitation and restlessness; experience fatigue and lack of energy; have a diminished ability to think or concentrate; be indecisive; and/or withdraw and isolate. The client might also limit engagement in conversation making it difficult to explore feelings, exhibit negative behaviors, and exhibit decline in other life tasks. This can be seen especially in children, who may be whiney, moody, angry, or tearful over little things. If suicidal ideation is expressed, the therapist must take appropriate actions, including informing other members of the treatment team. Areas of possible intervention include regular engagement in physical activity to reduce depressive symptoms, changing distorted thinking patterns using Cognitive Behavioral Therapy, implementing stress management and relaxation training, implementing strategies to help increase self-esteem and self-worth, making appropriate referrals to other team members for psychological evaluation and treatment, using structured successes in experiential learning to bolster self-esteem and self-confidence, and exploring what activities are personally meaningful to the client and designing treatment interventions to optimize participation in these activities.

Personal questioning: In this phase, the client often replays the accident or pre-diagnosis period over and over again in his/her mind in the hope of identifying what could have been done to avoid the current situation. The client will commonly ask, "Why did this happen to me" and "What did I do to deserve this?" The person may lose trust in the world and in his/her value systems. This type of questioning is both lonely and non-productive and often results in the person blaming himself/herself. People engage in this type of thinking to bring balance to their beliefs that now seem unbalanced. Holding oneself responsible is the price that is paid to maintain a belief that the world is not a random and unpredictable place. This compulsive search for causes and the unending questioning to find a meaning for the disability can impede treatment and the rehabilitation process. When always searching the past, the client never allows himself/herself to absorb the new and now, making it difficult to fully participate and learn from therapy sessions. The therapist should help the client understand the difference between what caused the disability (e.g., car accident, problem with the immune system) versus its meaning and purpose in the person's value system (e.g., "God gave this to me so I would take a different path in life."). The use of therapeutic responses, such as paraphrasing and clarifying, can be helpful in guiding the client through this realization. Therapists should refrain from answering questions about the meaning of the disability, as this is a personal process. If the client presses the therapist for his/her opinion, it is best to reflect the question back to the client, such as "I'm more interested in knowing what you think" or clarifying what caused the disability, such as "The car accident caused the injury." The therapist might also opt to use common sayings or phrases to highlight the positive. For example, "When I was growing up, my grandmother always told me that when a door closes, another door opens. Sometimes I don't always see the new door right away, or understand it, but I have faith that somewhere and at some time the door will open for me." Such statements, without being too personally revealing, might also help to strengthen the therapeutic relationship as it highlights the human side of the therapist and empathic understanding.

Anger: Anger is often a combination of feeling helpless, frustrated, fearful, and irritable. People often express anger when they feel out of control. Anger, when not expressed, can also result in depression. Anger might also be used by the client as a conscious or unconscious strategy to escape or avoid something, or in response to task anxiety. For example, when faced with a challenge the client does not want to perform, the client may become angry about it and storm out of the room to avoid the task. Anger

might also be the result of being unable to express needs. In therapy, the client might talk back, refuse to participate, degrade the therapist, act out, or exhibit violent, aggressive, or agitated behavior. The therapist should remain calm, acknowledge the client's behavior, and inquire about the cause of the behavior (e.g., "John, it seems like you are having a bad day, what's going on?"). If the therapist doesn't inquire about the behavior, it could continue to reinforce distorted thinking that no one truly cares about the client. On the other hand, the therapist must also fully recognize the situation and implement strategies to deescalate the client. If the underlying cause of the anger is identified (e.g., client is upset that he can't go to the bathroom on his own and the nurse took too long to answer the call bell resulting in a urinary accident), the therapist should help problem solve, focus on the positive to balance out negative, distorted thinking, provide increased opportunities for choice and control, help to identify anger triggers, structure successes, offer multi-modal ways to express anger in a healthy way, teach and implement stress management techniques, and educate the client about the impact of anger on health.

Growth/integration: A client reaches this phase when s/he understands and accepts the reality and implications of the disability, establishes new values and goals that do not conflict with the disability, and explores and utilizes his/her strengths and abilities. This phase may necessitate changes to the environment through changed interpersonal interactions or assistive technology and changes in role functioning for the client. The client assumes responsibility for the management of the disability and views disability as an opportunity for growth and learning. This phase is never complete because life always consists of challenges and demands that necessitate further changes. Clients at this phase might also advocate and support others with disabilities as a way to bring meaning and purpose to their own disability experience.

Transcendence: This phase is beyond acceptance and adjustment to disability. It is a combination of refusing to idealize normality (lack of disability), adopting a spiritual or philosophical orientation to disability, and embracing the experience. The disability is seen as a catalyst for the person to grow and develop, with the person feeling that s/he is a better person for having experienced the disability. Disability is viewed as a tool, an asset, and an opportunity.

Congenital Disability

Adjustment/response to a congenital disability typically follows a different pattern. Individuals who have a congenital disability tend to respond better to having a disability because there was no premorbid identity or functional loss. In addition, children with a congenital disability have not internalized society's prejudices and discriminations about disability. They haven't fully developed their body image and tend to have more cognitive and affective resilience and flexibility (Smart, 2001). This is not to say that individuals with congenital disabilities do not experience the same phases as those who have an acquired disability. They, too, will experience challenges in life that result in shock, questioning, anger, etc.

Individuals with congenital disabilities might also have atypical childhood experiences that impact disability adjustment/response, such as prolonged hospitalizations, early socialization into the role of patient, overprotection, relaxed discipline with increased tolerance for inappropriate behavior, engagement with numerous caregiving adults diminishing their ability to form reciprocal attachment bonds and increasing vulnerability to abuse. Parents are also affected, leading to depression due to loss of sleep and problems dealing with the child's problem behaviors, coping with the child's unusual appearance, adversity in the family, and overwhelming caregiving responsibilities. Parental issues may result in child abuse, neglect, and abandonment (Smart, 2001).

Overprotection and relaxation of discipline can result in lack of mastery, competence, and self-confidence, and can further result in isolation and poor social skills. This might not be apparent until the child enters school, when s/he begins to interact with peers and experience situations of prejudice and discrimination. Therapists should be aware of these possible background issues, screen for abuse or neglect regularly, address social skill deficits, encourage independence and locus of control to counter learned helplessness, set healthy limits on behavior in treatment sessions and encourage parents to do the same at home, and encourage developmental growth and/or adaptations in all health domains.

Approaches to Encourage Adjustment

In addition to the above treatment suggestions related to different phases of adjustment/response to disability, there are other therapeutic interventions and approaches that can be helpful. The therapist must first remember, however, that each client is an individual and that a cookie-cutter approach does not work. Clients come from a variety of backgrounds, experience different needs, and respond differently to interventions. Consequently, these ideas should be adapted and modified to meet the needs of the client.

Working on integration: Integrating clients back into the community is a vital step in the adjustment process. A client's readiness level will determine the environment and level of challenge for the outing. For example, a client may not find a trip to his home very threatening, yet he may consider a trip to the mall or to his place of work much harder. Do not force a client to go on an outing that s/he is not ready for, otherwise it may increase the client's anxiety and fear of the community environment. Some clients are receptive to sequential outings consisting of small steps (first a van, then a bus, then a train), while other clients want to jump right in and learn how to function in a challenging environment. The therapist can also consider the use of groups for outings to provide added support for the client. Occasionally it may be appropriate for the therapist to use the same equipment as the client during the outing, such as using a wheelchair alongside the client. Family and friends should also be included on integration outings for family training, as well as to provide support for the client. They should be instructed on how to assist the client to integrate back into the community after s/he is discharged from the facility, as the full integration process can take weeks to months to years. For the client in denial, who refuses to acknowledge deficits and limitations to the point where safety is a concern, the team may consider setting up a structured failure. In this situation the client will be faced with the direct results of his/her actions. For example a client may refuse to make phone calls to find out level of accessibility and the therapist purposely allows the client to plan an outing to a non-accessible facility. Integration can also be enhanced by allowing day or weekend passes with family and friends that have been adequately trained to assist the client, as long as these are approved by the physician and relevant insuring agency. Be aware that some health insurance policies will no longer pay for inpatient care if a client leaves the facility for more than a set number of hours.

Teaching relaxation techniques: Learning different techniques to relax assists with identification and awareness of stressors. Learning how to incorporate relaxation-training techniques as a problem-solving technique is an important skill that helps decrease anxiety and panic.

Healthy expression of emotions and feelings: Allow opportunities for expression of emotion. Clients may express anger, hostility, and frustration in negative ways (outbursts, stares, and attitude). Acknowledge the client's behavior (e.g., "Your stare makes me feel like you're angry. Is something upsetting you?"). Open the door to communication rather that allowing unhealthy behavior to continue. Assist the client in understanding feelings (e.g., "It must be really hard to deal with people like me asking you to do things when you're used to doing things on your own schedule."). Model good communication of feelings. Negative behavior will distance relationships, resulting in alienation rather than meeting the client's need for support. Allow opportunities for alternative modes of expressing and dealing with emotions, such as writing, propelling the wheelchair around an outdoor track, or weight training.

Fostering internal locus of control: Individuals who experience a disability are faced with the reality that there are things in their life that they are unable to control. Many of life's activities are controlled by others when a client is hospitalized, including meal times, appointments, assistance to use the bathroom, and privacy. Motivation and initiative are enhanced when internal locus of control is maximized. Allow as many opportunities for control as possible (e.g., therapy at 10 A.M. or 1 P.M., this activity or that activity, therapy inside or outside). Also allow opportunities for control that are outside of typical client parameters as appropriate to diminish the "patient" role. These may include eating in the staff cafeteria, open time in gym, and research on the Internet in the evening.

Encouraging independence: Hospital situations often foster dependence. Staff have a multitude of time-sensitive responsibilities, so they often provide the client with too much assistance to accomplish tasks rather than waiting a longer time for the client to complete the task alone or with minimal assis-

tance. It is quicker to put on the client's shoes than to wait for the client to put on his shoes, but it is not better for the client's ability to function after discharge. The client's treatment plan should include the goal of independence as appropriate throughout his/her whole day, not just in therapy. If the client can get to therapy sessions without help and set an alarm clock in the morning so s/he has enough time to dress independently, it provides success at being independent that will translate to experiences after discharge.

Providing active listening: Provide your full attention when the client expresses fears, concerns, anxieties, wishes, needs, and ideas. Reflect back to the client what you are hearing and convey understanding. Understanding means that you understand what the client is saying; it does not mean that you agree with it. You can gently offer guidance, as appropriate, but listening is therapy in and of itself. This does not mean that the therapist must abandon the treatment plan for the session and actively listen to the client. The therapist can sensitively redirect the client to the task at hand and encourage continuation of the discussion while completing the task. If the task is inappropriate given the situation, consideration should be given to change the focus of the treatment session. An example might be changing the session from making phone calls for an outing next week to outdoor wheelchair propulsion since the latter lends itself better to conversation with the therapist.

Accenting abilities and accomplishments: The rehabilitation process is fraught with attention to dysfunction. Although therapists highlight achievement over dysfunction, clients benefit from a focus on assets outside of dysfunction, such as intelligence, creativity, and stamina. Individuals who are praised, acknowledged, cared for, and respected will develop a good sense of self (image, confidence, esteem). One of the ways this is achieved is by accenting the client's strengths, abilities, and accomplishments, not only in the physical realm, but also in the emotional, cognitive, and social realms.

Clarifying values and attitudes: Helping a client explore values and attitudes will focus on his/her belief structure. A belief structure forms the foundation of actions. What does the client value in life: family, work, leisure, sitting in the yard? What attitudes does the client have about life tasks: strong work ethic, strong gender role identity, negative leisure attitudes? Understanding what the client values and the attitudes behind each value will assist the therapist in identifying a healthy activity pattern for the client. For example, if the client has a strong work ethic, then alternatives to work could be explored, such as enrolling for vocational rehab, finding volunteer work, or exploring career alternatives. Clients who are able to return to prior life roles and activities are more likely to successfully adjust to a disability. Clarifying values and attitudes will also open the door to changing past values and attitudes, which may lead to new ideas and thoughts that will positively influence the client's adjustment. For example, a middle-aged adult who has been focused on obtaining external rewards from work and career may be in the process of reviewing past choices. Clarifying values and attitudes may assist the client in finding new paths that will meet needs, thus assisting the client to move on to meet goals.

Enhancing a positive self-image: Disability often has a negative connotation, including unproductiveness, helplessness, and poor appearance. Although healthcare professionals know differently, individuals who have a disability may fall into the trap of viewing themselves negatively due to the disability and not evaluating themselves on who they really are. A positive self-image needs to be strengthened and stereotypes and myths need to be broken. Opportunities for attention to physical appearance, such as hairstyle or hair color, makeup, toenail polish, a new outfit, or teeth whitening, need to be provided, as well as opportunities to be independent and productive (e.g., help in designing accessible changes to home, organizing home care schedule).

Developing communication and interaction skills: Clients who are having difficulty expressing themselves in a healthy and appropriate manner benefit from learning how to communicate and interact with others effectively. In addition, clients who are newly disabled will need to interact with people in new situations. Among other things, they will need to inquire about accessibility, request assistance with retrieving items, and ask a store employee to alert others that there is someone of the opposite sex in the bathroom helping the client. Learning to be assertive in these situations may be required. Clients also need to be instructed on the various styles of conflict resolution (passive, aggressive, assertive) and understand the outcomes of each

style, as well as how to use new interaction and communication styles. Those that adopt assertiveness will be able to obtain resources and meet needs, thus impacting adjustment issues.

Engaging in problem solving: Initially the client's family and loved ones make the majority of decisions for the client, thus impacting the client's involvement in problem solving. The therapist will also make decisions and problem solve for many situations without the assistance of the client, for example changing the focus of treatment session because the client is having an emotionally challenging day. This type of behavior contributes to the client's lack of control and learned helplessness. Allowing the client to make decisions and solve problems contributes to internal locus of control, which directly contributes to psychosocial adjustment. The therapist should challenge clients to solve simple to complex issues (e.g., let me know on Tuesday where you want to go for our outing on Friday, draw a picture of the layout of your woodshop and come up with some adaptations that you think would work well for you). These skills must be enhanced as soon as possible. Otherwise the client may fall into the trap of learned helplessness, thinking that someone else must do everything for him/her.

Exploring new lifestyle options: "The patient's ability to adapt to disability is more certain when valued work, family and community roles, favorite activities, and membership in prized groups can be continued. Too great a variance between the premorbid and present life-styles may not be acceptable to the patient and will thus reduce intrinsic motivation to identify acceptable alternative roles and to retain belief in personal competence. These are generalizations, and much depends on the patient's range of interests, skills, past experiences, intelligence, and adaptability" (Trombly, 1989, p. 14). It can be difficult to accept that lifestyle changes may be needed in all aspects of life. Every effort should be made to integrate the client back into his/her premorbid lifestyle as long as it is healthy. Sometimes changes are necessary. For example, the client's wife files for divorce when the client is in rehab and now the client must find an accessible place to live prior to discharge: a place in which the client can function independently. Accepting the need for change is not always an easy task for the client. It can be equally difficult for the client to view his/her lifestyle any differently from what s/he already knows. Options should be available for the client to explore (e.g., integration outing to accessible apartment complex, research new career options). If a new lifestyle is needed and realistic options are identified with resourceful professionals, the client will be better prepared for the transition.

Opportunities for emotional support: Therapists and family provide the client with emotional support. However, support from someone who can personally relate to the client's situation can often be more helpful. Therapists and family can try to empathize with what the client is going through, but they may have never experienced it. A client may express this by saying, "You don't know what it's like," or "You say you understand, but you really don't." People who mean well when they offer encouragement and a positive outlook can be met with sarcasm and anger. Sometimes clients just need someone to sit in the mess with them, someone who can wallow in the mud hole, but who also knows how to pull himself out. Clients, however, are not always receptive to meeting with someone who has a disability, especially if they are trying to "run away" from the disability or they have a negative view of people who have a disability and think, "I am not like them." Do not push the client into a support group or force a meeting with a past client. Gently suggest that you know someone, preferably someone who is the same age as the client, who has been recovering for more than two years, who can relate to what the client is going through, and who can offer some ideas about how s/he handles certain problems. An informal approach can also be taken, where a mentor just stops by, happens to be visiting with the therapist at the time of the client's appointment, or shows up on an outing. Explain to the client that it is good to know someone who is in the same boat. One way to explain this is to say something like, "It's good to have a guy friend to talk with about guy stuff, right? Well, it can also be good to have a friend who has a spinal cord injury, so you can talk about spinal cord stuff."

Setting appropriately sized goals: Long-term goals can seem like they take forever to accomplish. Identification of short, concrete, realistic goals provides more immediate feedback of progress, enhancing a client's self-esteem and confidence in task accomplishment and ultimately impacting the client's ability to respond/adjust.

Providing different approaches to treatment: Each therapist has his/her own personality, some serious, others flexible. Therapists should be open to changing their approach, despite how comfortable the approach is for the therapist, to meet the needs of the client. Some clients will respond better to a sensitive and quiet therapist while others may respond to a straightforward and confident therapist. Some clients relate better to therapists that they can identify with on some level. Some clients prefer an easy-going therapist while others like a stick-to-the-textbook approach. Although clients will be thrust out into a world of many different personalities, in the rehabilitation process the therapist should make every attempt to adapt his/her approach to meet the needs of the client so as to bring out the best in the client. Therapists should be careful, however, not to accommodate the client so much that treatment goals are not reached. For example, therapist's flexibility should not allow the client to ignore certain tasks such as cathing in public restrooms.

Encouraging healthy responses by family and friends: Family and friends are also in a period of adjustment. It can be difficult to know what to say to loved ones, as well as how to say it. Sometimes, people want to help so much that they help too much, thus perpetuating learned helplessness. Sometimes family and friends become angry with the client due to the client's denial or lack of motivation or initiative, thus distancing their relationship at a time when the client needs them most. Family and friends, as appropriate, should be made aware of the adjustment/response process and ways to interact with the client to enhance progress. Counseling services should also be made available to the family and friends.

The primary ICF codes that are addressed by adjustment and response to disability are listed at the beginning of the chapter.

References

Doak, C. C., Doak, L. G., & Root, J. H. (1995). *Teaching patients with low literacy skills*. Baltimore, MD: Lippincott Williams & Wilkins.

Erikson, E. H. (1968). *Identity: youth and crisis*. New York: Norton.

Falvo, D. (2013). *Medical and psychosocial aspects of chronic illness and disability*. Burlington, MA: Jones & Bartlett Learning.

Smart, J. (2001). *Disability, society, and the individual*. Gaithersburg, MD: Aspen.

Stolov, W. & Clowers, M. (1981). *Handbook of severe disability*. Washington, DC: U.S. Department of Education.

Trombly, C. (1989). *Occupational therapy for physical dysfunction* (3rd ed.). Baltimore, MD: Williams & Wilkins.

3. Body Mechanics and Ergonomics

Heather R. Porter

Body mechanics describe the efficient use of the body to complete tasks and is closely tied with mechanical engineering principles. Ergonomics is the study of how to position the body and objects in the environment to maximize performance and decrease injury. This discussion takes into account physiology, psychology, and mechanical engineering.

Elements of Body Mechanics

There are seven basic elements that play a part in body mechanics. The therapist needs to know them for three reasons:

1. Often clients with impairments will have poor body mechanics. To help the client problem solve barriers to participation the therapist often needs to address at least one of the elements of body mechanics.

2. Other members of the treatment team discuss these elements during team meetings to describe impairments and precautions necessary for each client. To function as a member of the treatment team and to reduce potential risks to clients the recreational therapist will need to understand the elements of body mechanics.

3. To ensure the therapist's own safety, proper body mechanics must be utilized at all times, for example, when transferring a client or lifting supplies.

Timbly and Lewis (1992) list the seven elements of body mechanics as:

Gravity: The force that holds us on the earth and causes everything to move to the lowest possible level. It defines up and down.

Energy: The capacity for action. Energy is required to move things from one place to another, including the client moving his/her body. Energy is required to handle gravity, but the amount of energy required is less with good body mechanics.

Balance: A position of equilibrium or stability. To stay in balance, a person must keep the center of gravity over the base of support. Larger bases of support make it easier to move and stay in balance.

Center of gravity: The central point of the mass of an object. The center of gravity for a standing person is about two inches below the belly button, halfway from front to back and in the middle from side to side. Obesity tends to move the center of gravity forward from the place where the body structures are best able to handle weight.

Line of gravity: An imaginary line defined by the pull of gravity that goes straight up and down through the center of gravity. Good body mechanics requires other structures, such as the head, to also be on the line for lowest energy requirements.

Base of support: The part of an object in contact with the ground. The feet are the base of support when a person is in a standing position. Interactions with the center of gravity affect balance.

Alignment: The position of the parts of the body in relation to each other. We call the best body alignment good posture.

Body Mechanic and Ergonomic Techniques

Often, using good body mechanics is based on common sense tempered with self-discipline about how you move your body. Trombly (1989) makes the point by stating:

Use of correct body mechanics is absolutely necessary for anyone with chronic low back pain, but it is also recommended for all persons engaged in physical work inside or outside the home. The principles of good body mechanics elaborate on the ideas of joint alignment, use of large muscles instead of small, and working in harmony with gravity. Specifically, the principles are keep the head aligned with the trunk (tuck the chin); keep the shoulders and hips parallel (don't twist the trunk); maintain pelvic tilt (tuck the buttocks or keep one foot raised on a low stool while standing); maintain good balance (position the feet shoulder distance apart, one foot forward); keep the back straight (bend at the hip and knees simultaneously rather than bend over at the waist); and push before pulling and pull before lifting. If the person must lift and carry, he should keep the object close to the body to reduce the length of the resistance lever arm and subsequently the strain on trunk muscles and spinal ligaments (p. 412).

These principles can be applied not only in a static position (e.g., standing), but also in dynamic activity. For example, if you are walking past an item that you wish to retrieve, you should fully turn your feet, legs, hips, trunk, and shoulders to face the item rather than twisting your trunk.

One of the most common injuries due to poor body mechanics is lower back pain. However, muscle strains and sprains due to poor body mechanics are not limited to the lower back. The biggest risk factors for injury due to poor body mechanics include poor posture, being out of shape or overweight, and moving the body incorrectly. Individuals with physical disabilities may be at a higher risk of injury due to poor body mechanics because: (1) center of gravity, line of gravity, base of support, and alignment may be changed and compromised as a direct result of the impairment; (2) the client may lack knowledge or cognitive ability to understand good body mechanics based on the modified body structure; and (3) staff working with clients may not take into account a change in energy level, balance, center of gravity, line of gravity, base of support, or alignment when teaching the client new skills.

Good Body Mechanics

Some of the basics of good body mechanics, appropriate for both clients and therapists, include:

Bending and Leaning

Even though bending and leaning usually brings up the mental picture of someone bending over and touching his/her toes, proper bending and leaning involve the hips, knees, feet, and stomach muscles more than the back.

When bending to pick something up that is farther away than the length of your arms, the first action should be to step closer to the item so that it is within arm's length. If this is not possible, widen your base of support. This means standing with your feet shoulder-width apart with one foot slightly ahead of the other. Use (tighten) your stomach and thigh muscles as you lean forward. This helps your body maintain balance as it moves out of optimal alignment and is pulled forward.

When bending to pick up something that is lower than your hands, squat down by bending at the knees and hips instead of bending your back. Lower yourself using the strength in your thigh muscles. This helps maintain an alignment between your line of gravity and the body structures that are best suited to bear weight.

If seated in a wheelchair, the task of bending and leaning will vary depending on the abilities and limitations of the client. A client may have mobility limitations that restrict trunk flexion or rotation due to paralysis (e.g., tetraplegia), surgery (e.g., short-term back surgery parameters of limited trunk flexion and rotation, total hip precautions that prohibit bending more than 90°), or injury (e.g., back injury that causes pain with flexion or rotation). If a client sitting in a wheelchair is able to bend at the trunk to pick up an item from the floor, the first thing that s/he should do is to propel the wheelchair past the item and then back up so that the item is now on the side of the wheelchair. The reason for doing this is two-fold:

1. It properly aligns the caster wheels so that the front of the wheelchair is supported and does not tip forward when the client leans to pick up the item. When you back up the wheelchair, the caster wheels spin around so that the majority of the wheel is in front of the caster arm.

2. Reaching to the side to retrieve an item from the floor is safer than reaching forward because it minimizes the chance of the wheelchair tipping forward. Added supports for bending and leaning include the use of a reacher and other sturdy objects to assist with balance when bending and leaning. For example, people who have high-level paraplegia can

hook one arm around the wheelchair armrest to provide balance support.

Lifting Objects

Lifting incorrectly is the most common cause of back injury in healthcare workers. Healthcare workers lift as much weight as construction workers. Usually the best lifting technique involves keeping the object being lifted close to your body with your feet straddling the object. Bend with your knees and hips. It is important to keep your head in alignment with your back (don't lean forward) and your shoulders in alignment with your hips (don't twist). If you need to lift a heavy object above your waist try to lift it to waist level, place it on a secure table, change your grip, and lift again maintaining good alignment with an adequate base of support to maintain your balance. Remember that, when you hold an object, your center of gravity shifts to the center of mass for you and what you are holding.

These techniques can also be used for clients who do not have lifting or movement restrictions. Lifting techniques will need to be modified for those who have restrictions such as weight limits, range of motion impairments, paralysis, or joint protection precautions.

Client Transfers

In this case, client transfer refers to a therapist or caregiver physically moving a client from one location to another, not a transfer done by a client. Communication is the most critical element. You must make sure that you use the correct transfer for the client (check the medical chart) because using the wrong transfer technique may injure both you and the client. Communicate with the client to determine how much the client will be able to help you with the transfer. (Does the client understand what to do? Does the client have the skills or strength to help out?) And, if you are doing a two-person transfer, communicate with the other person to make sure that the transfer goes smoothly.

If you are moving a client in bed, point your feet in the direction that you plan to move the client. It is common for clients who need assistance with bed mobility to have a "draw sheet" under their torso. A draw sheet is a stout piece of fabric that usually measures two to three feet by five to six feet. If you put a sheet of plastic under the draw sheet, the sheet

will slide more easily. Talk with the client and other staff who may be helping you to coordinate efforts.

If you are helping a client go from sitting on the side of the bed to standing, make sure that your knees are braced against the client's knees. This provides a counterbalance, brings your mutual line of gravity closer to the muscles that need to support the weight, and provides a wider dynamic base of support for you as you lift the client. These dynamics only work well when the client has slip-resistant foot coverings.

A mechanical lifting device such as a Hoyer lift should be used when a client requires maximum assistance (or is dependent) to transfer.

Posture

Having good posture for the back is the basis of good body mechanics. The back normally has three gentle curves that help distribute stress throughout the vertebra and discs. The three gentle curves in the back are at the neck (slight curve forward), the shoulders (slight curve backward), and the lower back (slight curve forward). Maintaining these curves through most activities will reduce strain on the back.

Pushing and Pulling

Whenever possible push an item instead of pulling. People can usually push twice as much weight as they can pull before musculoskeletal damage occurs. When pushing an object, make sure to stay close to the weight of the load without leaning forward. Use arm, stomach, and leg muscles to move items.

Repetitive Motion

Repetitive motions can cause damage to the moving body parts unless precautions are taken. Try to take breaks, vary the movements, move light loads, and turn the entire body instead of twisting at the waist when possible.

Sitting

Sitting is almost twice as hard on back muscles as standing (Coastal Healthcare, 1993). Part of the reason for this is the beneficial curves in the spine are straightened out by sitting in some chairs. The lumbar curve is especially at risk to be reduced. This reduction in the curve modifies the center of gravity, line of gravity, and base of support. Chair height is also important in helping maintain beneficial spinal curves, base of support, and line of gravity. When sitting, your knees should be at the same height as your hips. If someone has a loss of sensation and sits in a way that reduces the lumbar spinal curve, base of support, or unbalances the line of gravity, cumulative damage may be occurring to the spine and associated muscles without the typical warning signs of lower back pain.

Standing

Standing, especially static standing without moving around, increases the stress on back muscles. To help relieve some of the stress it is a good idea to stand with one foot in front of the other and supported on a slightly raised footstool. Switch the forward foot every five or ten minutes.

Transfer Belts

In a treatment setting almost all types of transfers should be done with the client wearing a transfer belt. A transfer belt is a cotton or nylon belt that is about three inches wide and five feet long. This is placed around the client's waist on top of all clothing and tightened with only a little extra slack so that the therapist's hand can comfortably hold the belt firmly. Transfer belts are for both the therapist's and the client's safety. If the client were to start falling, the therapist does not have to catch the client to stop the fall. S/he can use the belt to safely guide the client to the floor bending at the hips and knees and not the back. If the client becomes slightly off balance, the therapist can help the client regain balance by providing a steadying pull on the transfer belt.

Fine Hand Use Ergonomics

How the environment is structured has an effect on the client's ability to perform tasks that require fine hand skills. It is the therapist's responsibility to create an environment that maximizes the client's potential.

Grandjean (1988) lists ten ways to improve a client's performance on tasks that require fine hand use skills. By setting up activities so that they comply with these ten principles, the therapist ensures that a client's performance is based on the client's skill level and that the client is not handicapped by the environment. The ten principles are

Elbow position: The activity should be set up so that the client's elbows are generally slightly lower than the wrists with an angle of between 85° to 110° at the elbow.

Visual distance: For activities with small details that require good eye-hand coordination, bring the work closer to the client. The client's body position should have only a slight bend in the neck and head while leaning forward. The idea is to allow the activity to be placed close enough to the client to allow the client to see well while not requiring the client to assume an uncomfortable position that taxes the body's muscles. It is a good idea for the therapist to ask a client if s/he is able to see the object clearly. Often clients are admitted to facilities without their glasses or contact lenses or lose them once they are admitted. Adaptive devices for vision should be provided for the client so that s/he is able to work in an appropriate position.

Muscle loading: Muscle loading is increasing the amount of strength the muscles are required to exert to maintain the activity. Muscle loading can be holding a heavy load in an uncomfortable position or holding a heavy load in the same position longer than the muscles are able to maintain adequate strength. An example of muscle loading is holding a gallon of milk straight out in front of you, a position that tires the arm muscles fairly quickly. Holding the gallon of milk at rib height close to the body with the elbow lower than the wrist limits the muscle loading required to hold the milk. Muscles that have a heavy muscle load are difficult to control or to coordinate. Position both the client and the activity to reduce the amount of force that causes muscle loading. This may mean that the client uses slings, elbow supports, or lightweight equipment to help reduce muscle loading.

Diversity of fine motor activity: Performance on fine hand tasks tends to increase if the client is required to perform only one fine hand use task at a time. An example of this principle is the old sewing machines versus the more modern ones. Older sewing machines required that one hand be used to start or stop the flywheel that made the needle go up and down while also guiding the fabric through the machine. Today's sewing machines tend to use foot pedals to start and stop the needle allowing both hands to move the fabric through the machine. Another example is in beading activities. If a client is stringing beads to make a necklace, it is not uncommon for the client to have to place a bead on the thread and then look around to select the next bead.

Beading trays allow a client to select all the beads needed for the necklace, place them in the tray trough in the desired order, and then string the already selected beads. For clients with significant impairment of one hand and arm (e.g., after a stroke), taping drawing paper to the table instead of requiring the client to stabilize the paper while drawing also helps limit the number of fine hand movements required at any one time.

Activity setup: The setup for the activity should help the activity flow from one step to the next and the materials selected should increase (instead of decrease) the client's chance of success. For example, in a painting activity the paper should be in front of the client, the paintbrush rinse water at two o'clock, the paper towel to help dry the brush after cleaning at one o'clock and the paints at twelve o'clock above the paper. (This placement is mirrored for a client who is left-handed.) Fausek-Steinbach (2002) discusses how to select the materials for a drawing activity.

> The materials one selects to work with are just as important as the process they are used in. Drawing materials can vary from expensive colored pencils to crayons. The way the materials are perceived, as well as how they perform, are very important when presenting them to your clients. I try to use oil pastels instead of wax crayons whenever possible only because crayons are perceived as "kid's toys" by teens and adults and quickly raise a red flag in the hesitant artist's mind. Avoid smudgy chalks or charcoal pencils for drawings, as the unintended smudges will frustrate your clients and give them an excuse to give up. Opt for smudge free pencils or markers when asking them to draw (p. 73).

Client-determined activity rhythm: The speed and pace of an activity freely chosen by the client is, in most cases, preferable to a pace selected by the therapist. By being able to self-pace an activity, the client can concentrate on the activity at hand instead of being worried about complying with someone else's timing and pace. This principle usually does not apply to clients with severe or profound intellectual disability, clients with dementia, or clients who have other significant cognitive impairments that interfere with activity initiation or carry through.

Activity in front of the client: Fine hand function tends to improve if the activity is placed immediately in front of and close to the client. When the activity requires the use of both hands at once, the therapist should structure the activity so that each sequence begins with both hands working symmetrically when possible. For example, when fly-casting (fishing) and reeling in the line, the move should start with one hand on the base of the fly rod and the other on the rod near the reel. The fly is cast and then the two hands work together holding up the rod and reeling in the line.

Arc of activity: A client's fine hand function will be best if the activity takes place within the first two-thirds of the arm's range of motion arc. This arc extends both vertically and horizontally from the position of the elbows being at the side of the body. The further the arms extend from this position, the more impaired the fine hand function will become.

Horizontal versus vertical movement: Horizontal and circular movements tend to allow better fine hand control than vertical or zigzag movements. For clients with fine hand movement impairments try to modify the activity to use horizontal or circular movements. As the client's ability increases, add vertical or zigzag movements to expand capability.

Handle and tool size: Handles to tools should fit easily in the client's hands without causing muscle loading and fatigue. This may require that the grips be modified to better fit the client's hands and ability. Gripping strength increases when the hand that is holding the tool is held in line with the client's forearm. For example, there are many gardening tools that have "trigger grips." These work well for clients with arthritis or weak grips.

Ergonomic Risk Factors

burlingame (2001) discusses seven risk factors that increase damage to the body and should be considered when evaluating a client's activities to ensure that no further harm is done. The seven risk factors are

Duration: Duration refers to the length of time that the body is exposed to a stress in the environment. Increased length of exposure can lead to increased impact on the immediate area of exposure and increased general fatigue response. Generally, the greater the duration of exposure to a stressful risk factor, the greater the length of time it takes the body to revert to its baseline function.

Force: The greater the force needed to complete the task, the greater the physiological stress to the body's muscles, tendons, and joints.

Mechanical compression or contact stress: Mechanical compression refers to pressure points created when an object places uneven pressure on the body such as a garden shovel would place extra stress on the tissue in the palm at the points that the handle of the shovel contacts the hand. Mechanical compression can impede blood flow and interfere with nerve function.

Posture: Awkward postures place stress on joints and surrounding tissue. This leads to extra muscle and tendon fatigue and joint soreness. The added stress is thought to contribute to an increased likelihood of musculoskeletal disorders.

Repetition: A repetitive motion is an action that is repeated many times with a cycle time of less than 30 seconds or when the basic cycle accounts for 50% or more of the total work cycle (OSHA, 1995). This repetitive action can lead to accelerated muscle fatigue and increased risk of muscle-tendon damage. Tasks that are very repetitive do not allow time for adequate tissue recovery.

Temperature: The lower a temperature goes, the greater the loss of dexterity, sensitivity, and grip force. Also, a lower temperature can make the impact of vibration worse. OSHA (1995) recommends that metal surfaces be above 59°F as temperatures below this point decrease dexterity. Metal surfaces below 44.6°F may lead to numbness. The American Conference of Governmental Industrial Hygienists (1995) recommends the following exposure limits: for sedentary work, 60°F; for light work, 40°F; and for moderate work (fine motor dexterity not required), 20°F.

Vibration: Vibration types can be impact, oscillation, or combined impact and oscillation. Vibration can also be categorized as localized (e.g., vibration of the hand) or whole body (e.g., riding on a motorcycle). National vibration threshold standards have been set for some aspects of the workplace to limit the neurological and fatigue factors associated with vibration.

Documenting Ergonomic Skills

Many clients need education on correct body mechanics. Therapists document the specific problem that the client is having with body mechanics or ergonomics (e.g., client's computer station setup is not ergonomically correct contributing to lower back and neck pain), recommendations (e.g., recommended to raise computer monitor to eye height), ability to apply proper body mechanics and ergonomics (usually measured as a percentage), and areas where the client needs assistance (e.g., requires moderate verbal cues to maintain good body posture during table games).

Clients increase their skills for using good body mechanics through observation of the therapist modeling the desired skills, education, and practice. If a client has difficulty performing proper body mechanics because of a specific disability, the therapist encourages the client to come as close as possible to good body mechanics. For example, a client with kyphosis would be asked to stand as upright as possible. Activities can also be modified to increase a client's ability to maintain good posture. For example, placing a box on top of the table and placing the activity on top of the box raises the height of the activity and encourages the client to stand upright.

ICF Connections

ICF codes that might require use of the information about body mechanics and ergonomics include b235 Vestibular Functions, b455 Exercise Tolerance Functions, many of the codes in b7 Neuromusculoskeletal and Movement-Related Functions, and s7 Structures Related to Movement. Deficits in d4 Mobility, especially d410 - d429 Changing and Maintaining Body Position, d430 Lifting and Carrying Objects, d435 Moving Objects with Lower Extremities, d440 Fine Hand Use, d445 Hand and Arm Use, and d455 Moving Around, will be addressed using principles discussed in this chapter. Concerns with d5 Self-Care, d6 Domestic Life, d8 Major Life Areas, and d9 Community, Social, and Civic Life may all have a component that requires consideration of body mechanics and ergonomics.

References

American Conference of Governmental Industrial Hygienists. (1995). Threshold limits for chemical substances and physical agents and biological exposure indices. Cincinnati, OH: ACGIH.

burlingame, j. (2001). *Idyll Arbor's therapy dictionary* (2nd ed.). Ravensdale, WA: Idyll Arbor, Inc.

Coastal Healthcare. (1993). *Protecting your back.* Virginia Beach, VA: author.

Fausek-Steinbach, D. (2002). *Art activities for groups: Providing therapy, fun, and function.* Ravensdale, WA: Idyll Arbor, Inc.

Grandjean, E. (1988). *Fitting the task to the man: A textbook of occupational ergonomics.* New York: Taylor & Francis.

Occupational Safety and Health Administration. (1995). Ergonomic protection standard (draft). Washington, DC: Government Printing Office.

Timbly, B. & Lewis, L. (1992). *Fundamental skills and concepts in patient care* (5th ed.). Philadelphia, PA: Lippincott Company.

Trombly, C. (1989). *Occupational therapy for physical dysfunction* (3rd ed.). Baltimore, MD: Williams & Wilkins.

4. Consequences of Inactivity

Heather R. Porter

Staying in bed or being inactive for long periods of time can be dangerous to a client's health. Recreational therapists need to have a full understanding of the secondary complications from inactivity and educate clients and caregivers about them.

Although knowledge does not always equal action, it is still a valuable component in formulating lifestyle change. In some situations, educating the client first about the consequences of inactivity can be helpful for clients to understand the benefits of recreational therapy (e.g., "Recreational activities can help reduce risks of developing these secondary conditions and I really don't want these problems because it will impact my ability to do [something that is meaningful to the client].").

Linking problems to their effect on activities that are meaningful to a client can make a profound impact (e.g., "If I don't become more active, I am at risk of losing more functioning and then I will need more help and possibly not be able to live alone anymore … and I don't want that because I value my independence." "I love to do things with my grandchildren so I need to stay active to be a part of their activities."). Taking this approach means that the recreational therapist:

1. Begins by talking with a client about his/her lifestyle.

2. Finds out what is meaningful to the client. Possibilities include health and recovery, ability to take care of himself/herself independently, spending time with friends, going back to school, or playing with other children.

3. Then ties together the effect of how a sedentary or inactive lifestyle could negatively impact the client's ability to participate in activities that are meaningful to the client.

There are many complications associated with inactivity and bed rest. Here are some of the important ones that recreational therapists address.

Contractures

As the old saying goes, "Use it or lose it." Muscles need to be stretched and joints moved through their full range so that they do not contract. If muscles are not stretched, they shorten and tighten, affecting the mobility (range of motion) of the joint. Prolonged inactivity of muscles can cause contractures (shortening of muscles that severely restrict range of motion). Once contractures occur, they are difficult to undo.

Typical treatment for contractures is serial casting. The joint or limb is stretched as much as possible and then a cast is applied to hold the stretch for a period of time to lengthen the muscle. The cast is then removed and the process is repeated until full range or optimal range is obtained. Contractures are common problems for people who spend a great amount of time in a fixed position. For example, hip and knee contractures happen to someone who spends too much time in a sitting position. Wrist and elbow contractures can occur in a paralyzed limb that is not routinely ranged.

Contractures can cause problems with self-care and life activities. Examples include inability to put on a shirt independently because of upper extremity contractures, difficulty standing upright due to hip and knee contractures, contractures in a paralyzed upper extremity preventing the client from using the limb as an assist during activities, or hip and knee contractures can make walking difficult.

Preventative measures can reduce the risk of contractures even when the client is relatively inactive. The care plan should make sure that the client moves each joint through its full range of motion at least once every eight hours, intermittently lies on the abdomen to help prevent hip flexion contractures, changes position often, and is involved in physically active self-care along with movement-related vocational, recreational, and community activities that hold meaning for the client.

Atrophy

Muscle fibers deteriorate from inactivity resulting in decreased strength. Total disuse of a muscle, as a result of paralysis, tendon tear, plaster casting, or severe pain on motion, will lead to the loss of about one-eighth of its strength each week. If paralysis exists, external electrical stimulation of the muscles is sometimes used to help prevent atrophy. If that is not the treatment of choice, the client must at least do range of motion exercises to prevent contractures. All clients who have had prolonged illness or inactivity will have some degree of disuse atrophy of their muscles. Backache and fatigue during periods of inactivity may be caused by atrophied muscles.

The heart is also a muscle, and it undergoes disuse atrophy just like other muscles when a person is inactive. If the heart muscle atrophies, it must work harder to do the same job as before. As a result, the client may experience shortness of breath, easy fatigability, palpitations, and/or lightheadedness with exertion. Trying to perform vigorous activities that are above current strength level can cause strains, pains, accidents, falls, and injury. This can limit independence, functioning, and quality of life.

Prevention involves strengthening muscles regularly through therapeutic exercise, self-care activities, and recreational and community activities.

Osteoporosis and Kidney Stones

When weight bearing through the arms and legs and when muscles pull and stretch at their connections, the body deposits and absorbs calcium in the bones. Bed rest and inactivity eliminate most of these stresses. Within three days of bed rest there are measurable increases in the amount of calcium in the urine because the bones are losing it. The bones then soften and weaken (osteoporosis), and even ordinary forces such as those encountered during transfers, therapy activities, or minor falls may cause bone fractures. Fractured vertebras are the most common result of osteoporosis in older persons. Ordinary x-rays do not show evidence of osteoporosis until more than 50% of the bone mineral has been lost.

Along with the loss of bone mass, there is the danger of kidney stones resulting from the increased calcium in the urinary system.

Prevention of osteoporosis requires weight bearing through the arms and legs. For example, standing at a table and performing an activity that requires the client to use the upper extremities for support, such as weight bearing through the left arm to provide support to be able to reach with the right hand. Weight bearing can be promoted through therapeutic exercise, self-care activities, vocational activities, and recreation and community activities.

Prevention of kidney stones requires drinking enough fluids to yield 1.5-2 liters of urine output a day. Increased activity level increases thirst, encouraging the client to drink more fluids. Increased fluid intake causes increased urination, helping to reduce stagnant urine in the bladder.

Urinary Tract Infection (UTI)

Emptying the bladder while lying down can prevent the bladder from fully emptying. The urine left over in the bladder can become stagnant, grow bacteria, and cause infection.

Prevention of UTIs involves drinking urine acidifiers such as cranberry juice or vitamin C to decrease bacteria growth in the urine and emptying the bladder in a standing or sitting position whenever possible. Increased activity level increases thirst, encouraging the client to drink more fluids. Increased fluid intake causes increased urination, helping to reduce stagnant urine in the bladder.

Deep Vein Thrombosis (DVT)

A DVT is a blood clot. It usually forms in the legs of people who are inactive for periods of time, sometimes as little as a few hours. Due to poor blood circulation, blood tends to pool in the lower extremities and blood clots form. The danger is that the blood clot could break loose and lead to an embolism (a blood clot blocking an artery) in the heart, lungs, or brain causing a heart attack, death, or stroke.

Prevention involves moving around frequently and varying positions to promote blood circulation (e.g., sit, stand, lie down, raise legs). Raising the legs can help to decrease edema (swelling due to fluid pooling in the legs from inactivity) and promote blood flow toward the heart. Compression stockings (thick elastic stockings) may be worn on the legs to help push fluid and blood toward the heart and keep it from pooling in the legs. Performing leg exercises when sitting or lying for long periods of time will reduce the risk of a DVT. Possible exercises include ankle flexion and extension, knee raises, knee flexion and extension, marching, and abduction and adduction of the hips.

Orthostatic Hypotension

Bed rest and inactivity, even after one to two weeks, can cause blood pressure to drop when the client is moving from one position to another position after having been in one position for an extended period of time, such as a client who has been lying down in bed standing up. Blood pressure that drops with a change in body position is called orthostatic hypotension.

When a person has been in one position for an extended period of time and the body position is changed, blood pools to the legs and abdomen. The circulatory system needs to respond quickly to the change in body position to make sure the blood is available to the brain. If it does not respond quickly enough, because of inactivity, the blood pressure drop causes the client to feel dizzy, weak, or faint. Orthostatic hypotension is rarely a chronic problem. With increased movement and changes in body positioning, the body learns to adjust the blood pressure quickly. However, for clients who stay in bed at home or sit for prolonged periods of time, orthostatic hypotension can be the cause of falls and injuries that could impact the client's ability to function and be independent.

Prevention involves changing body positions frequently throughout the day. This can be promoted through self-care or vocational, recreational, and community activities.

Pneumonia

Prolonged bed rest increases the risk for pneumonia. Lying down and poor posture, such as rounded shoulders with chin tucked when sitting in a wheelchair or being propped up in bed, result in a poor cough reflex and also make it difficult to take deep breaths. Air passages start to shut down and harmful bacteria begin to grow. Bacterial infections

can affect other body functions and, in clients whose health is already compromised, death can result.

Prevention requires changing body positions frequently throughout the day. This can be promoted through self-care or vocational, recreational, and community activities. Other preventative measures include having the client sit upright and breathe deeply at regular intervals. The therapist can use activities to stimulate coughing, breathing, and movement of secretions.

Malnutrition

Inactivity and prolonged bed rest can take a toll on a client's nutrition. It can be difficult to eat in a reclined position in bed or eat a proper meal when propped on up on the sofa. Consequently, clients tend to eat too much junk food and improperly balanced meals. Sedentary behavior can also increase food intake because there are less distractions and typically the television is on, which may cause the client not to realize how much food s/he is consuming. For some clients, decreased activity causes lack of appetite, also resulting in poor nutritional intake. Proper nutrition is necessary for the body to heal, repair, and maintain functioning.

Prevention requires, when possible, that the client cooperate in food-related activities. The client should be part of planning healthy meals and eat with other people. The client should not eat in bed or sitting in front of the television. Eating while sitting up at the table increases awareness of what is being eaten. Exercise stimulates appetite. This can be promoted through self-care or vocational, recreational, and community activities. The therapist should seek help from a nutritionist, if needed.

Constipation

Inactivity and bed rest can cause constipation. Whole body movements interact with the digestive system to stimulate the intestines. Food choices, as discussed earlier, may be less healthful when a client is on bed rest. Lack of proper hydration, which can also lead to constipation, may also occur during bed rest and inactivity.

Prevention requires the client to change body positions frequently throughout the day and engage in physical activity. Both can be promoted through self-care or vocational, recreational, and community activities. The client should be sure to eat a healthy diet with foods that have sufficient fiber and drink sufficient amounts of fluids.

Skin Breakdown

Prolonged pressure on the skin over boney processes can result in the development of decubitus ulcers. When pressure over a boney process, especially hipbones, elbows, and heels, is not relieved, blood circulation to the skin and underlying body tissue is impaired. Lack of oxygenated blood to the area causes damage to the cells and a skin breakdown. In some cases, a client may feel the discomfort but be unable to move into another position to relieve the pressure due to impaired mobility skills. In other cases, such as complete spinal cord injury, clients lack the sensation to feel the discomfort and must compensate by performing weight shifts every 20-30 minutes.

Prevention involves using special wheelchair cushions and bed mattresses designed to relieve pressure over boney processes, frequent changes of body position, and keeping the skin dry at all times because moisture increases fragility of the skin, quickening skin breakdown.

Emotional and Social Health

Inactivity and bed rest can take a toll on more than just the physical functioning of the body. Anxiety, depression, hostility, social isolation, and learned helplessness can occur. This could be because fewer activities allow for an increased focus on negative thoughts. For example, the client may have concerns about self-care or activities that need to be done by other people because the client is unable to perform them, such as whether or not a sibling will follow through and go to the bank for him/her today. Other possible problems include hostility and anger due to poor coping strategies and heightened stress, social isolation due to decreased community activities, and friends and family who tend to visit less often after the immediate health crisis is over. One important

consideration is learned helplessness due to over-helpful caregivers who cause the client to feel helpless or fearful related to his/her ability to perform certain tasks.

Prevention has several aspects:

Emotional and social health can be affected by many other variables in addition to inactivity and bed rest. For example, social networks and support can be helpful in offering advice, comfort, motivation, and coping skills. This can be promoted through social activities inside and outside the home, including recreational and vocational activities.

The client should, as much as possible, keep a healthy routine including a regular sleep pattern, meaningful activities, regular exercise, and healthy eating. See Activity Pattern Development in the Techniques and Interventions section.

Expressing feelings in a healthy manner is also important. Counseling services can be offered and the recreational therapist can help the client explore healthy coping strategies through interventions such as spirituality, exercise, meditation, and talking with a trusted friend. See Stress Management and Coping, as well as Leisure-Based Stress Coping in the Techniques and Interventions section.

The therapist should also encourage self-reliance and independence with appropriate tasks.

ICF Connections

ICF codes where deficits raise concerns about inactivity include b110 Consciousness Functions, b130 Energy and Drive Functions, b280 Sensation of Pain, b455 Exercise Tolerance Functions, b710 Mobility of Joint Functions, b730 - b749 Muscle Functions, b750 - b789 Movement Functions, s1 Structures of the Nervous System (where paralysis is a concern), s410 Structure of Cardiovascular System, s430 Structure of Respiratory System, s7 Structures Related to Movement, and d4 Mobility.

5. Education and Counseling

Heather R. Porter

To better understand the distinction between education and counseling it helps to review their definitions. Education is the process of acquiring skills and knowledge. It is largely based on information giving. Counseling is the process of facilitating growth and exploration. Although acquiring skills and knowledge can facilitate self-awareness, it is not the primary goal of education and, although personal growth and exploration can facilitate learning new skills, it is not the primary goal of counseling. We can agree that their common element is the desired outcome of positive change, that they do affect each other, and that they are commonly integrated, but they have two separate orientations.

In the past, the field of recreational therapy had a distinction between counseling and education. However, more recent literature (Austin, 2004; Stumbo & Peterson, 2004) suggests that leisure counseling is part of the continuum of leisure education rather than a separate service. This debate is sure to continue and we urge recreational therapy researchers, professors, and authors to consider the impact of the ICF in our developing profession. Furthermore, we would like to note that becoming aware of leisure benefits and acquiring new leisure skills (education) and understanding personal values (counseling) does not always result in the client embracing and incorporating it into his/her way of living by actually leading a more healthy life. Saying it and doing it are two different things. Often the short-term nature of the therapist/client relationship means that the therapist does not know whether the client made changes. Defining and differentiating between education and counseling helps to develop better testing tools, making the impact of our services easier to measure.

Education and Counseling and the ICF

Education and counseling are interventions. The ICF does not list interventions. Therefore the therapist must think about education and counseling interventions from the following perspectives when deciding where to document issues related to them:

*Specific activity-related intervention*s: If the intervention is being provided to assist a client in activity participation, the therapist scores the specific activity for which the intervention is being provided. For example, if a client is having difficulty using public transportation because of a lack of knowledge about how to identity and utilize wheelchair accessible buses, then the therapist would score the level of difficulty that the client is having utilizing public transportation (d4702 Using Public Motorized Transportation). The therapist would then provide education and counseling interventions to the client on how to identify and use wheelchair accessible buses as one of his/her interventions to assist the client in improving activity performance with using public buses. Using a specific activity code puts more of an emphasis on the activity, rather than a health behavior as described next in *specific health-related education.*

Specific health-related intervention: If the intervention revolves around health practices, the therapist should consider using the relevant health code in the ICF including d570 Looking After One's Health, d5701 Managing Diet and Fitness, d5702 Maintaining One's Health, and d240 Handling Stress and Other Psychological Demands. Good questions to ask when deciding what code to use are "Why am I providing this specific intervention? What is the desired activity behavior that I wish to see in my client?" The specific activity behavior desired (e.g., d570 Looking After One's Health) would then be scored and the education and counseling intervention would be provided to positively impact the specific activity behavior. Using a specific, health-related code puts more emphasis on the health behavior, rather than on a specific activity as described previously in *specific activity-related intervention.*

Learning and applying knowledge: One caution about using ICF codes is to be careful about reading the codes accurately. It may seem like the therapist can use d198 Learning and Applying Knowledge, Other Specified for documenting education or counseling interventions. However, this is not usually the case. The patient would have to have a diagnosis documenting a deficit in the ability to acquire or use knowledge before it would be appropriate to use this code as a treatment intervention. An appropriate intervention under this code would be something like creating and rehearsing a script to perform an activity the client could not otherwise remember how to do. For example, if the therapist develops a script for identifying and locating wheelchair accessible buses, the script part of the treatment would be documented as treatment for the diagnosis of d198 Learning and Applying Knowledge, Other Specified. What the client is able to do after learning how to follow the script would then treat a deficit in d4702 Using Public Motorized Transportation.

Use of environmental codes: Environmental codes, also called e-codes, can be used to reflect the extent that a particular resource in the environment is a barrier or facilitator for an activity. Changing the extent of a barrier or facilitator in a positive direction may require education or counseling. Using this approach, the specific deficit in the environment, as described in the diagnosis, is selected as the basis for treatment. For example, if a client does not have the adaptive equipment required for a craft activity, the therapist would note e1401 Assistive Products and Technology for Culture, Recreation, and Sport. During the assessment process, this e-code may be scored as a barrier due to lack of knowledge, availability, or use of the adaptive piece of equipment. Educating the client about the piece of equipment, ordering the equipment, and teaching her how to use it, will resolve the deficit in the ICF code. Counseling might be required to make the client comfortable with using adaptive equipment that wasn't necessary before the current change in health. The new equipment and related skills optimally will become a

facilitator for some other ICF code, such as d9202 Arts and Culture. Using an e-code to show a reason for an intervention is appropriate when the intervention revolves around deficits in ICF codes e1 Products and Technology, e2 Natural Environment and Human-Made Changes to Environment, e3 Support and Relationships, e4 Attitudes, or e5 Services, Systems, and Policies (the five chapters of Environmental Factors).

Education

The kind of education most often practiced by recreational therapists is called "leisure education." Recreational therapists commonly use this term to describe any form of education that pertains to leisure activity such as resource education, benefits of leisure education, leisure skills education (e.g., rules of playing an adaptive sport), community skills education (e.g., teaching a client about accessibility rights under the Americans with Disabilities Act), social skills education (e.g., how to respond in certain situations), and leisure appreciation education. Leisure appreciation is the act of realistically estimating an activity's worth and the amount of enjoyment it brings. It involves making a judgment and having a sensitive awareness of the emotional and physical benefits of an action, individual, group, or object. Nurturing leisure appreciation is the process of teaching clients about leisure and the health benefits of leisure participation and having the client apply the information by creating a healthy activity plan. Education about the benefits of leisure and fostering leisure appreciation are often interlinked.

The list of leisure education topics could go on, but the basic idea is that the topic of education is broad and the context for which recreational therapists use the term leisure education encompasses a wide array of categories and topics. Note, also, that the kinds of information presented to clients go far beyond simple leisure skills and many of what appear to be leisure skills are also useful in other areas of the client's life. Recreational therapists would do well to keep this in mind when they are discussing the kind of work they do.

Because the terms "education" and "leisure education" are broad, it benefits the therapist, and those who read the therapist's notes, to clearly document the specific education needed, measured, and provided.

Counseling

As previously discussed, counseling is different from education in that counseling is the process of facilitating growth and exploration, whereas education is the process of acquiring skills and knowledge. Many therapists use the term "leisure counseling" to denote a portion of the total scope of recreational therapy counseling. However recreational therapy practice expands past this term and utilizes a variety of counseling approaches and techniques to address a multitude of issues including psychosocial adjustment to disability and illness; clarification of values, beliefs, and attitudes; management of specific problems, such as anxiety, pain, and anger; facilitation of personal growth and exploration that affect health practices and quality of life; relationship building; change in behaviors and thinking patterns; and understanding different perspectives.

Counseling can be provided in various formats (e.g., informal vs. formal, individual vs. group) and to various people by role or location (e.g., client, caregiver, support group, senior center). For example, in family training, attention is given to the needs of the caregivers to maximize compliance with recommendations. Some examples include: a family may requiring counseling about the value of activity to understand its role in recovery and health promotion, a mother of a disabled child who comes to a therapy session lacking sleep and breakfast may benefit from brief informal counseling on the importance of caring for herself related to her ability to help her child, or a caregiver that exhibits anxious behavior when learning how to assist her spouse in doing a car transfer may benefit from suspending the task for a moment and receiving counseling from the therapist on the value of relaxation training techniques in decreasing performance anxiety, thus maximizing her assistance.

Recreational therapists also expand counseling to include people in the community. For example, a camp director may require counseling about reasonable accommodations under the Americans with Disabilities Act to be persuaded to make accommodations for a client. Recreational therapists may also provide counseling to community groups to promote health and optimal living, for example, in a senior center.

To best understand the use of counseling in recreational therapy it is necessary to distinguish among forms of therapy, psychotherapy theory and approaches, and counseling techniques. Forms of therapy refer to the broad therapy topic of practice, such as family therapy, drug and alcohol counseling, and leisure counseling. Psychotherapy theory and approaches refer to the specific orientations from which the therapist practices his/her form of therapy, such as cognitive behavioral therapy or existential therapy. Some therapists follow one specific theory or approach, such as a family therapist who only uses psychoanalytic therapy, whereas others use and sometimes combine a variety of theories and approaches in what is called an eclectic approach. Recreational therapists follow an eclectic approach. Lastly, counseling techniques refer to specific techniques or interventions that are used by therapists to promote change. Common counseling techniques can be found across many different theories and approaches, as described in the rest of this chapter.

Psychotherapy Theories and Approaches

There are many psychotherapy theories and approaches. Entire textbooks are devoted to them. For the purpose of this section, we will review three of the most common found in recreational therapy practice: psychoanalytic therapy or supportive-expressive therapy, cognitive-behavioral therapy, and existential counseling.

Supportive-Expressive Therapy (SE)

Psychoanalytic therapy is often referred to as supportive-expressive therapy. The therapist is *supportive* of the client's feelings and thoughts "so that the [client] will feel secure enough to venture to try to undo the restrictions in functioning" (Luborsky, 1984, p. 71). The therapist also encourages the client to *express* himself/herself by setting "the stage for the [client] to express thoughts and feelings and to listen and to reflect on them, with the aim of understanding and changing what needs to be changed" (p. 90).

The therapist gives support to the client by conveying though words and manners a sense of understanding, respect, acceptance, hope, and a we-bond with the therapist and client working towards a goal. Therapists highlight strengths of a client, give review and recognition of accomplishments, especially when the client applies learned information, and encourage discussions (at times) about topics of interest other than exploratory topics to reflect genuine interest in the client.

To encourage the client to talk (express thoughts and feelings) the therapist first needs to employ active listening. This required eye contact, engaged body posture, and silence. Periods of silence can be very uncomfortable for new therapists, but it is in the silence that connections are made. Therefore, therapists should not be quick to fill in the empty space with talk. When the therapist understands in part or whole what the client is trying to convey, the therapist shares his/her insight with the client in terms that the client understands. The therapist then resumes active listening and listens for the client's reaction to the feedback in addition to new information shared.

Cognitive-Behavioral Therapy (CBT)

Cognitive-Behavioral Therapy (CBT) is also referred to as Rational Emotive Behavior Therapy (REBT). CBT stems from the premise that people's interpretations, reactions, and beliefs are a result of conditioning. They are learned behaviors. Working on thinking and acting rather than feelings and emotions changes these distorted thinking patterns. The client is taught new ways of thinking and behaving. Skills are taught and practiced until new and healthy thinking patterns overtake the previously held distorted thinking patterns.

The A-B-C Theory of Personality is central to REBT. The belief is that an event does not cause an emotional or behavioral response. It is the person's belief that affects how the person responds to the event. The same event (e.g., traumatic spinal cord injury) does not result in the same emotional or behavior response for all individuals. The variable that influences the response is the person's belief system. If the person's beliefs are causing an unhealthy emotional or behavioral response, then the therapist will act by providing modalities that dispute the person's irrational belief system. For example, this may include education on quality of life for clients who sustain spinal cord injuries. The therapist will point out faults in the client's belief system such as, "I will never be able to go skiing now that I have a spinal cord injury." This belief can be disputed by providing information on adaptive skiing, setting up a meeting with another person who has a spinal cord injury who skis, or viewing videos of adaptive skiing.

The therapist challenges the client's irrational beliefs by asking questions (e.g., "Why is it terrible or horrible if life is not the way you want it to be?").

"Through a series of refutations, therapists are instrumental in raising the consciousness of their clients to a more rational (self-helping) level" (Corey, 1996, p. 328).

Examples of Verbal Challenges:

1. Challenging dogmatic beliefs (should, ought, must): Client, "I must transfer without a transfer board." Therapist, "Why MUST you?" Client, "Because I have to show progress." Therapist, "What do you think will happen if you can't?" Client, "I'll be discharged." Therapist, "And why is that a bad thing?"

2. Challenging self/other ratings (I'm or s/he is worthless, bad): Client, "I am worthless." Therapist, "What makes you say that?" Client, "Because I can't do anything." Therapist, "What do your children say?" Client, "They tell me that I'm doing just fine, that they love me, and can't wait until I come home." Therapist, "That doesn't sound like 'worthless' to me."

3. Replacing negative thoughts with positive thoughts: Client, "This is so hard to do. I can't do it." Therapist, "If you think you can't, then you won't. But if you think you can, you will. Think positive. At the very least, allow yourself to try." Client, "Ok, I'll try, but no guarantee that I can do it."

4. Challenging awfulizing and low frustration tolerance with humor (I can't stand it, I need it): Client, "This entire situation is terrible." Therapist, "Is everything terrible?" Client, "Yes, everything!" Therapist, "Yesterday you did a fantastic job in therapy." Client, "Well, that was yesterday. Today is different." Therapist, "Ok, then we can agree that not everything in terrible … just today (small laugh)."

Other interventions include individual work (homework) in which clients are challenged to look at their beliefs rationally; replace negative thoughts with positive thoughts; develop and participate in an action plan that refutes irrational beliefs; change "should," "ought," and "must" language to preferences; and change absolutes to more flexible terms. The therapist might additionally use humor to "show absurdity of certain ideas that clients steadfastly maintain" (Corey, 1996, p. 330). Practical examples of interventions include assisting the client in performing a task that s/he thought s/he could never do, regularly praising the client for a job well done, and reviewing progress after each session to combat negative thinking. Language modification includes changing never/always to sometimes, changing "I can't" to "I'll try," and changing "I ought/should" to "I would like to." Some additional techniques that can help in refuting irrational beliefs include role-playing, relaxation techniques, modeling, systematic desensitization, self-management principles, and operant conditioning. It may help to find humor in conversation, incorporating funny or exaggerated gestures related to what you are asking the client to do, and using fun or make-believe items, such as magic fairy dust for kids — "Now you can!" Most important is for the therapist to be a model of positive/rational thinking for the client.

In summary, CBT interventions can have an effect on the person's belief structure, thus resulting in a new feeling toward the current activating event. CBT is commonly used in recreational therapy, especially trying to change an individual's perspective on how his/her lifestyle has a direct effect on health, how s/he can still lead an optimal and personally meaningful life, obtain personal goals, develop internal locus of control, and adjust to disability in a community setting. Disability, unfortunately, is fraught with many negative connotations and many of these must be tackled head on by the therapist in order to facilitate change and growth.

Existential Counseling

Existential counseling is the process of searching for value and meaning in life and encouraging clients to explore options for creating a meaningful existence. Clients are encouraged to become aware of their own power in making life changes rather than being a victim of circumstance. The client is the architect of his/her life. The choices that s/he makes not only determine the life that s/he leads but also the person that s/he becomes. To become aware of this power and make positive life changes based on this awareness is the focus of existential counseling.

As humans, we often seek answers to life questions, such as "What is life all about? Why am I here? What is my purpose?" These questions are answered by reflecting on what we know and what we sense and feel psychologically and emotionally. The answers to these questions bring meaning, stability, and order to our lives. It gives us a sense of purpose and a foundation to stand on when we set our life goals. From this, we form a mental picture of our life in our mind's eye. This picture is referred to as a "life

scheme." It ties together our past, present, and future events into a logical whole oriented around our life goals. For example, a client may think, "After college, I'm going to move to the country and help make a difference in the lives of people who have disabilities. Later, I want to settle down, marry, and raise a happy family."

Unfortunately, our live scheme doesn't always go as planned. Things that we "knew" and "felt" can be turned upside down by illness, disability, death of a loved one, loss of a job, betrayal, and other unexpected life events. Our lives might not make sense any more because life goals may now be in doubt. Unplanned events can cause identity changes, plummeting self-esteem, unpredictable and chaotic events, and loss of order or purpose. It shakes the person's very foundation.

As humans, we do not like chaos and uncertainty and try to find balance again in our lives, as described by Balance Theory. It is in this struggle that we search for meaning and begin to answer our life questions, again (e.g., "What's the point of living. I thought I knew, but now I don't. Why am I here in this world?"). This can be a very difficult and uncomfortable place for someone to be emotionally. As a therapist, you can't answer these questions for the client. It is a process of personal discovery, where previous thoughts and ideas may need to be adapted or replaced. In the end, the client must come to terms with the present situation and seek to re-build his/her life scheme in order to regain a life of meaning, purpose, and balance.

Developing a life scheme, much less reconstructing a new life scheme, can be very difficult. If a person fails in his/her attempt to reconstruct meaning, or struggles for a time in the search for meaning, then an existential vacuum occurs, characterized by identity crisis, loss of order, and purposelessness. In relation to leisure, if leisure activities fail to provide meaning because they are boring, redundant, non-stimulating, the above crisis can ensue leading to maintaining or exacerbating secondary health conditions in all domains of health.

There are no specific techniques that are well defined for existential counseling; however Corey (1996) outlines three phases in the therapeutic process:

Initial phase: Therapists help clients to explore their assumptions about the world (What is life about?) and their perceived value and purpose in the world (Why am I here?). Clients are challenged to consider the validity of these beliefs. This can be difficult for some clients, especially those who have an external locus of control. Clients are encouraged to examine their own role in designing their life.

Middle phase: Clients are encouraged to more fully examine their own role in designing their life (Who is really in control? Who has authority?) and what is truly valued as meaningful in their lives. This process typically leads to new insights and some restructuring of attitudes and values. Clients begin to develop a clearer picture of the life they wish to lead.

Final phase: The goal of this phase is to enable clients to concretely implement changes in their lives to reflect new insights and values, thus leading to more purposeful lives.

As a recreational therapist, you can help your clients find meaning again through play, leisure, recreation, and community activities. Facilitate engagement in activities that allow the client to gather up desired meanings, such as a sense of belonging, an opportunity to express identity, and a purpose in life, such as engaging in family leisure activities that help the individual realize his/her purpose in being a role-model for his/her children.

After developing a therapeutic relationship with the client, engage the client in activities and discussions that help the client express feelings about his/her life, such as using a gardening activity as a catalyst for talking about life growing in new and different directions. Provide activities that promote insight, contemplation, expression, and new perspectives, such as journaling and repetitive activities such as walking or beading that allow the client's mind to wander in thought. Re-involve the client in pre-injury activities that promote a sense of the client's old self. Provide leisure education and counseling about the role of leisure in "living life to its fullest" and achieving personal meaning, and then assist the client in engaging in activities to achieve a sense of fulfillment, purpose, and meaning.

Recreational therapists have their own existential question, "What is the reason for rehabilitating a person?" The unique place of recreational therapy in the rehabilitation process is that it attunes itself to the whole person. Recreational therapy does not act exclusively to bring about functional change, but seeks to enhance engagement in activities that allow the individual to find meanings that are important to him/her, which strengthens quality of life. After all, isn't this what life's all about?

Positive Psychology

Positive psychology is a strengths-based approach. It is defined this way in the *Oxford Handbook of Positive Psychology* (Lopez & Snyder, 2009).

> [Positive psychology] is the "scientific" study of what makes life most worth living. It is a call for psychological science and practice to be as concerned with strength as with weakness; as interested in building the best things in life as in repairing the worst; and as concerned with making the lives of normal people fulfilling as with healing pathology. Nowhere does this definition say or imply that psychology should ignore or dismiss the very real problems that people experience. Nowhere does it say or imply that the rest of psychology needs to be discarded or replaced. The value of positive psychology is to complement and extend the problem-focused psychology that has been dominant for many decades. (p. xxiii)

The field of positive psychology is underpinned by three truisms (Lopez & Snyder, 2009, p. xxiii): (1) What is good in life is as genuine as what is bad. It is not secondary, non-existent, or illusory. It is real and deserves to be recognized as such. (2) What is good in life is not simply the absence of what is problematic. Just because a person does not have a problem, does not automatically result in the attainment of a good life. (3) The good life requires its own explanation, "not simply a theory of disorder stood sideways or flipped on its head" (p. xxiii).

Common areas of focus in positive psychology include positive emotions, character strengths, resilience, happiness, life satisfaction, wisdom, well-being, flow, self-esteem, emotional intelligence, creativity, mindfulness, optimism, hope, self-efficacy, self-determination, courage, curiosity, closeness with others, compassion, empathy, altruism, forgiveness, gratitude, love, humility, distinctiveness, flexibility, social support, hardiness, meditation, spirituality, storytelling, benefit-finding, growth, and meaning-making (Lopez & Snyder, 2009). Positive psychology is utilized by various health professions, not just psychologists, and has been integrated into various non-healthcare settings such as schools, family life, and the workplace.

Positive psychology has been, and continues to be, an integral component of recreational therapy practice (e.g., Anderson & Heyne, 2013; Anderson & Heyne, 2012a; Anderson & Heyne, 2012b; Carruthers & Hood, 2007; Carruthers & Hood, 2004; Dattilo, 2015; Dattilo, Kleiber, & Williams, 1998; Heyne & Anderson, 2012; Hood & Carruthers, 2013; Kleiber, Hutchinson, & Williams, 2002). Two practice models steeped in positive psychology have been developed. The first is the Leisure and Well-Being Model (Carruthers & Hood, 2007; Hood & Carruthers, 2007). See the chapter on Theories, Models, and Concepts for information about this model. The second is the Flourishing through Leisure Model (Anderson & Heyne, 2012b). The Flourishing through Leisure Model is an extension of the Leisure and Well-Being Model and outlines the scope of recreational therapy practice as facilitation of spiritual strengths and resources, physical strengths and resources, social strengths and resources, cognitive strengths and resources, and psychological strengths and resources, along with enhancing the leisure experience through facilitation of leisure skills and knowledge and facilitation of leisure environments. All of these are based on the client's goals, dreams, and aspirations. As a result, a flourishing life in all domains (spiritual, social, psychological, leisure, cognitive, and physical) occurs leading to well-being, a state of successful, satisfying, and productive engagement in life. The model is based on seven principles that guide the strengths-based approach to recreational therapy practice (Anderson & Heyne, 2012b, p. 133):

- The client is at the center of recreational therapy services.
- The client's goals, dreams, and aspirations drive the recreational therapy process.
- The client is seen within the rich context of the environments in which s/he participates.
- The recreational therapist considers all aspects of the client holistically: psychological, emotional, social, cognitive, physical, spiritual, as well as leisure, which permeate all domains.
- Both the client's individual strengths and the environmental strengths and resources are taken into account during the recreational therapy process.

- The client's strengths and the environmental strengths and resources nourish and flourish life.
- Recreational therapy services are outcome based and reflect the multidimensionality of human well-being and quality of life.

Recreational therapists employing a strengths-based approach can use these two models to guide practice. They are encouraged consult positive psychology literature on particular techniques for fostering growth in particular areas, such as resiliency or hope, as this is beyond the scope of this brief introduction.

Education and Counseling Techniques

How the recreational therapist does education and counseling is as important as the kinds of education and counseling the therapist does. A therapist can have the perfect information or technique for a client, but it has no value if it is presented in a way that the client can't understand or if it is presented in a way that the client actively or passively resists. The next part of this chapter will look at some of the ways a therapist can improve the client-therapist interaction.

Many of these techniques are common practice in the therapeutic milieu. They become almost second nature to the therapist who systemically addresses multiple issues in a treatment session. It is not uncommon for a therapist to delicately balance his/her relationship with the client while providing instruction and counseling around a particular issue. With experience, multi-tasking becomes easier and integrating these skills into a treatment session becomes instinctive — just as the therapist learns to adjust the client-therapist interaction into what the client needs to obtain maximal growth.

Some of the issues of counseling that are important to recreational therapists include relationship building, understanding actions and motivations, and dealing with loss and crisis. Here are some techniques that are effective for dealing with these issues:

Relationship Building

Interaction cannot be void of social-emotional contact, no matter what the basis of interaction. At the most basic level, pleasantries are shared (or not shared) and an attitude or perception of the person is formed. The therapist is judged on not only what was said or not said, but also how it was said, when it was said, who it was said to, and why it was said. The therapist is also judged on his/her appearance. Clients initially desire someone who looks professional, takes a genuine interest, is pleasant and friendly, and appears competent and trustworthy. How a client assesses a therapist is not consistent. Still, how the therapist is perceived has a great impact on the relationship.

The therapeutic relationship builds a foundation for treatment. It not only fosters the client's personal growth, but also directly influences physical and cognitive performance. For example, a client who perceives a therapist to be preoccupied and disinterested will be less likely to open up emotionally to the therapist. If this results in ill feelings towards the therapist, the client may in turn reflect his/her dislike for the therapist behaviorally, including not performing a task at the level requested. This type of behavior will not only negatively affect the client's physical skill development, but also stunt the client's emotional growth and adjustment to disability. The client may also deal with cognitive challenges apathetically because s/he thinks the therapist doesn't care. The therapist must be constantly aware that the mind and body work together to form a sensitive and highly complex system that reacts to input in an integrated way. Consequently, the client-therapist relationship is much more than just an exchange of pleasantries. It is a catalyst for systemic change.

The employment of counseling techniques, along with a genuine and caring attitude, opens the door to growth. Luborsky (1984) recommends five steps for opening psychoanalytic therapy. These steps are also relevant for a variety of allied health professions. Incorporating these steps into the evaluation process will encourage the therapist to attend to relationship issues, which may otherwise be minimized because insuring agencies tend to focus attention on physical outcomes.

1. Listen in order to establish what the client's problems are and let the client try to cast these as goals in the client's order of importance. Document the deficits in abilities and attitudes found during these discussions.

2. Explain and demonstrate to the patient what the role of the recreational therapist is.

3. Make explicit arrangements about the treatment, including time and place.

4. Allow a relationship of trust and rapport to be developed through genuine interest and concern.

5. Begin the process of formulating the basis for the main relationship, including problems and associated symptoms. This must be done because client-therapist relationship issues (e.g., client says that therapist doesn't understand his situation as a teenager) and manifestations of the issues in the client-therapist relationship (e.g., client is emotionally non-disclosing and repeats belief of therapist's lack of understanding) may allow the client to retreat from emotionally charged discussions.

A sixth step would be to form a relationship treatment plan, especially if deficits are discovered in ICF codes d5702 Maintaining One's Health, d710 Basic Interpersonal Interactions, d720 Complex Interpersonal Interactions, or d740 Formal Relationships. The therapist develops and implements planned interventions to enhance the client-therapist relationship, with the full understanding that positive relationship changes can enhance function in all domains, as well as contribute to the client's adjustment and integration.

Understanding Actions and Motivations

There are many things a therapist can do to improve the therapy interaction. One of the important ones is helping a client better understand his/her actions and motivations. Brammer (1988) identifies seven helping skills that the therapist can use to promote the client's understanding of himself/herself.

Listening Skills

The therapist actively attends to what is verbally and non-verbally expressed by the client. Words, context, emotions, body language, and mannerisms form a total perception of what the client is experiencing. This process is sometimes referred to as "listening with the third ear." Listening can be broken down into the following subcategories.

Attending: Genuine, warm eye contact is used to convey caring and understanding, as well as to hold the attention of the client and evaluate the nonverbal messages conveyed through the client's eyes (e.g., looking away, tearful, shut tight, hard stare). The therapist exhibits engaged social posture and gestures (leaning forward, arms uncrossed, etc.) and offers non-directional verbal comments (e.g., "I understand.") as appropriate to convey active attention.

Paraphrasing: When there is an appropriate conversational pause, the therapist reiterates in concise terms what s/he is "hearing" verbally and non-verbally from the client (e.g., "Being here really makes you angry." or "You appreciate your mom's helpfulness, but I detect from your sarcasm that it bothers you sometimes." or "You say that you are fine but I detect that you are feeling a bit angry given that your arms and legs are crossed and folded tightly."). It is important to note whether the client confirms or denies what the therapist says.

Clarifying: The therapist poses questions to the client to clarify understanding (e.g., "I'm not sure I understand what you mean. Can you explain that to me again?") or states in more concise terms what s/he thinks the client is trying to communicate (e.g., "Are you trying to say that you are afraid?").

Perception checking: This is the process of determining if the perception that the therapist holds is correct. It is different from paraphrasing or clarifying because a perception reflects the therapist's awareness of a large amount of material shared by the client rather than the last few sentences. For example, "I think I hear you saying two different things. On one hand you feel frustrated and yet on the other hand you feel relieved. Is this correct?"

Leading

The therapist anticipants the direction of the client's thoughts and offers his/her insight to the direction. Leading techniques encourage the client to talk.

Indirect leading: Indirect leading encourages the client to talk (e.g., "What do you think that means?" or "How does that make you feel?"). It is a general question that is purposely vague. Following the question the therapist pauses in silence in anticipation of the client's response.

Direct leading: Direct leading provides more direction for the client, yet it still encourages the client to assume responsibility for the conversation (e.g., "Tell me more about what you like about hiking." or "What do you mean by 'it makes you feel icky'?").

Focusing: Focusing helps the client to explore a particular aspect of the conversation. Therapists challenge the client to focus when it behooves the client therapeutically (e.g., "You've been talking a lot about all of the things that scare you. Tell me, what makes you feel confident."). Therapists may also find it helpful to use just one word like "but?" or "so?" or "and?" to encourage the client to focus more on the particular aspect of the conversation.

Questioning: Avoid the question "why?" because it comes across as being accusatory and often puts the client on the defensive. For example, instead of saying, "Why don't you like hiking?", ask "What is it about hiking that you don't like?" Ask open-ended questions that require a client to answer through explanation rather than with a yes or no answer. These facilitate exploration of feelings or help the client to clarify thoughts.

Reflecting

This expresses to the client that the therapist understands the client's frame of mind. The therapist reflects how s/he understands the feelings of the client, the experience of the client, and the content that the client is trying to express.

Summarizing

Brammer (1988) says that summarizing gives the client a "feeling of movement in exploring ideas and feelings, as well as awareness of progress in learning and problem solving" (p. 79). For example, "Let review what we have talked about so far." or "Let's take a look at the progress you have made."

Confronting

Confronting a client may put the therapy at risk because the technique can result in a negative or defensive reaction from the client. It is a useful technique in certain circumstances, though, because it challenges the client and encourages open communication. Confronting the client allows the therapist to share with the client what s/he feels or thinks is going on. For example, the therapist may say, "I believe that you are underestimating yourself. Based on your performance in the clinic, I think that you will need very little physical assistance when you're out in the community."

Interpreting

This helps clients see their problems in new ways and encourages clients to explore new ways of looking at life problems on their own without the help of a therapist.

Informing

This is part of the education process. Providing the client with information that impacts his/her ability to handle stress, maintain or improve health, or maximize functioning and independence is an essential component of helping skills.

Dealing with Loss and Crisis

Brammer (1988) explains that "dealing with people in crisis calls for flexibility of response, rapid and creative intervening with alternatives, and setting limited goals for getting the person functional" (p. 95). The client's ability to deal with stress and crisis depends on many factors including his/her values, beliefs, attitudes, culture, experiences, and personality. Examples of a significant loss or crisis include death of a loved one, disaster, divorce, imprisonment, disability, or loss of a job.

Zuckerman (2000) recommends that therapists working with clients who are in crisis acknowledge and validate the client's distress, despite the therapist's own interpretation of the event, and encourage the client to express his/her feelings. The client and family should be reassured that the therapist and/or other identified health professionals are readily available and willing to help. When positive expressions are observed (e.g., a smile, verbalizing a positive feeling) the therapist is to acknowledge, support, and reinforce these responses. The availability and encouragement to engage in healthy coping activities, such as expressive writing, meditation, or physical exercise, is another helpful intervention. For clients who have a strong likelihood of making the current situation worse by making impulsive decisions clouded by stress, written or verbal behavior contracts may be helpful. This also holds true for the client who has a strong likelihood to engage in unhealthy behaviors when feeling down and depressed. (Substance abuse, suicide, and the decision to sell everything and move into a shack in the mountains are probably not the best choices.) Finally, Zuckerman recommends that therapists provide ongoing support and reassurance until the crisis is resolved or able to be managed in a healthy way.

Singer (2001) proposes a different model for dealing with crisis. She suggests that the client should avoid thinking about or dealing with any aspect of the crisis until most of the details of normal life are restored. Some losses, such as losing a home during a fire, are so great that thinking about the loss can consume all of the survivor's limited energy. It is better to not think about the loss and concentrate that energy on getting life back together. She offers six tactics for survivors of emotional shock:

1. People who go through emotional shock need more than a bed for sleeping. Calm, un-cluttered surroundings convey order and safety, which survivors need to mentally rest.

2. Return to basic routines as quickly as possible. This means regular mealtimes and bedtimes. In the first weeks, you should limit, if possible, unnecessary changes such as shuttling from one hotel to another.

3. Friends and helpers can give practical help with cleanup, food, telephone calls, and replacing survivor's toiletries with familiar brands and scents.

4. The anxiety triggered by emotional shock interferes with the survivor's ability to retain information. Let a helper take notes at meetings with FEMA, insurance adjusters, and bank officers.

5. Familiar faces of friends, neighbors, store clerks, and librarians stabilize and reassure survivors.

6. Steer away from replays of the fire, earthquake, or any other disturbing event as they can reawaken impressions of the all-to-recent catastrophe and rekindle emotional distress (p. 18).

Lucas (2004) points out that there are two kinds of loss or trauma and that it is important to differentiate between them when deciding on a course of treatment. One kind of loss occurs in a way that is outside the client's control. This is most commonly seen in natural disasters such as fires, floods, and hurricanes. For this kind of loss, there is no reason for the client to spend any time or energy thinking about what happened. There is no way to change it, and other issues are more pressing. The second kind of loss occurs because of something that is in the client's control such as abuse of a child by an alcoholic partner. In this case the client can end the ongoing trauma by leaving the relationship. Ongoing counseling to look at the bad relationship is appropriate in these cases because the client will need to think about the problem every day to avoid falling back into the old relationship or starting a new, equally destructive one.

While "processing" or "talking through" trauma is the generally accepted approach to all trauma cases, there are some situations where it makes the situation worse. The therapist needs to distinguish between the two kinds of loss or trauma and advise the client appropriately.

Experiential Learning

Experiential learning is a technique that can be applied in many situations. It is the process of learning through experiences. It relates to several old sayings, "I need to see it with my own eyes," "I need to experience it myself," and "Seeing is believing." Therapists are wonderful educators, and they are also wonderful craftsmen and craftswomen. Therapists carefully design situations, environments, and events so that experiential learning opportunities provide education and counseling. Such learning opportunities may be structured in a community environment where the client is challenged to carry over learned skills from the clinic or in a group situation where the client may be challenged to assert himself/herself in a healthy manner. Unless clients are challenged to actually practice and apply skills they have learned, they will be unlikely to do them on their own after discharge.

Common Psychotherapy Terms

Common psychotherapy terms often used in recreational therapy counseling literature are discussed below. Many of the issues discussed are not acknowledged in the ICF, because they are not universally accepted or defined in all cultures (e.g., one culture may promote autonomy while another culture does not). Consequently, if the therapist wants to note the extent of impairment of these functions in the ICF, it is recommended that therapists score the specific skill or activity that is being affected by the function and write a notation to the right of the scored code (e.g., d5702 Maintaining One's Health — affected by impaired self-efficacy). If the ICF does list a specific function described below, you will be directed to the correct code.

Autonomy

Autonomy is the extent to which a client feels free to make decisions and choices. Loss of autonomy is common for clients in healthcare settings, often contributing to symptoms of depression. To maintain autonomy, clients should be given as many decisions and choices as possible, such as choosing one of the two treatments modalities available for the session or contributing to therapy schedule development.

Self-Efficacy

Self-efficacy is how well the person feels that s/he can perform a particular behavior or action in a defined setting given all of the probable constraints and facilitators. In other words, to what extent does the person feel that s/he can accomplish the task at hand? "Clients' expectations of themselves largely determine how willing they will be to deal with their problems, how much effort they will be willing to expend, and whether they will make a perseverant effort. Those who are self-doubters are likely to express little effort and will give up quickly if their initial efforts are not productive. Those with high efficacy expectations are apt to face their difficulties with determination, to exert maximum effort, and to persevere even when frustration is encountered" (Austin, 2004, p 409). Bandura (1986) identifies four sources of information that affect self-efficacy.

Performance: Successful (and repetitive) accomplishment of an action, task, or behavior that the client perceives to be successful. The concept of success is defined by the person's interpretation of his/her performance. Despite the interpretation of others, if the person does not view his/her performance as a success, it will not contribute to perceived self-efficacy. Recreational therapists provide clients with tasks that can be completed successfully and then gradually increase the complexity of the task as self-efficacy grows. For example, instead of the therapist asking a client with a newly acquired spinal cord injury to try to do a full wheelie, s/he shows the client how to pop the front caster wheels one inch off the ground and has the client perform this skill as a precursor skill to learning how to do a full wheelie.

Vicarious experience: Observing other people who are similar to ourselves succeed at a desired action, task, or behavior contributes to feelings of self-efficacy. It can be viewed as a source of motivation and a model of encouragement. The though may be, "If he can do it, then I can do it." In some cases, the recreational therapist is an appropriate model. However, in other instances a more similar peer would provide better self-efficacy outcomes. For example, the client may be somewhat motivated by watching her overweight therapist exercise on her lunch hour. However, observing the unstructured-time exercise of a fellow client who is more similar in age, injury, and abilities may instill a deeper feeling of self-efficacy. The use of peer counselors is another common intervention. This may involve asking a former client who has the same, or nearly the same, injury and life characteristics to meet with the current client who is experiencing a problem or concern that the former client also experienced and worked through successfully.

Verbal persuasion: Positive remarks about performance from a respected and trusted person can affect perceived self-efficacy (e.g., "You are a strong person and I am proud of you. Keep going."). The best person to meet this need for the client will vary, and the therapist may need to be creative in finding a person the client responds well to. Therapists encourage positive remarks by modeling the behavior in front of the identified person. Therapists may also meet with the identified person separately and encourage the sharing of positive remarks with the client.

Physiological arousal: Some level of physiological arousal is helpful. The client saying something like, "I was feeling a little nervous, but I did it," shows that the client's ability to work through feelings of anxiousness contributed to self-efficacy. If stress and anxiety are too high, however, it can be detrimental to performance. It does not improve self-efficacy when the reaction is "I'm too nervous to do it. There is no way I'm going to do that." Finding a balance is key. Recreational therapists provide clients with tasks where success is expected and challenges are realistically achievable.

Self-Awareness

Self-awareness is the extent to which the client is aware of his/her strengths, weaknesses, preferences, beliefs, attitudes, and values. A realistic appraisal of self and some level of acceptance of personal attributes is a good foundation for developing a healthy leisure lifestyle. Austin (2004) defines education in leisure self-awareness as helping "clients examine their leisure lifestyles so that they may become aware of values, patterns, and behaviors reflected in their lifestyles, as well as barriers to achieving the leisure lifestyle they seek. Having such an understanding allows clients to plan and make alteration in their leisure lifestyle" (p. 66). The ICF doesn't use the term self-awareness because it is not a concept that is universally held in all cultures. However, there are numerous categories in the ICF that relate to aspects of self-awareness including b11420 Orientation to

Self, b1644 Insight, b180 Experience of Self and Time Functions, d570 Looking After One's Health, d710 Basic Interpersonal Interactions, and d720 Complex Interpersonal Interactions.

Self-Esteem

Self-esteem is the extent that a client feels good about his/her attributes and the amount of positive regard a client has for himself/herself. How a client feels about himself/herself can positively or negatively affect many life activities. Self-esteem that affects life activities in a negative manner can have a direct impact on health. For example, a client who has poor self-esteem may not give herself permission to care for her own needs ("I'm not worth it."). Lack of self-care could then impact her physical, emotional, social, spiritual, and mental health. Recreational therapists recognize that a basic sense of self-esteem is a fundamental building block to good health. For without self-esteem, optimal self-care will not happen.

Self-esteem is a complicated topic. It is difficult to measure and there are several theories on its development. A popular theory of self-esteem, "perceived adequacy," as discussed by Feldman and Elliott (1990), is based on how adequately the person performs in domains that are considered important by the person. Therefore, success in areas judged unimportant by the person would have little impact on his/her self-esteem. It is the discrepancy between the person's expectations of himself/herself (the ideal self) and the person's perceived adequacy that affects self-esteem. So if the client doesn't place value on schoolwork, then poor academic scores would not affect his/her self-esteem. For a client who does value schoolwork, poor academic scores would affect self-esteem. Although this is a very individualistic approach, the researchers did find common themes that affect self-esteem. The strongest influence on self-esteem from infancy through adulthood was how a person judges his/her physical appearance. The second strongest influence on self-esteem was social acceptance by peers. For children, however, parental attitudes have a greater impact on self-esteem than peers. In adolescence, attitudes of classmates are the greatest predictors of self-esteem although parental attitudes still weigh in at a significant second. In the college years, peers far outweigh parental attitudes.

Scholastic competence, athletic competence, and conduct follow behind.

Another theory ("the looking-glass self") is that a person imitates the attitudes that significant others reflect about him or her. For example, a young child who receives negative verbal and non-verbal messages from his parents about himself takes on those negative attributes. The basic idea is that a person's self-esteem is defined by what is mirrored to him/her, hence the "looking glass" (the mirrored image). The client looks to others to define his/her self-esteem.

Feldman and Elliott (1990) make some additional notes about self-esteem that are important for therapists to be aware of regarding the relationship of self-esteem to depression and delinquent behavior. The risk of developing depression and suicidal ideation increases when the client fails to meet his/her standards in domains that the client judges as important (including domains that are important to the client's parents) and when peer support seems unattainable (especially when support is contingent on meeting parental expectations or conforming to peer demands). This can lead to feelings of hopelessness.

Another concern related to self-esteem is delinquent behavior in adolescents. Feldman and Elliott (1990) report that failure to meet the expectations of the dominant membership group, which could be family, peers, club members, or others, leads to negative self-attitudes. In turn the client seeks out adolescent groups where dominant standards are ignored and delinquent behaviors are admired. The client receives the benefit of increased self-esteem in this group from engaging in anti-social actions. Adolescent boys with low self-esteem are at a larger risk for delinquent behavior than girls. In adult males, self-esteem is often measured by success, toughness, and sexual prowess.

Combining these two thoughts on self-esteem helps to guide the therapist in developing a treatment plan. Recreational therapists can:

1. Design activities that encourage exploration of feelings about self-esteem. One idea is to ask the client to make a picture frame and write all of the positive things that s/he feels about himself/herself on the frame and then place the client's picture inside. Another is to write the client's name down the side of a piece of paper and then ask the client to write a positive affirmation for each letter in his/her name such as "A" stands for "achieves good grades," "attractive," "athletic."

2. Explore alternative leisure activities with the objective of broadening the client's awareness of leisure options that could positively affect self-esteem. An example is Alphabet Leisure: write the letters of the alphabet down the right hand side of a sheet of paper hung on the wall. Clients shout out leisure activities that begin with each letter. The therapist writes the ideas next to the letter. This is best done in a group to obtain a variety of ideas.

3. Involve the client in activities that will enhance positive feelings in areas that are important to the client. For example, if a client values intellect and enjoys helping others, involve the client in a group that designs and implements community service projects.

4. Address precursor skills, such as social skills or teambuilding skills, that inhibit the client's ability to achieve success in valued areas of self-esteem.

5. Consider who has the greatest impact on the client's self-esteem and implement a plan accordingly. If parental attitudes have the greatest impact on self-esteem, assess whether or not the parents would benefit from education about their role and what they can do to facilitate positive self-esteem in their child. If attitudes of peers have the greatest impact, steer the client towards positive peer groups that highlight competences of the client.

6. Provide opportunities for personal autonomy and freedom of choice to help enhance self-esteem.

Self-esteem is a feeling about oneself that is not understood or recognized in all cultures, so it is not part of the ICF. However, b1266 Confidence is part of the ICF and is defined as "mental functions that produce a personal disposition that is self-assured, bold, and assertive, as contrasted to being timid, insecure, and self-effacing." Other ICF codes related to aspects of self-esteem might be found in b126 Temperament and Personality Functions, b130 Energy and Drive Functions, and d710 Basic Interpersonal Interactions.

Setting measurable objectives for self-esteem can be difficult because it is not easily defined. Although it is an internal thought process rather than an external skill, it can still be measured through its reflection in specific behaviors such as positive self-statements, posture, tone of voice, interactions with others, initiation, communication, assertiveness versus passivity, taking time for self-care behaviors, acceptance of positive remarks made by others, and engagement in self-nurturing activities. To put this into practice, a goal for self-esteem may be a simple as "Improve self-esteem." The treatment objectives that fall under this goal could be: State three positive self-attributes during self-exploratory clinic activity; sit upright throughout group sessions with minimal cueing; verbally thank others independently for positive remarks made during group sessions; plan structured activities for self-nurturing as part of daily rehab routine with moderate assistance; or engage in planned self-nurturing activities at home independently.

Locus of Control

Internal locus of control is the extent to which a client believes and behaves in a manner that reflects a feeling of control over his/her life, choices, and actions. The person feels like s/he is in control of himself/herself. External locus of control is the extent to which a client believes and behaves in a manner that reflects a feeling of lack of control over his/her life, choice, and actions. The person feels like s/he is being controlled by outside forces, often including family, relationships, and work. Giving a client the kinds of experiences and choices discussed in the sections on self-determination, self-efficacy, and autonomy will allow the client to experience a more internal locus of control.

The ICF does not have references to locus of control because cultures do not agree on which locus of control is most appropriate, but specific aspects of maintaining control of oneself are reflected in ICF codes such as d5 Self-Care.

Self-Determination

Self-determination is being in control of one's behavior by acting based on one's values and beliefs instead of society's norms. Dattilo and Williams (2000) define self-determination as "being in control of the course a life takes" (p. 169). The concept of self-determination is another of the concepts used in recreation and leisure that has a cultural bias. Self-determination tends to be a strongly held belief in the United States, but it is not a universally accepted concept (Reber, 1995). Reber points out that self-determination tends to be supported by theorists with an existentialist orientation. Self-determination is not

contained in the ICF model but probably falls under the heading of making decisions (d177 Making Decisions). Austin (2004) reports that leisure self-determination is an attribute required for a person to experience leisure. He feels that leisure requires the attitude, "I create my own life. I choose my actions. I design my destiny." Achieving self-determination and promoting control over his/her leisure lifestyle is a complex process that varies from client to client based on the client's current beliefs, experiences, and learned behaviors. Experiential learning through tasks in which the client experiences control, existential counseling, and cognitive-behavioral interventions to change distorted thinking patterns are common techniques used to promote and develop self-determination.

Attitude

Attitude is a low intensity emotional state that is relatively short-lived (burlingame & Blaschko, 2010). Attitudes are often influenced by culture, religion, peers, life experiences, situations, and desired outcomes. Attitudes are hard to measure because they are not visible actions. The measurement of attitudes relies heavily on the client's report through valid assessment tools. burlingame and Blaschko (2010) report that using a solid testing tool for measuring attitudes is important because "attitudes can clearly be barriers to developing and nurturing relationships, being willing to risk new experiences to allow use of one's community, or even participating in treatment" (p. 208). Additionally, attitudes help the therapist identify a direction of treatment (e.g., need for education, need for further assessment, doesn't need counseling on general benefits of leisure and can move on to assessment of leisure lifestyle). This is particularly important for the recreational therapist because attitudes and beliefs are typically assessed and addressed prior to implementation of other interventions. A full understanding of the benefits of leisure by the client along with the understanding by the therapist of the client's beliefs and attitudes forms the basis for developing a leisure lifestyle plan. burlingame and Blaschko (2010) discuss seven complete testing tools for attitudes. The most important ones are the *Cooperation and Trust Scale, Free Time Boredom,* the four subscales of the *Idyll Arbor Leisure Battery,* and the *Life Satisfaction Scale.*

Values

"Values are deeply held attitudes and beliefs we have about the truth, beauty, or worth of a person, object, action, or idea. One criterion of a 'true' value is that it has become a part of a pattern of a person's life. In other words, values must not only be identified, but embraced and expressed" (Purtilo & Haddad, 2002, p. 5).

Recreational therapists help clients explore what holds meaning in their lives, what holds importance, and what is cherished. It may be a specific action, such as spending time with grandchildren, a concept like peace and calm, a person, an attribute, such as honesty, or a variety of other things. Clients are asked to look closely at how they spend their time and lead their lives to evaluate the degree of expression of those things in their life. If they are reflected minimally or are absent from the client's lifestyle, the therapist and client explore ways for the client to experience and incorporate these ideals into his/her life, thus contributing to life satisfaction. Austin (2004) cautions therapists "not to impose a value or course of action on participants but to encourage them to look at alternatives and their consequences" (p. 70). Facilitating this insight is also educational. It highlights characteristics of activities, use of time, and personal values, all of which increase understanding of leisure and heighten awareness of personal control. Questions that can be asked include, "Are you living and expressing your life in a way that you want to? What control do you have over changing it? How would you go about changing it?" Different cultures have different attitudes about whether the person or society should control the goals in life, but, as Holland (2014) points out, both ask the question. "Are you living the kind of life you value?" See Values Clarification in the Techniques and Interventions section for more information.

Beliefs

A belief is an emotional acceptance of a statement or position that cannot be supported by observable evidence (burlingame & Blaschko, 2002). Like values, beliefs are often influenced by culture, religion, and life experiences. It is the recreational therapist's responsibility to understand the client's beliefs. There are some serious ethical issues that arise when beliefs are involved, especially in the area of religion. Some religions believe that God is the only appropri-

ate healer and that medical interventions are never appropriate. This leads to cases where parents refuse life-saving care for their children. Often the courts become involved to force the parents to allow the care. Whether it is appropriate for a therapist, a medical team, or the courts to try to change a client's beliefs or force a client to go against his/her beliefs is a complex ethical issue that is beyond the scope of this book.

References

Anderson, L. S. & Heyne, L. A. (2013). A strengths approach to assessment in therapeutic recreation: Tools for positive change. *Therapeutic Recreation Journal, 47*(2), 89-108.

Anderson, L. S. & Heyne, L. A. (2012a). Flourishing through leisure: An ecological extension of the leisure and well-being model in therapeutic recreation strengths-based practice. *Therapeutic Recreation Journal, 46*(2), 129-152.

Anderson, L. & Heyne, L. A. (2012b). *Therapeutic recreation practice: A strengths based approach.* State College, PA: Venture Publishing.

Austin, D. (2004). *Therapeutic recreation processes and techniques* (5th ed.). Champaign, IL: Sagamore Publishing.

Bandura, A. (1986). *Social foundations of thought and action: A social cognitive theory.* Englewood Cliffs, NJ: Prentice-Hall, Inc.

Brammer, L. (1988). *The helping relationship: Process and skills* (4th ed.). Englewood Cliffs, NJ: Prentice Hall.

burlingame, j. & Blaschko, T. M. (2010). *Assessment tools for recreational therapy and related fields* (4th ed.). Enumclaw, WA: Idyll Arbor.

Carruthers, C. & Hood, C. D. (2007). Building a life of meaning through therapeutic recreation: The leisure and well-being model, part I. *Therapeutic Recreation Journal, 41*(4), 276-297.

Carruthers, C. & Hood, C. D. (2004). The power of the positive: Leisure and well-being. *Therapeutic Recreation Journal, 38*(2), 225-245.

Corey, G. (1996). *Theory and practice of counseling and psychotherapy* (5th ed.). Pacific Grove, CA: Books/Cole Publishing Company.

Dattilo, J. (2015). Positive psychology and leisure education: A balanced and systemic service delivery model. *Therapeutic Recreation Journal, XLIX*(2), 148-165.

Dattilo, J., Kleiber, D., & Williams, R. (1998). Self-determination and enjoyment enhancement: A psychologically based service delivery model for therapeutic recreation. *Therapeutic Recreation Journal, 32*(4), 258-271.

Dattilo, J. & Williams, R. (2000). Leisure education. In J. Dattilo (Ed.), *Facilitation techniques in therapeutic recreation*. State College, PA: Venture Publishing, Inc.

Feldman, S. & Elliott, G. (1990). *At the threshold: The developing adolescent.* Cambridge, MA: Harvard University Press.

Heyne, L. A. & Anderson, L. S. (2012). Theories that support strengths-based practice in therapeutic recreation. *Therapeutic Recreation Journal, 46*(2), 106-128.

Holland, J. (2014). *Cultural Competence in Recreational Therapy.* Enumclaw, WA: Idyll Arbor.

Hood, C. D. & Carruthers, C. (2013). Mindfulness-based therapeutic recreation intervention. *Annual in Therapeutic Recreation, 21*, 73.

Kleiber, D. A., Hutchinson, S. L., & Williams, R. (2002). Leisure as a resource in transcending negative life events: Self-protection, self-restoration, and personal transformation. *Leisure Sciences, 24*(2), 219-235.

Luborsky, L. (1984*). Principles of psychoanalytic psychotherapy: A manual for supportive expressive treatment*. New York: Basic Books.

Lucas, K. (2004). Private communication.

Purtilo, R. & Haddad, A. (2002). *Health professional and patient interaction* (6th ed.). Philadelphia, PA: W. B. Saunders Company.

Reber, A. (1995). *Implicit learning and tacit knowledge: An essay on the cognitive unconscious*. New York, NY: Oxford University Press.

Singer, I. (2001). *Emotional recovery after natural disaster: How to get back to normal life*. Ravensdale, WA: Idyll Arbor, Inc.

Stumbo, N. & Peterson, C. (2004*). Therapeutic recreation program design: Principles and procedures* (4th ed.). San Francisco, CA: Pearson Benjamin Cummings.

Zuckerman, E (2000). *Clinician's thesaurus* (5th ed.). New York, New York: Guilford Press.

6. Parameters and Precautions

Heather R. Porter

Whether conducting an assessment, implementing a treatment session, or planning post-discharge activities for a client, the recreational therapist must be aware of the precautions and parameters set by the physician in the medical record. The precautions and parameters guide the therapist's clinical decisions about appropriate activities and meeting client needs. They also inform the therapist of monitoring, such as blood pressure, that needs to be done during sessions for the purpose of minimizing risk and maximizing outcomes. At times, the recreational therapist may wish to implement a specific modality that taxes particular body systems. Understanding whether this is appropriate may require a conversation with the physician to seek activity participation clearance and obtain any additional precautions or parameters related to the activity. Some of the most common precautions and parameters encountered in healthcare are reviewed in this chapter. The therapist is also required to understand other precautions and parameters that are important in the therapist's treatment setting.

Cardiac Precautions

For individuals with cardiac conditions, such as coronary artery disease, myocardial infarction, or coronary artery bypass graph, the client's surgeon or physician will set specific cardiac precautions that must be followed during therapy sessions including a set of vital signs (systolic blood pressure, diastolic blood pressure, heart rate, respiration rate), oxygen levels, MET ranges, and fatigue. Each is discussed in this chapter. If the client presents outside of the prescribed parameters, appropriate interventions or responses are taken, such as seeking immediate assistance from primary nurse/physician, increasing oxygen level, initiating pursed lip breathing, etc. The interventions and responses will vary by client. It is

the responsibility of the therapist to fully understand the correct protocols. ICF codes that indicate a need for cardiac precautions are found in b4 Functions of the Cardiovascular, Hematological, Immunological, and Respiratory Systems, especially the areas b410 - b429 Functions of the Cardiovascular System, b440 - b449 Functions of the Respiratory System, and b455 Exercise Tolerance Functions.

Diet and Swallowing Precautions

Ingestion functions can be impaired as a result of brain injury, such as a cerebrovascular accident that impairs muscular functions related to swallowing, mouth impairments, such as missing teeth, damage to the esophagus from burns or other trauma, and surgery, including a wired jaw.

A common problem is dysphagia. Dysphagia is defined as difficulty swallowing due to impaired neurological functions from, for example, a cerebrovascular accident, traumatic brain injury, or from some obstruction of the esophagus, such as an esophageal tumor. Obstructions generally allow swallowing liquids; impaired neurological function may prevent swallowing both solids and liquids. If a client has difficulty swallowing, s/he could choke or aspirate food and liquids.

The speech language pathologist evaluates the client's ingestion functions through a swallowing study that allows the therapist to see how the client bites, chews, manipulates, and swallows food. The results of the study will indicate to the therapist the type of diet the client should follow. There are four common food levels (pureed, mechanical soft, chopped, and regular) and four common fluid consistencies (one called thin and three with varying levels of thickness).

Pureed foods are blenderized.

Mechanical soft foods are those that require little or no chewing such as mashed potatoes, short flat noodles, and cooked carrots.

Chopped diet consists of foods that require some, but not rigorous chewing, such as cubed chicken, chopped lasagna, and chopped string beans.

Regular diet has no food texture restrictions.

Thin liquids include water, iced tea, coffee, and lemonade.

Thick liquids are those with significant solid material in the liquid. They come in three consistencies (UPMC, 2014). Nectar-thick liquids are easily pourable and are comparable to apricot nectar or thicker cream soups. Honey-thick liquids are slightly thicker, are less pourable, and drizzle from a cup or bowl. Pudding-thick liquids hold their own shape. They are not pourable and are usually eaten with a spoon. A product called Thick It is commonly used to thicken thin liquids. As per the product's label, a certain amount of the Thick It powder is stirred into the thin liquid to make it the desired consistency.

In addition to determining the diet level, the speech language pathologist will recommend specific swallowing techniques to decrease risk of aspiration such as thorough chewing, tucking in the chin, and swallowing twice.

People who do not have dysphagia, but who do have other difficulties with chewing and swallowing, such as missing teeth, burned esophagus, or wired jaw, will also have specific recommendations. Individuals who are missing moderate numbers of teeth may have difficulty chewing and manipulating food resulting in the recommendation of eating mechanical soft and chopped foods. Certain foods may irritate a burned esophagus and, depending on the extent of damage to the esophagus, a feeding tube may be needed. A person who has a wired jaw will typically be allowed to eat small amounts of pureed foods and thin liquids through a straw.

Therapists document the type of diet the client is following (e.g., mechanical soft and thins), causes of swallowing impairments (e.g., client requires a mechanical soft diet secondary to missing teeth), ability of the client to adhere to special diet in real-life settings (e.g., client requires moderate cues to adhere to dietary restrictions in a community dining setting), ability of the client to follow swallowing techniques in real-life settings (e.g., client demonstrates modified independence secondary to increased

time to integrate swallowing techniques into social dining), and any other restrictions or adaptations that are required by impairments in functioning (e.g., client needs additional liquid when eating because of minimal saliva production).

The recreational therapist needs to be aware of diet levels (both food and liquid) and recommended swallowing techniques for several reasons:

1. The therapist needs to know what a client is allowed and not allowed to have during a therapy session (e.g., client asks for a glass of water; client wants to eat a cookie that was made in the therapy kitchen; when out in the community the client wants to order a specific food or liquid).

2. The therapist is responsible for problem solving for the impact that diet levels have on activity participation (e.g., client refuses to engage in community socializing activities because food and drink are often available and the client does not want to use thickener in front of his peers).

3. The therapist must reinforce proper food choice in a real-life community environment (e.g., what items on the menu are considered mechanical soft).

4. The therapist must also reinforce proper swallowing techniques in a real-life community environment (e.g., using swallowing techniques at a restaurant).

Clients may also have other special diet restrictions or precautions. The recreational therapist must be aware of these and control food interactions during sessions. The restrictions may be medical such as a diabetic diet, low salt diet, or involve specific food allergies. The restrictions may also be a personal choice of the client such as vegetarian or vegan diets.

ICF codes that indicate the possible need for diet and swallowing precautions include b5 Functions of the Digestive, Metabolic, and Endocrine Systems, especially b510 Ingestion Functions and b540 General Metabolic Functions.

Exercise Precautions

Prior to exercise participation, clearance for participation must be obtained from the physician, along with an order that outlines specific parameters and precautions to be followed during exercise. Parameters typically revolve around vital signs, such as blood pressure and heart rate. However, additional parameters (e.g., glucose level, MET level) and precautions (e.g., fatigue, fluid intake, heat) might be set depending upon the client's health condition. ICF codes that indicate the need for exercise precautions include b4 Functions of the Cardiovascular, Hematological, Immunological, and Respiratory Systems, b545 Water, Mineral, and Electrolyte Balance Functions, b540 General Metabolic Functions, b550 Thermoregulatory Functions, and b7 Neuromusculoskeletal and Movement-Related Functions. As an example, information on exercise precautions for individuals with diabetes is provided below.

Exercise Precautions for Diabetes

Blood sugar (glucose) levels must be monitored before, during, and after exercise for hypoglycemia (low blood sugar; glucose levels < 45 mg/dl) or hyperglycemia (high blood sugar; glucose levels > 180 mg/dl) (Cleveland Clinic Foundation, 2011a & 2011b). Symptoms of hypoglycemia include weakness, shakiness, irritability, dizziness, hunger, headache, confusion, cold sweat, and blurry vision (severe cases can cause coma or death) (Cleveland Clinic Foundation, 2011b). To raise glucose levels ingest 15 grams of carbohydrates (e.g., half cup fruit juice, two to four glucose tablets) and recheck glucose in 15 minutes (the 15-15 rule) (Lane, 2012). Symptoms of hyperglycemia include increased thirst, frequent urination, tingling in hands or feet, slow-healing sores, feeling tired, stomach pain or nausea, dry or itchy skin, and frequent infections (Cleveland Clinic Foundation, 2011a). Contact doctor if glucose levels are > 180 mg/dl for more than one week or have two consecutive readings > 300 mg/dl. If glucose levels remain high, damage can occur to nerves, blood vessels, and body organs (Cleveland Clinic Foundation, 2011a). Lane (2012) and Cistian (2012) recommend the following related to exercise:

Before exercise: Check blood sugar before exercise. Blood sugar drops about 50 points for every 30 minutes of exercise. If blood sugar is 100 mg/dl or less, client must eat one carbohydrate snack, such as a piece of bread, fruit, or granola bar, to decrease risk of hypoglycemia.

During or after exercise: Vigorous exercise can cause blood sugar to rise temporarily. If this occurs, retest again in 30 minutes. If exercising for a long period of time, check blood sugars during the workout to monitor any dangerous swings in glucose levels. If blood sugar drops to 70 mg/dl or lower

drink a carbohydrate, such as fruit juice, or eat two to five glucose tablets.

If the glucose level is 240 mg/dl or higher, checking for ketones is required. Vigorous exercise when ketones are present can raise glucose levels, which may lead to ketoacidosis, a life-threatening condition (American Diabetes Association, 2104).

Falls Precautions

Falls account for approximately 70% of all inpatient accidents and can cause serious injury affecting quality of life, length of stay, need for medical care, and healthcare costs (Payson & Haviley, 2005). In older adults, falls account for 40% of injury-related deaths and are the leading cause of injury-related hospitalizations. Fifty-six percent of falls occur outside the home (in the garden, street, sidewalks, shops) and 44% occur at various locations inside the home (Lord et al., 2007). Consequently, clients are routinely assessed for risk of falls. If a client is determined to be a falls risk, falls precautions are implemented. Healthcare agencies have specific falls precaution policies and protocols so therapists will need to inquire about these at their particular facility. Typically, if a client is assessed to be a falls risk, an order for "falls precaution" is written by the physician and all treating healthcare professionals then follow the specific falls precautions. Common indicators for risk of falls include (Boltz, 2012; Lord et al., 2007; Joint Commission Resources, 2008; Payson & Haviley, 2005):

- nursing home or extended care facility transfer (deconditioning)
- history of falls
- confusion or delirium
- altered level of consciousness
- disorganized thinking, confusion, or anxiety
- memory or cognitive impairments that could impair safety judgment
- impaired insight about deficits
- ataxia, unsteadiness, shuffling gait
- assistance required for ambulation or unable to ambulate and transfer
- balance impairment or vertigo
- unstable glucose levels
- shortness of breath
- new CVA
- new amputee
- bleeding disorder

- osteoporosis
- withdrawal (might not ask for help when needed)
- bowel or bladder urgency or frequency
- incontinence
- visual perceptual impairment
- postural hypotension
- medications, illegal drugs, or alcohol use that can cause any of the above

Many ICF codes are directly tied to risks of falls. These include ICF codes in b1 Mental Functions, b2 Sensory Functions and Pain, b4 Functions of the Cardiovascular, Hematological, Immunological, and Respiratory Systems, and b7 Neuromusculoskeletal and Movement-Related Functions.

The number and extent of falls precautions taken are dependent upon the number and extent of impairments putting the client at risk for falls. Specific falls precautions to reduce the client's risk of falling might include (Boltz, 2012; Lord et al., 2007; Joint Commission Resources, 2008; Payson & Haviley, 2005):

- orientation to room and call button
- bed wheels locked
- bed in low position
- clutter removed from room
- personal items within client's reach
- adequate lighting (including night lights)
- client/family education about falls precautions
- falls risk sign or symbol (e.g., purple dot) placed on client's door and/or wrist band
- direct supervision
- assistance offered regularly (e.g., assistance to use the bathroom offered every hour)
- safe footwear (e.g., footies with rubber bottom or flat rubber soled shoes)
- safety bed (e.g., enclosed bed)
- chair and bed alarms to monitor client movement
- close proximity to the nursing station
- bed side rails are up and locked
- wheelchair seat belt or restraint

If a client continues to be at risk for falls upon discharge, recommendations are made to reduce the risk of falling in the discharge environment. Such precautions might include:

Adaptive devices: Prescribing adaptive devices, including self-care equipment and mobility equipment.

Modifications: Teaching the client how to modify his/her home and other frequently used environments to decrease falls risk. This may include removing throw rugs, keeping items off the stairs, picking up items that are left in pathways, eliminating furniture that is seldom used, removing stacks of things on the floor that could topple over or take up needed walking areas, eliminating or moving electrical cords and phone cords so they are not tripping hazards, wearing flat shoes that neither grab nor slip, installing railings on staircases, installing tub and toilet grab bars, moving commonly used items to waist height to decrease bending and reaching, using brighter light bulbs in areas where there isn't much light or in places where the surface is uneven, and using nightlights, especially in the bedroom, hallway, and bathroom.

Medical monitoring: Subscribing to a home medical monitoring system, especially if the client will be alone at times. This is usually a necklace with a push button that automatically connects to a medical monitoring service that then contacts the local emergency center.

Phone: Having a phone on the client's person at all times when left alone. For example, have the client wear an apron, a canvas tool pouch, or a fanny pack to hold the phone so it is easily at hand should client fall and need assistance. Choose a phone that has large buttons that are easy to see and push and not so many buttons that they confuse the client.

Precautions that can help the client in a community setting include the following possibilities:

Cell phone: Have a cell phone for emergencies that occur in the community. Some counties have a senior or low-income program that provides free cell phones to individuals. These are used phones that are turned in by community members. Choose a phone with a simple design and few buttons to limit confusion.

Alertness: Be extra careful and alert when walking on uneven or slippery surfaces.

Mobility equipment: Use mobility equipment that provides more support (e.g., uses a single point cane at home, but uses a rolling walker in the community to provide increased mobility support).

Energy conservation: Use energy conservation techniques to avoid fatigue, which can increase risk for falls. The client should park close to the door, plan out a walking route at the store to limit over-walking, use an electric scooter at the store, take frequent rest breaks, etc.

Metabolic Equivalents

Metabolic equivalents are used to provide a standardized measure of the amount of energy used to do common tasks. A metabolic equivalent (MET) is the ratio of the work metabolic rate to the resting metabolic rate. One MET is defined as one kcal/kg/hour and is roughly equivalent to the energy cost of sitting quietly. A MET is also defined as a level of oxygen uptake of 3.5 ml/kg/min. As with the energy definition, one MET equals the oxygen cost of sitting quietly. The ICF code most closely tied to METs is b455 Exercise Tolerance Functions.

There is a Compendium of Physical Activities that lists the MET values for many common activities. Activities are classified by a 5-digit code that identifies the category (heading) as the first two digits and type (description) of activity as the last three digits. An example is

Code: 01010

Heading: 01 - bicycling

Description: 010 - Bicycling, < 10 mph, leisure, to work or for pleasure (Taylor Code 115)

MET: 4.0

Recreational therapists can use the Compendium as a way to determine the relative intensity of activities. Recreational therapists, especially those who work on an inpatient cardiac unit, may have physician orders that require the therapist to use only activities that fall within a specific MET range (e.g., 1.0-2.5). Therefore, it is necessary for therapists to be familiar with the MET levels of certain activities. The Compendium can be found at http://prevention.sph.sc.edu/tools/compendium.htm

There are some significant limitations on the MET numbers that the therapist needs to keep in mind. The Compendium was not developed to determine the precise energy cost of physical activity for a particular individual. Even the ratios of the activities will be different depending on characteristics such as body mass, adiposity, age, sex, efficiency of movement, geography, and environmental conditions in which the activities are performed. Individual differences in energy expenditure for the same activity can be large and the true energy cost for an individual may or may not be close to the stated mean MET level as presented in the Compendium.

Consequently, therapists use the Compendium of Physical Activities to identify, in a general sense, activities that tend to correlate with a specific MET level, knowing that clients with health conditions will use more METs than the number listed in the Compendium. Vital signs, such as blood pressure, pulse, and oxygen saturation levels, and observation are more important in evaluating a client's response to activity than MET numbers.

Example: A physician's order for a client with a cardiac condition states the MET range (e.g., 1.0-2.5), blood pressure parameters (no change in systolic or diastolic blood pressure greater than 20), oxygen saturation level (if oxygen levels drop below 94%, stop activity, if levels do not rise with cessation of activity and application of breathing techniques, client is to be put on two liters of oxygen and reassessed), and pulse parameters (stop activity if change from resting heart rate is greater than 20). The therapist refers to the Compendium of Physical Activities to identify activities with a MET level of 1.0-2.5. Because a client with health conditions will expend more energy for activities than reflected in the Compendium, higher MET-level activities outside of the MET level orders are never attempted without physician clearance. The client is asked to perform an activity with the lowest MET first (e.g., standing activity with minimal movements at 1.4 MET). The therapist monitors the client's vital signs to see if the client can participate in the activity while maintaining precautions and parameters. If the client is unable to maintain precautions and parameters, the activity is stopped and the therapist follows the orders of the physician. Depending on the severity of the client's reaction to activity, immediate assistance may be warranted. If the client is able to participate and stay within precautions and parameters, the activity is upgraded to one with a higher MET level (e.g., standing activity with moderate movement). Again, vital signs are monitored along with observation to assess the client's physiological response to activity.

Pulmonary (Oxygen and Oxygen Saturation Levels)

For individuals with pulmonary conditions, such as COPD, specific oxygen saturation levels indicated by the treating physician must be maintained or complications can arise. Normal oxygen saturation levels are 94-100% in adults and full term neonates

(Shilling, 2002). In general, oxygen saturation levels below 60% are typically associated with cardiac decompensation; below 53%, with lactic acidosis; below 32%, with unconsciousness; and below 20%, with permanent cellular damage (Shilling, 2002, p. 355). For individuals with health issues, normal oxygen saturation levels may be lower then the norm. Consequently, the treating physician will write an order in the medical chart that lists the baseline level for the specific client (e.g., O2 Sat ≥ 90). ICF codes that may indicate pulmonary issues include b440 - b449 Functions of the Respiratory System and b455 Exercise Tolerance Functions.

Oxygen saturation levels are measured using a pulse oximeter, which consists of a clip attached to an index finger kept at the level of the heart. Oxygen saturation levels are monitored and documented before, during, and after activity. If levels fall slightly with exercise, initiate a rest break and implement techniques to help increase oxygen saturation levels, such as pursed lip breathing, and then reassess. If levels do not rise, or they continue to drop or drop dramatically, the primary nurse or physician must be alerted immediately to determine the next steps.

Measuring Oxygen Saturation

There are two primary ways to measure oxygen saturation: an arterial blood sample and a pulse oximeter.

The most accurate test for measuring oxygen saturation is an arterial blood gas test. A small sample of blood is drawn directly out of an artery (instead of a vein). The blood is directly tested for its oxygen level. Other tests, such as the level of carbon dioxide and the pH of the blood, can be done at the same time. A recreational therapist will rarely be responsible for taking a blood sample, so this topic will concentrate on using an oximeter and observing other signs of too much or too little oxygen.

The pulse oximeter (PulseOx) measures the client's peripheral oxygen saturation. A small clip is placed at the end of the client's finger or on the client's earlobe. The clip usually has a pair of small light-emitting diodes (LEDs) on one side and a device to measure the amount of light received on the other side. One LED is red, with wavelength of 660 nm. The other is infrared at 910 nm. Hemoglobin (the part of the blood cell that carries oxygen) absorbs the light differently when it has oxygen and when it

doesn't. From the difference in absorption, the oximeter can calculate the level of oxygen saturation. The latest generation of pulse oximeters use advanced digital signal processing to make accurate measurements in clinical conditions that used to be impossible, including when the patient is moving, when there is not much blood flowing, in bright ambient light, and when there is electrical interference. The devices are not perfect, however. Therapists need to make sure, among other things, that the client is not wearing red nail polish or something else that might block the light or affect the reading.

A normal blood saturation level is greater than 95%. If the saturation level is below the parameter set by the physician (e.g., client's level is 90 and the parameter set by the physician is >95), the therapist has the client stop the activity, and engage in pursed lip breathing as described below to raise the saturation level.

Table 1: Pursed Lip Breathing

Breathe in through the nose for the count of two and out of the mouth for the count of four with pursed lips, as if causing a candle to flicker. This creates backpressure in the lungs which helps to open the airways to release built up carbon dioxide. Breathing rate slows and each breath is more efficient.

After a few minutes, the therapist takes the saturation level again. If the level does not rise, the therapist contacts the client's primary nurse and reports the situation to determine the next course of action (e.g., nurse instructs therapist to bump up oxygen by one liter, bring client back to nursing station, physician to be paged).

If the client's level is far below or far above the parameter or if s/he is exhibiting signs of oxygen deprivation or toxicity (as discussed later), the therapist needs to call the client's primary nurse immediately. If the nurse is not available, the therapist needs to immediately call a physician.

If a client is on oxygen and will be engaging in a sedentary activity, the therapist is to take the oxygen saturation level of the client when the client enters the treatment room at the start of the session and then every 15 to 30 minutes throughout the duration of the session. If the client will be engaging in physical activity, the therapist is to take the saturation level prior to the start of the session and every five to ten minutes during the physical activity.

Therapists who will be working with clients in a community setting that will not have immediate access to a physician, nurse, or respiratory therapist, must receive in-house training on changing oxygen tanks. The therapist should have an oximeter to monitor the client's oxygen saturation levels and a cell phone to contact the client's primary nurse, physician, or respiratory therapist should questions or concerns arise that do not warrant an emergency call to 911 and taking the client immediately to the closest emergency room. An extra oxygen tank should be taken in case of an emergency, such as a client who requires the oxygen level to be increased so the tank does not last as long as required.

In addition to the oximeter, there are other signs the recreational therapist can use to detect oxygen saturation that is too high (toxicity) or too low (deprivation).

Table 2: Signs and Symptoms of Oxygen Toxicity

Chest pain: with the pain generalized under the sternum.
Dry cough: initially, with a moist cough developing as lung tissue is damaged by too much oxygen.
Nausea and vomiting.
Restlessness: "ants in the pants" restlessness; an inability to sit quietly.
Stuffiness of the nose.

Table 3: Symptoms of Oxygen Deprivation

Dyspnea: shortness of breath; not being able to get enough oxygen into the blood to meet the body's need for oxygen. Dyspnea is not necessarily due to a disease process. When someone runs a mile faster than his/her physical condition is ready for, it is normal for the person to be "out of breath." The recreational therapist will want to watch for clients being more out of breath than would be expected given their current physical condition.
Hypoxia: an inadequate saturation of oxygen at the cellular level.
Fatigue: When the blood is not able to carry enough oxygen to meet the body's physical needs, the person becomes too tired to engage in normal activity.

Cyanosis: bluish discoloration seen in the skin and lips.

Oxygen Therapy

For a variety of reasons clients with pulmonary conditions will be using oxygen therapy equipment during leisure activities. The advent of more portable oxygen equipment allows clients to be more mobile and less constrained in where they can live and play. For that reason it is as likely that a recreational therapist will work with clients who use oxygen therapy equipment in the community.

Oxygen therapy is a physician-prescribed treatment that specifies the method of administration of the oxygen and the amount of oxygen to be given. Because the delivery of oxygen is a prescription, the recreational therapist should not change the delivery rate or method of delivery without written orders from the physician, nor should the therapist encourage the client to do so. (This is assuming that the recreational therapist is trained and approved to make changes with the physician's permission.) Too little oxygen can cause brain damage and too much oxygen can be toxic. Because clients may be more physically active during leisure, the therapist should watch for signs of low oxygenation and work closely with the client's physician to develop a regimen of oxygen therapy that describes when and how the flow of oxygen may be changed to accommodate activity.

Oxygen is prescribed in percentages but the flow meters for oxygen are often measured using liters of oxygen per minute. The type of equipment used to deliver the oxygen to the client makes a difference in the actual amount of oxygen received by the client. For example, at 6 L/min (liters per minute) a nasal cannula delivers around 44% oxygen, a simple mask delivers around 50%, a partial re-breather mask delivers 35%, and a non-re-breather mask delivers 55-60% oxygen (Timbly & Lewis, 1992). Room air typically has about 20% oxygen.

Methods of Delivering Oxygen

There are numerous ways to deliver oxygen to the client. The most common methods that a recreational therapist will see are the nasal cannula, nasal catheter, oxygen mask, and direct delivery into a trachea. In rare cases the therapist may work with clients who are in oxygen tents.

Nasal cannula: A nasal cannula is a narrow, flexible, clear plastic tube that extends from the oxygen flow meter to the client. At the client end, the tube splits into a loop that lets the tubing be placed just below the client's nose, looped behind the client's head, with the tubing being tucked over each ear and then joined back together under the client's chin. At the portion of the tube that is placed under the nose there are two short stubs of tubing that are placed inside the nostrils. The nasal cannula allows the client the greatest freedom to engage in leisure activities of any of the oxygen delivery options. Its other advantage is that it is less visible and does not interfere with talking, eating, or drinking. The length of the tube from the flow meter to the client varies. If the length of the tube is too short for the client to engage in activities, the recreational therapist should ask the physician if it is medically appropriate for the client to have a longer tube. Some tubes can be ten feet or more in length. Tubes can also be too long, causing a tripping hazard. The recreational therapist can provide feedback to the physician as to appropriate tubing length.

Nasal catheter: A nasal catheter is a flexible plastic tube that is inserted into the client's nose all the way to the nasopharynx (near the back of the throat). The nasal catheter is secured into place by taping it to the client's nose. This is a very efficient means of getting oxygen into the client's lungs while still allowing the client to eat, drink, and talk. However, it is fairly uncomfortable to have the tube placed up the client's nose and, unlike the nasal cannula, it is not easy to remove for short periods of time.

Oxygen mask: There are many different types of oxygen masks. Oxygen masks cannot be used when eating or drinking and interfere with talking. They are used primarily when the client is very ill and needs to have high percentages of oxygen delivered to the lungs. Clients often complain of feeling claustrophobic (fear of being closed in a small space). Clients may also develop skin problems where the mask touches the skin if masks are used for very long. Masks are often used with clients who have pneumonia, smoke inhalation, or carbon monoxide poisoning. When oxygen masks are taken off to eat, the client often needs to use a nasal cannula to ensure adequate oxygen saturation.

Transtracheal oxygen: For clients with a long-term need to be on oxygen, some choose to have the oxygen delivered through a tracheal opening (an opening surgically cut into the throat at the trachea). The tube that is placed into the opening is called a catheter. The catheter is held in place by a thin chain that goes around the neck. Both the tracheal catheter and the necklace type chain can be hidden under a collar or scarf. Depending on the amount of mucus that the client has, the tracheal catheter may need to be replaced many times a day or only once or twice a week. A clogged tracheal catheter can be a life-threatening situation. Therapists who take clients with tracheal catheters into the community need to be trained in how to clean them out in case they become clogged.

Oxygen tent: An oxygen tent is a portable, lightweight, clear plastic structure that fits over the client's head and chest while s/he is in bed. There is a motorized unit that provides oxygen at the desired rate while keeping the temperature in the tent comfortable for the client. Oxygen tents are seldom used anymore for adults but they may be used for young children or cognitively impaired adults who need humidified air and who tend to pick at and pull out cannulas or catheters.

Activity and Oxygen Delivery

There are a few aspects of providing treatment and leisure activities for clients on oxygen that the therapist will need to take into account.

Infection control: By far the most prevalent method of providing enhanced oxygen levels to clients is the cannula. Most people do not like to have a nasal cannula in their nostrils so they fiddle with them, sometimes taking them off for short periods of time. The stems on the nasal cannula from which the oxygen flows are placed inside the client's nose. That means that if the client takes the cannula off for a short period of time and places it on his/her lap while in bed, the germ-filled mucus on the cannula will deposit germs on the client's blankets. When the therapist places a game board or other shared recreational equipment on the client's bed, the equipment itself becomes contaminated. If this equipment is used by other staff or clients before it is appropriately cleaned, it becomes a transmission source for germs. And, if the recreation equipment is not cleaned before being placed on the client's bed, the cannula will then pick up the germs when it is taken off. When the cannula is repositioned, it puts the germs into the client's nose and lungs, both excellent ways to transmit an infection.

Oxygen supply: When the client is an inpatient, his/her oxygen tubing is likely to be hooked up to the oxygen port located in the wall of the room near the head of the client's bed. Occasionally the tubing becomes kinked when the client raises or lowers his/her bed. The therapist should check the integrity of the oxygen tubing each time the client repositions himself/herself or changes the position of the bed. Most recreational therapy activity rooms do not have oxygen in the wall. When the client goes to the activity room (or to the hospital cafeteria, outside the building, etc.) the client will be switched to a portable oxygen tank on a small cart. The portable oxygen tank has a gauge on the tank outlet that indicates how much oxygen remains in the tank. The therapist should watch the gauge and make sure that the client does not run out of oxygen. The recreational therapy department can usually work out an arrangement with respiratory therapy (the department that usually exchanges oxygen tanks) to replace the tank right in the activity room if enough notice is given.

Cognitively impaired clients: Clients with cognitive impairments often fiddle with the oxygen gauges. It is a good policy for the recreational therapist to know what level of oxygen the client should be getting. This information should be written down in the recreational therapist's notes about the client and updated daily. When the therapist first greets a client who is on oxygen, s/he should read the level of oxygen being provided. If the level does not match what the therapist understood the prescribed level to be, s/he should immediately call the nurses' station to double check. The therapist should visually check the gauges once every ten to fifteen minutes throughout the activity, more often if the client is seen handling the gauge or is known to handle the gauge.

Open mouth: With a nasal cannula, when the client's mouth is open (for talking, mouth breathing, or the mouth is positioned so that the lips do not seal), air comes in the mouth as well as the nose. Because the air coming in through the client's mouth is not as rich in oxygen as the air coming in through the nose, the client is not getting the prescribed amount of oxygen delivered to his/her lungs. The problem can occur because a client may appear quiet and with-

drawn in his/her room (as an inpatient) or in the doctor's office (as an outpatient having oxygen saturation measured). The amount of oxygen prescribed is based on the level of activity those situations. If the client becomes more physically active during recreational therapy, experiences increased activity levels at the community center, or has hours of conversation with friends, the amount of time with an open mouth may increase and his/her oxygen saturation may drop to sub-therapeutic levels fairly quickly. If the therapist feels that the client's activities do not match the activity level that the oxygen percentage was set for, the therapist should work with the physician to get a more realistic oxygen therapy regime.

Increased restlessness and irritability: Whenever a client, especially an elderly client, has increased restlessness or irritability, the client's oxygen and carbon dioxide levels should be measured. Increased restlessness and irritability are signs of both oxygen deprivation and oxygen toxicity. Carbon dioxide narcosis is a cognitive state of being confused or disoriented because of high levels of carbon dioxide in the blood.

Anaerobic pathway by-products: If there is not enough oxygen in the blood, the body starts pulling energy from a secondary (and less efficient) source, the anaerobic pathway. Normally, when a client breathes in oxygen, the body uses the oxygen and produces carbon dioxide as the by-product. When the cells are required to pull energy from the anaerobic pathway, a different set of by-products is produced. The parts of the body that are most susceptible to injury from the anaerobic pathway by-products are the brain, heart, pulmonary vessels, and the liver (Anderson, Anderson, & Glanze, 1994). If a client is receiving too high of a percentage of oxygen (oxygen toxicity), the brain decreases the respiratory stimulus and the client's breathing rate and volume decrease. With reduced respiration the client's body begins to retain carbon dioxide, causing the same symptoms as too little oxygen.

Precautions for Activities and Supplies

Oxygen enhances combustion of other material that can burn, so if it is exposed to spark, open flame, or lit cigarettes, there is a chance of an explosion. Here are some of the devices to watch out for:

Electrical devices: Electrical devices, including hair dryers, electric saws, drills, and sanders, may produce enough of a spark in their engines to ignite a fire.

Glue guns: Many of the glue guns used in arts and crafts activities are low heat glue guns that require low heat glue. This type of hot glue gun is preferable to the higher temperature glue guns.

Open flames: Open flames are inappropriate for clients using oxygen therapy. This includes being anywhere near the barbeque during picnics, use of candles, and campfires.

Petroleum products: Petroleum products such as oil paints, rubbing alcohol, epoxy glues, oil-based face paints, and oil-based stains should not be used near oxygen.

Smoking: There should be no smoking near clients with oxygen. In the United States almost every type of treatment facility and most recreation centers are now smoke free. However, there are places that a client can go and still be exposed to lit cigarettes. For example, if an inpatient on oxygen is going to sit outside of the hospital cafeteria with his family to enjoy the sunshine, he may end up sitting next to someone who is smoking. And, in fact, some clients on oxygen still smoke — a very dangerous situation.

Static electricity: Static electricity from fabrics could cause an explosion. Some facilities have policies that prohibit staff from wearing uniforms or clothing made of materials that are highly susceptible to producing static electricity. When using fabrics for activities (even the use of parachutes for activities), the therapist will want to select fabrics that are less susceptible to producing static electricity. Cotton fabrics tend to not produce static electricity.

Equipment that is of special concern to therapists of clients on oxygen therapy includes:

Oxygen tanks: When the client is receiving oxygen from a metal container, the therapist should ensure that the activities do not cause the tank to tip over or to be harmed. Tanks are usually secured in a carrying cart. Even without heat sources close by, if a tank tips over and the seal to the flow meter is broken, the therapist can have an explosive situation. The gas inside the tank is under a lot of pressure. The larger tanks will have internal pressures greater than 2000 pounds per square inch. When the cap or flow meter covering the tank outlet is cracked or broken off, the tank acts like a rocket, propelled by the pressurized gas in the tank. It could very easily go through a brick wall.

Tubing integrity: It is important that the tubing not be kinked or blocked during activity. The therapist should regularly check to make sure that the wheels of the tank cart are not on top of the tubing, that no one is standing on the tubing, that no books or other supplies are sitting on top of the tubing, and that no blockages are occurring. The clear tubing is often hard to see, especially for clients who have impaired vision, such as in nursing homes. The therapist should make sure that there is no room for anyone to walk between the client and his/her oxygen supply.

Seizure Precautions

If a client is at risk for having a seizure, seizure precautions are taken to reduce the likelihood of a seizure, as well as keep the client safe should a seizure occur. The ICF codes that indicate a need for seizure precautions are b110 Consciousness Functions and s110 Structure of Brain.

To reduce the likelihood of a seizure, the therapist talks with the client and treating physician to find out if there are any particular seizure triggers. If triggers are identified, steps are taken to avoid or minimize exposure. Triggers may include: missed medication; adding or removing medications or supplements; hormone fluctuations; excessive use or withdrawal from alcohol or drugs; emotional stressors, especially if combined with fatigue or chronic sleep loss; external stimuli such as flashing lights, circles, stripes, or other patterns usually of high contrast; TV and electronic screen games that flicker; sensory stimuli such as light touch, tapping, or soaking in hot water; and/or complex mental processes such as mathematical calculations (Epilepsy Foundation, 2012a). If a client has a seizure, follow the specific policy of the agency and take the following safety precautions: place something soft under the head, loosen tight clothing, clear area of sharp or hard objects, do not force objects into the person's mouth, do not restrain the person's movements (unless they place the person in danger), turn the person on his/her side to open the airway and allow secretions to drain, stay with the person until the seizure ends, do not pour any liquids into the person mouth or offer any food, drink, or medication until the person is fully awake, begin CPR if the person does not resume breathing after the seizure, let the person rest until fully awake, and be reassuring and supportive when consciousness returns (Epilepsy Foundation, 2012b).

Sternal Precautions

Following a sternotomy, sternal precautions must be followed to avoid undue stress to the healing sternum. The precautions are followed until clearance is provided by the surgeon (typically six to eight weeks). The ICF code that indicates a need for sternal precautions is s760 Structure of Trunk. Sternal precautions (Cistian, 2012; Choi et al., 2003; Gogelova, 2011; Gonzalez-Fernandez & Friedman, 2011) include:

- No pushing, pulling, or lifting objects greater than five to ten pounds.
- Do not use a bed trapeze or bed ladder.
- Don't pull on stair rails when going up or down stairs.
- No wheelchair propulsion.
- No pushing up with bilateral arms to get out of bed. Use a "side-rolling" (also called "log-rolling") maneuver for getting out of bed to avoid strong contraction of the abdominal muscles.
- No bilateral reaching overhead. Active bilateral shoulder flexion must be less than 90 degrees; active bilateral shoulder abduction must be less than 90 degrees. Encourage unilateral upper extremity active range of motion to facilitate functional mobility and reduce the risk of shoulder active range of motion impairment and muscle weakness.
- Avoid full weight bearing through upper extremities, such as pushing up with arms during transfers from sit to stand or reaching back before sitting down.
- If using a walker, weight-bear mostly through legs. Do not weight-bear through arms.
- Avoid activities that could cause a Valsalva maneuver, such as heavy lifting, forceful coughing, or straining on the toilet. If the client needs to cough or sneeze, s/he should hold a small pillow over the chest. Stool softeners are commonly prescribed to avoid bowel straining.
- No driving or sitting in a passenger seat with an airbag.

Suicide Precautions

If the client is found to be at risk for committing suicide, the client is placed on suicide precautions. ICF codes that might indicate a need for suicide precautions include b126 Temperament and Personality Functions, b130 Energy and Drive Functions, b134 Sleep Functions, b152 Emotional Functions, b160 Thought Functions, b180 Experience of Self and Time Functions, d163 Thinking, d240 Handling Stress and Other Psychological Demands, d5 Self-Care, d7 Interpersonal Interactions and Relationships, and d9 Community, Social, and Civic Life.

When suicide precautions are initiated, staff are alerted to the precaution as outlined in the agency policy. This might include an order in the medical record or a purple sticker on client's wristband and door. The suicide precaution policy that staff follow will vary by agency, but generally it consists of a systematic team approach including (Sanchez, 2010; Simon & Hales, 2012):

Removal of potential environmental hazards that the client could use to inflict self-harm: The U.S. Department of Veterans Affairs developed the Environmental Programs Service Mental Health Guide (a pdf document) to use in mental health facilities to assess environmental hazards that increase the chance of patient suicide or self-harm. It is an excellent resource and is available for free at www.patientsafety.va.gov/docs/joe/eps_mental_health_guide.pdf.

Monitoring of the client and implementing care: The type and frequency of monitoring and care varies by client need (e.g., 24-hour direct supervision; all staff in contact with client monitoring for suicidal thoughts and behavior; referral for psychotherapy, etc.).

The suicide risk is continually reassessed. An assessment commonly consists of:

Analysis of current episode: Duration of preceding suicidality, amount of planning and forethought for attempt, client's hope for outcome or attempt, manner (if any) by which attempt came to attention of others, how client feels about attempt now.

Dynamic risk assessment: Housing, recent breakup, unemployment, anniversary of death or loss, relapse into substance use.

Static risk factors: age, race, marital status, gender.

Cultural factors: Religious prohibitions against suicide, cultural view on suicide, cultural understanding of mental illness, belief in afterlife or punishment.

Modifiable factors that led to attempt (if there was an attempt): alcohol use, drug use, lapse in medication, relationship stressors.

New stressors due to current hospitalization: anxiety, insomnia, inability to attend job or school, loss of housing, isolation from social support.

Total Hip Precautions (THP)

After a total hip replacement or hip fracture with a closed reduction, total hip precautions (THP) must be followed until the soft tissue has healed adequately and the surgeon discharges the THP (typically about 12 weeks post surgery) (Zachazewski & Quillen, 2008). THP are designed to protect the hip joint and avoid injury, such as dislocation. ICF codes that indicate a need for THP are s740 Structure of Pelvic Region and s750 Structure of Lower Extremity. The usual precautions include (Cooper, 2006; Kennon, 2008):

Do not flex involved hip beyond 90°. The client will have to sit on elevated chairs or toilet seats to maintain this precaution and cannot bend over from the hips to reach objects or tie shoes. The client should use a reacher instead.

Do not rotate the hip internally. Do not turn the leg inwards.

Do not rotate the trunk in a way that may result in internal hip rotation.

Do not turn the feet excessively inward or outward, including not pivoting on the operated leg.

Do not cross the legs at the ankles or knees.

Do not lie or roll onto the uninvolved side.

Place a pillow between the legs when lying on the involved side.

An abduction wedge pillow is commonly used during waking hours to prevent internal rotation of the hip. The "V" shaped abduction pillow is placed between the legs and Velcroed around the thighs to hold it in place. Sometimes clients are instructed to wear it when sleeping to prevent breaking hip precautions.

For some clients, individualized precautions may be prescribed by the surgeon. Inpatient rehab therapists must be diligent about checking the client-specific THP set by the surgeon.

Vital Signs

Vital signs consist of a person's temperature, pulse, respiration, and blood pressure. They are also called cardinal signs. Vital sign changes indicate physiological changes in the body, so regular and consistent vital-sign monitoring provides insight into a client's health. It is not within the practice of recreational therapy to determine the extent of vital-sign impairment. However, recreational therapists do monitor vital signs. The need to monitor vital signs may be triggered by deficits in ICF codes that are part of b4 Functions of the Cardiovascular, Hematological, Immunological, and Respiratory Systems and b5 Functions of the Digestive, Metabolic, and Endocrine Systems.

The contribution of the recreational therapist about a client's vital signs is valuable because it (1) monitors the client's physiological functioning in different environments, activities, and times; (2) ensures the safety of the client by making sure the client does not exceed parameters activities, and (3) assists with identifying the effectiveness of treatment plans and the client's response to a specific intervention. For example, recreational therapy documentation could show that the client was able to stay within pulse parameters during 15 minutes of light cardiovascular activity compared to last week when client was only able to participate in eight minutes of light cardiovascular activity prior to exceeding pulse parameters.

Vital signs have a standard range (e.g., normal blood pressure for an adult is below 120/80). However, depending on the age and health of the individual, the desired range may change. For example, a physician may desire a client to maintain a blood pressure that does not rise above 140/90 during exercise. Vital signs will also fluctuate. This is expected. Vital signs can change with time of day (e.g., pulse is quicker in the morning than in the evening), time of the month (e.g., body temperature rises with ovulation), exercise (vital signs rise with aerobic activity), age (e.g., a healthy resting pulse for a child is quicker than a healthy resting pulse for an adult), sex (e.g., males typically have fewer respirations per minute due to greater vital capacity), weight (e.g., weight increases blood pressure), metabolic conditions (e.g., any activity that increases metabolic rate increases vital signs), general health status (e.g., temperature rises when fighting infection), pain (e.g., pain increases heart rate and blood pressure), and medications or illegal drugs (e.g., cocaine increases blood pressure, specific medications can be prescribed that decrease blood pressure).

When documenting vital signs, include the following qualifiers: date, time of day, location, activity, and vital-sign reading. If a response to a vital sign was needed, document the specific response taken and the outcomes of the action. For example, actions for low oxygen levels could be documented with something like "O2 Sat level increased from 89 to 94 after three minutes of pursed lip breathing."

Body Temperature

Body temperature measures the internal temperature of the body. Humans are warm blooded. Unlike cold-blooded animals, such as reptiles, whose internal body temperature changes with the temperature of the environment, human beings regulate their internal body temperature. A constant body temperature optimizes cell and organ functioning. A normal body temperature is 98.6°F. Because of the various factors that influence body temperature, a slight deviation from the norm may be acceptable and appropriate.

Factors that Influence Body Temperature

Time of day: Body temperatures are typically lower in the early morning and higher in the late afternoon and early evening.

Age: Younger children typically have higher body temperatures because they (1) are more susceptible to temperature changes in the environment due to the immaturity of their thermoregulatory system and (2) have a higher level of physical activity and metabolic rate. Conversely, older adults typically have lower than normal body temperatures due to decreased physical activity and metabolic rates, as well as less subcutaneous tissue to provide insulation to protect against heat loss.

Emotions: Extremes in emotion, whether joyous, sad, excited, or other, increase body temperature.

Exercise: Exercise increases metabolic rates thus increasing body temperature.

Menstrual cycle: During ovulation the body temperature rises slightly.

Pregnancy: During pregnancy, the metabolic rate increases causing the body temperature to slightly elevate.

External environment: On hot and humid days, the body temperature becomes slightly elevated. The

outside temperature increases body temperature and the humidity impairs evaporation of sweat making it difficult for the body to cool down. On cold days the body temperature may be slightly lower due to the external environment cooling down the body.

Clothing: Loose fitting cotton clothing allows the body temperature to cool down on warm days because it allows for the escape of body heat, compared to heavy, layered clothing that traps body heat and is optimal for cold days.

Location of measurement: Rectal temperatures are slightly higher than oral temperatures and axillary temperatures (under the arm) are slightly lower than oral temperatures.

Ingestion of cold or warm foods and smoking: Cold and warm foods, as well as smoking, can affect the recorded body temperature when taken orally. It is recommended that people refrain from the above 15-30 minutes prior to taking oral temperature readings.

Measurement

Oral temperature: Temperatures are commonly assessed in the hospital environment using an electronic thermometer. To take an oral body temperature, the thermometer is placed under the client's tongue in the back to the left or right of the frenulum (where the tongue connects to the bottom of the mouth). Ask the client to close his/her lips (not teeth) to hold it in place. The length of time will vary depending on the specific electronic thermometer. It can range from 10-45 seconds for a large hospital model to two to four minutes for a handheld battery operated unit. They will beep when the proper amount of time has elapsed.

Axillary temperature: Axillary temperatures are less accurate than oral temperatures, so they are typically used only when oral temperatures are contraindicated. Contraindications include dyspnea (difficult or labored breathing), surgical procedures involving the mouth or throat, very young children, and delirious or irrational patients (O'Sullivan & Schmitz, 1988). Clinical glass thermometers are typically used. Pat the underside of the arm and the side of the trunk dry if needed. Do not rub or it will increase body temperature. Place the thermometer between the upper arm and the trunk about two inches down from the armpit and ask the client to hold the thermometer in place by pulling the arm across his/her chest. In some instances the therapist may need to hold the thermometer in place (e.g., young child, poor upper arm control). When recording the temperature, note that it was an axillary temperature.

Rectal temperature: Rectal temperatures are typically used only with young children and infants when an oral or axillary temperature reading is difficult or contraindicated. Place the infant or child in a prone position (on stomach). Put a dab of Vaseline on the end of a digital thermometer and insert the tip of the thermometer into the anus about ¼ of an inch. When the digital thermometer beeps, remove it and record the reading.

Ear thermometer: An ear thermometer measures body temperature through the tympanic membrane in the ear. To use an ear thermometer, place a disposable cover on the ear thermometer, open up the client's ear canal by gently pulling the ear up and back, gently insert the covered tip into the ear canal, press the button to turn on the thermometer, continue to hold the button until it beeps, remove the thermometer from the ear, read the temperature on the display, and then discard the disposable cover. If the client has an increased build up of wax in the ear, readings can be inaccurate. Consequently, remove excessive built-up wax prior to using the ear thermometer.

Temporal artery thermometer: A temporal thermometer is an infrared thermometer that measures the surface temperature of the temporal artery on the forehead. To use a temporal thermometer, remove the cap, turn on the device, press the button (and continue to hold the button), place the device in the center of the client's forehead, quickly slide it horizontally across the forehead to the hairline, release the button, and then read the temperature on the display. Readings can be affected by sweat. Consequently, if the client's forehead is sweaty, readings can be taken by sliding the device horizontally across the carotid artery. To ensure the temperature is correct, repeat the horizontal slide three times and record the highest reading. Temporal artery thermometers are helpful when a client is congested causing difficulty breathing through the nose and is therefore unable to keep his/her mouth closed to take an oral temperature. Temporal artery thermometers may also be used when there are concerns about the safety of other temperature taking methods. These concerns include fear that the client will bite the oral electronic thermometer or when the client exhibits a poor behavioral response to the sensation of having temperature taken via an ear thermometer.

Pulse

When the left ventricle contracts it sends a wave of blood through the arterial system. The measure of these waves it called a pulse. A newborn's pulse can range from 70-170 beats per minute (average is 120) and continues to slow down as a person grows older. In a healthy adult, a pulse of 70 beats per minute is average (range is 50-100).

Factors that Influence Pulse

Pulse rate is typically a bit lower in males than females. There are also external variables that affect pulse rate including emotions, exercise (to meet increased oxygen demands), and systemic or local heat (fever or the use of a hot pack causes vasodilatation of peripheral vessels to dissipate heat).

Measurement

The pulse can be palpated in several areas. Arteries that are close to the skin (superficial arteries) in front of a bony surface are the easiest to feel because the artery can be sandwiched between the fingers and the bony surface. These areas are called pulse points. Guidelines for common pulse points are

Radial (on the wrist at the base of the thumb): The radial pulse is the most frequently used for monitoring pulse.

Temporal (top of the cheekbone, in front of the ear): The temporal pulse is used if the radial pulse is difficult to feel or if it is contraindicated or unavailable because of casting. It is the second most common pulse point for pulse monitoring.

Carotid (on the side of the neck): The carotid pulse is used in cardiac arrest. It is also commonly used for infants due to the difficulty in feeling a radial pulse and for monitoring blood flow to the brain.

Brachial (the inside bend of the arm): Although the brachial pulse can be used to monitor pulse rate, it is most commonly used as a pulse point to measure blood pressure.

Popliteal (behind the knee, easier to palpate when the knee is slightly flexed): The popliteal pulse is used to monitor lower extremity circulation. It can also be used for measuring blood pressure.

Pedal (on top of the foot between the big toe and the second toe, about three inches from the toes): The pedal pulse is used to monitor lower extremity circulation.

To palpate a pulse point, place the tips of the first two or three fingers on the pulse point and press firmly enough to feel the pulse. If you press too firmly the artery will become occluded and a pulse will not be felt. Once the pulse is detected, look at a watch or clock with a second hand and count the number of beats felt for one full minute. This is the pulse rate. The therapist can also take the pulse for 15 seconds and multiply it by four or take it for 30 seconds and double it. Taking a pulse rate for the full minute is the most accurate.

If the pulse points are difficult to palpate or they are contraindicated for medical reasons, the therapist can listen to (instead of feeling) the pulse. This is called an apical pulse. A stethoscope is placed directly over the top portion of the heart. Count the number of beats heard in a minute to obtain the pulse rate.

When monitoring a client's pulse, a therapist feels for rate, rhythm, and volume. Rate is the number of beats per minute. Rhythm describes the regularity of the beats. If the amount of time between each beat is the same, it is said to be regular or constant, as contrasted with an irregular or erratic rhythm. Volume refers to the force of each beat. The force of each pulse beat should be equal. When feeling the pulse, pay attention to how easily the pulse can be halted by applying pressure. If blood volume is high it will be difficult to halt the pulse (a bounding or full pulse). If blood volume is low it will be easy to halt the pulse (a weak or thready pulse). Therapists may also note the quality or feel of the arterial wall. The vessel should feel soft, smooth, flexible, and elastic, compared to vessels that feel hard, rigid, patchy, or cordlike. Sclerotic changes of the vessels are common as part of the aging process resulting in decreased smoothness and elasticity of vessels.

Respiration

Respiration rate is the number of inhalations per minute. Baseline respiration rates are taken in a relaxed state. Respiration rates can also be taken during exercise to monitor levels of exertion.

Factors that Influence Respiration

Exercise/metabolic rate: Exercise and any other event that increases the metabolic rate increases respiration rate due to the increased oxygen demand.

Age: The respiration rate for a newborn is between 30 and 60 per minute. It gradually slows down until adulthood when the average respiration rate reaches a minimum of 12 to 18 a minute. In older adults, the respiration rate may be slightly higher due to decreased lung functioning associated with the aging process. There may be decreased elasticity of the lung and decreased efficiency of exchange.

Sex and body type: Men, as well as people who are tall and thin, typically have a greater vital capacity (ability to hold more air in the lungs) than women or people who are short and overweight. People with greater vital capacity need fewer respirations per minute.

Emotions: Extreme emotions, such as fear and anxiety, can raise respiratory rate.

Measurement

To measure the base respiration rate, the person should be in a relaxed and normal state. The person must not know that respiration rates are being counted. If the person is aware that respiration rate is being recorded, the person may inadvertently or purposefully alter his/her breathing resulting in a skewed measure. Typically, vital signs are taken one after another (temperature, blood pressure, pulse, and then respiration), so a common trick is to continue acting as if you are taking the pulse but count the respirations instead. It is recommended that the person's chest be exposed so the therapist can assess the depth of breath (shallow or deep) and easily see respirations by the rise and fall of the chest. If this is not possible, a technique that can be helpful is to take the client's pulse on the wrist that is furthest from you so that the client has to cross his/her arm across the chest. The person's arm will rise and fall to indicate respirations. Inhalations or exhalations are counted for a full minute or for 30 seconds and then doubled. If a 30-second measure seems irregular (e.g., faster or slower than expected), it indicates the need to do a full minute count. When monitoring respirations, the therapist assesses the depth of breathing (by looking at the chest for a full rise and fall to note whether breathing appears to be deep or shallow), the rhythm of breathing (same amount of time between each breath; regular or irregular rhythm), and the character of the respirations (the amount of effort and the sound of the respirations). Some common terms used to describe the character of respirations include (O'Sullivan & Schmitz, 1988):

Dyspnea: labored or difficult breathing.

Wheezing: a whistling sound produced by air passing through narrowed bronchi or bronchioles. It may be heard on both inspiration and expiration but is more prominent on expiration. Apparent with emphysema and asthmatic patients.

Stridor: a harsh, high-pitched, crowing sound that occurs with upper airway obstructions caused by narrowing of the glottis or trachea. Possible causes are tracheal stenosis or presence of a foreign object.

Rales: rattling, bubbling, or crackling sounds that occur because of secretions in the air passages of the respiratory tract. They may be heard with the ear but are most accurately assessed by use of a stethoscope.

Sigh: a deep inspiration followed by a prolonged, audible expiration. Occasional sighs are normal and function to expand alveoli. Frequent sighs are abnormal and may indicate emotional stress.

Stertorous sounds: a snoring sound from secretions in the trachea and large bronchi.

Blood Pressure

Blood pressure is the force that the blood exerts against the wall of a vessel.

Factors that Influence Blood Pressure

Blood volume: Blood loss will lower blood pressure and increased blood volume, such as with a blood transfusion, will raise blood pressure.

Exercise: Physical activity raises systolic blood pressure because there is a greater cardiac output.

Body position: If the person is in a position other than those reviewed, it must be reflected in the documentation because different body positions can affect blood pressure readings by as much as 20 mmHg. When taking a brachial blood pressure, the person is seated with the arm supported at heart level (about four inches higher than a standard chair armrest). This type of chair is common at a blood-testing lab but is not usually available in a standard therapy environment. Therapists typically rest a person's arm on a tabletop, counter, adjustable rolling bed, or therapy table to raise the arm into this position. When taking a popliteal blood pressure, the client is placed into a prone position with the knee slightly flexed.

Emotions: Emotional stress such as fear, anxiety, anger, excitement, and upset can raise blood pressure.

Measurement

Blood pressure is measured using a sphygmomanometer, a blood pressure cuff, and a stethoscope.

Brachial blood pressure: The cuff is wrapped around the upper arm about an inch above the bend of the arm. The correct cuff size must be used to get a proper reading. Sizes include infant, pediatric, adult, extra wide for popliteal blood pressure or for a client who is morbidly obese. The cuff should fit snugly but comfortably. The center of the cuff is lined up with the brachial artery on the inside bend of the arm. Most cuffs have an arrow on the cuff to help identify the center of the cuff. Put on the stethoscope. With one hand, place the stethoscope on top of the brachial artery below the cuff. With the other hand, close the valve on the bulb of the blood pressure cuff and squeeze it continuously until the needle (or mercury) on the meter rises about 20 mmHg above the anticipated systolic pressure. For example, if the anticipated blood pressure reading is 120/80, pump the needle up to 140. Very slowly open the valve on the bulb to release a little bit of air. The needle will begin to fall. Readjust the valve (tighten or loosen) if needed. For example, if the needle is falling too quickly to be able to accurately read the pressure at the first heartbeat, the therapist closes the valve a bit more to slow down the fall of the needle. Listen for the first audible heartbeat through the stethoscope. The number that the needle is on when the first audible heartbeat is heard is the systolic blood pressure reading (highest pressure against the arterial wall). Continue listening until the heartbeat is no longer heard. The number that the needle is on when the last heartbeat is heard is the diastolic pressure reading (lowest pressure against the arterial wall). If there is difficulty hearing a heartbeat, readjust the stethoscope and/or re-tighten the bulb valve and gently give it a pump or two to raise the needle a bit higher past the point of uncertainty. For example if you are at 120 and are not sure if the heartbeat started at 125 or 130, close the valve, pump it back up to 140, gently loosen the valve to let out a small amount of air and re-listen for the heartbeat. Once the systolic and diastolic pressures are identified, fully open the valve of the bulb to totally deflate the blood pressure cuff. Remove the cuff and clean the stethoscope with an alcohol swab.

Popliteal blood pressure: If taking a brachial blood pressure is contraindicated or if a comparison of upper and lower blood pressures is needed, for example, to monitor peripheral vascular disease, a popliteal (behind the knee) blood pressure can be taken. The person is placed into a prone position (on the stomach). A wide blood pressure cuff is wrapped around the lower third of the thigh and centered on the popliteal artery. The person is asked to slightly flex the knee of the leg to be used by raising the foot about six inches. The stethoscope is placed on the popliteal artery below the cuff and the same measurement procedure is followed as in the brachial blood pressure reading.

Weight Bearing Precautions

Weight-bearing precautions are set by the surgeon or physician for a variety of conditions, such as total hip or knee replacements, fractures, or sprains. ICF codes that indicate a need for weight-bearing precautions are s740 Structure of Pelvic Region and s750 Structure of Lower Extremity. Specific weight-bearing precautions are written in the client's medical record and must be followed to prevent injury and promote healing. Changes will be made to weight-bearing precautions as healing occurs. There are five levels of weight bearing (Cooper, 2006):

Non-weight bearing (NWB): Unable to put any weight on the identified extremities. If the restriction involves both lower extremities, activity is limited to those completed while sitting or in bed. May complete transfers using a transfer board.

Touchdown weight bearing (TDWB) or *toe-touch weight bearing* (TTWB): The majority of the client's weight bearing must be through the client's arms on the walking device and the unaffected extremity. Approximately 10% of normal weight bearing may go on the affected leg. Physical therapists recommend strategies for safe walking and prescribe a mobility device to help clients adhere to weight-bearing precautions. Close collaboration between the physical therapist and other allied health professionals working with the client is essential so that the client is able to engage in functional activity safely and effectively while using the device. Weight bearing on the involved extremity is limited to using toes to make contact with the floor, primarily to maintain balance. Note that TTWB is not as much weight as the client can carry on his/her toes.

Partial weight bearing (PWB): This typically refers to bearing 50% of the client's body weight on the involved extremity. It is frequently estimated by the client and therapist and requires sustained effort and attention. Note that when walking, a normal gait puts 100% of the client's weight on the extremity when it is the only limb on the ground. This would not be allowed with partial weight bearing.

Weight bearing as tolerated (WBAT): The amount of weight put on the extremity is left to the discretion of the client based on his/her level of comfort.

Full weight bearing (FWB): No restrictions on amount of weight put on the extremity. Client can fully weight-bear through the extremity.

References

American Diabetes Association. (2104). Hyperglycemia (High blood glucose). Accessed via website www.diabetes.org/living-with-diabetes/treatment-and-care/blood-glucose-control/hyperglycemia.html.

Anderson, K., Anderson, L., & Glanze, W. (Eds.). (1994). *Mosby's medical, nursing, and allied health dictionary* (4th ed.). St. Louis, MO: Mosby.

Boltz, M. (2012). *Evidence-based geriatric nursing protocols for best practice.* New York: Springer.

Choi, H., Sugar, R., Fish, D. E., Shatzer, M., & Krabak, B. (2003). *Physical medicine and rehabilitation pocketpedia.* Philadelphia, PA: Lippincott Williams & Wilkins.

Cistian, A. (2012). *Patient safety in rehabilitation medicine: An issue of physical medicine and rehabilitation clinics.* Philadelphia, PA: Elsevier Health Sciences.

Cleveland Clinic Foundation. (2011a). Hyperglycemia. Accessed via website http://my.clevelandclinic.org/disorders/diabetes_mellitus/hic _hyperglycemia_and_diabetes.aspx.

Cleveland Clinic Foundation. (2011b). Hypoglycemia. Accessed via website http://my.clevelandclinic.org/disorders/hypoglycemia/endo_d efault.aspx.

Cooper, G. (2006). *Essential physical medicine and rehabilitation.* New York: Springer.

Epilepsy Foundation. (2012a). Seizure provoking triggers. Accessed via website www.epilepsyfoundation.org/aboutepilepsy/Diagnosis/seizur eprovokingtriggers.cfm.

Epilepsy Foundation. (2012b). First aid for generalized tonic-clinic seizures. Accessed via website www.epilepsyfoundation.org/aboutepilepsy/seizures/genconv ulsive/tonicseizures.cfm.

Gogelova, H. (2011). *Anglictina pro fyzioterapeuty.* Prague: Grada Publishing.

Gonzalez-Fernandez, M. & Friedman, J. D. (2011). *Physical medicine and rehabilitation pocket companion.* New York: Demos Medical Publishing.

Kennon, R. (2008). *Hip and knee surgery: A patient's guide to hip replacement, hip resurfacing, knee replacement, and knee arthroscopy.* Raleigh, NC: Lulu.com.

Lane, J. T. (2012). *The type 2 diabetes handbook: Six rules for staying healthy with type 2 diabetes.* Omaha, NE: Addicus Books.

Lord, S., Sherrington, C., Menz, H., & Close, J. (2007). *Falls in older people: Risk factors and strategies for prevention.* New York: Cambridge.

Joint Commission Resources. (2008). *Reducing the risk of patient harm resulting from falls: Toolkit for implementing national Patient Safety Goal 9.* Oakbrook Terrace, IL: Joint Commission Resources.

O'Sullivan, S. & Schmitz, T. (1988). *Physical rehabilitation: Assessment and treatment* (2ⁿᵈ ed.). Philadelphia, PA: F. A. Davis Company.

Payson, C. A. & Haviley, C. A. (2005). *Falls assessment and prevention: Strategies and tools to apply with JCAHO.* Danvers, MA: HC Pro, Inc.

Sanchez, F. (2010). *Understanding suicide and its prevention: A neuropsychological approach.* Bloomington, IN: Xlibris Corporation.

Schilling, J. A. (2002). *Illustrated manual of nursing practice* (3ʳᵈ ed.). Philadelphia, PA: Lippincott Williams & Wilkins.

Simon, R. I. & Hales, R. E. (2012). *The American psychiatric publishing textbook of suicide assessment and management.* Arlington, VA: American Psychiatric Publishing.

Timbly, B. & Lewis, L. (1992). *Fundamental skills and concepts in patient care* (5ᵗʰ ed.). Philadelphia, PA: Lippincott Company.

UPMC. (2014). Thickened Liquids: Nectar-Thick. Accessed via website www.upmc.com/patients-visitors/education/nutrition/pages/thickened-liquids-nectar-thick.aspx.

Zachazewski, J. E. & Quillen, W. S. (2008). *Pathology and intervention in musculoskeletal rehabilitation.* Philadelphia, PA: Elsevier Health Sciences.

7. Participation

Heather R. Porter

Recreational therapists do not view participation in an activity as an either/or scenario (either the client participated or s/he did not). Recreational therapists study participation patterns (also called levels). Evaluation of a client's participation level clarifies the client's quality of participation in an activity. It is important to form a baseline of the client's participation pattern, to note changes, and to formulate and measure attainment of goals. The quality of participation in an activity deserves special attention since the quality of participation brings with it specific health benefits. For example, the health benefits of being a spectator are very different from the benefits of active participation in a physical activity.

Dehn's Leisure Step Up model (Dehn, 1995) provides a hierarchy of healthy leisure participation levels. burlingame's (2001) clarification of the differences between attendance and participation was developed to help therapists and researchers clarify client participation levels and patterns in a way that leads to a better understanding of how activities affect the client's life. In both cases, the quality of participation can be seen by looking at the involvement of the client.

Attendance

Attendance is defined as how many times or how often a client shows up for an activity. Attendance does not measure effort, quality of participation, emotional involvement, behavior, or attitude. It only measures if the client was there or not. Attendance is a good measure for monitoring use of an activity, facility, or equipment to help determine staffing, budget, and maintenance needs. Attendance is also used to measure the very basic skill of showing up at an activity. This may be a good way to measure progress in a client who has trouble with compliance or follow-through issues. For clients with these issues, just showing up at an activity can be progress. The ICF is not concerned with attendance though. The ICF goal is to measure the level of the client's abilities, therefore the term "attendance" is not used in the ICF codes. The definition of attendance is provided in this section to give the therapist a clear understanding of its difference from participation.

Participation

Participation measures the quality of the client's actions and the amount of effort that the client puts into the activity. Recreational therapists view participation along a continuum and measure participation on a spectrum from healthy (beneficial to self and others) to unhealthy (harmful to self or others). Recreational therapists most commonly use the nine levels of participation described in the Leisure Step Up Program (Dehn, 1995) to quantify the level of a client's participation in recreation, leisure, and community activities. The levels consist of five positive levels, one neutral level, and three negative levels. The levels are described as:

Cathartic level: This level is described as the ultimate level of leisure participation. The client has a high level of emotional involvement in the activity and it acts as a catalyst for growth in the client's lifestyle. Not everyone reaches this level of participation.

Level 4 (Creative Participation): Emotions are expressed. Participation in the activity does not follow a plan, pattern, or instruction. The client puts a part of himself/herself into the activity and the finished activity reflects what the client has given (making a clay sculpture, writing music or poetry). Creativity can be learned and practiced; it is not solely an innate skill.

Level 3 (Active Participation): The client is a player rather than a spectator. Clients at this level think of recreation in terms of activity (there are instructions, rules, a plan, etc.) and it requires physical, cognitive, and/or social components for participation. The activities must reflect a balance of physical, social, and cognitive components. Not all have to be reflected in one activity but in the client's activity pattern as a whole.

Level 2 (Involved Spectator): The spectator is emotionally involved in the activity. The client is interested in the activity and expresses or experiences emotions related to the activity. This type of participation provides emotional and/or cognitive health benefits, but it does not fulfill all of our leisure needs. Examples would include attending an opera where the songs and acting move you or getting charged up over watching a football game on television.

Level 1 (Uninvolved Spectator): There is no emotional involvement. The client often lacks a personal investment in participating in positive leisure activities. Examples would include staring at the television without any real interest in the storyline or sitting outside watching the cars drive by. Dehn points out that our mind, body, and emotions can become fatigued and that the need to just do nothing (and not feel guilty about it) is a form of healthy participation. Although this level of participation is on the healthy side of leisure, it does not fulfill all of our leisure needs. Clients should be encouraged to strive for higher participation levels.

Level 0 (Preoccupied): This level is neither positive nor negative. The client is present at the activity, goes through the motions, but is too preoccupied with other things to fully experience the activity. Examples would include going camping at a beautiful lake but being so preoccupied with a troubled relationship that the client doesn't truly experience the beauty of the lake. Participating in activities that are used as a therapeutic means to cope with a problem that is preoccupying the individual is also considered to fall into this level. Such examples include going for a walk when feeling angry or journaling to help express feelings of sorrow. Clients who participate at this level usually have high levels of stress, frustration, and/or depression. At first glance, it looks like Level 0 might be the same as "attendance," but, in reality, each of the levels in Dehn's model requires attendance. Attendance only measures where the body is. To record what the client is experiencing, we must describe where the mind and emotions are, too.

Level -1 (Harm to Self): It is the first level in the unhealthy direction of leisure participation. An activity at this level either puts the client at high risk of harm or causes actual physical, mental, or emotional damage. Examples include smoking, not getting enough sleep, not eating a well-balanced diet, talking down to one's self (e.g., "I look stupid", "I'll never do this right"), and participating in dangerous high risk activities without proper training and safety measures.

Level -2 (Harm to Others): The leisure actions of the person have inflicted physical, emotional, or mental harm to others, such as hurting animals, ignoring family, substance abuse, gambling, stealing, destroying property, and gossiping. People at this level may deny that these things are hurtful and say they are just having fun. People at this level are often in need of developing basic social skills and an awareness of their risk to spiral downwards towards Lost Freedom.

Lost Freedom: People at this level have been voluntarily or involuntarily committed to an institution that places constraints on the type and amount of leisure that is available (e.g., prison, mental health facility, juvenile delinquency facility) or have lost their freedom (mentally and emotionally) because of trauma (e.g., a victim of rape or a person in profound mourning whose leisure activities are constrained by thoughts and feelings of rage, guilt, fear, or depression). Participation at this level has a drastic effect on the person, as well as other people who are around the person. People at this level are often preoccupied with suicidal thoughts, suffer from extreme depression and loss of interest, or have a total disregard for the self and others (e.g., gang fighting with no concern for self or others, infecting others with HIV, suicide attempts). Clients at this level are in need of developing leisure patterns that promote health. Counseling by a variety of disciplines is often required for the client to begin moving in a positive direction.

Clients may exhibit different levels of participation among various activities. For example a client may be at Level 2 when watching sports on TV and at Level -1 when riding a dirt bike. Measurement of the level of participation is vitally important when assessing the impact that leisure participation has on a client's health and well-being. For example, individuals who actively participate in social conversations and activities (Level 3) will not doubt receive different benefits compared to an individual who chooses to be an uninvolved spectator (Level 1) during social conversation and activities. The level of participation is determined through a clinical interview with the client (and others as appropriate), as well as observation of the client's behavior, attitude, and demeanor during specific activities.

Participation and the ICF

In the ICF, participation is defined as "involvement in a life situation" (World Health Organization, 2007, xvi). When considering an activity, the ICF is concerned with two aspects of participation. The first is the person's ability to perform the activity itself. The second is other characteristics the person demonstrates during participation.

For scoring the ability, there is an entire section of Activities and Participation codes. For each of the codes in the Activities and Participation section, the therapist scores the level of difficulty that a client has performing the specific task in a standardized environment. For example, after observation of a crafts activity the therapist would score the level of difficulty a client has engaging in a clinic setting when assistance is provided and when assistance is not provided. The ICF also allows the therapist to score the level of difficulty that a client has performing the specific task in a real-life setting. The second pair of scores reflect the level of difficulty a client has engaging in crafts at the client's community senior center when assistance is provided and when assistance is not provided. These scores are totally unrelated to Dehn's levels of participation.

The characteristics a person shows while doing an activity relate directly to Dehn's model. The ICF is far more specific about the findings, so that a Level -1 in Dehn's model is recorded as a set of specific deficits in ICF codes. Some of the important ICF codes to consider include those under b126 Temperament and Personality Functions, b130 Energy and Drive Functions, b152 Emotional Functions, b164 Higher-Level Cognitive Functions, d570 Looking After One's Health, d710 Basic Interpersonal Interactions, d910 Community Life, d920 Recreation and Leisure, and d930 Religion and Spirituality. When considering the negative levels on Dehn's scale, activities such as gambling or drug use may also involve ICF codes d760 Family Relationships, d770 Intimate Relationships, and d845 Acquiring, Keeping, and Terminating a Job, along with other interpersonal codes. Consider the following example:

Sam is a 15-year-old boy with conduct disorder. He enjoys riding his motorized dirt bike at a local field in his neighborhood. The field is not sanctioned for such riding and those caught riding there can be ticketed and have their bike impounded. Sam doesn't wear a helmet or protective gear, he rides predominantly by himself (and doesn't have a cell phone for safety), and boasts about "ripping up the property" with his bike and his ability to get his bike up to 15 feet off the ground when jumping the dirt hills. Sam also shared with the recreational therapist that sometimes there are other kids on the field when he is riding his dirt bike and he likes to scare them by riding close to where they are playing. The ICF code for riding a motorcycle is d4751 Driving Motorized Vehicles. When scoring this code, the therapist indicates that he has "no difficulty" engaging in this task. But that is not the end of the story. Sam's Leisure Step Up score is Level -2. Finding the appropriate ICF codes might look like this: First, he is not of legal age to be riding a motorcycle (b1267 Trustworthiness). Second, he is disobeying the local law by riding in a field that is not sanctioned for such riding (b1262 Conscientiousness), and doesn't seem to care that he is breaking the law (b1267 Trustworthiness, b1645 Judgment, d2501 Responding to Demands). Third, he isn't adhering to basic safety needs (d2400 Handling Responsibilities, d5702 Maintaining One's Health). Fourth, he is destroying property (d910 Community Life). And, fifth, he is putting his own life, as well as the lives of the other children playing on the field, in danger (b1261 Agreeableness, b1645 Judgment, d5702 Maintaining One's Health, d710 Basic Interpersonal Interactions, d910 Community Life). Also consider ICF codes b1263 Psychic Stability, b1304 Impulse Control, b152 Emotional Functions, and d240 Handling Stress and Other Psychological Demands as other possibilities for itemizing the reasons for the Level -2 score.

References

burlingame, j. (2001). *Idyll Arbor's therapy dictionary* (2nd ed.). Ravensdale, WA: Idyll Arbor.

Dehn, D. (1995). *Leisure step up*. Ravensdale, WA: Idyll Arbor.

World Health Organization. (2001). *International classification of functioning, disability, and health*. Geneva, Switzerland: World Health Organization.

8. Psychoneuroimmunology

Heather R. Porter

The connection between the mind and the body is not a new concept. The Greeks, more than two thousand years ago, "understood intuitively that emotions and health are one" (Sternberg, 2000, p. 3). Hippocrates, whose oath still underlies the principles of modern medicine, taught that health lay in a balance among a healthy diet, pure waters, exercise, and the support of friends and family, as well as soothing activities that calmed the person such as music, sleep, and prayer. "So integral to the healing of the body was the mind that the god of medicine carried a staff with the symbols both intertwined: Asclepius carried in his left hand the caduceus, a wooden staff with a serpent curled around it, an ancient symbol of body and soul, and today the universally recognized symbol of medicine" (Sternberg, 2000, p. 2).

Many traditional and alternative health professionals witness the power of the mind in healing the body and many behavioral studies have documented the connection between mind, emotions, activity, and health. Despite how convincing and exciting these studies have been, the medical community desires concrete biochemical evidence that such a connection exists. A relatively new discipline, psychoneuroimmunology (PNI), is now providing that evidence. PNI is the study of the interrelationships between the central nervous system (s1 Structures of the Nervous System) and the immune system (b435 Immunological System Functions).

PNI has shown that the brain and the immune system are a bi-directional circuit. They are in constant communication with each other. Simply put, emotions and demands from the immune system trigger certain hormonal and chemical changes in the body. These biological changes travel throughout the body and affect bodily processes, including the immune system, which directly influences the proc-ess of disease in a positive or negative direction. In one study, Candace Pert, a neuropharmacologist at the National Institute of Mental Health, found that individuals who were made to feel helpless by using loud noise to prevent concentration on a puzzle had slower than usual macrophage movement. (Macrophages surround and consume infection and rebuild damaged tissues.) Thus she speculated that the client who gives up hope might fare worse than the client who is optimistic. The client who is optimistic will have macrophages that keep moving while the client who gives up will have macrophages that slow down. She goes on to say that, "The more I look, the more I'm convinced that emotions are running the show" (Weschsler, 1987, p. 55).

Although we don't expect the medical community to shift totally from a conventional approach to a holistic approach, we do expect that medical practice will become more holistically focused, taking into consideration the client's emotional, social, and spiritual health, aspects that are already included in the ICF. For recreational therapists, this branch of research also adds more validity to what we do for our clients. Our focus on helping our clients achieve optimal emotional and social health does, indeed, have a direct influence on our clients' recovery and disease process. Not only does this focus improve the quality of their lives, but it also contributes to the biomedical approach to eradicating disease.

Thoughts, Feelings, and Emotions

Since we are now aware that thoughts, feelings, and emotions influence our physical health, we need to ask the question, "What is it, exactly, that influences our thoughts and feelings?" This is an important question since healthy emotional responses are optimal in the recovery process. Is it our perception and interpretation of a situation? Is it hormonal and chemical changes in the body as a result of disease? Is it activity that triggers hormonal and chemical changes? Is it life experiences? Yes, yes, yes, and yes. All of these influence our thoughts and feelings. Our world and our selves are complex systems functioning within systems of systems. All are interrelated and interdependent. Why should our thoughts and feelings be any different? As recreational therapists, we are keenly aware of the many interventions that can be implemented to optimize emotional health both directly and indirectly.

Perceptions and Interpretations

"Our thoughts create the context that determines our feelings. In thinking about health, and especially in trying to change the consequences of an illness or the behavior that leads to it, an awareness of context — or what I have come to call 'mindfulness' — is crucial" (Langer, 1989, p. 48). If one thinks negatively, one's emotional response will be fear and high anxiety. If one thinks positively and realistically, one's emotional response will be hopeful with a controlled sense of calm. Our "perceptions and interpretations influence the ways in which our bodies respond to information in the world. If we automatically — 'mindlessly' — accept preconceived notions of the context of a particular situation, we can jeopardize the body's ability to handle that situation, we can jeopardize the body's ability to need to place our perceptions intentionally, that is, mindfully in a different context" (Langer, 1989, p. 48).

Recreational therapists can enhance their client's perceptions and interpretations of situations through a variety of counseling techniques. Many chapters in this book contain counseling information, such as Education and Counseling; Theories, Models, and Concepts; Cognitive Behavioral Counseling; Leisure Education and Counseling; and Sexual Well-Being.

Hormonal and Chemical Changes

As reviewed earlier, PNI research indicates that the brain and the immune system are bi-directional. Therefore, it is not a far stretch to think that the immune system could affect emotions controlled by the brain.

Signals from the immune system may even reach the emotional and rational centers of the brain, which may explain why people get irrita-

ble when they're sick, and why mental capacity often deteriorates at the same time as resistance to infection (Weschsler, 1987, p. 53).

You have probably heard a family member of a client say, "I don't know why he's acting that way. That's not like him." Sometimes a client may even recognize the changes and make the same observation. Chances are the family member and client are right. It's probably not the typical behavior or emotional response of the client, but the illness or disease process that is triggering the release of certain hormones and chemicals that are affecting his/her behavior and/or emotions. The recreational therapist may be able to influence this process indirectly by enhancing macrophage movement. By fostering the client's emotional health in a positive direction, for example with increased locus of control, achievement, or esteem, macrophage movement may increase, thus optimizing the body's defenses to combat disease and rebuild tissue. The therapist can also assist the client in developing skills for managing unwanted emotional responses by using, for example, relaxation techniques for anxiety and thought stopping for negative thinking cycles.

However, if the illness or trauma directly affects the functioning of the brain, as with stroke, the changes in the client's behavior and personality may be better attributed to brain damage.

Activity

Activity, in and of itself, can cause the release of hormones and other chemicals that enhance mood. For example, a "runners high" is explained by the release of endorphins, the body's natural painkillers. After a run, people often report feeling uplifted, relaxed, and recharged. Those who practice yoga report feelings of inner peace and strength and those who participate in an activity that highlights personal skills may exhibit increased self-worth. All of these positive and healthy emotions result in hormonal and chemical changes in the body.

One must question, however, if it is the activity, in and of itself, that is the primary cause of the emotional response, or if it is the secondary benefits of the activity. For example, was it the beauty of nature that invoked a sense of relaxation from the run, was it the music that generated feelings of strength from yoga exercises, or was it the recognition of one's personal skills that fostered a sense of self-worth from the activity? How one achieves emotional change varies from person to person and it is difficult, if not impossible, to tease out the specific things that fostered change, because, chances are, it was a coming together of many complex systems, of which activity is a part.

Activities that have been shown to enhance a client's emotional state include meditation, prayer, popping bubble-wrap, hypnosis, biofeedback, placebos, imagery, relaxation techniques, friends, pets, music, art, humor, and anything that provides a "thrill" (a subtle nervous tremor caused by intense emotion or excitement — climatic music, great beauty in nature or art, sexual activity, watching emotional interactions between other people). Knowing this, therapists educate clients on the positive and negative influence of the immune system on mood and work with clients to determine what activities are realistic as part of the clients' activity patterns. See the chapter on Activity Pattern Development for more information.

Life Experiences

One's past and present life experiences shape beliefs, attitudes, opinions, and actions — all of which influence emotional health, thus positively or negatively affecting the immune system. If one experiences betrayal, then one may mistrust. If one experiences unconditional love, then one may feel accepted. Who we are and what we have become are shaped by many things in our lives: our family, our friends, our accomplishments, our failures, our hopes and dreams, as well as our disappointments and struggles. These experiences give shape to how we interpret situations, cope, and live our lives. Therapists should not be blind to a client's life experiences and focus only on the present situation, for in the past one may find answers. For example:

A 32-year-old female client is angry and bitter since being diagnosed with cancer. Being unable to move past these emotions is affecting many of her life activities. The client shares with you that her mother died from cancer when she was young. You learn that she swore to herself that she would never leave her children as her mother did and yet she now finds herself in the same situation. The anger from her mother's death has still not been resolved and her own promise to herself will now be broken. The rec-

reational therapist makes a referral to counseling services and designs an RT treatment program for developing healthy coping strategies.

A client who has been diagnosed with multiple sclerosis for 10 years is exhibiting signs of depression. At least once a year, he experiences an exacerbation. Rehabilitation following each exacerbation has improved his functioning moderately, but the exacerbations continue. In the beginning, he exercised regularly, controlled his stress level, ate a healthy diet, and did not push himself past fatigue. Over time, his efforts have not yielded the results he had hoped for, thus extinguishing his internal locus of control. He now comes to you, after his 10th exacerbation, depressed, and in "learned helplessness" mode. He has no motivation or initiative and just wants to sit in front of the television. This client's past life experiences have reinforced that no matter what he does it doesn't matter, despite how unrealistic this interpretation may be. The recreational therapist educates and counsels the client about the relation of activity to exacerbation management and helps the client to better understand what his past actions "have" done rather than what they "have not" done for his health.

Other considerations that influence the client's life experiences include cultural and religious beliefs and practices. For example, some cultures believe that it is unacceptable to share or show emotions, while other cultures belittle a man who is unable to fulfill the traditional male role of being the provider, and certain faiths promote the idea that one is afflicted with disease due to bad behavior. All of these influence the client's emotional state, thus positively or negatively affecting the immune system, as well as affecting the client's ability to develop healthy coping skills. Therapists must be aware of their client's life experiences as they affect his/her current situation in order to best understand the client's emotional state and implement appropriate interventions to enhance emotional health.

Research

"There is a growing body of evidence to support the effect of the psyche — stress, in particular — on immune responses…. The effects of stress on shifting the immune response are not completely understood; however, research has shown that stress modifies the delicate balance between health and disease.... Seeking alternative interventions can only enhance our ability to treat patients" (Tausk et al., 2008, p. 27). Some supportive research is provided below:

Adverse Childhood Events

The more adverse childhood events a person experiences, the greater the relationship to adult diseases, including heart disease, cancer, chronic lung disease, skeletal fractures, and liver disease (Dube et al., 2001; Felitti et al., 1998).

Antibodies

Antibodies to an orally ingested antigen were found to be higher on days when the participant reported more positive mood, and lower on days when more negative mood was reported (Stone et al., 1994).

Cancer

Men with depression had increased incidence of cancer at 10-year follow-up and increased mortality from cancer at 10- and 20-year follow-ups (Shekelle et al., 1981). Increased risk of breast cancer was found to be associated with major negative life events, such as death of a loved one or divorce (Lillberg et al., 2007).

Healing from Surgery

A systematic review by Mavros et al. (2011), found that feelings of anxiety, anger, avoidance coping, subclinical depression, and intramarital hostility appear to complicate recovery from surgery, whereas optimism, religiousness, anger control, and low pain expectations seemed to promote healing.

HIV/AIDS

People with AIDS who survived longer than others had a significantly higher score on *Kobasa's Hardiness Measure* (the ability to gain personal growth and benefit from stressful situations through control, commitment, and challenge) (Soloman et al., 1987). Greater anger in HIV-positive men was found to be associated with faster progression to AIDS (Leserman et al., 2002).

Infections

Students were found to have more infectious illnesses during exam periods (Glaser et al., 1987).

Maternal Stress

Maternal stress may produce lasting effects on the infant's health status, immune system, and neuro-cognitive development (Ruiz & Avant, 2005).

Mortality Risk

Middle-aged Swedish men who experienced significant life events within the year and lacked perceived emotional support were found to exhibit higher mortality risk (Rosengred et al., 1993).

Natural Killer Cell Activity

Among women, negative mood throughout the day was associated with reduced natural killer cell activity (Valdimarsdottir & Bovbjerg, 1997). Intrusive thoughts were found to be associated with lower levels of natural killer cell activity among hurricane victims (Ironson et al., 1997).

Skin Disease

Based on a review of the literature by Tausk and colleagues (2008), "[e]motional stressors have been linked to the development or evolution of a variety of cutaneous diseases including acne, vitiligo, alopecia areata, lichen planus, seborrheic dermatitis, herpes simplex infections, pemphigus, urticarial, psoriasis, and atopic eczema" (p. 26).

Wound Healing

Individuals in marriages with hostile interactions had dermal blister wounds heal a median time of two days longer than individuals in marital relationship with non-hostile interactions (Keicolt-Glaser, Loving, Stowell, et al., 2005). In punch wound biopsy studies, students healed faster during vacation time compared to exam time (Marucha et al., 1998). Individuals caring for others (a stressed population) took longer to heal (Kiecolt-Glaser et al., 1995).

Intervention Evidence

In regards to interventions,

There is good observational evidence that certain psychological and social factors can influence the onset and progression of disease. However … [t]here are many challenges ahead. These include gaining a greater understanding of the mechanisms underlying these relationships; continuing to examine whether relationships observed in tightly controlled experimental settings are upheld in naturalistic contexts, such as caregiving, bereavement, etc.; a greater focus on the clinical relevance of indicators of immunocompetence; and finally expanding the research agency to include a wider range of psychological and social factors (e.g., the assessment of both positive and negative mood states). These developments are important if we are to develop interventions to reduce psychological burden, not only for the positive effects this has, *per se*, but also to harness the effects of the mind on the body (Byrne-Davis & Vedhara, 2008, p. 761).

A sampling of research related to interventions follows:

Relaxation training, T'ai Chi training, and spiritual growth groups were found to significantly improve immune function in individuals with HIV suggesting that "findings of improved immune function have important clinical implications, particularly for person with immune-mediated illness" (McCain et al., 2008, p. 431).

Relaxation training was shown to improve natural killer cell activity (Glaser et al., 1986; Keicolt-Glaser et al., 1984).

Healthy students who participated in hypnosis and relaxation had increased T helper cells (Kiecolt-Glaser et al., 1995).

Therapeutic Touch in postoperative surgical patients resulted in higher natural killer cells, as well as lower cortisol and pain levels (Coakley & Duffy, 2010).

Older adults who engaged in an exercise intervention three days a week with 30 minute of cardiovascular activity healed a 3.5 mm dermal wound significantly faster than participants who did not engage in the exercise intervention (Emery et al., 2005).

Women with breast cancer who used expressive writing to describe traumatic or upsetting experiences (20 minutes a day on four consecutive days) self-reported less symptoms at three-month follow-up (Stanton et al., 2002).

Women with breast cancer were found to live longer if involved in a support group (Spiegel et al., 1989).

A review of the literature (81 studies) by Uchino, Cacioppo, and Kiecolt-Glaser (1996) found that "social support was reliably related to beneficial effects on aspects of the cardiovascular, endocrine, and immune systems" (p. 488).

Individuals with metastatic melanoma who receive psychosocial interventions exhibited increased survival rates (Fawzy et al., 1993).

Despite the evidence listed above, Ziemssen and Kern (2007) remind us, "Many different kinds of behavioural interventions are more or less effective in improving mood, quality of life, health behavior and in altering neuroendocrine and immune functions. However, the question remains as to whether these latter effects are sufficiently large or last long enough to contribute to one's health status, or if they are even relevant to the development of a specific disease. Unfortunately, we have not yet reached the stage where the selection of a behavioural intervention is based on its ability to change those parameters of physiological function that are relevant to the progression of specific disease processes" (Ziemssen, & Kern, 2007, p. 11).

ICF Connections

The need to work on PNI issues to improve bodily health will show up in deficits in b1 Mental Functions, especially b126 Temperament and Personality Functions, b130 Energy and Drive Functions, b134 Sleep Functions, b152 Emotional Functions, and b180 Experience of Self and Time Functions. The results of using the concepts of PNI will most likely be scored with Body Function codes in b2 Sensory Functions and Pain, b4 Functions of the Cardiovascular, Hematological, Immunological, and Respiratory Systems, b5 Functions of the Digestive, Metabolic, and Endocrine Systems, b6 Genitourinary and Reproductive Functions, b7 Neuromusculoskeletal and Movement-Related Functions, b8 Functions of the Skin and Related Structures, and any of the Body Structure codes.

Conclusion

The mind and the body, our being, is an interrelated complex system where behavior, emotions, and health are constantly seeking a biological balance. No longer are one's emotions and beliefs secondary in the healing process. It has been validated via psychoneuroimmunology (PNI) that our emotions directly influence illness and disease processes. Recreational therapists should use this information to add professional validation for the field, as well as to educate clients on the value of emotional health on functioning and recovery. As Asclepius's staff symbolizes the coming together of body and soul, so should we, as health professionals, uphold this belief and instill it in our clients.

References

Byrne-Davis, L. M. & Vedhara, K. (2008). Psychoneuroimmunology. *Social and Personality Psychology Compass, 2*(2), 751-764.

Coakley, A. B. & Duffy, M. E. (2010). The effect of therapeutic touch on postoperative patients. *Journal of Holistic Nursing, 28*(3), 193-200.

Dube, S. R., Anda, R. F., Felitti, V. J., Chapman, D. P., Williamson, D. F., & Giles, W. H. (2001). Childhood abuse, household dysfunction, and the risk of attempted suicide throughout the life span: Findings from the adverse childhood experiences study. *Journal of American Medical Association, 286*, 3086-3096.

Emery, C. F., Kiecolt-Glaser, J. K., Glaser, R., Malarky, W. B., & Frid, D. J. (2005). Exercise accelerates wound healing among healthy older adults: A preliminary investigation. *Journal of Gerontology, 60A*(11), 1432-1436.

Fawzy, F. I., Fawzy, N. W., Hyun, C. S., Elashoff, R., Guthrie, D., Fahey, J. L., & Morton, D. L. (1993). Malignant melanoma: Effects of an early structured psychiatric intervention, coping, and affective state on recurrence and survival 6 years later. *Archives of General Psychiatry, 50*(9), 681-689.

Felitti, R. F., Anda, D., Nordenberg, D., Williamson, D. F., Spitz, A. M., Edwards, V. Koss, M. P., & Marks, J. S. (1998). Relationship of childhood abuse and household dysfunction to many of the leading causes of death in adults: The adverse childhood experience (ACE) study. *American Journal of Preventative Medicine, 14*(4), 245-258.

Glaser, R., Rice, J., Sheridan, J., Fertel, R., Stout, J., Speicher, C., Pinsky, D., & Kiecolt-Glaser, J. (1987). Stress-related immune suppression: Health implications. *Brain, Behavior, and Immunity, 1*(1), 7-20.

Glaser, R., Rice, J., Speicher, C. E., Stout, J. C., & Kiecolt-Glaser, J. K. (1986). Stress depresses interferon production by leukocytes concomitant with a decrease in natural killer cell activity. *Behavioral Neuroscience, 100*(5), 675-678.

Ironson, G., Wynings, C., Schneiderman, N., Baum, A., Rodriguez, M., Greenwood, D., Benight, C., Antoni, M., LaPerriere, A., Huang, H., Klimas, N., & Fletcher, M. (1997). Posttraumatic stress symptoms, intrusive thoughts, loss, and immune function after Hurricane Andrew. *Psychosomatic Medicine, 59*(2), 128-141.

Kiecolt-Glaser, J. K., Garner, W., Speicher, C., Penn, G. M., Holliday, J., & Glaser, R. (1984). Psychosocial modifiers of immunocompetence in medical students. *Psychosomatic Medicine, 46*(1), 7-14.

Keicolt-Glaser, J. K., Loving, T. J., Stowell, J. R., Malarkey, W. B., Lemeshow, S., Dickinson, S. L., & Glaser, R. (2005). Hostile marital interactions, proinflammatory cytokine production, and wound healing. *Archives of General Psychiatry, 62*(12), 1377-1384.

Kiecolt-Glasser, J. K., Marucha, P. T., Mercado, D. M., Malarkey, W. B., & Glaser, R. (1995). Slowing of wound healing by psychological stress. *The Lancet, 346*(8984), 1194-1196.

Langer, E. (1989). The mindset of health. *Psychology Today, 23*(4):48.

Leserman, J., Petitto, J. M., Gu, H., Gaynes, B. N., Barroso, J., Golden, R. N., Perkins, O., Folds, J. D., & Evans, D. L. (2002). Progression to AIDS, a clinical AIDS condition and mortality: Psychosocial and physiological predictors. *Psychological Medicine, 32*(6), 1059-1073.

Lillberg, K., Verkasolo, P. K., Kaprio, J., Teppo, L., Helenius, H., & Koskenvuo, M. (2007). Stressful life events and risks of breast cancer in 10,808 women: A cohort study. *American Journal of Epidemiology, 157*(5), 415-423.

Marucha, P. T., Kiecolt-Glaser, J. K., & Favagehi, M. (1998). Mucosal wound healing is impaired by examination of stress. *Psychosomatic Medicine, 60*(3), 362-365.

Mavros, M. N., Athanasiou, S., Gkegkes, I. D., Polyzos, K. A., Peppas, G., & Falagas, M. E. (2011). Do psychological variables affect early surgical recovery? *PLoS ONE, 6*(5), e20306.

McCain, N. L., Gray, P., Elswick, R. K., Robins, J. W., Tuck, I., Walter, J. M., Rausch, S. M., & Ketchum, J. (2008). A randomized clinical trial of alternative stress management interventions in persons with HIV infection. *Journal of Consulting and Clinical Psychology, 76*(3), 431-441.

Rosengred, A., Orth-Gomer, K., Wedel, H., & Wilhelmsen, L. (1993). Stressful life events, social support, and mortality in men born in 1933. *British Medical Journal, 307*(6912), 1102-1105.

Ruiz, R. J. & Avant, K. C. (2005). Effects of maternal prenatal stress on infant outcomes: A synthesis of the literature. *Advances in Nursing Science, 28*(4), 345-355.

Shekelle, R. B., Raynor, W. J., Ostfeld, A. M., Garran, D. C., Bieliauskas, L. A., Liu, S. C., Maliza, C., & Paul, O. (1981). Psychological depression and 17-year risk of death from cancer. *Psychosomatic Medicine, 43*(2), 117-125.

Soloman, G. F., Temoshok, L., O'Leary, A., & Zich, J. (1987). An intensive psychoimmunological study of long term surviving persons with AIDS. *Annals of the New York Academy of Sciences, 496*(1), 647-655.

Spiegel, D., Bloom, J. R., Kraemer, H. C., & Gottheil, E., (1989). Effects of psychosocial treatment on survival of patients with metastatic breast cancer. *The Lancet, 334*(8668), 888-891.

Stanton, A. L., Danoff-Burg, S., Sworowski, L. A., Collins, C. A., Branstetter, A. D., Rodrigues-Hanley, A. Kirk, S. B., & Austenfeld, J. L. (2002). Randomized, controlled trial of written emotional expression and benefit finding in breast cancer patients. *Journal of Clinical Oncology, 20*(20), 4160-4168.

Sternberg, E. (2000). *The balance within: The science connecting health and emotions.* New York, NY: W. H. Freeman and Company.

Stone, A. A., Neale, J. M., Cox, D. S., Napoli, A., Valdimarsdottir, H., & Kennedy-Moore, E. (1994). Daily events are associated with a secretory immune response to an oral antigen in men. *Health Psychology, 13*(5), 440-446.

Tausk, F., Elenkov, I., & Moynihan, J. (2008). Psychoneuroimmunology. *Dermatologic Therapy, 21*(1), 22-31.

Uchino, B. N., Cacioppo, J. T., & Kiecolt-Glaser, J. K. (1996). Relationship between social support and physiological processes: A review with emphasis on underlying mechanisms and implications for health. *Psychological Bulletin, 119*(3), 488-531.

Valdimarsdottir, H. B. & Bovbjerg, D. H. (1997). Positive and negative mood: Association with natural killer cell activity. *Psychology and Health, 12*(3), 319-327.

Weschsler, R. (1987). A new prescription: Mind over malady. *Discover (February),* 51-61.

Ziemssen, T. & Kern, S. (2007). Psychoneuroimmunology: Cross-talk between the immune and nervous systems. *Journal of* *Neurology, 254*(Suppl 2), 11/8-11/11.

9. Stress

Heather R. Porter

Stress is a natural and healthy feeling, although it can turn into a big problem if it becomes excessive, unrelenting, or unmanaged. Unfortunately, people often don't give stress the attention it deserves. Stressful events and situations are typically viewed as things that one has little control over. There is a feeling of "That's just the way life goes." along with an acceptance of an external locus of control. When someone talks about managing stress, the common reaction is, "yeah, right" along with a laugh.

The word "stress" is a part of our everyday vocabulary. It doesn't have a shock value like the word "cancer." People joke about it, put funny pictures on mugs about it, and depict daily stressors in the Sunday comics. Those things are funny because many of us can relate to them, but they may cause us to forget the potentially devastating effects that unmanaged stress can have on our lives.

There are many sources of stress: environment, occupation, health, relationships, finances, etc. Changes of any kind can be sources of stress. Obviously there is a great deal of overlap in the areas of stress described. Sources of stress are not universal either. What is stressful for one person may not be stressful for another. How the event is perceived has a lot to do with whether it is classified as stressful. In dealing with stress, it is important to see the problem from the client's perspective.

Types of Stress

Acute Stress

An acute stressor is one that lasts minutes to hours (Dhabhar & McEwen, 1997). When a person experiences a short-term stressor, the body reacts by activating the sympathetic nervous system in a "fight-or-flight" response. This process prepares to the body to fight the stressor physical, verbally, and/or emo-

tionally or run from it by physically running away, withdrawing, or some other method of escape. Epinephrine and norepinephrine, also referred to as catecholamines, are released by the adrenal glands in response to the physical or emotional stress. Catecholamines increase heart rate to increase movement of blood and increase power, increase blood sugar to increase muscle energy, shift blood volume from the digestive organs to skeletal muscles to increase power, speed up the blood clotting process in event of a wound, widen pupils for greater awareness and visual acuity, increase breathing rate to increase oxygen supply to vital organs, and cue the brain to release endorphins to decrease sensitivity to pain (Finan, Zautra, & Wershba, 2010; Elliot, 1994).

The specific stressor doesn't matter. The body responds this way whether the actual stressor is something minimal like forgetting an appointment or something major like being in a car accident. In all animals this response is required at times for survival. For individuals who have health impairments and illnesses, aspects of the fight-or-flight response can be concerning, such as raised blood sugar in someone who has diabetes or increased blood pressure for someone who has a cardiac condition. However, once the stressor is removed, the body systems return to normal functioning. Problems occur when small issues cause major stress leaving the person feeling stressed all the time. It's one thing to deal with a tiger attacking once a month. Bodies can handle that. If the same level of stress occurs when the person is stuck in traffic for hours every day, the person goes into a chronic stress condition, which can cause many significant problems, as discussed in the next section.

Chronic Stress

Chronic stress occurs when a person experiences stress (whether real or perceived) over a long period of time, for several hours per day for weeks or months (Dhabhar & McEwen, 1997). When this happens, the body prepares to deal with the stressor for the long term and activates the hypothalamic-pituitary-adrenal (HPA) axis, which stimulates the production of cortisol (Finan et al., 2010). To maximize the amount of physical energy needed to deal with the stressor, the body suppresses other essential bodily functions in addition to continuing the initial bodily reactions to stress. Some of the resultant outcomes of chronic stress include:

- Suppression, weakening, and dysregulation of the immune system (Davis, Eshelman, & McKay, 2000; Cooper, 2013; Contrada & Baum, 2010; Dhabhar, 2010), reproductive system (Davis, Eshelman, & McKay, 2000), digestive system (Davis, Eshelman, & McKay, 2000), tissue repair and growth (Davis, Eshelman, & McKay, 2000), and inflammatory system (Davis, Eshelman, & McKay, 2000).
- Increased susceptibility to infections and cancer (Dhabhar, 2010).
- Exacerbation of asthma and allergic, autoimmune, and inflammatory diseases (Dhabhar, 2010).
- Increased frequency of colds (Cooper, 2013; Contrada & Baum, 2010).
- Increased vulnerability of previously injured areas (Cooper, 2013; Contrada & Baum, 2010) and worsening of currently health conditions or onset of new problems (Cooper, 2013; Contrada & Baum, 2010).
- Changes in cognition, including lapses in memory, racing thoughts, poor concentration and judgment (Cooper, 2013; Contrada & Baum, 2010), and hyperalertness (Eliot, 1994; Finan et al., 2010; Mayo Clinic Staff, 2013).
- Changes in the physical domain, including apathy, changes in weight, muscle tension, chronic fatigue, and shuttering (Cooper, 2013; Contrada & Baum, 2010).
- Increased cholesterol levels (Eliot, 1994; Finan et al., 2010; Mayo Clinic Staff, 2013).
- Slowed heart beat (Eliot, 1994; Finan et al., 2010; Mayo Clinic Staff, 2013).
- Raised blood pressure, which resets to a new normal at the higher pressure (Cooper, 2013; Contrada & Baum, 2010; Eliot, 1994; Finan et al., 2010; Mayo Clinic Staff, 2013).

- Reduced metabolism, resulting in increased storage of fats (Eliot, 1994; Finan et al., 2010; Mayo Clinic Staff, 2013).
- Formation of blood clots from the increased supply of platelets (Eliot, 1994; Finan et al., 2010; Mayo Clinic Staff, 2013).
- Headaches (Cooper, 2013; Contrada & Baum, 2010).
- Induction of negative psychological, emotional, and social responses, such as feelings of emptiness, hopelessness, loss of direction, hostility towards others, and feelings of anxiety, anger, depression, (Cooper, 2013; Contrada & Baum, 2010; Eliot, 1994, Finan et al., 2010, Mayo Clinic Staff, 2013), as well as irritability (Eliot, 1994; Finan et al., 2010; Mayo Clinic Staff, 2013).

Emotional responses also negatively impact health. For example, negative mood is associated with reduced natural killer cell (NKC) activity, inhibition of the immune system, lowered percent of T-lymphocytes, cardiovascular problems, such as coronary heart disease, increased incidence of all-cause mortality, and increased pain and inflammatory processes. Anxiety is associated with mortality, especially in people after coronary artery bypass surgery. Anger has been associated with heightened pain reactivity. All of these indirectly contribute to the development of chronic pain symptoms through their effect on adipose tissue distribution and muscle tension (Finan et al., 2010).

There is also a unique body of research that is exploring the body's reaction to different types of emotional stress. For example, stressors that have a social aspect that induces a feeling of shame appear to be associated with greater salivary cortisol response (Gruenewald et al., 2004, as cited in Finan et al., 2010) and greater tumor necrosis activity (Peters et al., 1999, as cited in Finan et al., 2010).

In contract, positive emotions appear to undo the stimulating effects of negative emotions and aid in returning the body to homeostasis. For example, inducing a sense of calm and serenity through yoga mantra and rosary prayer induced healthier cardiovascular rhythms (Bernardi et al., 2001) and individuals experiencing a feeling of joy after the experience of a stressful event showed quicker cardiovascular recovery (Fredrickson et al., 2000). It is thought that positive emotions, might therefore serve as a buffer to the effects of negative mood (Finan et al., 2010).

In the field of psychoneuroimmunology that studies the interrelationships between the nervous system and the immune system, research has shown that feelings of social rejection and social isolation (a source of stress) trigger the activity of pro-inflammatory immune cells (Slavich et al., 2010). Cognitive behavioral therapy, meditation, T'ai Chi, and yoga help to decrease disease activity in patients with inflammatory disorders such as rheumatoid arthritis (Cousins Center, 2011).

Emotional symptoms manifested by stress, such as depression, fearfulness, and anxiety, can also negatively impact adherence to treatment regimens and quality of life (Garrido et al., 2010). It is consequently recommended that healthcare practitioners take an active role in identifying and addressing the underling cause of the distress rather than just treating the resultant outcomes, such as depression. A review of the literature by Garrido et al. (2010) found that the following four pathways appear to link the experience of chronic disease to distress: (1) the experience of pain that severely compromises functional abilities, (2) receiving a specific chronic disease diagnosis and receiving related treatment (distress is less in those who are undiagnosed and do not receive related treatment), (3) the client's perspective related to treatments and lifestyle behaviors, and (4) disruption of social roles and relationships that lower feelings of self-efficacy and self-worth. The authors recommend that clinicians explore these four areas with clients to identify and subsequently address related perceptions, cognitions, and behavioral responses.

It is important to note that chronic stress can become a vicious cycle that continues to affect a person's physical, mental, social, and emotional functioning. As previously reviewed, it impacts life tasks and gives rise to further stressors. Stressors exacerbate problems and then problems heighten stressors. Ultimately a person can become emotionally and/or physically disabled from untreated chronic stress.

Eustress

Not all stress is bad. Eustress, also referred to as good stress, is when a demand is placed on a person in which the person experiences a high degree of control, the person desires to meet the demand, and the ability to meet the demand is viewed as being important (Cooper, 2013). It is thought that eustress gives a person a break from ongoing negative stressors and provides an opportunity for creative problem solving that re-energizes the person to continue to cope with other stressors (Cooper, 2013; Lazarus et al., 1980). It might also indirectly facilitate health through fostering feelings of mastery, control, self-efficacy, and optimism, which can act as a buffer for future stressful events (Cooper, 2013).

Sources of Stress

Some areas of life can be especially stressful. The cause of the stress can affect the type of treatment the therapist uses. Here are some considerations for particular areas of stress.

Emotional and psychological: Feelings about self, the sources for meeting emotional needs, and awareness about emotional needs can all be sources of stress. For example, low self-esteem, pessimism, and external locus of control promote poor coping strategies. Looking towards others to provide direction for living restricts a person from looking inward, identifying his/her own values, and living a "true" life that aims to reach personal aspirations instead of the aspirations of others. For the client facing a new disability or a health crisis, many emotional and psychological issues surface, contributing to stress. For example, a client may not see self-esteem as a source of stress, but a therapist knows that self-esteem is an integral component of being able to respond to life's stressors in a healthy manner. The same is true for a client who has not "found himself." Meaning, that he isn't really clear on what he values in life, what he wants out of life, and where he fits in life. A client who is not self-assured and grounded will be influenced by others and searching for validation to define himself/herself. Trying on many roles to find the one that fits is a common developmental stage for adolescents and sometimes a person who was once self-assured becomes insecure when his/her life changes drastically.

Environment: The environment has a huge impact on stress. Stressors include noise, crowding, lighting, signs, odors, colors, and litter. Clients who identify their work, neighborhood, school, or home environments as stressful work with therapists to find ways to alter these environments. In some cases, clients opt to move from an urban to a rural environment in an attempt to escape these stressors. Clients must be careful to fully evaluate this move since a rural area may have inherent stressors that the client is unaware of such as lack of transportation, loss of current social relationships, or loss of close conveniences like a nearby bank and grocery store. In the hospital setting, a clean and sterile environment often lacks the comfort and relaxing atmosphere of a home. Noises, including nurses and carts going up and down the hall, people crying or screaming, or a roommate that has the television on all night long, can cause significant stress. Odors, changes in schedules, unfamiliar food, and many other things are also stressors. Clients who find the hospital environment stressful should be encouraged to ask loved ones to bring in familiar items from home as appropriate.

Finances: Money is one of the top stressors. Not making enough money and not having enough money are constant stressors in most lower and middle class families. It is also a stressor for many people who are experiencing a dramatic change in their income due to disability. Money issues can cause arguments, and an inability to pay the bills can cause tremendous stress. Therapists often avoid this topic believing that it is the personal business of the client, and some clients refuse to discuss it. Therapists, however, should not avoid this topic. Instead they should approach the subject with the client in a caring and helpful manner. It is not possible for a therapist to know and understand the full context of a client's finances, nor is it appropriate to do so. However, asking the client if s/he is on a tight budget and expressing an understanding of the difficult situation encourages a client to share information. Getting a sense of the client's finances helps to identify a need for assistance and lets the therapist point the client in the right direction to find help. Many people do not like to talk about money and therefore do not receive the support that they are entitled to. Having a sense of the client's finances also helps the therapist identify activities that are within the client's budget. The identification of financial assistance and exploration of tasks that are within the client's budget can be helpful in reducing stress related to finances. Some clients also benefit from existential counseling about the meaning of life because sometimes people get so caught up in keeping up with the Joneses that they don't really look at what they truly value and want in their life. Addressing money issues is not forbidden.

Recreational therapists address money management issues when it is necessary for the client's independence or successful task engagement. For example, a client with multiple sclerosis may have trouble with her memory and vision and need help designing a new system to manage her checkbook or a client who is blind needs help to design a system of identifying money in his wallet.

Health: Good health does not precipitate stress unless the client is preoccupied with his/her health and fears health problems (e.g., cancerous tumor has been removed and client is now in remission, however client's fear of cancer growing back is a significant source of stress). People who have health problems, however, do not always perceive their health as a source of stress. If a problem is well managed and does not significantly impact functioning, quality of life, and independence, it may not be a source of stress. The same holds true for clients who have adapted well to limitations imposed by health conditions and have a strong internal locus of control. Even so, therapists who work with clients in a health-care setting will often find that the clients report their current health condition as a source of high stress. Therapists help clients to adjust to disability and address the client's primary concerns to foster functioning, independence, and quality of life.

Life crises: Major life changes, whether good or bad, are sources of stress. This could include death of a loved one, change of job, disability, moving to a new home, or having a child. Therapists ask the client to tell him/her about any changes that have occurred during the last year. The more changes, the more stress. Therapists cannot control change, but they can help clients adapt and cope with change. The interventions will vary depending on the changes. Examples of interventions include a referral for grief counseling for loss of spouse, developing a circle of friends because of a move, general relaxation training to combat anxiousness about anticipated changes.

Relationships: Dynamics occurring in relationships can be sources of stress. Issues that may cause stress include, but are not limited to, inadequate quality time with a spouse, caring for an elderly parent, and lack of positive feelings such as appreciation and respect. If a client is having relationship trouble that requires outside intervention, such as when abuse is happening, appropriate referrals are made. Recreational therapists commonly address issues related to quality of time and positive and healthy communication by identifying activities and interactions that improve quality of time, as well as teach positive and healthy communication skills to promote growth and connectedness in relationships. Looking at another part of the issue, those who lack friendship, close relationships, and connectedness have higher mortality rates. Recreational therapists help clients to develop or enhance healthy relationships by identifying and integrating clients into social opportunities and addressing issues within the scope of recreational therapy practice that impact the ability to participate in social environments (e.g., communication skills, self-esteem, self-confidence, anxiety). In the hospital setting, therapists are aware of relationship changes regarding access to primary relationships for support and the need for continuing relationships in the hospital. This is especially important for prolonged hospitalization, such as waiting for a heart transplant. Therapists encourage family and friends to continue to provide support and provide them with methods to do so, as appropriate, including videos, e-mails, phone calls, cards, banners, and quality time alone with a spouse. Therapists also identify alternative supports and facilitate them, such as introducing one client to another client who is also waiting for a heart transplant or providing a social environment for clients to meet, talk, and engage in activity.

Time: Feeling crunched for time can occur because the client has more responsibilities than she can accomplish in a set amount of time or because s/he lacks the ability to cope with time demands. Both contribute to stress. A client may feel stressed because of lack of time, and the resultant feeling of being unable to control his/her life can exacerbate certain behaviors and feelings that impact the ability to deal with stress. It's harder to cope when a person is short fused, irritable, frustrated, or anxious. These feelings can also be exacerbated in a hospital setting when therapies and care needs are scheduled without a break. Therapists evaluate responsibilities, demands, and desires of the client and compare them with the time available to decide if the client needs more skills related to time management. In the hospital setting, therapists try to alter the client's therapy and nursing care schedules so that the client and staff do not feel stressed about time.

Work: Work can be a source of stress for many different reasons. Some include the relationship with a boss, the type of work, work conditions, or the commute. If work is a significant source of stress and the stress cannot be remedied, the client may want to explore a new worksite or a change in career. People who have disabilities may need to make worksite or career changes depending on their abilities and limitations. People who anticipate problems returning to work because of a disability or who are unable to return to their career because they are now unable to perform the required skills are referred to the Office of Vocational Rehabilitation (OVR). OVR is a state program that assesses a client's ability to return to work and facilitates the client's ability to become part of the workforce. OVR will assist clients financially to return to school or obtain needed equipment related to return to work, such as hand controls for a car or ramp to enter and exit a place of business. A social worker or case manager refers clients to OVR. Clients are put on a waiting list and are usually called in a few months. The goal is to find the client a career that matches his/her interests and abilities. Therapists also educate clients about their rights under the Americans with Disabilities Act as it pertains to employment. In some facilities recreational therapists perform worksite evaluations and assist the client and employer in identifying needed changes. Recreational therapy is beginning to do more in this area (worksite evaluations, work skills, employer ADA training, worksite integration) because of the rising older adult population who are choosing to work for pleasure rather than as a necessary life task to pay the bills.

Contributors to Stress

When assessing sources of stress, and subsequently considering a specific stress management or coping intervention, therapists should consider the following contributors to stress:

Alcohol: Alcohol is a CNS depressant. Short-term behavioral effects can include disinhibition, relaxation, or anger and violence. Alcohol affects physical coordination, memory, concentration, and insight. Alcohol use can cause stress for an individual who feels pressured to drink or is trying to quit and is experiencing related frustration. Reactions of others in the home or at work to the amount of alcohol the client is drinking can also be a source of stress. Therapists address this issue by teaching the client assertiveness skills, relaxation training, and stress management skills, as well as addressing issues related to susceptibility to peer pressure, such as low self-esteem. Alcohol use can also impact the client's ability to deal with stress effectively. Alcohol-induced violent behavior, for example, impacts the response to the immediate stressor and negatively perceived alcohol-induced actions can continue to cause problems after the alcohol is no longer in the system. Although alcohol is a legal drug, therapists discourage its use when resultant cognitive and behavioral changes contribute to emotional and physical stress. Clients who wish to cease social alcohol consumption and find it difficult to do so explore the payoffs of social drinking, such as relaxation, stress reduction, social atmosphere, and fitting in with peers. They address each issue with a therapist to find alterative ways to meet these needs. Treatment for abuse of alcohol or alcoholism is not the same as reducing social drinking. The therapist needs to apply different techniques, and abstinence is generally considered to be a requirement for the client.

Body weight: Clients who are overweight are putting a significant amount of stress on their body's cardiovascular, muscular, pulmonary, and skeletal systems, putting themselves at increased risk for disease, dysfunction, and health-related problems related to inactivity. A client who has a current health condition should be particularly concerned about his/her body weight because it often plays a large role in the development of secondary problems that affect functioning, independence, and quality of life. For example, excess body weight contributes to the pain level of a client with chronic back problems because it adds pressure on the back when the stomach accentuates the lumbar curve by pulling it forward. Pain causes the client to sit or lie down to reduce the pain. Prolonged periods of inactivity contribute to further problems, causing the client to lose function. Loss of function may require the client to seek assistance from others, thus impacting his/her level of independence. Needing assistance from others combined with decreased functioning can significantly impact the client's ability to perform desired life tasks that contribute to quality of life. Excess body weight can also be a source of emotional stress if the client is trying to lose weight and is experiencing frustration with the task or is the target of jokes

and ridicule. Therapists help clients to meet their ideal body weight determined by the Body Mass Index and/or the recommendation of the physician. Therapists help clients reduce body weight by encouraging regular physical activity and a proper diet. Therapists must receive approval from the physician to begin an exercise program, as well as an order that describes additional information about precautions and parameters relevant to participation. Therapists identify activities that are enjoyed by the client that have the potential to be a form of physical exercise. For example, if a client enjoys talking and socializing, involvement in an exercise program like a walking club that promotes talking and socializing might be well received. A form of exercise that does not promote such interactions like walking on a treadmill without an exercise partner may not be acceptable. Of course, the therapist must fully evaluate how realistic the exercise choice is, the resources available to the client, the client's current health status as it relates to performance of the task, and the client's willingness and motivation to participate in the activity. The report, Healthy People 2010, recommends that people participate in moderate physical activity three to five times a week for a period of 20-30 minutes. This recommendation is for people who do not have a current health condition. People who have health conditions must seek medical clearance from their physician and guidelines for exercise participation to avoid further injury or harm. Therapists must also be aware of other problems, such as depression or metabolism problems, that can cause an increase in body weight requiring assistance from other health professionals.

Caffeine: Caffeine is a central nervous system stimulant found in coffee, tea, chocolate, and some sodas. After it is ingested, effects are experienced in about 30 minutes and maximum levels are reached within two hours (Julien, 2004). Caffeine increases mental alertness so quality and amount of sleep can be affected. Heavy consumption of caffeine (12 plus cups per day) causes agitation, anxiety, tremors, rapid breathing, and insomnia (Julien, 2004). Behavioral responses of agitation and anxiety can affect a client's ability to implement healthy coping mechanisms. Lack of sleep affects concentration, attention, mental alertness, and stress tolerance compounding the problem when caffeine is no longer in the system. Clients may not view caffeine intake as a stressor, but it can significantly impact the client's ability to cope and deal with stress. Caffeine is not a nutritional requirement so it should be eliminated from diets unless it is prescribed by a physician. (It may be prescribed for migraine headaches.) Withdrawal symptoms from caffeine can include headache, irritability, fatigue, dysphoric mood changes, muscle pain and stiffness, flu-like feelings, nausea, and craving for caffeine products. Clients should be encouraged to reduce caffeine intake in increments until it is fully eliminated from the diet to help minimize withdrawal symptoms. Therapists also assist clients to identify alternative contributors to mental alertness, such as physical exercise, quality and amount of sleep, proper diet, stress reduction, and relaxation training.

Diet: Inadequate nutrition can lead to health and behavioral problems that can contribute to or affect the ability to manage stress. Lack of a proper diet can affect mental and physical energy levels possibly making the level of effort that is needed to cope with stress difficult. Therapists need to understand the basic food pyramid and make recommendations consistent with the American Dietetic Association's balanced diet. Therapists should know the nutritional recommendations from the client's physician and/or dietician and the acceptable consistency of foods from the speech therapist. If a therapist believes that a client is not eating a well-balanced and healthy diet, a consult should be made to a nutritionist for a full evaluation. Recommendations from the nutritionist are incorporated into the client's lifestyle with the help of the recreational therapist. Clients who present with an eating disorder require more intense treatment from an eating disorder specialist.

Lack of exercise: Lack of exercise can contribute to secondary problems that cause stress, especially if there is a pre-existing health condition. Exercise is also a very effective intervention for managing stress because it induces a relaxation response, clears thinking, and expends energy.

Nicotine: Nicotine increases blood pressure, increases heart rate, and stimulates the release of adrenaline that produces a fight-or-flight response as discussed above. Smoking, or the use of any tobacco product that contains nicotine, may also be a source of stress if the person is trying to quit and is frustrated with this task. Therapists do not condone smoking and encourage clients to quit since it

adversely affects health. If the physician recommends that the client stop smoking, it is helpful for both the therapist and the physician to have a meeting with the client. The physician explains to the client why s/he should quit smoking, prescribes something to assist the client with smoking cessation, if needed and appropriate, and explains to the client that nicotine withdrawal typically takes two to four weeks, although full withdrawal can take six months or longer (Julien, 2004). The client will also have to combat the psychological dependence and social components of smoking. The physician makes clear to the client that these two issues are just as important as nicotine withdrawal to successfully quit smoking and that s/he has ordered a recreational therapy consult to address these issues and integrate them into a post-discharge plan. Once the meeting is over, the recreational therapist schedules a separate session to evaluate when, where, and why the client smokes and identifies strategies for combating the desire. This could include making small changes in routine to decrease associations, increasing activity levels, learning healthy coping strategies for stress triggers, identifying non-prescription external aids that can help the client quit smoking (e.g., chewing gum), and providing education on the benefits of activity with particular attention to the power of relaxation and distraction for smoking cessation. Therapists also discuss the social consequences of not smoking that are concerns of the client. All of identified interventions are then reflected in the client's activity pattern. (See Activity Pattern Development in the Techniques section.)

Sleep: Lack of sleep or impaired quality of sleep can lead to problems paying attention, concentrating, and tolerating stressful situations. Therapists help clients improve sleep by identifying and addressing causes of sleep problems, which may include frequent urination in the middle of the night, stress, caffeine, or depression. Further evaluation and sleep studies may also need to be conducted if conditions such as sleep apnea or PTSD are suspected.

Telephone and other electronic communication devices: Constantly being wired into interactions with others can be intrusive and demand attention. In the hospital setting, a ringing telephone can prompt a client to move too quickly to retrieve the call; it can be upsetting when the client receives yet another message asking for an explanation about the current situation; and it can be bothersome when trying to rest. Clients can request to have the hospital telephone removed from their room and might consider doing the same with their cell phone. They certainly should turn off the ringer when they need to rest. Clients can also tell family and friends to only call between certain hours or designate a person or two to pass along information to others instead of each person calling the client. Once at home, the client can continue this by turning off the ringer and answering messages at his/her convenience. A cordless or cell phone in a pant's pocket or apron pocket to use in case of an emergency and to answer phone calls without having to rush to the phone can help, but the constant demands a cell phone can make need to be handled to reduce stress.

Work ethic: With the high work ethic in the North American culture, the choice to play, relax, have fun, and laugh is often given second place to other responsibilities at the sacrifice of emotional, physical, social, and cognitive health. Recreational therapists heighten the client's awareness of the relationship between leisure and health and help to bring balance to the client's life. Engagement in tasks that offer relaxation and leisure experiences is imperative for good health. Recreational therapists need to have a full understanding of the benefits of leisure and help clients who are not leading a healthy leisure lifestyle to develop one. Engagement in activities that are enjoyable and relaxing opens the mind to new ideas and thoughts that help us cope with stress.

Defense Mechanisms

The American Psychological Association (APA, 1994) supplies an even more detailed description of some of the common coping styles that people use. The APA refers to them as defense mechanisms, which means that they are probably not looking at positive stress in their evaluation. Defense mechanisms are automatic psychological processes of which the person may or may not be aware that protect the client from stress, anxiety, and psychological harm. Many defense mechanisms can be both healthy and unhealthy depending on (1) the severity of the adaptation (e.g., a client uses the defense mechanism of humor to cope with stressors too often and it is now affecting his relationship with his spouse, "He never takes anything seriously."), (2) the psychological state of the client (e.g., the defense

mechanism of anticipation is relatively a good coping strategy — looking ahead and planning a response — however, a client who has generalized anxiety disorder may heighten her anxiety with anticipation), and (3) the specific stressor involved (e.g., it may not be appropriate to assert one's feelings of frustration to a parent who has Alzheimer's disease).

Although many defense mechanisms can be both healthy and unhealthy, some defense mechanisms are clearly healthy. These include asserting feelings in a non-confrontational style, provided that the other person is mentally and emotionally stable. Others are clearly unhealthy, such as denial of stress. Therapists are aware of defense mechanisms and are careful not to quickly attribute behavioral changes to biological changes that might be caused by the client's disease. Attention to a client's defense mechanisms is helpful in measuring positive or negative changes in a client's coping abilities. When maladaptive defense mechanisms are suspected, the therapist attempts to identify the particular stressor, alleviate the stressor, and teach the client healthier coping styles through counseling and experiential interventions.

Defense mechanisms, as outlined in the *Defensive Functioning Scale*, include seven levels that are defined below (American Psychiatric Association [APA], 1994; Dziegielewski, 2013; Aldwin, 2012; Sadock & Sadock, 2003, 2008).

High Adaptive Level

Optimal adaptation due to conscious awareness of feelings.

Anticipation: The client thoughtfully considers the possible stressors that may occur, the possible emotional feelings that could result, and the strategies that s/he could employ to minimize the stressor and its related emotional outcomes. For example, the mother of three young children anticipates the death of her husband due to terminal cancer and makes plans to ensure financial security and emotional support for the family.

Affiliation: The client seeks assistance such as advice and support from others. The client does not necessarily seek to have others take responsibility for the problems.

Altruism: The client copes with stressors by seeking to negate the negative feelings through pleasing and helping others. This gives the client a sense of fulfillment and pleasure.

Humor: The client copes by accentuating the comical and ironic features of the stressor.

Self-assertion: The client asserts his/her thoughts and feelings appropriately.

Self-observation: The client reflects on his/her own actions, motivation, feelings, and thoughts about a specific conflict or stressor and carefully plans an appropriate course of action.

Sublimation: The client directs negative energy caused by conflict and stress into socially appropriate behaviors or actions.

Suppression: When stress and conflict become overwhelming, the client purposely chooses to ignore and avoid feelings or thoughts about the stressor or conflict.

Mental Inhibitions (Compromise Formation) Level

Used to keep potentially threatening thoughts out of awareness.

Displacement: This is when a client transfers stressful feelings and thoughts to a less threatening source.

Dissociation: The client detaches himself/herself from reality to escape the stressor. This is a common coping mechanism for abuse. The client blocks out the situation and "goes somewhere else." The client may not be able to recall the situation and may have a distorted perception of self, the environment, and sensory and motor behavior.

Intellectualization: The client excessively intellectualizes the stressor or conflict to control the severity of the emotional impact. Thoughts are used to take the place of feelings.

Isolation of affect: The client emotionally separates from the event. The client is able to recall and describe the event in detail but it is void of emotional connection. For example, a client was terrified and anxious during a rape yet now describes the event in detail and feels no emotion about it.

Reaction formation: The client adopts behaviors, thoughts, or feelings that are the utter and complete opposite of his/her unacceptable thoughts or feelings. For example, a client may bend over backwards to please a boss that, objectively, should be reported to the police.

Repression: The client blocks stressful events from his/her conscious awareness. The client is unable to recall the event, yet is often conscious of the feelings and emotions resultant from the event.

For example, the client feels angry but does not consciously remember the childhood trauma that is the root of the anger.

Undoing: The client deals with conflict or external stress with actions intended to negate in part a previous action or communication. An example is a spouse who brings home flowers after having a lunchtime affair. It may be related to the magical thinking of childhood.

Minor Image-Distorting Level

Distortions in the image of the self, body, or others to regulate one's self-esteem.

Devaluation: The client overstates the negative qualities of himself/herself or others to manage stressful events.

Idealization: The client overstates the positive qualities of others to manage stressful events.

Omnipotence: The client feels and acts as if s/he is better than everyone else and has special qualities that others do not possess.

Disavowal Level

Keeping stressors out of awareness with or without a misattribution to external causes

Denial: The client does not acknowledge the emotional impact of a stressor even though it is apparent to others.

Projection: The client falsely attributes negative feelings and behavior caused by stress and conflict to another person or event rather than taking ownership for his/her feelings.

Rationalization: The client devises reasons why actions, thoughts, and feelings are justified in order to conceal his/her real motivations.

Major Image-Distorting Level

Gross distortion or misattribution of self or others.

Autistic fantasy: When stressors and conflicts arise, the client daydreams to avoid interaction with others, effective action, or problem solving.

Projective identification: This is similar to "projection" except that the client reacts to the projected feelings, often leading the other person to actually experiencing the feelings that were projected. It can be confusing as to who is doing what to whom. For example, a client who says to someone, "You really don't like me." can lead to the person really not liking the client, if the client is insistent enough.

Splitting of self-image or image of others: The client deals with stressors or conflicts by splitting and alternating his/her self-image or the image of others into polar opposites of positive and negative qualities. Because the person is unable to simultaneously be aware of both the positive and negative qualities of himself/herself or others, unrealistic views are held.

Action Level

Dealing with stressors through action or withdrawal.

Acting out: The client responds to stressors or conflicts through actions instead of emotional reflection. Defensive acting out behavior is not necessarily bad, but it usually means that the client is not finding a way to deal with his stress by understanding it.

Apathetic withdrawal: A pattern of behavior indicating indifference in which the person removes himself/herself and demonstrates an under-response or a lack of reactivity to a situation that should cause a response.

Help-rejecting complaining: The client deals with stressors or conflicts by complaining and continuing to ask for help. It disguises covert feelings of anger and blame. When assistance is given, the client rejects it. Complaints and requests for help can be related to a physical, emotional, or life task.

Passive aggression: The client acts as is s/he is complying with what is requested, but the compliance masks covert resistance, resentment, or hostility. The resistance expresses itself in an indirect, non-violent manner such as obstructionism, procrastination, inefficiency, stubbornness, and forgetfulness. It may be adaptive for individuals in subordinate positions who have no other way to express their feelings more overtly.

Level of Defensive Dysregulation

Failure of defense regulation to contain reaction to stress, resulting in a break with reality.

Delusional projection: The client alters reality in response to the projection, which removes feelings of guilt and anxiety (often persecutory in nature).

Psychotic denial: The client refuses to perceive or consciously acknowledge unpleasant aspects of reality because it is too threatening, which decreases emotional conflict and anxiety.

Psychotic distortion: The client grossly reshapes external reality to meet internal needs.

Stress and the ICF

The ICF has several codes that can be used to document stress and its effects on the client. The primary code is d240 Handling Stress and Other Psychological Demands. Other codes can be used to describe aspects of the client's personality that lead to stress. These include b126 Temperament and Personality Functions, b130 Energy and Drive Functions, and b180 Experience of Self and Time Functions. Other codes that indicated causes of stress include b280 Sensation of Pain, d210 Undertaking a Single Task, d220 Undertaking Multiple Tasks, d230 Carrying Out Daily Routine, d4 Mobility, d7 Interpersonal Interactions and Relationships, d8 Major Life Areas, and d9 Community, Social, and Civic Life.

Different codes can be used to describe the effects stress is having on the client. These codes include b134 Sleep Functions, b140 - b189 Specific Mental Functions, b4 Functions of the Cardiovascular, Hematological, Immunological, and Respiratory Systems, b5 Functions of the Digestive, Metabolic, and Endocrine Systems, b6 Genitourinary and Reproductive Functions, d160 Focusing Attention, d570 Looking After One's Health, d8 Major Life Areas, and d9 Community, Social, and Civic Life.

References

Aldwin, C. M. (2012). *Stress, coping, and development: An integrative perspective* (2nd ed.). Guilford Press.

American Psychiatric Association. (1994). *Diagnostic and statistical manual of mental disorders, IV edition*. Washington, DC: American Psychiatric Association.

Antoni, M. H., Lehman, J. M., Kilbourn, K. M., Boyers, A. E., Culver, J. L., Alferi, S. M., et al. (2001). Cognitive-behavioral stress management intervention decreases prevalence of depression and enhances benefit finding among women under treatment for early-stage breast cancer. *Health Psychology, 20*, 20-32.

Antoni, M. H., Wimberly, S. R., Lechner, S. C., Kazi, A., Sifre, T., Urcuyo, K. R., et al. (2006). Reduction of cancer specific thought intrusions and anxiety symptoms with a stress management intervention among women undergoing treatment for breast cancer. *American Journal of Psychiatry, 163*, 1791-1797.

Bernardi, L., Sleight, P., Bandinelli, G., Cencetti, S., Fattorini, L., Wdowczyc-Szulc, J., et al. (2001). Effect of rosary prayer and yoga mantras on autonomics cardiovascular rhythms: A comparative study. *British Medical Journal, 323*, 1446-1449.

Carruthers, C. & Hood, C. (2007). Building a life of meaning through therapeutic recreation: The Leisure and Well-Being

Model, Part I. *Therapeutic Recreation Journal, 41*(4), 276-297.

Carver, C. (2010). Coping. In Contrada, R. & Baum, A. *The handbook of stress science: Biology, psychology, and health.* New York, NY: Springer Publishing Company.

Chesney, M. A., Chambers, D. B., Taylor, J. M., Johnson, L. S., & Folkman, S. (2003). Coping effectiveness training for men living with HIV: Results from a randomized clinical trial testing a group-based intervention. *Psychosomatic Medicine, 65*, 1038-1046.

Contrada, R. & Baum, A. (2010). *The handbook of stress science: Biology, psychology, and health.* New York, NY: Springer Publishing Company.

Cooper, C. L. (2013). *From stress to wellbeing: Volume 1: The theory and research on occupational stress and wellbeing.* New York, NY: Palgrave Macmillan.

Cousins Center. (2011). Research highlights 2007-2012. Accessed via website www.semel.ucla.edu/cousins/research.

Cruess, D. G., Antoni, M. H., McGregor, B. A., Kilbourn, K. M., Boyers, A., Alferi, S. M., et al. (2000). Cognitive-behavioral stress management reduces serum cortisol by enhancing benefit finding among women being treated for early stage breast cancer. *Psychosomatic Medicine, 62*, 304-308.

Davis, M., Eshelman, E. R., & McKay, M. (2000). *Relaxation & stress reduction workbook* (5th ed.). Oakland, CA: New Harbinger.

Dhabhar, F. S. (2010). Effects of stress on immune function: Implications for immunoprotection and immunopathology. In Contrada, R. & Baum, A. *The handbook of stress science: Biology, psychology, and health.* New York, NY: Springer Publishing Company.

Dhabhar, F. S. & McEwen, B. S. (1997). Acute stress enhances while chronic stress suppresses immune function in vivo: A potential role for leukocyte trafficking. *Brain, Behavior, & Immunity, 11*, 286-306.

Dziegielewski, S. F. (2013). *DMS-IV-TR in action: Includes DSM-5 update chapter.* John Wiley & Sons.

Edenfield, T. M. & Blumenthal, J. A. (2010). Exercise and stress reduction. In Contrada, R. & Baum, A. *The handbook of stress science: Biology, psychology, and health.* New York, NY: Springer Publishing Company.

Eliot, R. (1994). *From stress to strength.* New York, NY: Bantam Books.

Fawzy, F. I., Fawzy, N. W., & Canada, A. L. (2001). Psychoeducational intervention programs for patients with cancer. In A. Baum & B. L. Anderson (Eds.). *Psychosocial interventions for cancer* (pp. 235-267). Washington, DC: American Psychological Association.

Finan, P. H., Zautra, A. J., & Wershba, R. (2010). The dynamics of emotion in adaptation to stress. In Contrada, R. & Baum, A. *The handbook of stress science: Biology, psychology, and health.* New York, NY: Springer Publishing Company.

Fredrickson, B. L., Mancuso, R. A., Branigan, C., & Tugade, M. M. (2000). The undoing effect of positive emotions. *Motivation and Emotion, 24*, 237-258.

Garrido, M. M., Hash-Converse, J. M., Leventhal, H., & Leventhal, E. A. (2010). Stress and chronic disease management. In Contrada, R. & Baum, A. *The handbook of stress science: Biology, psychology, and health.* New York, NY: Springer Publishing Company.

Glanz, K., Rimer, B., & Lewis, F. (2002). *Health behavior and health education: Theory, research, and practice.* Indianapolis, IN: Jossey-Bass.

Gruenewald, T. L., Kemeny, M. E., Aziz, N., & Fahey, J. L. (2004). Acute threat to the social self: Shame, social self-esteem, and cortisol activity. *Psychosomatic Medicine, 66*, 915-924.

Grunberg, N. E., Berger, S. S., & Hamilton, K. R. (2010). Stress and drug use. In Contrada, R. & Baum, A. *The handbook of stress science: Biology, psychology, and health.* New York, NY: Springer Publishing Company.

Hamilton, N. A., Kitzman, H., & Guyotte, S. (2006). Enhancing health and emotion: Mindfulness as a missing link between cognitive therapy and positive psychology. *Journal of Cognitive Psychotherapy: An Internationally Quarterly, 20*, 123-134.

Hood, C. & Carruthers, C. (2007). Enhancing leisure experience and developing resources: The Leisure and Well-Being Model, Part II. *Therapeutic Recreation Journal, 41*(4), 298-325.

Iwasaki, Y. (2008). Leisure and quality of life in an international and multicultural context: What are major pathways linking leisure to quality of life? *Social Indicators Research, 82*(2), 233-264.

Iwasaki, Y., Coyle, C., Shank, J., Messina, E., & Porter, H. (2013). Leisure-generated meanings and active living for persons with mental illness. *Rehabilitation Counseling Bulletin, 57*, 46-56.

Julien, R. (2004). *A Primer of Drug Action, 10th edition.* New York: Worth Publishers.

Kabat-Zinn, J. (1990). *Full catastrophe living: Using the wisdom of your body and mind to face stress, pain, and illness.* New York: Delacorte.

Lazarus, R. S., Cohen, J. B., Folkman, S., Kanner, A., & Schaefer, C. (1980). Psychological stress and adaptation: Some unresolved issues. In H. Seyle (Ed.). *Seyle's Guide to Stress Research*, pp 90-217. New York: Academic Press.

Mayo Clinic Staff. (2013). Chronic stress puts your health at risk. Accessed via website www.mayoclinic.org/healthy-living/stress-management/in-depth/stress/art-20046037.

McGregor, B. A., Antoni, M. H., Boyers, A., Alferi, S. M., Blomberg, B. B., & Carver, C. S. (2004). Cognitive-behavioral stress management increases benefit finding and immune functioning among women with early stage breast cancer. *Journal of Psychosomatic Research, 56*, 1-8.

Nezu, A. M., Nezu, C. M., & Xanthopoulos, M. S. (2010). Stress reduction in chronically ill patients. In Contrada, R. & Baum, A. *The handbook of stress science: Biology, psychology, and health.* New York, NY: Springer Publishing Company.

Pandey, A., Quick, J. C., Rossi, A. M., Nelson, D. L., & Martin, W. (2010). Stress and the workplace: 10 years of science, 1997-2007. In Contrada, R. & Baum, A. *The handbook of stress science: Biology, psychology, and health.* New York, NY: Springer Publishing Company.

Peters, M. L., Godaert, G. L. R., Baleiux. R. E., Brosschot, J. F., Sweep, F. C., & Swinkels, L. M. (1999). Immune responses to experimental stress: Effects of mental effort and uncontrollability. *Psychosomatic Medicine, 61*, 513-524.

Porter, H. (2009). Developing a Leisure Meanings Gained and Outcomes Scale (LMGOS) and exploring associations of leisure meanings to leisure time physical activity adherence among adults with type 2 diabetes. ProQuest #3359696.

Porter, H. & burlingame, j. (2006). *Recreational therapy handbook of practice.* Enumclaw, WA: Idyll Arbor, Inc.

Porter, H., Iwasaki, Y., & Shank, J. (2011). Conceptualizing meaning-making through leisure experiences. *Society & Leisure, 33*(2), 167-194.

Porter, H., Shank, J., & Iwasaki, Y. (2012). Promoting a collaborative approach with recreational therapy to improve physical activity engagement in type 2 diabetes. *Therapeutic Recreation Journal, Special Issue Part I: Collaborative Practices and Physical Activity, XLVI*(3), 202-217.

Rook, K. S., August, K. J., & Sorkin, D. H. (2010). Social network functions and health. In Contrada, R. & Baum, A. *The handbook of stress science: Biology, psychology, and health.* New York, NY: Springer Publishing Company.

Sadock, J. & Sadock, V. (2003). *Kaplan & Sadock's synopsis of psychiatry* (9th ed.). Philadelphia, PA: Lippincott Williams & Wilkins.

Sadock, J. & Sadock, V. (2008). *Kaplan & Sadock's concise textbook of clinical psychiatry* (3rd ed.). Lippincott Williams & Wilkins.

Slavich, G. M., O'Donovan, A., Epel, E. S., & Kemeny, M. E. (2010). Black sheet gets the blues: A psychobiological model of social rejection and depression. *Neuroscience and Biobehavioral Reviews, 35*(1) 39-45.

Taylor, S. E. & Master, S. L. (2010). Social responses to stress: The tend-and-befriend model. In Contrada, R. & Baum, A. *The handbook of stress science: Biology, psychology, and health*. New York, NY: Springer Publishing Company.

Uchino, B. N. & Birmingham, W. (2010). Stress and support processes. In Contrada, R. & Baum, A. *The handbook of stress science: Biology, psychology, and health*. New York, NY: Springer Publishing Company.

World Health Organization. (1998). *Coping mechanisms*. Geneva, Switzerland: WHO.

10. Theories, Models, and Concepts

Heather R. Porter

What exactly causes change to happen in the treatment process? It's not the number of hours of therapy received or the particular intervention, but rather the ingredients within the intervention (Dijkers, 2014).

For example, consider two clients who have identical health situations. Both clients receive the same number of recreational therapy sessions (four 30-minute sessions a week) and the same intervention (cognitive rehabilitation), but therapist A's client has better outcomes than therapist B's client. Why does this happen?

We can reason that there are multiple variables that affect treatment outcomes, such as the client's level of motivation, level of social support, and so on, but how closely have we looked at what is actually occurring within the interventions. For example, during the cognitive rehabilitation sessions, therapist A might have facilitated the sessions in a quiet environment to foster concentration, used activities that held personal meaning for the client to facilitate more minutes of engagement, and graded the tasks in a manner that induced a sense of self-efficacy. Therapist B may not have had access to a quiet environment, may have chosen standard cognitive rehabilitation tasks that didn't necessarily hold personal meaning for the client, and might not have graded the activities in a manner that achieved optimal levels of self-efficacy.

It is not enough to educate therapy students and practitioners "about" interventions, such as basic cognitive rehabilitation principles. They need to understand the ingredients in interventions that bring about change. In order to do this we must identify what the ingredients are.

In 2008, Mount Sinai Hospital and Moss Rehabilitation Hospital received a grant from the National Institute on Disability Rehabilitation Research (NIDRR) to explore such ingredients (Dijkers, 2014). The end goal of the research grant is to not only explore and identify the ingredients, but to develop a conceptual framework for a classification system that can be used as a cross-disciplinary rehabilitation treatment taxonomy (RTT). The taxonomy itself is still under development, but the conceptual framework on which the taxonomy is built is available. An illustration and full explanation of the conceptual framework can be found in Dijkers at al. (2014). At the most basic level, the conceptual model can be divided into two parts (p. S47):

Treatment Theory: Treatment theory is hypothesized linkages between components of the tripartite structure consisting of ingredients, mechanism of action, and target.

- *Ingredients*: Observable measurable actions, chemicals, devices, or forms of energy that are selected or delivered by a clinician. Includes active ingredients that are considered essential [defining a particular treatment and distinguishing it from other treatments] as well as other active ingredients that moderate treatment effects but may be common to multiple treatments. Appended to ingredient codes there may be optional codes to designate: (1) skill or knowledge, attitudes, beliefs, and domains, (2) deficit being compensated by activities of daily living, etc. and (3) exercises assigned in "homework."
- *Mechanism of action*: Processes by which the essential ingredients induce change in the object of treatment.
- *Target*: Measurable aspects of the treatment recipient's functioning or personal factors that are predicted to be DIRECTLY changed by the treatment and are functionally

relevant. Targets are grouped into four domains: structural tissue properties, organ functions, skilled performances, and cognitive and affective representations.

Enablement/Disablement Theory: Direct and indirect effects (positive or negative, at a "higher" or "lower" level) of changes in one aspect of a client's functioning. "Changes in the target of treatment can have repercussions for other aspects of functioning (as specified by enablement theory), which may be a clinical aim(s) downstream from the target of treatment" (p. S46).

To illustrate this, consider the following: The treatment *target* is to improve voluntary control of the right upper extremity. The recreational therapist chooses to utilize Modified Constraint-Induced Movement Therapy (MCIMT) principles. The *ingredients* would be the specific things that the therapist does in the MCIMT sessions. This might include guiding movements, providing performance feedback, gradual decreases in the size of the objects, and gradual increases in the range of the activity. The *mechanism of action* is a description of what exactly is taking place during the MCIMT sessions that is causing the change. One example might be neuroplasticity theory, which suggests these ingredients will lead to strengthening old neural connections in the brain and forming new ones to facilitate function. Note that neuroplasticity theory is referred to as a *treatment theory* because it predicts the effects of a specific form of treatment on the target.

The therapy sessions can also cause direct and indirect effects in other aspects of the client's functioning and life. For example, improved voluntary control of the right upper extremity may have improved the client's ability to hold and operate a fishing pole (direct effect — called an *aim*), which subsequently enhanced the client's standing tolerance because he is now fishing from a standing position more often due to the improvement in functioning. The standing tolerance would be an indirect effect — also called an *aim.* Given that fishing is a personally meaningful activity for the client, let's say that the client experiences positive emotions when engaging in the activity. This will motivate his continued engagement in the activity and may also lead him to try new leisure activities because the positive emo-

tions increase his openness to new ideas. This sequence of behavior is reflected in the Broaden-and-Build Theory of Positive Emotions, which is part of *enablement/disablement theory* because it specifies how a change in one aspects of the client's functioning can influence changes in another aspect of the client's functioning.

Dijkers and colleges (2014) note that the identification and development of theories, as well as ingredients and mechanisms of action, are necessary to advance rehabilitation research and related treatment. And, that although "[t]he ICF categories may be useful in partially describing the target of treatment, or in identifying distal treatment aims ... they do not describe what the therapist [does] to eliminate or reduce the deficit — the ingredients that [are] delivered ... [and that it] may be, that for use in taxonomizing rehabilitation treatment session, an all-new classification of human functions, or a specific modification to the ICF, will be needed" (p. S50).

This also highlights the need for recreational therapists to be keenly aware of theories that guide treatment decisions and interventions. Conceptual models that illustrate the relationship among factors and clearly defined terms also contribute. To this end, the remainder of this chapter provides a description of common theories, models, and concepts in recreational therapy that practitioners can use to inform their practice and research. Keep in mind that there are many more theories, models, and concepts in recreational therapy practice and that this chapter reflects a few of the most widely used ones.

Theories and Models

Disability, Health, and Human Services

Medical Model

Disability is viewed as a medical problem that resides within the individual. Examples include a problem that occurred during fetal development causing spina bifida, a problem in growth hormones resulting in dwarfism, and a problem in the immune system causing multiple sclerosis.

Adapted from: Cardoso and Chronister, 2009; World Health Organization, 2001.

Environmental Model (also referred to as the Minority Model or Social Model)

Disability is viewed as a social construction. The problems lie not within the person with a disability but in the environment that fails to accommodate people with disabilities and in the negative attitudes of people without disabilities. People with disabilities are seen as a minority group.

Adapted from: Cardoso and Chronister, 2009; Hammell, 2006.

Moral Model

Disability is viewed as a defect caused by a moral lapse or sin. Examples of this type of thinking can be "God did this to me. This is my punishment for living the kind of life I lead." "What did I do wrong to deserve this?"

Adapted from: Hammell, 2006.

Functional Model

Disability is defined by the individual and based on the extent that it hinders his/her ability to perform meaningful tasks. For example, a classical pianist who has a finger amputated may define herself as having a disability, whereas a psychotherapist who has a finger amputated may not.

Adapted from: Cardoso and Chronister, 2009.

Biopsychosocial Model

Disability is a combination of biology, psychology, and social factors. The biology includes body structures and functions, as in the Medical Model. Psychological functioning includes thoughts, emotions, and behavior, as in the Moral Model and Functional Model. Social factors include personal and environmental factors, such as attitudes and accessibility of buildings, as in the Environmental Model. The International Classification of Functioning, Disability, and Health (ICF) is a biopsychosocial model and classification system.

Adapted from: World Health Organization, 2001.

Health Behavior Change

Changing a health behavior can be difficult, especially when it has become engrained in the person's day-to-day life in actions such as smoking, isolating from others, and making poor food choices. Recreational therapists assist clients in making positive health behavior changes, such as engaging in leisure time physical activity; making healthy food choices during leisure activities; ceasing use of tobacco, drugs, and alcohol; developing and improving interpersonal relationships; engaging in healthy coping mechanisms to manage stress; and getting quality sleep. Other changes may include looking out for personal safety by, for example, using safety equipment during recreation, engaging in safe sex, and avoiding situations and behaviors that put the person or others at risk for harm or injury, and performing behaviors that reduce health conditions, such as performing regular weight shifts or checking insulin levels.

Health Belief Model

The Health Belief Model (HBM) theorizes that an individual will take action to prevent, screen for, and control ill-health conditions and behaviors if the person believes s/he is susceptible to the condition, that potentially serious consequences could occur, that a course of action available would be beneficial in reducing susceptibility to, or the severity of, the condition, and the anticipated barriers to or costs of taking the action are outweighed by the benefits. One example would be a person with type-2 diabetes who is concerned about limb amputation or loss of vision. The person will increase leisure time physical activity with the goal of achieving a healthy body weight as long as time and transportation are available.

Various strategies, called "cues to action," can be helpful to activate the person's readiness to make a behavior change. These include leisure education and counseling, posters, and brochures. It is also recommended that therapists employ interventions that aid in improving the person's confidence in self-efficacy for behavior change through direct training and instruction, use of progressive goal setting, providing verbal praise and other reinforcement, and modeling the desired health behavior change.

Adapted from: Glanz, Rimer, and Lewis, 2002.

Social Networks and Social Support

Social networks (the person's web of social relationships) can be described by reciprocity (extent of give-and-take), intensity (extent of emotional closeness), complexity (extent to which the relationship serves many functions), density (extent to which members know and interact with each other), homogeneity (extent to which members are demographically similar), and geographic dispersion (extent to which members live in close proximity to one another). Social support (the assistance exchanged through social relationships) can be described by emotional support, instrumental support through tangible aid or service, informational support, and appraisal support, which is information that is useful for self-evaluation. Together, both social networks and social support can influence health and health behavior through five pathways.

Pathway 1: Simply "by meeting a person's basic human need for companionship, intimacy, a sense of belonging, and reassurance of one's worth as a person, supportive ties may enhance well-being and health regardless of stress levels" (Glanz, Rimer, & Lewis, 2002, p. 189).

Pathway 2: Social networks and social support can impact health and health behavior by strengthening the person's coping resources, including adding to his/her problem-solving abilities, providing access to new contacts and information, and increasing perceived control.

Pathway 3: Social networks and social support can influence the frequency and duration of exposure to stressors, thus impacting health and health behavior.

Pathway 4: Social networks and social support can strengthen community resources, including its empowerment and competence, thus impacting health and health behavior of the community.

Pathway 5: Social networks and social support can influence preventative health behavior, such as going to annual check-ups, illness behavior, such as encouragement to take care of oneself, and sick-role behavior, such as encouragement to take responsibility for getting better, thus impacting the incidence of, and recovery from, disease.

Adapted from: Glanz, Rimer, and Lewis, 2002.

The Transtheoretical Model and Stages of Change

The Transtheoretical Model (TTM) theorizes that change is a process that occurs over time, rather than as a one-time occurrence. The model outlines five stages of change.

Precontemplation: The person has no intention to take action within the next six months. At this stage, the pros of engaging in the current behavior seem to outweigh the cons and there is little to no perceived

reason to make a change. The therapist can utilize several strategies to help move the client to the next stage: (1) Consciousness raising (getting the facts) is the process of helping the client find new information or ideas (e.g., causes, consequences, cures) that support behavior change. (2) Dramatic relief (paying attention to feelings) is the process of increasing emotional experiences, such as fear and anxiety, related to the poor behavior, as well as positive emotions related to taking action, such as feeling inspired by others who have made the specific health behavior change. (3) Environmental reevaluation (also called self-reevaluation — creating a new self-image) is the process of realizing the negative impact of one's behavior on others in the environment, as well as the positive impact one can have on others by making the health behavior change and being a role model. (4) Social liberation (noticing public support) is the process of helping the client realizes that the social norms are changing in the direction of supporting the healthy behavior change.

Contemplation: The person intends to take action within the next six months. At this stage, the cons of engaging in the healthy behavior begin to decrease and there is a glimmer of self-efficacy. Self-reevaluation, by discovering that the behavior change might be an important part of the client's identity, can be helpful in assisting the person to move from contemplation to preparation.

Preparation: The person intends to take action within the next 30 days and has taken some behavioral steps in this direction. At this stage, the cons of engaging in the healthy behavior decrease and the pros for engaging in the healthy behavior rise. The person's belief in self-efficacy begins to strengthen. Three factors can help the client move from preparation to action: Self-liberation involves making a firm commitment to the behavior change. Helping relationships provide social support for the healthy behavior change. Counterconditioning can substitute healthier alternative behaviors and cognitions for the unhealthy behavior.

Action: The person has changed overt behavior for less than six months. At this stage, the pros for engaging in the healthy behavior outweigh the cons and self-efficacy continues to strengthen with successful experiences. Self-liberation, helping relationships, and counterconditioning continue to be helpful. Two other actions assist the person to move from action to maintenance. Reinforcement management increases the rewards for the positive behavior change and decreases the rewards of the unhealthy behavior. Stimulus control adds reminders and cues to engage in the healthy behavior and removes reminders and cues to engage in the unhealthy behavior.

Maintenance: The person has changed overt behavior for more than six months.

Adapted from: Glanz, Rimer, and Lewis, 2002.

The Transactional Model of Stress and Coping

The Transactional Model of Stress and Coping is a framework for evaluating the process in which people cope with stressful events. When a stressful event occurs, a person does a primary appraisal to evaluate the potential threat and a secondary appraisal to evaluate the ability to handle the stressor. The primary appraisal is about problem management by finding strategies directed at changing the situation. The secondary appraisal looks at emotional regulation by seeking strategies aimed at changing the way the person thinks or feels about the situation. These appraisals affect the person's coping effort and subsequent outcomes. The framework also acknowledges that the person's dispositional coping style and social support can influence each process in the framework, and if the person experiences positive emotions through the chosen coping effort and subsequent outcomes, it will help to sustain the coping process.

Adapted from: Glanz, Rimer, and Lewis, 2002.

Theory of Reasoned Action and Theory of Planned Behavior

The Theory of Reasoned Action (TRA) postulates that a person's *attitude* towards a health behavior and the person's *subjective perception* of the norm about the behavior influence behavioral intention and subsequent action. Attitude is defined as a belief that a behavior is associated with outcomes and that each outcome has a certain value to the person. Subjective perception is defined as the person's belief about whether the norm approves or disapproves of the behavior and the person's motivation to do what the norm thinks.

The Theory of Planned Behavior (TPB) is an extension of the TRA. It is not a separate theory. It adds the concept of *perceived behavioral control*, which

looks at the perceived likelihood that each facilitating and constraining condition will occur and the perceived effect of each condition in making behavioral performance difficult or easy. The TPB stipulates that the person's perceived behavioral control additionally influences behavioral intention and subsequent action.

Adapted from: Glanz, Rimer, and Lewis, 2002.

Play, Leisure, and Recreation

Play and Recreation as a Way to Manage Energy

Surplus Energy Theory: Individuals have excess energy that needs to be burned off once basic needs are met in order to obtain balance. Consequently, individuals engage in play and recreation to burn off this energy and achieve balance. An example of this is children chasing each other around the playground.

Relaxation or Recreation Theory: Play, leisure, and recreation are ways to restore and renew energy that is depleted through work. It is an activity or behavior that emerges from the need to relax.

The two theories combine to provide insight into how people maintain an optimal level of energy, and how they can use play and recreation for both gaining and burning off energy.

Adapted from: Elsevier, 2006; Hayes, 2000; Hughes, 2009; Kamlesh, 2011; Russell, 2009; Saracho, 2013; Sluss, 2015; Tomlin, 2007.

Play, Leisure, and Recreation as an Instinct

Practice or Pre-exercise Theory (also referred to as *Anticipation Theory*): Play is a medium by which children reproduce and carry out adults roles to prepare for adult life, such as when playing house or doctor.

Recapitulation Theory: In early times, people had to hunt for food and hide from predators. This required people to climb, strike, jump over obstacles, run fast, and duck and cover. Children's play mirrors these movements, which are believed to be part of our ancestral instincts.

Instinct Practice Theory: Play is instinctive and allows children to learn and grow, as well as find gratification. Play is considered to be a reflection of the child's pre-mature ripening of instincts. During play children express these pre-mature instincts through games that involve, for example, construction and destruction of block towers, combat, and self-assertion of playing cops and robbers. It provides an environment for practicing skills that are needed in later life, such as cooperation and communication.

"Play-is-Life" Theory: All organic living beings, including humans, are in a constant state of activity, as activity is the very essence of life and takes many forms, including physical, cognitive, social, emotional, and recreational.

Adapted from: Elsevier, 2006; Hayes, 2000; Hughes, 2009; Hurd and Anderson, 2010; Kamlesh, 2011; Russell, 2009; Saracho, 2013; Sluss, 2015; Tomlin, 2007.

Play for Development

Psychoanalytic Theory: Play is utilized to master or conquer negative events or thoughts to achieve emotional equilibrium, as well as express feelings, of which the child may not be aware. Play provides a sense of control over the world, thus reducing anxiety.

Cognitive Theory: Play is used to foster cognitive development by providing opportunities to consolidate already learned material, as well as opportunities for new learning.

Competence/Effectance Theory: Play is used to meet a person's developmental need to acquire competency and control in the environment. It shows the person's effect on things.

Ego-Expanding Theory: Play is nature's way of forming, building, and expressing the ego, which in turn develops cognitive skills and aids in the emergence of additional skills.

Conflict Enculturation Theory: Play is an opportunity to experience and learn new behaviors, such as cooperation, competition, and social skills in a safe environment. In play this can be done without taking a lot of emotional risk or experiencing serious consequences if the concepts are misunderstood.

Developmental Tool Theory: Play is a developmental tool and therefore reflects the developmental level of the person.

Adapted from: Elsevier, 2006; Hayes, 2000; Hughes, 2009; Hurd and Anderson, 2010; Kamlesh, 2011; Russell, 2009; Saracho, 2013; Sluss, 2015; Tomlin, 2007.

Play, Leisure, and Recreation for Expression and Coping

Catharsis Theory: Play, leisure, and recreation are used to release or express bottled-up emotions.

Self-Expression Theory: Play, leisure, and recreation result from the need for self-expression, as in expressing personality, ability, feelings, and identity.

Arousal Modulation Theory: Also called Optimal Arousal Theory or Stimulus-Arousal Theory. Optimal stimulation is needed to ward off stress and boredom. Consequently, engagement in play, leisure, and recreation provides varied stimuli to maintain arousal.

Adapted from: Elsevier, 2006; Hayes, 2000; Hughes, 2009; Hurd and Anderson, 2010; Kamlesh, 2011; Russell, 2009; Saracho, 2013; Sluss, 2015; Tomlin, 2007.

Play, Leisure, and Recreation for Desired Personal Outcomes

Diversion Theory: People engage in play, leisure, and recreation purely for the sake of amusement.

Autotelic Theory: Play, leisure, and recreation are done for their own sake with the reward residing in the process itself.

Compensation Theory: Play, leisure, and recreation are utilized to fulfill a person's needs that are not met through work.

Adapted from: Elsevier, 2006; Hayes, 2000; Hughes, 2009; Russell, 2009; Saracho, 2013; Sluss, 2015; Tomlin, 2007.

Play, Leisure, and Recreation for Life Balance

Core Plus Balance Theory: People have a need for balance in their lives. In the theory, core activities represent continuity and balance activities represent change. Core activities are play, leisure, and recreation activities that are woven into everyday life, such as easily accessible and low-cost activities like TV, visiting with friends and family, reading, walking, and shopping. Balance activities are play, leisure, and recreation experiences that add uniqueness to everyday life. These are things that aren't done regularly, such as going horseback riding on a day trip to the mountains or playing a game of volleyball on the beach during a summer vacation. As people's lives change, they seek different activities outside of the core. The balance activities "balance out" our lives.

Adapted from: Hurd and Anderson, 2010.

Classification Theory of Play

Mildred Parten created a classification system for observing children during play, called *Parten's Social Levels of Play*. Parten theorized that children progress through six levels of play. "It should be noted that children do not 'pass through' stages of play … [r]ather these types of play persist as more advanced forms of play are added to the child's repertoire" (Brain & Mukherji, 2005, p. 134). The six stages of play are

Unoccupied behavior: The child watches and responds to things in the environment that catch his attention, such as sounds, colors, movements, and sensations.

Onlooker behavior: The child does not engage in play, but rather watches other children play.

Solitary play: The child prefers to play alone and does not interact or show interest in interacting with others, despite opportunities to do so. The child, however, may grab toys from others when the opportunity presents itself.

Parallel play: The child plays next to others, but does not attempt to communicate or share toys or materials with others. For example, while sitting next to other children who are building towers out of blocks, the child builds his own tower from his own pile of blocks. He doesn't interact with the other children or attempt to borrow or use blocks that the other children are using.

Associative play: The child plays next to others who are doing the same activity, and takes, lends, and borrows toys and materials from others. For example, during an individual art project, the child sits at a table with other children who are also completing the same individual art project, such as making paper and popsicle-stick butterflies. During the activity, the child borrows supplies from other children.

Cooperative play: The child plays with others to accomplish the same task or goal. For example, children working together to build a single tower out of blocks or working together by kicking a soccer ball to other players to make a goal.

Adapted from: Brain and Mukherji, 2005; Sluss, 2015.

Theory of Teaching through Play

Montessori Method: Maria Montessori developed the Montessori Method for teaching that focuses on development of a child's independence and cognitive ability through hands-on activities. The theory behind the method consists of four principles: choosing materials, choosing activities, progressions, and leading. See the chapter on the Montessori Method for more information.

Adapted from: Sluss, 2015.

Stages of Play Theory

Piaget's stages of play and *Smilansky's stages of play*: Jean Piaget identified three stages of play. Piaget believed that a child's intellectual development was evident through play. Consequently, Piaget's stages of play align with Piaget's stages of development. Sara Smilansky expanded upon Piaget's stage of play and added a fourth stage, constructive play. See Table 4.

Table 4: Stages of Play

Sensorimotor Stage: 0-2 years old
Piaget: Practice or Functional Play
Smilansky: Practice or Functional Play
Interprets sensory information, gains mastery over the environment, and learns to coordinate muscles and actions through the manipulation of objects.

Pre-Operational Stage: 2-7 years old
Piaget: Symbolic or Dramatic Play
Smilansky: Symbolic or Dramatic Play
Engages in make-believe and pretend play.

Smilansky: Constructive Play
Making things with objects.

Concrete Operational Stage: 7-11 years old
Piaget: Games with Rules
Smilansky: Games with Rules
Engages in activities that are bound by rules that offer competition and achievement.

Adapted from: Hayes, 2000; Kamlesh, 2011; Sluss, 2015; The Play and Playground Encyclopedia, 2015.

Play, Leisure, and Recreation as Continuation of Work

Spillover Theory: This theory explains that play, leisure, and recreation might reflect the type of work that people do in their everyday life. People typically choose jobs that contain tasks that are enjoyable. A person who likes to read might gravitate towards jobs that have a reading component, such as editing. A person who likes to socialize might gravitate towards jobs that have a socialization component, such as sales. In play, leisure, and recreation people continue to participate in similar activities.

Adapted from: Hurd and Anderson, 2010.

Leisure and Recreation as Attainment of the "Good Life"

Classic Leisure Theory: Classic Leisure Theory comes from the classical Greek era, such as Plato and Aristotle. The theory states that leisure reflects the attainment of the good life, which allows for the acquisition of knowledge through writing, reading, and other scholarly pursuits.

Adapted from: Hurd and Anderson, 2010.

Leisure and Recreation Categorized by Societal Values

Nash's Pyramid Theory: Nash's Pyramid Theory is a hierarchy of leisure pursuits based on societal values. It contains six levels (lowest to highest): (Subzero) Acts performed against society: Leisure pursuits that damage society, such as painting graffiti in public spaces. (Zero) Injury or detriment to self: Leisure pursuits that have the potential to cause harm to the self, such as drinking alcohol, smoking cigarettes, and increased sedentary behavior. (1) Entertainment, amusement, escape from monotony, killing time: Leisure pursuits that don't require much energy or engagement, such as watching television or reading a magazine. (2) Emotional participation: Leisure pursuits that activate psychological arousal, such as cheering for a team or playing a competitive game. (3) Active participation: Leisure pursuits that require active physical participation, such as playing a sport. (4) Creative participation: Leisure pursuits that require creativity, such as painting and pottery.

Adapted from: Hurd and Anderson, 2010.

Leisure and Recreation as Serious Activity

Serious Leisure Theory: Casual leisure is immediately intrinsically rewarding but relatively short-lived pleasurable activity requiring little or no special training to enjoy. Its main types are play, relaxation, passive entertainment, active entertainment, sociable conversation, and sensory stimulation. It is considered less substantial and offers no career of the sort found in serious leisure.

Serious leisure is the systematic pursuit of deep satisfaction through an amateur, hobbyist, or volunteer activity that participants find so substantial and interesting that, in the typical case, they launch themselves on a (non-work) career centered on acquiring and expressing its special skills, knowledge, and experiences. Serious leisure is defined by its six distinguishing qualities: (1) perseverance, which typically generates positive feelings about the activity by conquering adversity, (2) sense of (non-work) career, which is shaped by its own special contingencies, turning points, and stages of achievement or involvement, (3) substantial personal effort, based upon specially acquired knowledge, training, and/or skills (4) durable benefits and outcomes, particularly self-actualization, self-enrichment, self-expression, regeneration and renewal of the self, feelings of accomplishment, enhancement of self-image, social interaction and belongingness, self-gratification, and lasting physical products of the activity, (5) a unique ethos and social world, and (6) personal and social identity including a strong identification with the chosen pursuit. Examples of serious leisure include intense involvement in dog breeding and competitive dog shows; social causes, such as Habitat for Humanity; and researching, organizing, labeling, and finding collections.

Adapted from: Hurd and Anderson, 2010; Stebbins, 1999; Stebbins, 2000.

Leisure and Recreation Influenced by Social Frameworks

Sociological Leisure Theory: The theory stipulates that people often choose their leisure activities based on the social contexts of their lives. "That is, the meaningfulness of a leisure experience must be contextualized within social frameworks such as community, family, and friends. In addition, the degree of freedom a person has in the leisure experience or activity influences meaningfulness; the freedom is very often tied directly into the social frameworks that surround the activity. Freedom can be either high or low, and meaning can range from intrinsic (i.e., internal) to social as it is related to family, community, relationships with others, and so on" (Hurd & Anderson, 2010, p. 12). Sociological Leisure Theory consists of four components:

Unconditional leisure: Satisfying in and of itself; unconstrained by family or other social roles; is intrinsically chosen; predominant in childhood and later adulthood and retirement; has intrinsic meaning, with high freedom. Examples include children playing with friends and retired individuals going to the recreation center to swim.

Compensatory and recuperative leisure: Allows for rest and recovery from work; predominant in early and middle adulthood; has intrinsic meaning, with low freedom. Examples include watching television or going for a walk in the evening after work.

Relational leisure: Allows for the expression and building of relationships; chosen with little perception of role constraints; predominant in early and middle adulthood; has social meaning, with high freedom. Examples include going to a club to socialize with friends or taking a cooking class to meet new people.

Role-determined leisure: Leisure chosen in response to role expectations, such as family; predominant in early and middle adulthood; has social meaning, with low freedom. Examples include taking the kids to the playground and going on family vacations.

Adapted from: Hurd and Anderson, 2010; Kelly, 1972.

Recreational Therapy/Therapeutic Recreation Models

Leisure Ability Model by Gunn and Peterson

This is the oldest and most commonly referenced practice model. The primary focus of the model is the development of a self-satisfying and healthy leisure lifestyle. It is based on three assumptions (1) everyone needs, wants, and deserves leisure, (2) most people experience barriers to satisfying leisure, and (3) people with disabilities or illnesses may experience more frequent, severe, or lasting barriers. Consequently, people with disabilities may need recreational therapy to help eliminate, reduce, overcome, or compensate for leisure barriers. The model is a continuum consisting of three levels: (1) functional interventions that address skills in all domains that interfere and are necessary for leisure engagement; (2) leisure education that develops leisure awareness, skills, and resources to maximize leisure engagement; and (3) recreation participation with opportunities for fun, enjoyment, and self-expression. The client can enter the continuum at any level and moves in a linear fashion to the next level as each level is accomplished. As a client progresses from functional intervention, to leisure education, to recreation participation, the therapist's degree of control lessens and the client's degree of freedom increases. In this model, recreation participation is the outcome goal. Leisure is an end rather than a means.

Adapted from: Carter and Van Andel, 2011; Peterson and Gunn, 1984; Ross and Ashton-Shaeffer, 2009; Sylvester, Voelkl, and Ellis, 2001.

Health Protection/Health Promotion Model by Austin

The goal of this model is to obtain the highest level of health, where the recreational therapist helps a client recover from a health threat (health protection) and achieve optimal health (health promotion). There are two underlying principles of the model: (1) a humanistic perspective that humans have an innate or inherent drive for health and wellness that can be nurtured by non-judgmental, caring professionals, and (2) a balance theory that says that humans seek stabilization, so when there is a threat to health, people have a natural tendency to move towards growth-enhancing behaviors that lead to health promotion. This theory looks at barriers to health, not barriers to recreation, as in the Leisure Ability Model. Recreational therapists use three means to help people overcome barriers and grow toward their highest levels of health and wellness:

Prescriptive activity: These are activities predominantly chosen by the therapist to "energize" clients in poor health so they can begin to experience control over the situation and overcome feelings of helplessness and depression

Recreation: As clients begin to experience feelings of mastery and self-efficacy, they become motivated to pursue therapeutic outcomes and form a partnership with the therapist. Together, they choose and participate in recreation activities that are restorative and have the potential to reduce their symptoms and optimize their health.

Leisure: Clients engage in self-directed leisure pursuits that allow for the progression to an optimum level of health and wellness, leading to feelings of self-efficacy, empowerment, excitement, and enjoyment.

A client can enter the continuum at any point and may receive services from more than one of the means at the same time. As clients move through the health continuum to optimal health, their control and freedom to choose activities increases and the therapist's role and control decreases. In this model, health and wellness are the outcome goals and recreation and leisure are the means to achieve health and wellness. Leisure is a means rather than an end.

Adapted from: Carter and Van Andel, 2011; Ross and Ashton-Shaeffer, 2009; Sylvester, Voelkl, and Ellis, 2001.

Optimizing Lifelong Health through Therapeutic Recreation by Wilhite, Keller, and Caldwell

The goal of this model is to assist clients in achieving and maintaining a leisure lifestyle that will enhance their health and well-being across the life course. The recreational therapist helps facilitate the adoption of a healthy leisure lifestyle that prevents or minimizes the impact of disabling or dysfunctional conditions and secondary complications while promoting optimal health and well-being. The model consists of four basic elements:

Selecting: The therapist assists clients in setting goals that focus on their capabilities, skills, and motivations in all domains that will help them to achieve a healthy leisure lifestyle. The goals must be realistic, meaning that the clients' environment must support the effort to achieve, maintain, or regain a healthy leisure lifestyle. All of the Environmental Factors in the ICF should be considered.

Optimizing: This is a process that uses educational strategies to assist clients in selecting activities that maximize the use of their personal and environmental resources and meet their leisure goals.

Compensating: This involves assisting clients in using psychological or social efforts, and/or assistive technology to compensate for loss of ability or skill. This can include training in coping skills, working with friends, activity substitution, and/or adaptations so the activity can be accomplished. In this element there is no focus on functional skill restoration.

Evaluating: This part of the process involves making decisions regarding the costs and benefits of selecting, optimizing, and compensating. The therapist and client work together to achieve a healthy level of interdependence (a balance between independence and dependence).

There are also four inputs that impact selecting, optimizing, compensating, and evaluating: (1) client needs; (2) resources, opportunities, and environments; (3) health and human service systems; and (4) the health of the person's leisure lifestyle. Each of the four basic elements is completed in the sequential order.

The model is based on successful adaptation to aging. In this model, health and well-being are the outcome goals and recreation and leisure are the means to achieve health and well-being. Leisure is a means rather than an end.

Adapted from: Carter and Van Andel, 2011; Ross and Ashton-Shaeffer, 2009; Sylvester, Voelkl, and Ellis, 2001.

Self-Determination and Enjoyment Enhancement Model by Dattilo, Kleiber, and Williams

The goal of the model is functional improvement. The recreational therapist supports clients in achieving the goals of self-determination, enjoyment, and, ultimately, functional improvement. There are six outcome components in the model:

Self-determination: This involves the client making his/her own choices and decisions free from external influence or interference. When people are able to be in control of their free time, they are more likely to experience enjoyment.

Intrinsic motivation: A person engages in the activity because of his/her internal drive.

Perception of manageable challenge: The client is aware of the challenge being presented, along with his/her ability to meet the challenge. Successful experiences are necessary in order to perceive that challenging experiences can be managed.

Investment of attention: The person is willing to invest attention to the task. It involves concentration, effort, and a sense of control, which are obtained when goals are clear, feedback is relevant, and challenges and skills are in balance. There is a feeling of being in a state of flow.

Enjoyment: Enjoyment is more than just fun. It entails psychological involvement that results in positive feelings.

Functional improvement: When an individual is intrinsically motivated to engage in the activity, it provides the client with feelings of challenge, freedom, and enjoyment, which increases involvement with resultant functional improvement.

The model begins with self-determination. With the assistance of the therapist, self-determination is enhanced as the client gains a sense of control and choice. This leads to intrinsic motivation. This then prompts a perception of manageable change and the feeling of "I can do this." This results in an investment of attention and feeling of enjoyment, which serves as a stimulus for extra effort in functional areas of behavior resulting in functional gains. In this model, functional improvement is the outcome goal and recreation and leisure are the means to achieve functional improvement. Leisure is a means rather than an end.

Adapted from: Carter and Van Andel, 2011; Ross and Ashton-Shaeffer, 2009; Sylvester, Voelkl, and Ellis, 2001.

Aristotelian Good Life Model by Widmer and Ellis

The goal of the model is to achieve happiness, which is referred to as the "good life." The model contains four major elements:

Afflictions and oppression: These are challenges a client experiences that might lead him/her to seek services from a recreational therapist. These may include an illness or disability that inhibits freedom; failure to follow the "principle of enough" leading to substance abuse or addictions; discrimination; and focusing on goods that have limited potential to contribute to the good life, such as fast food and too much reality TV.

Aristotelian goods: These are elements that are necessary for a good life. They include primary goods and secondary goods. Primary goods satisfy biological needs, mobility, functional skills, and subsistence needs. Secondary goods promote learning, creating, and developing meaningful relationships and help approach *summum bonum* (Latin for the highest good). Secondary goods include leisure and gaining intellectual virtues of art, knowledge, understanding, and wisdom.

Freedom and responsibility: As individuals overcome afflictions and oppression, freedom increases and primary goods give way to secondary goods and, ultimately and ideally, to eudemonia, which is Greek for happiness, human flourishing, and well-being. Greater freedom through treatment also implies greater individual responsibility to the self, family, and community.

Progression of the therapist's role: The therapist's role changes during the process of achieving the good life. There is a therapist role for helping clients overcome afflictions and oppression and an educator role for helping clients attain primary and secondary goods. The additional facilitator and resource roles also help clients attain secondary goods. And, the resource and advocate roles help clients approach eudemonia.

In this model, happiness is the outcome goal and recreation and leisure are the means to achieve happiness. With that said, however, leisure is also identified as one of the highest goods, depicting that leisure within the model is also an end.

Adapted from: Widmer and Ellis, 1998.

Therapeutic Recreation Outcome Model and Therapeutic Recreation Service Delivery Model both developed by Van Andel

The Therapeutic Recreation Outcome Model (TROM) was designed to be an extension of the Therapeutic Recreation Service Delivery Model (TRSDM). The goal of the TROM is to assist clients in achieving the highest possible level of health and well-being through leisure and non-leisure experiences. The model has three primary components: (1) Functional Capacities/Potential in all domains of health, (2) Health Status/Wellness, and (3) Quality of Life.

The model stipulates that quality of life with feelings of satisfaction, joy, self-determination, well-being, and mastery are affected by a person's functional capacities and wellness. In other words, when functional capabilities go up and "health status/wellness" goes up, then quality of life goes up. They are all interrelated. Therefore, the purpose of recreational therapy is to facilitate outcomes related to functional capacity and health/wellness to drive up quality of life.

The goal of the TRSDM is to empower clients to achieve desired goals towards the development of a lifestyle that supports health. The model has three components: (1) scope of therapeutic recreation services, (2) nature of services, and (3) nature of the therapist/client interaction.

The model also has four sub-categories:

Diagnosis/needs assessment: Assessment techniques are utilized to determine the client's abilities, strengths, and limitations.

Treatment/rehabilitation: This involves restoring or stabilizing the client's health or functional abilities.

Client education: Strategies are used to develop the attitudes, values, and skills needed to function more effectively in society, to improve overall health, and achieve a higher quality of life.

Prevention and health promotion: Activities, such as stress management and exercise are used to protect or promote healthy lifestyles.

The therapist begins by conducting a diagnosis and needs assessment. The therapist then provides planned interventions that are goal oriented to assist in moving the client towards empowerment so that s/he takes control of his/her leisure experiences that promote health, as well as allow for the experience of fulfillment, satisfaction, and well-being. Along the continuum the client's degree of dependence lessens and the therapist's degree of control lessens. Clients can enter the continuum at any point and may be receiving interventions in more than one part of the continuum at the same time.

How do the TROM and TRSDM work together? The TROM illustrates how functional abilities (which are addressed in the TRSDM) and a healthy leisure lifestyle (which the therapist is striving for in the TRSDM) interact with each other and affect quality of life.

In the models, leisure is illustrated as both a means and an end. In the TROM, the goal is to assist clients in achieving the highest possible level of health and well-being through leisure and non-leisure experiences, using leisure as a means. In the TRSDM, the goal is to empower clients to achieve desired goals towards the development of a lifestyle that supports health, viewing healthy leisure engagement as an end. This illustrates that both leisure as an end and as a means can co-exist in practice.

Adapted from: Carter and Van Andel, 2011; Ross and Ashton-Shaeffer, 2009; Sylvester, Voelkl, and Ellis, 2001.

Recreation Service Model by burlingame

The International Classification of Functioning, Disability, and Health (ICF) was previously called The International Classification of Impairments, Disabilities, and Handicaps (ICIDH). Within the ICIDH the terms disease, impairment, disability, and handicap were defined. The Recreation Service Model (RSM) utilized these four definitions as a framework to develop a taxonomy for related recreational therapy interventions. At the disease level, recreational therapists seek to address issues related to disease prevention, infection control, and immediate health needs, such as autonomic dysreflexia. At the impairment level, the recreational therapist seeks to enhance functional ability at the systems level, such as cognitive retraining and strength. At the disability level, the recreational therapist seeks to enhance performance of skills that are required as part of an activity, such as social skills and anger management. And, at the handicap level, the recreational therapist seeks to facilitate the use of skills within a community setting, such as identifying and using community resources or eliminating barriers to participation in the community. Throughout each level, the recreational therapist helps to promote competency, mastery, confidence, and pleasure to encourage self-efficacy, empowerment, enjoyment, and intrinsic motivation. The model also includes a "Promotion of Wellness" level that consists of the provision of education to enhance skills, techniques, and knowledge, such as learning how to swim or play golf, followed by facilitation of recreation engagement, including provision of facilities and staff, leading to independent activity engagement where no direct recreational therapy services are provided.

Adapted from: burlingame, 1998

Leisure-Spiritual Coping Model by Heintzman

The goal of the model is well-being, of which spirituality is considered an integral component. The model is used with clients who experience stress to enable them to cope with, adapt to, and transcend life challenges; promote mental health; and enhance quality of life. According to the model, when clients first experience a stressor, such as disability, death of a loved one, or poverty, they appraise the situation in one of three spiritual contexts:

Attributions: They attribute their stress to a spiritual player, such as God.

Primary appraisal: They evaluate how the event negatively affects their relationship with their spiritual player or other sacred aspects of their life, such as "My relationship with God will never be the same because this happened to me. I have lost my faith."

Secondary appraisal: They consider whether spiritual coping strategies may be helpful in dealing with the stressor, such as "Maybe if I pray, I will find the answer that I need."

In addition to the spiritual appraisals, there are also person factors that guide an individual in his/her interpretation, understanding, and response to the stressful experience. These include religious orientation, worldviews, and degree of hope. Depending on the spiritual appraisals and person factors, leisure may be utilized by the individual in various ways:

Leisure spiritual coping behaviors: These are traditional and non-traditional activities that have a spiritual dimension, including activities that allow a person to be sensitive to the sacred such as meditation, jogging, gardening, or tai chi. It may also include activities that allow for contemplation; promote being open and aware of spiritual possibilities; allow for spiritual time and space, such as spiritual holidays and rituals; and allow a person to get away from the everyday environment.

Leisure-spiritual connections: Leisure is used to feel a special spiritual connection with nature, others, spirits, etc.

Leisure-spiritual meaning-making: Leisure experiences are used to discover meaning in a stressful situation, as well as being a way to express spirituality.

In this model, well-being is the outcome goal and recreation and leisure are the means to achieve well-being. Leisure is a means rather than an end. Leisure is being used as a context to make, strengthen, and explore spiritual connections, employ coping techniques, and find meaning, all of which contribute to the end goal of well-being.

Adapted from: Heintzman, 2008; Ross and Ashton-Shaeffer, 2009.

Hierarchical Dimensions of Leisure Stress Coping Model by Iwasaki and Mannell

This model conceptualizes the relationship among leisure, stress, and health. The model is divided into two components: Leisure Coping Beliefs and Leisure Coping Strategies, each with separate subcomponents. With respect to Leisure Coping Beliefs, people have varying degrees of beliefs about the role of leisure as an opportunity to strengthen friendships and personal autonomy. Friendships provide emotional support, esteem support, tangible aid, and/or informational support. Personal autonomy strengthens as leisure develops personality charac-

teristics that allow people to effectively cope with stress.

Leisure autonomy is also divided into the subcomponents of self-determination, disposition, and empowerment. Disposition is the belief that leisure behavior is freely chosen and under one's control. Empowerment is the extent to which people believe that they are entitled to leisure and that leisure provides them with the opportunity for self-expression. Depending upon these beliefs, people use varying degrees of the following Leisure Coping Strategies to deal with stress:

Leisure companionship: This is the use of leisure to provide discretionary and enjoyable shared experiences as a form of social support.

Leisure palliative coping: This is the use of leisure as an escape-oriented coping strategy to keep the mind busy and temporarily escape the stressful event.

Leisure mood enhancement: This is the use of leisure to enhance positive mood and reduce negative mood.

In this model, stress coping is the outcome goal and recreation and leisure are the means to achieve stress coping. Leisure is a means rather than an end.

Adapted from: Iwasaki and Mannell, 2000.

Leisure Facilitators and Constraints Model by Raymore

Raymore adapted Crawford, Jackson, and Godbey's leisure constraints model to include facilitators. The purpose of the model is to illustrate the layers of leisure facilitators and constraints that impact recreation and leisure participation. The model contains three layers: (1) intrapersonal facilitators and constraints (individual characteristics, traits, and beliefs), (2) interpersonal facilitators and constraints (individuals and groups), and (3) structural facilitators and constraints (societal institutions, organizations, and beliefs). In this model, leisure participation or nonparticipation is the outcome. Leisure is an end rather than a means.

Adapted from: Raymore, 2002.

Leisure Buffering Model by Coleman and Iso-Ahola

The model conceptualizes the relationship among leisure, stress, and health. The model stipulates that leisure-generated self-determination disposition and leisure-generated social support can buffer against stress. If buffering effects occur, physical and mental health are maintained, which in turn facilitates continued leisure participation. If the buffering effects are not experienced, physical and mental health deteriorate, which in turn increases the likelihood of negative events that could further increase stress. The model also indicates that leisure-generated social support, despite having the ability to provide a buffering effect, can, in some cases, cause increased life stress, as when there are unwanted or obligatory social contacts. In this model, stress buffering is the outcome goal and recreation and leisure are the means to achieve stress buffering.

Adapted from: Coleman and Iso-Ahola, 1993.

Healthy Living through Leisure by Shank and Coyle

The model "presents a schematic model ... that integrates concepts of health, wellness, and leisure and can be used to create health promotion and leisure education programs that assist clients with behavior change" (Shank & Coyle, 2002, p. 155). The model consists of four parts:

Becoming informed: This part increases a person's awareness about health and wellness and the role of leisure, understanding health and wellness, understanding lifestyle issues, understanding leisure influences, and assessing oneself. It asks the question, "How well am I?"

Motivation and readiness: This part examines a client's motivation and readiness for change, which can lead to establishing meaningful and realistic goals.

Decision-making and skill development: In this part the client and therapist create an action plan for behavior change that focuses "on lifestyle changes that promote health through recreation involvement" (p. 156). This can include choosing to be physically active, choosing to be socially connected, choosing to maintain balance, developing skills, negotiating barriers, and using resources.

Ensuring behavioral change: In this phase the therapist provides support, problem solves for setbacks, and uses rewards to promote continued change.

Adapted from: Shank and Coyle, 2002.

Leisure and Well-Being Model by Carruthers and Hood

The goal of this model is well-being, which is a state of successful, satisfying, and productive engagement with life and the realization of one's full potential in all domains. The model is based on positive psychology, which focuses on the development of a person's existing strengths and facilitation of the positive aspects of life rather than simply remediation of problem areas.

Well-being is developed through two mechanisms: (1) increasing the value of leisure in building resources, creating positive emotions, and cultivating potential and (2) providing psycho-educational interventions that facilitate resource development. The model has two major components: (1) developing psychological, social, cognitive, physical, and environmental resources and (2) enhancing leisure experiences as an avenue through which to support well-being. Leisure experiences are enhanced by facilitating five aspects of leisure:

Savoring leisure: This involves paying attention to the positive aspects of, and emotions associated with, leisure involvement and purposefully seeking leisure experiences that give rise to positive emotions.

Authentic leisure: This requires purposeful selection of leisure involvement that is reflective of essential aspects of the self.

Leisure gratification: These are leisure experiences that are optimally challenging and engaging. They lead to sustained personal effort and commitment to the experience and a feeling of flow.

Mindful leisure: These are leisure experiences that facilitate non-judgmental full engagement and conscious awareness of unfolding present experiences with a simultaneous disengagement from concerns about daily life, the past, or the future.

Virtuous leisure: This is the capacity to engage in leisure abilities in the service of something larger than oneself.

The recreational therapist focuses attention on the client's strengths so that they may be further developed and used by clients to improve their own lives and help clients construct a life of ongoing personal development and contribution to the world. In the process, the interventions develop a collaborative relationship between clients and therapists that encourages hope and inspires change, validates clients' experiences, and supports clients to mobilize their assets and capacities towards the desired end. The model does not have a starting point, but rather reflects the relationship among the components in the model. For this model, well-being is the outcome goal and recreation and leisure are the means to achieve well-being.

Adapted from: Carter and Van Andel, 2011; Ross and Ashton-Shaeffer, 2009; Sylvester, Voelkl, and Ellis, 2001.

Flourishing through Leisure Model by Anderson and Heyne

The Flourishing through Leisure Model is an extension of the Leisure Well-Being Model. The Leisure Well-Being Model has a strong focus on the individual, whereas the Flourishing through Leisure Model more firmly situates the individual within his/her environment, recognizing the impact that the environment has on well-being. It looks at the situation from an ecological perspective.

The model is divided into two sides, the left side and the right side. The left side of the model reflects what a recreational therapist "does." The therapist focuses on enhancing the person's leisure experiences through the facilitation of leisure skills and knowledge and facilitation of leisure environments. Leisure skills and knowledge include savoring leisure, authentic leisure, leisure gratifications, mindful leisure, virtuous leisure, interests and preferences, talents and abilities, skills and competencies, leisure knowledge, and aspirations. Facilitation of leisure environment includes real choices for leisure, typical lifestyle rhythms, social support, and inclusive environments.

The therapist also assists the individual in developing strengths and resources in psychological, emotional, cognitive, social, physical, and spiritual domains. The client's goals, dreams, and aspirations determine the specific areas of focus.

The right side of the model depicts the outcomes that the person experiences from the recreational therapy services provided, which include leisure, cognitive, physical, spiritual, social, psychological, and emotional well-being. These outcomes lead to an ultimate state of well-being, a state of successful, satisfying, and productive engagement with life. The growth of well-being propels a flourishing life, all of which is supported by environmental resources and

personal strengths that cultivate growth, adaptation, and inclusion.

Adapted from: Anderson and Heyne, 2012a; Anderson and Heyne, 2012b

Leisure Education and Counseling

Dattilo's Model of Leisure Education

Seven components comprise Dattilo's Model of Leisure Education:

Leisure appreciation: Increasing awareness of the concept and benefits of leisure.

Self-awareness: Examining values, patterns, barriers, and behaviors as they relate to and reflect leisure engagement.

Decision-making: Fostering decision-making skills related to leisure engagement, along with related skills such as goal setting and problem solving.

Self-determination: Identifying leisure preferences and taking control of engaging in a healthy leisure lifestyle. This also includes developing related skills such as assertiveness, self-esteem, and self-confidence, which influence a person's degree of self-determination.

Leisure activity skills: Developing skills that are needed to engage in leisure in order to broaden the client's leisure repertoire and maximize participation.

Community skills: Developing skills that are needed to participate in community leisure activities, such as money management and transportation.

Social skills: Developing social skills to foster healthy interactions with others within the context of leisure pursuits.

Leisure resources: Exploring personal and community resources to facilitate leisure participation.

Adapted from: Austin, 2004; Dattilo and McKenney, 2011; Stumbo and Wardlaw, 2011.

McDowell's Leisure Counseling Model

McDowell developed a leisure-counseling model that set forth specific leisure counseling components addressed by the therapist:

Leisure-related behavioral problems: Assist clients in resolving problem leisure behaviors, such as ineffective coping mechanisms resulting in poor leisure choices.

Leisure lifestyle awareness orientation: Assist clients in developing knowledge and understanding of leisure values, beliefs, and attitudes and how they influence leisure behavior.

Leisure resource guidance orientation: Assist clients in identifying personal and community leisure resources for leisure participation.

Leisure-related skills development orientation: Assist clients in developing leisure-related skills, such as social skills, transportation skills, and assertiveness skills.

Adapted from: Austin, 2004; Stumbo and Wardlaw, 2011.

Mundy's Scope and Sequence Model

"The goals for the model are that, as a result of leisure education, an individual will be able to (1) enhance the quality of life in leisure, (2) understand the opportunities, potentials, and challenges in leisure, (3) understand the impact of leisure on quality of life individually and the fabric of society, and (4) have the knowledge, skills, and appreciations that enable broad leisure choices" (Mundy, 1998, p. 50). The model is comprised of a horizontal axis consisting of six categories: (1) self-awareness, (2) leisure-awareness, (3) attitudes, (4) decision-making, (5) social interaction, and (6) leisure activity skills. Underneath each of these six categories, there is a vertical axis that consists of 107 progressive leisure education objectives that begin at pre-kindergarten and advance to retirement. The entire leisure education program/model is available in the appendix of Mundy (1998).

Adapted from: Mundy, 1998.

Mundy's Systems Approach Model

The model consists of four major components, which are further broken down into sub-components and behavioral outcomes:

Leisure awareness: The subcomponents are the definition of leisure, perceived freedom, internal motivation, self-selected experiences, self-responsibility, leisure experiences, relationship of leisure to life, lifestyle, quality of life, and time. The behavioral outcomes are that the client understands the concept of leisure and is able to apply it to his/her life, knows the concept of leisure and its relationship to other areas of his/her life, acknowledges and accepts personal responsibility for leisure, and identifies a variety of potential leisure experiences.

Self-awareness: The subcomponents are interest, values, attitudes, motivation, satisfaction, capabilities, needs, leisure expectations, goals, outcomes, and leisure constraints. The behavioral outcomes are that the client understands how his/her interests, values, attitudes, capabilities, and needs interact with and impact leisure experiences; identifies current level of leisure satisfaction and the factors that contribute to or detract from it; identifies realistic leisure expectations; determines and reconciles life with leisure goals; identifies and understands current and desired outcomes for leisure; and understands leisure constraints and ways to deal with them.

Leisure skills: The subcomponents are personnel, products, equipment, places, community, and environment. Behavioral outcomes are that the client utilizes decision-making, problem solving, planning, and evaluation processes to achieve leisure goals; clarifies value issues in relation to leisure goals; is competent to realistically plan for leisure and leisure experiences; possesses activity skills for self-selected leisure experiences; utilizes techniques to facilitate desired behavioral change; and possesses social interaction skills needed for leisure satisfaction.

Leisure resources: The client identifies and utilizes personal, community, and environmental resources for leisure and leisure experiences; evaluates and utilizes leisure products, equipment, and places for worth, usefulness, and their contribution to leisure goals.

Adapted from: Mundy, 1998.

Peterson and Gunn's Leisure Education Content Model

The Leisure Education Content Model is one of the three components of the Leisure Ability Model that was described earlier in this chapter. Leisure education includes four components:

Leisure awareness: Knowledge of leisure, self-awareness, leisure and play attitudes, and related participatory decision-making skills.

Leisure resources: Activity opportunities, personal resources, family and home resources, community resources, and state and national resources.

Social interaction skills: Shown in dual, small group, and large group activities.

Leisure activity skills: Both traditional and non-traditional.

Adapted from: Peterson and Gunn, 1984; Stumbo and Wardlaw, 2011.

Stumbo and Peterson Leisure Education Content Model

This model expands upon Peterson and Gunn's Leisure Education Content Model, described above. It keeps the same four components as Peterson and Gunn's Leisure Education Content Model, with the exception of the social interaction skills component. In Peterson and Gunn's Leisure Education Content Model, this component of the model consisted of three subcomponents to denote types of social groups: dual, small group, and large group. In the updated Stumbo and Peterson Leisure Education Content Model, the social interaction skills component now includes subcomponents that reflect skills, rather than types of social groups: communication skills, relationship-building skills, and self-presentation skills. In addition to this change, Stumbo and Peterson provide possible content for each of the four model components, some of which is divided by settings and diagnosis.

Adapted from: Stumbo and Wardlaw, 2011.

Leisure Behavior Model

Hutchinson and Robertson (2012) state that, "Understanding leisure behavior, and why individuals make the choices that they do during free time, informs the process of leisure education. In order to develop leisure education initiatives that will facilitate positive leisure functioning, one must first understand the decision process related to the use of free time" (p. 132). The model explains the process of how leisure engagement decisions are made. In general, people are not aware of this cognitive process and how it guides their leisure decision-making. The purpose of leisure education is to create a conscious awareness of this process, in order to identify areas for intervention that could enhance leisure functioning. The model consists of four components.

Needs: People have a range of needs and seek to satisfy the most dominant ones as they arise. Some individuals are not aware of their needs or how to select leisure pursuits to satisfy such needs while also enhancing health and well-being

Leisure repertoire: A broad repertoire of leisure activities is optimal to meet the person's multitude of needs. In order for an activity to become part of a person's leisure repertoire, it must be congruent with the person's values, attitudes, knowledge, interest, skills, and experience.

Intervening factors: When a person has one or more activities in his/her leisure repertoire to satisfy a risen need and intends to engage in the activity to meet that need, the person may have to deal with internal and external intervening factors. Internal intervening factors are constraints rooted in the individual including low self-efficacy and perceived social role. External intervening factors are constraints that are outside the individual and may include lack of time or finances, to name two.

Leisure behavior outcomes: Depending upon the success of negotiating the intervening factors, three outcomes may occur: 1) Engagement in the activity with the intention to satisfy the risen need. Ideally this satisfies not only the immediate need but also contributes to health and well-being. 2) No engagement in the desired activity, resulting in negative emotions, such as apathy, boredom, and frustration. This may lead to engagement in simple activities, such as television watching, as a form of escape. 3) If there is no leisure activity to meet the person's need in his or her leisure repertoire or the person is unable to negotiate the intervening constraints, but is motivated to action, the person is more likely to seek out alternative, deviant, delinquent, or unhealthy means to satisfy his/her needs.

Adapted from: Hutchinson and Robertson, 2012.

Aging and Activity

Disengagement Theory of Aging

Disengagement theory says that aging is a natural progressive process of gradual physical, psychological, and social withdrawal. A person slows down his/her activity level, shifts attention from the outer world to the inner world, and decreases interactions with people in society. This benefits both the individual and society. For the individual, the disengagement process provides opportunities for reflection, engagement in tasks and activities of interest, and decreases emotional investment in people and events. This allows for leaving the world peacefully knowing that social ties are minimal and obligations have been satisfied. For society, it transfers tasks from the older generation to the younger generation, making for a smooth transition from one generation to the next.

Adapted from: MacNeil and Teague, 1987; Moody and Sasser, 2014.

Activity Theory of Aging

Activity theory says that people have specific needs and values in life and they are reflected in the roles they play and the activities in which they engage. These needs and values continue throughout life, even as part of the aging process. Consequently, older adults do not seek to disengage from society, but rather strive to continue their roles and activities, as the more active people are, the more satisfied they are with life.

Adapted from: MacNeil and Teague, 1987; Moody and Sasser, 2014.

Continuity Theory of Aging

Continuity theory says that older adults seek to continue the same habits, activities, life role, style of life, personality, etc. that were developed in their adult life. Consequently, any disengagement from society is better explained by other variables, such as poor health or disability.

Adapted from: Moody and Sasser, 2014.

Attribution Theory of Aging

Attribution theory says that, as humans, we seek to find meaning in our behavior and the behaviors of others in an attempt to exercise control over our environment. People attribute behaviors to qualities that are inherent in the person or qualities inherent in the situation. When the person is primary, there is a focus on internal variables such as talents, skills, and knowledge. This is called dispositional attribution and fosters a sense of internal locus of control. When the situation is primary, there is a focus on external variables such as luck, weather, or culture. This is called environmental attribution and fosters an external locus of control. In general, young people and adults often seek dispositional attributions in behaviors to feel a sense of control over their environment. As people age, however, they are more often confronted with situations that imply environmental attributions resulting in a gradual unconscious shift from being in control of situations to being controlled by the situations, thus affecting the aging process.

Adapted from: MacNeil and Teague, 1987.

Selection, Optimization, and Compensation Model

This theory suggests that successful adaptation to aging includes:

Selective optimization of specific behaviors: The person chooses a few select behaviors to focus on, which requires the person to reduce the range of behaviors. The person then practices those few select behaviors to improve performance through effort and commitment to a goal.

Compensation of behaviors: When there is a loss or constraint, the optimization includes adaptation and modification to attain similar performance. For example, a person might use his vision to look for obstacles when walking due to decreased proprioception in the feet.

Adapted from: Baltes, 1996; Depp and Jeste, 2009.

Model of Successful Aging

Successful aging include three interactive components: a low probability for disease and disease-related disability; high cognitive and physical functional capacity, as these are required for activity; and active engagement with life. When these are in place, a person can continue to have meaningful interpersonal relationships and productive activity that creates societal value, such as caring for others and volunteer work.

Adapted from: Rowe and Kahn, 1997.

Community Interaction and Integration

See the chapter on Community Participation: Integration, Transitioning, and Inclusion for information on the following models: Acculturation Model, Functional Independence Model, and Normalization Model.

Rehabilitation

Many of the chapters in this book include intervention-specific theories, models, and concepts. Refer to the specific intervention chapter for information.

Strength-Based, Wellness, and Positive Psychology

Broaden-and-Build Theory of Positive Emotions by Frederickson

The theory stipulates that the experience of positive emotions, such as joy, happiness, and serenity, broadens momentary thought-action repertoires. Positive emotions allow the person to be more open to new thoughts and behaviors resulting in a willingness to think in new ways and try new things. When we think in new ways and try new things, we build resources, such as making new friends, learning new information, learning new things about ourselves, and gaining new skills. The building of such resources transforms people and produces upward spirals in their lives, which then circles back to create even more positive emotions (and the cycle continues).

Adapted from: Frederickson, 2001.

Well-Being Theory (PERMA) by Seligman

The theory stipulates that five elements are needed to obtain lasting well-being (PERMA): (1) Positive emotion, (2) Engagement, (3) Positive Relationships, (4) Meaning, and (5) Accomplishment/Achievement.

Adapted from: Seligman, 2011.

Character Strengths and Virtues Theory by Peterson and Seligman

The Character Strengths and Virtues Theory provides a theoretical framework for the measurement and classification of positive traits. The classification is intended to help practitioners develop practical applications. There are six classes of virtue that are comprised of 24 character strengths:

Wisdom and knowledge: comprised of creativity, curiosity, judgment, love of learning, and perspective.

Courage: comprised of bravery, persistence, honesty, and zest.

Humanity: comprised of love, kindness, and social intelligence.

Transcendence: compromised of appreciation of beauty, gratitude, hope, humor, and spirituality.

Justice: comprised of teamwork, fairness, and leadership.

Moderation: comprised of forgiveness, modesty, prudence, and self-control.

Adapted from: Peterson and Seligman, 2004.

Resiliency Theory

This theory explains why some youth grow up to be healthy adults despite having been exposed to adversity or risk, whereas other youth do not. For example, why do some children who have been exposed to traumatic experiences grow up to be psychological well adjusted, whereas others do not? The theory suggests that positive contextual, social, and individual variables (called promotive or protective factors) operate in opposition to risk factors, and therefore help children overcome the negative effects of the risk exposure. There are two types of promotive factors:

Assets: These are positive factors that reside within the individual, such as self-efficacy, self-confidence, and self-esteem.

Resources: These are positive factors that reside outside of the individual that provide opportunities to learn and practice skills, such as youth programs, family support, and mentors.

In some literature, resources are further broken down into family, close relationships, community, and organizations. The combination of assets and resources provides youth with the individual and contextual attributes that are needed for healthy development. Masten and colleagues (2009) provide a list of protective factors for psychosocial resilience in children and youth:

In the child: Important factors include problem-solving skills; self-regulation skills for self-control of attention, arousal, and impulses; easy temperament in infancy; adaptable personality later in development; positive self-perceptions of self-efficacy; faith and a sense of meaning in life; a positive outlook on life; talents valued by self and society; and general appeal or attractiveness to others.

In the family and close relationships: Important factors include positive attachment relationships; close relationships to competent, prosocial, supportive adults; authoritative parenting that is high on warmth and structured with appropriate monitoring and expectations; positive family climate with low discord between parents; organized home environment; postsecondary education of parents; parents with qualities listed as protective factors in the child; parents involved in child's education; socioeconomic advantages; connections to prosocial and rule-abiding peers; and romantic relationships with prosocial and well-adjusted partners.

In the community and relationships with organizations: Important factors include effective schools, ties to prosocial organizations, neighborhood with high "collective efficacy," high levels of public safety, good emergency social services, and good public health and health-care availability.

Adapted from: Masten et al., 2009; Zimmerman, 2013.

The Sustainable Happiness Model

In this model happiness is defined as frequent positive affect, infrequent negative affect, and high life satisfaction. Research shows that happiness results in larger social rewards; superior work outcomes; more activity, energy, and flow; greater self-control; better self-regulatory and coping abilities; stronger immune systems; longer life; and character traits that are more cooperative, pro-social, charitable, and "other-centered." Specifics include more successful marriages, more friends, stronger social support, richer social interactions, greater creativity, increased productivity, higher quality of work, and higher incomes. See Lyubomirsky, Sheldon, and Schkade (2005) for research.

"In summary, happy individuals appear more likely to be flourishing people, both inwardly and outwardly. Thus, we argue that enhancing people's happiness levels may indeed be a worthy scientific goal, especially after their basic physical and security needs are met" (Lyubomirsky, Sheldon, & Schkade, 2005. p. 112). The Sustainable Happiness Model focuses on chronic happiness rather than daily happiness. What is important is the level of happiness during a particular period in a person's life or enduring happiness. In the model there are three primary factors that influence chronic happiness:

Set point: A person's happiness set point is genetically determined, assumed to be fixed, stable over time, and immune to influence or control. Research supports that this accounts for 50% of a person's chronic happiness.

Circumstances: These include circumstances that are relatively stable facts of a person's life, such as demographic factors, personal history, and life status variables. Specific examples include martial status, occupational status, security, and income; health; religious affiliation; and the national, geographical, and cultural region where a person lives. Research supports that this accounts for 10% of a person's

chronic happiness and that changes in circumstance have limited potential for changing chronic happiness.

Intentional activity: These are specific behavior, cognitive, and volitional actions or practices chosen by the person. They require effort and include behaviors such as engaging in physical activity; cognitive behaviors such as practicing gratitude, hope, and forgiveness; and volitional behaviors such as pursuing self-generated personal goals. Research shows they account for 40% of a person's chronic happiness. The activities must remain fresh, meaningful, and positive; otherwise they will become part of Circumstance. "[I]tentional activity appears to offer the best prospects for increasing and sustaining happiness…. In other words, if anything can do it, intentional activity can" (Lyubomirsky, Sheldon, & Schkade, 2005, p. 121).

Adapted from: Lyubomirsky, Sheldon, and Schkade, 2005.

Other Psychological

Models of Emotional Intelligence

Emotional Intelligence (EI) "represents the ability to perceive, appraise, and express emotion accurately and adaptively; the ability to understand emotion and emotional knowledge; the ability to access and/or generate feelings when they facilitate cognitive activities and adaptive action; and the ability to regulate emotions in oneself and others. In other words, EI refers to the ability to process emotion-laden information competently and to use it to guide cognitive activities like problem solving and to focus energy on required behaviors" (Salovey et al., 2009, p. 237).

It is believed that EI can be learned and can be a relevant predictor of success in many facets of life, including personal relationships, family life, and work life. There are three competing models of EI. Mayer and Salovey (1997) present an ability-focused model based on mental ability. Bar-On (1997) and Goleman (1995) present mixed models based on mental ability and personality characteristics. The most popular is Mayer and Salovey's Model of EI, which has four components:

Perception and expression of emotion: This includes the ability to attend to, recognize, and interpret verbal and non-verbal emotional messages from cues in facial expression, tone of voice, body posture, etc. This is the first step in developing EI.

Assimilating emotion in thought: This is the ability to integrate the emotions a person feels or perceives from others into cognitive thought and harness that information for more effective problem solving, decision making, reasoning, etc. It forces a person to think more deeply about the situation and view the multi-dimensionality of the interaction.

Understanding and analyzing emotion: This includes the ability to understand the meaning of an emotion and blended emotions. The person understands causes, potential outcomes, triggers, how they blend together, and how they progress over time. For example, the person would be able to understand that frustration and anger could lead to aggression, that feelings of loneliness and sadness might result from long-term feelings of abandonment, or that feeling proud is experienced in contexts that can evoke feelings of mastery.

Reflective regulation of emotion: This is the ability to use techniques to regulate and control emotions in oneself and harness emotions in others. This can be done through activities such as exercising, socializing with others, listening to music, journaling, and reading to change mood. It also includes knowing when to self-disclose and when not to self-disclose and knowing how to foster or facilitate the attainment of emotions in others, such as how to help others feel a sense of security and love.

Adapted from: Mayer, Salovey, and Caruso, 2000; Salovey, Mayer, Caruso, and Yoo, 2009.

Flow Theory by Csíkszentmihályi

Flow refers to complete absorption in the present moment, where engagement in the activity becomes autotelic — the engagement, in and of itself, has purpose. It is a state of being between boredom and anxiety where the challenge of the activity matches the skills of the person. If the activity is too difficult, anxiety results. If the activity is too easy, boredom results. If the activity matches the skills of the person, flow results. Elements of flow include:

The activity is challenging and requires skill.

There is a merging of action and awareness that brings about a sense of being one with the activity.

Time transforms so it seems to fly by.

There are clear goals, structure, and feedback inherent within the activity.

The activity requires concentration on the task at hand.

There is a sense of personal control.

There is a loss of self-consciousness with a decreased awareness of self.

Adapted from: Csíkszentmihályi, 1990.

Activity Restriction Model of Depressed Affect by Williamson and Shaffer

The model stipulates that the degree to which a person's normal activities are restricted by a major life stressor mediates the degree of psychological adjustment. Individuals who experience major disruptions in normal activities have poorer mental health outcomes.

Adapted from: Williamson and Shaffer, 2000.

Learned Helplessness Theory

Learned helplessness is a result of a sufficient number of adverse occurrences to convince a person that s/he will not be able to escape an adverse situation, even if the person is capable of positive action. One example is a person who wants to propel his own wheelchair, but is not allowed to by his family. The adverse occurrences are family telling the person he is not capable and then taking control of the wheelchair. After hearing enough times that he is incapable, he finally gives up trying. The therapist will find it very difficult to break through this learned helplessness to convince the person that he really is capable of propelling his wheelchair independently.

When a person repetitively experiences adverse events, motivation to do things decreases. There is an external locus of control. Choosing to believe the constant negative messages, even when the person knows that they really aren't correct, can lead to depression or anxiety.

Adapted from: Maier and Seligman, 1976; Peterson, Maier, and Seligman, 1993.

Development

Erikson's Psychosocial Stages of Development

Erikson's theory of psychosocial development contains eight stages. Each stage consists of a specific psychosocial issue that must be resolved to successfully master the stage. Upon successful completion of each stage, the person attains a basic character strength, which Erikson calls a virtue.

Virtues in earlier stages are required to resolve subsequent issues. If a person does not successfully complete a stage, it can hinder the person's ability to advance through other stages, resulting in unhealthy behaviors and poor sense of self. The stages are associated with a particular age, but individuals can sometimes resolve unsuccessful stages later in life.

Table 5: Erikson's Stages of Development

Stage 1: Trust vs. Mistrust, Infancy (0-1.5 years)
Basic Virtue: Hope
If care is consistent, predictable, and reliable, a sense of trust and security will prevail, even when a crisis arises. The child believes that the world is a basically a safe place that can be trusted. If care is harsh, inconsistent, unpredictable, and unreliable, mistrust in the world will ensue resulting in fear, anxiety, and insecurity. The child believes the world and the people in it are basically unsafe and untrustworthy.

Stage 2: Autonomy vs. Shame and Doubt, Early Childhood (1.5-3 years)
Basic Virtue: Will
If a child is encouraged and supported to develop independence in age-appropriate tasks, such as toilet training, confidence and feelings of autonomy will ensue. The child will believe that s/he can effect change in the world, resulting in increased self-confidence. If a child is overly criticized or controlled, shame and doubt will ensue. The child will believe that s/he does not have the right to a place in the world and that what s/he wants doesn't matter.

Stage 3: Initiative vs. Guilt, Play Age (3-5)
Basic Virtue: Purpose
If a child is provided with opportunities to take initiative by planning activities or making up games, s/he will find the beginnings of a sense of purpose. If a child is not provided with these opportunities because others are overly critical, the child will stop trying to do things and will not develop the ability to find a purpose of his/her own.

Stage 4: Industry vs. Inferiority, School Age (5-12)
Basic Virtue: Competence
If a child is provided with opportunities to demonstrate his/her competence at tasks, s/he will continue to develop more skills and competencies. When the work that the child is doing is accepted by peers and adults, feelings of competence will ensue resulting in a sense of self-confidence and ability to achieve goals. If a child is consistently told that his/her efforts have no value, feelings of inferiority and doubt will ensue. The child will believe s/he is not competent and will not be able to be as effective in his/her life.

Stage 5: Ego Identity vs. Role Confusion, Adolescence (12-18)
Basic Virtue: Fidelity
An adolescent explores social, sexual, and occupational roles. If an adolescent is given enough freedom, s/he develops a sense of self and what s/he wants to be in life. If an adolescent doesn't have a sense of self and doesn't know what s/he wants to be in life, especially if the parents are trying to force particular roles on the adolescent, role confusion results. Fidelity, the virtue of this stage, speaks to being true to oneself. It is required to be true in relationships with others, too.

Stage 6: Intimacy vs. Isolation, Young Adult (18-40)
Basic Virtue: Love
Young adults seek intimacy with others outside of family. When a young adult develops an intimate relationship with someone, a sense of safety, commitment, and care ensues. If a young adult does not develop an intimate relationship with someone, the result is isolation and the negative emotions that go along with not belonging.

Stage 7: Generativity vs. Stagnation, Adulthood (40-65)
Basic Virtue: Care
In adulthood, people develop a sense of being a part of a bigger picture by contributing to society through careers, raising children, and involvement in the community. When these objectives are achieved, a sense of productiveness and purpose ensues. The person feels that s/he has generated something worthwhile. If these objectives are not met, a sense of unproductiveness and stagnation results.

Stage 8: Ego Integrity vs. Despair, Maturity (65+)
Basic Virtue: Wisdom
In older adulthood, people look back on their lives and evaluate the success of their lives. Older adults who feel their lives were productive and led to the accomplishment of meaningful goals get a sense of closure and completeness. Older adults who feel their lives were not productive, feel despair about their path in life. They are not able to close out their lives feeling like they did what they should have done.

Adapted from: Crain, 1992; McLeod, 2013.

Piaget's Cognitive Stages of Development

In Piaget's theory of child development a schema is the basic building block of intellectual development. Piaget defines a schema as knowledge that is linked together to make meaning of something or a cognitive pattern. A child builds schemata (plural of schema) through the process of assimilation and accommodation. In *assimilation*, the child uses an existing schema in a new situation. As long as the schema is effective, the child remains in a state of *equilibrium*. In accommodation, the current schema does not work, so the child enters a state of *disequilibrium* and develops a new schema. The continuation of the assimilation and accommodation process results in the development of more useful and more complex schemata as the child grows.

To illustrate this, let's look at an example of a child learning about animals. To start a parent might show a child a picture of a dog and tells the child it is a dog. From looking at the picture, the child creates a schema for identifying a dog as something with four legs, two ears, and a tail.

The child then sees something at the park that looks like a dog because it has four legs, two ears, and a tail, but it's also furry and barks. The child tries to actively construct meaning out of this new experience. He assimilates the additional information that dogs also include attributes of furry and barking into his schema of a dog. His mother confirms that addition to the schema.

Using this same example, let's look at accommodation. The child, although having constructed a schema for dogs, has not yet constructed a schema for cats. Consequently, when the child encounters a cat for the first time, he mentally compares his schema for a dog to the cat. Close enough, he thinks, and calls the animal a dog. The mother says that it is a cat, which causes disequilibrium, and prompts the child to process this new information. Accommodation occurs when the child changes his set of schemata for recognizing animals to include cats. Now that the conflict is resolved, the child re-enters a state of equilibrium.

The ongoing assimilation and accommodation process facilitates the movement from one developmental stage to the next when major accommodations occur that make the child's way of thinking qualitatively different.

Sensorimotor stage (0-2 years old): During this stage, the child develops an understanding that objects exist and events occur independent of his/her own actions. The child begins by behaving as if an object no longer exists when it is no longer seen, as when it is covered with a blanket or placed behind a person's back. Over time the child accommodates to a series of experiences with objects disappearing and coming back to realize the object continues to exist even when it can't be seen. The schema about objects that says a hidden object continues to exist is called object permanence. One demonstration that the child has developed object permanence is that the child will actively seek the object by lifting up a blanket or looking behind a person's back. This stage consists of six sub-stages:

- *Reflex acts* (first month of life): Innate reflex actions in response to external stimulation, such as the sucking reflex when the baby's lips are touched with a finger.
- *Primary circular reactions* (one to four months): Intentional actions centered on the body that result in pleasure, such as kicking feet or thumb sucking.
- *Secondary circular reactions* (four to 10 months): Intentional actions involving objects that result in pleasure, such as shaking a rattle.
- *Coordinating secondary schemes* (10-12 months): Utilizes knowledge to achieve a goal that brings about pleasure, such as pushing something out of the way to retrieve a desired object.
- *Tertiary circular reactions* (12-18 months): Intentional adaptations to specific situations. The child may have taken objects apart in the previous stage. In this stage the child will try to put the objects back together. Knocking over a block tower and restacking the blocks is another example.
- *Symbolic thought* (18-24 months): Demonstrates ability to visualize things that aren't physically present (object permanence).

Preoperational stage (two to seven years old): During this stage, the child develops the ability to mentally represent events and objects, and engage in symbolic play. Key features at this stage include:

- *Centration*: The child focuses on only one aspect of a situation at a time. During this stage the child has difficulty decentering so that s/he can focus on more than one aspects of a situation.
- *Egocentrism*: The child views situations only from his/her perspective. S/he is unable to see another person's point of view and believes that others feel, see, and hear and same as the child.
- *Play*: The child engages in parallel play, absorbed in his/her own private world. Speech at this stage is mostly used to communicate what the child is thinking rather than communicate with others. S/he hasn't grasped the social function of language or rules.
- *Symbolic representation*: The child has the ability to make a word or object stand for something other than itself.
- *Pretend or symbolic play*: The child engages in pretend play by pretending to be someone else or using objects to support the role-playing. A child might tuck a blanket in the back of his shirt and pretending he is a superhero.
- *Animism*: The child believes that inanimate objects have human feelings. There is a progression away from this belief. Up until four or five years old the child believes almost everything is alive and has a purpose. Between five and seven the child believes only objects that move are alive and have a purpose. At seven to nine years old the child believes only objects that move spontaneously are alive and have a purpose. After this age, the child believes that only plants and animals are alive and have a purpose.
- *Artificialism*: The child believes that certain aspects of the environment, such as clouds, are made by people.
- *Irreversibility*: The child is unable to reverse the direction of a sequence of events to their starting point.

Concrete operational stage (seven to 11 years old): During this stage, the child gains an understanding of conservation. Conservation is the schema that says redistributing materials does not affect their number, volume, or length. Below are examples for each type of conservation:

- *Conservation of liquid* (volume): The child realizes that the amount of liquid is the same, regardless of the shape of the containers. A tall thin glass doesn't have more liquid than a short wide glass just because it is taller. The child realizes that the liquid takes different forms in each glass but its volume remains the same.
- *Conservation of number*: The child realizes that the number of items placed on a table (A...B...C...D) doesn't change when the items are farther apart (A........B........C........D). The child no longer thinks that there are more items because the items take up more space on the table.
- *Conservation of length*: An item that measures a certain length is still the same length even if it is placed in a different manner (e.g., horizontal vs. vertical, straight vs. curved).

Thinking becomes more organized and rational, but the child at this stage continues to have difficulty in thinking abstractly or hypothetically. A child at this stage also progresses in ability to classify objects (an apple, banana, and pear are all fruit), seriation (ability to arrange items according to a specific dimension, such as height), reversibility (ability to reverse the direction of a sequence of events to their starting point), decentering (ability to take the perspective of others), and transitivity (ability to recognize relationships among various things).

Formal operational stage (11 to adulthood): Young people gain the ability to think abstractly. They can manipulate ideas in their head, think creatively, and hypothesize outcomes. The can perform higher-ordered reasoning and combine and classify items in a more advanced manner. They also develop inferential reasoning, which is drawing conclusions that are based on information that is not directly expressed, such as "If A is older than B, and B is older than C, who is the oldest?".

Adapted from: Crain, 1992; McLeod, 2015; Wadsworth, 2005.

Vygotsky's Social Development Theory

This theory argues that social interaction precedes development and that consciousness and cognition are the result of socialization and social behavior. Communication is the process that facilitates meaning-making, which subsequently develops cognition. The development of cognition through socialization is facilitated by the More Knowledgeable Other (MKO) who is a person who knows more than the learner. Vygotsky also developed the concept of the Zone of Proximal Development. The Zone of Proximal Development is the area where the person receives guidance and encouragement from the MKO to move from what is not known to what is known. For example, if a child does not know how to catch a ball, a parent, acting as an MKO, can provide sensitive instruction, guidance, and encouragement to the child about how to catch a ball, in an effort to move the child from not knowing how to catch a ball to knowing how to catch a ball. The child moves from what is not known to what is known. In this example, the instruction, guidance, and encouragement provided by the parent are referred to as the Zone of Proximal Development.

Adapted from: Crain, 1992; McLeod, 2014b.

Kohlberg's Stages of Moral Development

Moral development is difficult to define, as children are taught very different cultural and family moral values through upbringing and life experiences. Despite this, Kohlberg found that the way people made moral decisions changed as people grew older, resulting in three levels of morality, each with two sublevels. Kohlberg's stages are linear, meaning that people can only pass through the stages in the specific sequential order outlined. Each new stage replaces the reasoning utilized at the previous stage.

Table 6: Kohlberg's Stages of Moral Development

Level I: Pre-conventional Morality

Stage 1: Obedience and Punishment Orientation
The person believes that authority must be obeyed. If rules are not followed, punishment will ensue. The person does not speak as a member of society. If the person is punished, that is all the evidence the person needs to know that s/he did something wrong.

Stage 2: Individualism and Exchange
The person recognizes that there is not a single right or wrong view. Punishment is seen as a risk that one tries to avoid and there is a strong focus on fairness.

Level II: Conventional Morality

Stage 3: Good Interpersonal Relationships
The person believes that s/he should live up to expectations and be "good." Good behavior is based on having good motives and interpersonal feelings, such as love, empathy, trust, and concern for others.

Stage 4: Maintaining the Social Order

The person becomes more concerned with society as a whole rather than with individuals. The person obeys laws to keep social order. The person-centered reasoning in Stage 3 changes to reasoning based on a set of rules.

Level III: Post-Conventional Morality

Stage 5: Social Contract and Individual Rights
The person begins to ask, "What makes a good society?" The person understands the value of laws, but considers the justness of the laws themselves in making moral decisions. The spirit of the law becomes more important than the letter of the law.

Stage 6: Universal Principles
The concept of justice is believed and practiced. Justice ensures that individual rights and the dignity of others are respected. Everyone is entitled to be treated fairly and therefore justice is universal. At this level, the person supports laws that help all people, not ones that help some but hurt others. The principles of justice are a guide for making decisions.

Adapted from: Crain, 1992.

Bronfenbrenner's Ecological Theory

The theory states that multiple layers of the person's environment influence a person's development. The theory is depicted as multiple concentric rings. At the center, lies the individual with the person's unique qualities, such as age, sex, health, attitudes, and beliefs. The second ring, called the microsystem, represents the most immediate environmental influences on the child, such as family, peers, school, and church. The third ring, called the mesosystem, refers to the interactions that occur within the microsystem, such as interactions between family and church or peers and school. The fourth ring, called the exosystem, represents more distant environmental influences such as friends of family, neighbors, mass media, and parents' employers. The last ring, called the macrosystem, refers to the culture in which the child lives. This includes attitudes and ideologies of the many cultures influencing the child, such as family culture and school culture. There is also a chronosystem in the theory that states that the patterns of when and how often events occur and transitions during life, such as moving to another city or death of a loved one, are also environmental influences that affect development.

Adapted from: Shaffer, 2008.

Roger's Theory of Personality Development

A person's notion of self (self-concept) is composed of three components: (1) self-worth and self-esteem (what we think about ourselves), (2) self-image (how we see ourselves, which influences how we think and behave in the world), and (3) ideal self (the person we want to be). Our ideal self is always changing. When a person's self-image is different from the ideal self, there is incongruence, and self-actualization will be difficult. When a person's self-image and ideal self are similar, there is congruence, resulting in the ability to self-actualize and fulfill one's full potential. A fully functioning person who reaches self-actualization possesses the characteristics of being open to experience; appreciating the present (existential living); trusting feelings and instincts; seeking new experiences, thinking creatively, and taking risks (creativity); and feeling happy and satisfied (a fulfilled life).

In order for a person to grow, the person needs an environment that provides genuineness, acceptance, and empathy. Genuineness allows a person to be open and authentic, express feelings and ideas freely, and have honest communication without a false front. Acceptance happens when there is a deep, genuine, and unconditional care for the person. The person is accepted without placing stipulations on the acceptance, such as "I'll only accept you if...." Empathy means that the person feels that s/he is being listened to and understood. In treatment this means that the therapist sees things from the client's perspective.

Adapted from: Corey, 1996; McLeod, 2014a.

Learning

Bandura's Social Learning Theory (also called Social Cognitive Theory)

The theory states that people learn by observing the behavior of others in the context of social interactions and experiences. They can vicariously learn the consequences of the behavior by observing whether or not the behavior was reinforced or punished. This is referred to as observational learning. For example, a person might observe another person

talk back to someone and observe the negative consequences that resulted. The person then learns that talking back to someone could cause the other person to feel angry. Part of the observer's decision-making process, when the opportunity to talk back occurs, is based on this observation.

Adapted from: Sigelman and Rider, 2014.

See the chapter on Behavior Strategies and Interventions for more information on learning and behavior theories.

Motivation

Self-Determination Theory by Deci and Ryan

The theory postulates that people have an inner drive for growth, but in order to achieve growth people need to have three basic psychological needs met: competence, relatedness, and autonomy. Competence means that the person needs to have the skills to accomplish the task. Relatedness refers to interacting and connecting with others. Autonomy is having a sense of free will and being able to act based the person's own interests and values. When people experience these three things, they have enhanced mental health, become self-determined, and are intrinsically motivated to pursue things in life. If any of these three needs are not met, it leads to diminished motivation and well-being.

Adapted from: Deci and Ryan, 2002; Ryan and Deci, 2000.

Competing Response Theory

This theory states that intrinsic motivation is reduced when external rewards are provided. Internal motivation comes from an activity or accomplishment in and of itself. External rewards, such as a prize or award, are extrinsic reinforcements that reduce intrinsic motivation. They act as a competing response that can distract from or interfere with responses that facilitate internal motivation. In many therapy situations it's best to use intrinsic rewards because they allow the client to generalize a behavior to a wider range of situations.

Adapted from: Oxford University Press, 2015.

Maslow's Hierarchy of Needs

Maslow proposed that people are motivated to obtain certain needs before other needs, creating a hierarchy of needs. The hierarchy of needs is illustrated as a pyramid. When it comes to meeting needs, people start at the bottom of the hierarchy and move up. There are five levels. At the very bottom there are the physiological needs for air, water, food, sex, sleep, shelter, and warmth. Above the physiological needs are safety needs for protection from harm, security, order, law, limits, and stability. The third level has love and belongingness needs that can be fulfilled by affiliation with others and acceptance by others, family, affection, and relationships. The fourth level consists of esteem needs, such as achievement, status, responsibility, reputation, competency, gaining approval, and recognition. The top level is self-actualization, which is achieved through personal growth to fulfill a person's unique potential.

The first four needs are referred to as basic needs or deficiency needs (D-needs) and the fifth need (self-actualization) is referred to as a growth need or being need (B-need). In therapy a client who is hungry will be motivated to find something to eat before wanting to engage in social conversation. Likewise, if someone doesn't feel safe in their environment, they won't be motivated by achievement-oriented tasks. Although individuals meet needs in a hierarchical manner, people continue to go up and down the ladder throughout life and can have needs on different levels at the same time. For self-actualization, people are motivated to satisfy 14 meta-needs to develop their personal potential: wholeness, perfection, completion, justice, richness, simplicity, aliveness, beauty, goodness, uniqueness, playfulness, truth, autonomy, and meaningfulness. In his later years, Maslow explored a further dimension of growth needs that expanded the concept of self-actualization. He called this level self-transcendence and stated it was reached when people connect to something beyond the ego by giving themselves to some higher goal outside themselves through altruism and spirituality.

Adapted from: Coon and Mitterer, 2015.

Group Dynamics and Group Identity

There are several models related to group dynamics and group identity. There are similarities between the models that suggest an agreement on the basic stages with small differences in how finely the stages are divided.

Cog's Ladder Model

In Cog's ladder model group development occurs through five stages. If a new member is introduced to the group at any time in the process, the group will regress to earlier stages.

Polite: There are superficial interactions, surface issue conversations, and stereotyping of members.

Why we're here: Movement to this stage occurs when there is a shift from focusing on individuals to focusing on common goals and objectives. Hidden agendas appear, cliques strengthen, the need for approval diminishes, conflicts are perceived, and leadership and guidance from the group leader is sought.

Bid for power: Members try to influence each other and cliques are used to wield power. Group dynamics are challenging because some people become more aggressive. In the process, listening decreases, members take sides, and there is a struggle for informal leadership within the group. Hidden agendas become clearly visible, solutions begin to emerge, and members consciously and unconsciously adopt group roles, which include dominators, aggressors, followers, harmonizers, compromisers, and gatekeepers.

Constructive: Members realize that decisions must be made and problems must be solved. Active listening occurs because active questioning and trust emerges. A team spirit begins to replace cliques. Leadership is shared, participation is more even, and conflicts are viewed as a team problem instead of a win-lose battle. In processing, high creativity is exhibited, and better solutions emerge due to teamwork. There is also social loafing where some members let others do the work.

Esprit: The emergence of empathy is triggered by trust, behaviors, and successes. High morale is achieved and there is intense group loyalty. Members admire individuality. Hidden agendas are fully visible and respected. Cliques dissolve and feelings of freedom, warmth, and group identity emerge. Structure becomes irrelevant. Synergy is high, and members often achieve more than is expected due to the collective talents of the members.

Adapted from: Bolea and Atwater, 2014.

Tuckerman's Stages of Group Development

In Tuckerman's model, group development goes through five stages:

Forming: There are guarded interactions and superficial communication. Members begin sharing information with others as they try to figure out norms and roles.

Storming: Tension surrounding the development of group goals, roles, norms, decisions, and leadership builds. Conflict-related behaviors such as defensiveness and distrust emerge.

Norming: Stabilization of relationships among members occurs as group norms for behavior, communication, and decisions are developed. Group members become committed to the group as members turn to focusing on the task at hand and the group becomes more organized.

Performing: Tasks are completed and the group operates effectively and efficiently.

Adjourning: The group disperses, which can cause negative feelings if members aren't ready to disband.

Adapted from: O'Connell and Cuthbertson, 2009.

Fisher's Phases of Group Development

Fisher proposes four stages of group development:

Orientation: Members get to know each other through interpersonal communication and become aware of others' opinions of the task.

Conflict: Members debate and discuss possible solutions.

Emergence: Members collaborate, compromise, and listen to others to find a solution.

Reinforcement: Members agree on a decision and defend or implement the outcome.

Adapted from: O'Connell and Cuthbertson, 2009.

Johnson and Johnson's Group Development Theory

In this model a designated group leader facilitates group development through seven stages:

- Defining and structuring procedures.
- Conforming to procedures and getting acquainted.
- Recognizing mutuality and building trust.
- Rebelling and differentiating.
- Committing to and taking ownership of goals, procedures, and other members.
- Functioning maturely and productively.
- Terminating.

Adapted from: O'Connell and Cuthbertson, 2009.

Optimal Distinctiveness Theory by Brewer

The Optimal Distinctiveness Theory says that within and among groups, a person desires to obtain a balance between assimilation and distinctiveness. Assimilation is the need to be included and to be perceived as the same as the rest of the group. Distinctiveness is the need to differentiate and to be different. When there is too much of one desire, the other motive needs to increase. In other words, when a person feels too much like everyone else, s/he will seek to be different in some way. If someone feels too different from everyone else, s/he will seek to be more like everyone else by finding commonalities. The basic tenets of the model include:

Social identification will be the strongest for social groups or categories at that level of inclusiveness, which resolves the conflict between needs for differentiation of the self and assimilation with others.

Optimal distinctiveness is independent of the evaluative implications of group membership, although, other things being equal, individuals will prefer positive group identities to negative identities.

Distinctiveness of a given social identity is context-specific. It depends on the frame of reference within which possible social identities are defined at a particular time. These can range from participants in a specific social gathering to the entire human race.

Optimal level of category distinctiveness or inclusion is a function of the relative strength of the opposing drives for assimilation and differentiation. For any individual, the relative strength of the two needs is determined by cultural norms, individual socialization, and recent experience. Brewer additionally notes that too much distinctiveness in a group can create stigma, negative self-concept or self-esteem, and undesirable social identity.

Adapted from: Brewer, 1991.

Social Identity Theory by Tajfel

Social identity is a person's sense of self based on the groups to which s/he belongs. Group membership fosters a sense of pride, self-esteem, and belonging. To increase self-image, people inflate the status of the group to which they belong and often simultaneously degrade groups to which they do not belong and/or seek to find negative aspects of those groups to which they do not belong. Consequently, people divide the world into "us" (in-group) and "them" (out-group). Such stereotyping comes from the instinct to group things together. This type of thinking can also lead to prejudices. There are three cognitive processes that a person undergoes when evaluating in-groups vs. out-groups:

Social categorization: This process assigns people into categories, such as Group A and Group B.

Social identification: In this process group members adopt the identity of a group to which they believe they belong.

Social comparison: Groups compare themselves to other groups.

The theory states that once two groups have identified themselves as being rivals, they are forced to compete in order to maintain self-esteem and identity.

Adapted by: McLeod, 2008; Tajfel and Turner, 1979.

Terms and Concepts

Community integration: The process of integrating into all aspects of community life (Sander, Clark, & Pappadis, 2010).

Community reintegration: The terms community integration and community reintegration are often used interchangeably. However, the prefix "re" means "back" or "again." Consequently, the term community reintegration can be understood as the process of integrating into a community where the individual was previously integrated.

Deviant leisure: Leisure behavior that violates criminal and noncriminal moral norms (Williams, 2009).

Inclusion: A planning process in which individuals with disabilities have the opportunity to participate fully in activities offered to people without disabilities. It requires providing the necessary framework for adaptations, accommodations, and supports so that individuals can benefit equally from an experience (National Council for Therapeutic Recreation Certification, 2015).

Leisure: The term leisure can be defined as a subjective state of mind, activity, and/or time. State of mind is the experience of freedom and enjoyment which motivates participation. Activity can be any

sort of activity. Since leisure is not a particular type of activity, any activity could provide a context for leisure. Time for leisure is defined as the time left over after work and other responsibilities (Dattilo & McKenney, 2011; Godbey, 2003; Mobily & Ostiguy, 2004).

Leisure lifestyle: "Lifestyle is a term that has been used extensively in the leisure studies literature, often with different meanings or with no apparent definition at all" (Jenkins & Pigram, 2004, p. 288). This book defines leisure lifestyle as the pattern of leisure in one's life, such as the client leads an active leisure lifestyle, sedentary leisure lifestyle, or well-balanced leisure lifestyle.

Leisure meaning-making: The processes of gaining something important or valuable in life through leisure (Iwasaki, 2008).

Leisure time physical activity: Physical activity during one's leisure time.

Play: Play is most commonly defined as behavior that is intrinsically motivated, more focused on means than ends, distinct from exploratory behavior, nonliteral with an element of make-believe or distortion of reality, free from externally imposed rules, and actively engaged in either physically and psychologically (Rubin, Fein, & Vandenberg, 1983).

Recreation: Most commonly associated with organized activity that people do for enjoyment, such as arts and crafts, boating, archery, bowling, or skiing (Dattilo & McKenney, 2011).

Therapeutic Recreation vs. Recreational Therapy: Therapeutic recreation is the field. Recreational therapy is the practice. "A treatment service designed to restore, remediate, and rehabilitate a person's level of functioning and independence in life activities, to promote health and wellness as well as reduce or eliminate the activity limitations and restrictions to participation in life situations caused by an illness or disabling condition" (American Therapeutic Recreation Association, 2015b). Recreational therapists are the practitioners. The CTRS (Certified Therapeutic Recreation Specialist) is the qualified provider (American Therapeutic Recreation Association, 2015a).

Quality of Life (QOL) and Health Related QOL (HRQOL): QOL means something different to every person or group, but basically it is includes subjective evaluations of both positive and negative aspects of life. HRQOL are those aspects of overall QOL that can be clearly shown to affect either physical or mental health (Centers for Disease Control, 2011).

Well-being: A general term encompassing the total universe of human life domains, including physical, mental, and social aspects that make up what can be called a "good life" (World Health Organization, 2001).

References

American Therapeutic Recreation Association (ATRA). (2015a). *ATRA summer 2015 newsletter*. Hattiesburg, MS: ATRA.

American Therapeutic Recreation Association (ATRA). (2015b). *FAQ about RT/TR*. Retrieved from https://www.atra-online.com/what/FAQ.

Anderson, L. S. & Heyne, L. A. (2012a). Flourishing through leisure: An ecological extension of the leisure and well-being model in therapeutic recreation strengths-based practice. *Therapeutic Recreation Journal, XLVI*(2), 129-152.

Anderson, L. S. & Heyne, L. A. (2012b). *Therapeutic recreation practice: A strengths approach*. State College, PA: Venture Publishing, Inc.

Austin, D. R. (2004). *Therapeutic Recreation: Processes and techniques* (5th ed.). Champaign, IL: Sagamore Publishing.

Baltes, P. B. (1996). On the incomplete architecture of human ontogeny: Selection, optimization, and compensation as foundation of developmental theory. *American Psychologist, 52*(4), 366-380.

Bar-On, R. (1997). *The emotional quotient inventory (EQ-i): Technical manual*. Toronto, Canada: Multi-Health Systems.

Bolea, A. & Atwater, L. (2014). *Applied leadership development: From conceptual to personal*. London: Routledge.

Brain, C. & Mukherji, P. (2005). *Understanding child psychology*. New York: Oxford University Press.

Brewer, M. B. (1991). The social self: On being the same and different at the same time. *Personality and Social Psychology Bulletin, 17*(5), 475-482.

burlingame, j. (1998). Chapter 5: Clinical practice models. In F. Brasile, T. Skalko, & j. burlingame (Eds.). *Perspectives in recreational therapy: Issues of a dynamic profession* (pp. 83-106). Ravensdale, WA: Idyll Arbor, Inc.

Cardoso, E. & Chronister, J. (2009). *Understanding psychosocial adjustment to chronic illness and disability: A handbook for evidence-based practitioners in rehabilitation*. New York: Springer Publishing Company.

Carter, M. J. & Van Andel, G. E. (2011). *Therapeutic recreation: A practical approach* (4th ed.). Long Grove, IL: Waveland Press.

Centers for Disease Control (2011). *HRQOL concepts*. Retrieved from www.cdc.gov/hrqol/concept.htm.

Coleman, D. & Iso-Ahola, S. E. (1993). Leisure and health: The role of social support and self-determination. *Journal of Leisure Research, 25*(2), 111-128.

Coon, D. & Mitterer, J. (2015). *Introduction to psychology: Gateways to mind and behavior*. Boston, MA: Cengage Learning.

Corey, G. (1996). *Theory and practice of counseling and psychotherapy* (5th ed.). New York: Brooks/Cole Publishing Company.

Crain, W. (1992). *Theories of development: Concepts and applications* (3rd ed.). Englewood Cliffs, NJ: Prentice Hall.

Csíkszentmihályi, M. (1990). *Flow: The psychology of optimal experiences*. New York: Harper and Row.

Dattilo, J. & McKenney, A. (2011). *Facilitation techniques in therapeutic recreation* (2nd ed.). State College, PA: Venture Publishing.

Deci, E. L. & Ryan, R. M. (2002). *Handbook of self-determination research*. New York: University of Rochester Press.

Depp, C. A. & Jeste, D. V. (2009). *Successful cognitive and emotional aging*. Arlington, VA: American Psychiatric Publishing.

Dijkers, M. P. (2014). Rehabilitation treatment taxonomy: Establishing common ground. *Archives of Physical Medicine and Rehabilitation, 95*(1 Suppl), S1-S5.

Dijkers, M. P., Hart, T., Whyte, J., Zanca, J. M., Packel, A., & Tsaousides, T. (2014). Rehabilitation treatment taxonomy: Implication and continuations. *Archives of Physical Medicine and Rehabilitation, 95*(1 Suppl), S45-54.

Elsevier. (2006). *Theories of play*. In Elsevier's dictionary of psychological theories. Accessed via http://search.credoreference.com.libproxy.temple.edu/content/entry/estpsyctheory/play_theories_of/0.

Fredrickson, B (2001). The role of positive emotions in positive psychology: The broaden-and-build theory of positive emotions. *American Psychologist, 56*(3), 218-226.

Glanz, K., Rimer, B. K., & Lewis, F. M. (2002). *Health behavior and health education: Theory, research, and practice*. San Francisco, CA: Jossey-Bass.

Godbey, G. (2003). *Leisure in your life: An exploration* (6th ed.). State College, PA: Venture Publishing.

Goleman, D. (1995). *Emotional intelligence*. New York: Bantam Books.

Hammell, K. W. (2006) *Perspectives on disability and rehabilitation: Contesting assumptions, challenging practice*. Philadelphia, PA: Elsevier Health Sciences.

Hayes, N. (2000). *Foundations of psychology*. Boston, MA: Cengage Learning.

Heintzman, P. (2008). Leisure spiritual coping: A model for therapeutic recreation and leisure services. *Therapeutic Recreation Journal, XLII*(1), 56-73.

Hughes, F. P. (2009). *Children, play, and development*. Thousand Oaks, CA: Sage.

Hurd, A. R. & Anderson, D. M. (2010). *The park and recreation professional's handbook*. Champaign, IL: Human Kinetics.

Hutchinson, S. & Robertson, B. (2012). Leisure education: A new goal for an old idea whose time has come. *Pedagogia Social, 19*, 127-139.

Iwasaki, Y. (2008). Pathways to meaning-making through leisure-life pursuits in global contexts. *Journal of Leisure Research, 40*(2), 231-249.

Iwasaki, Y. & Mannell, R. (2000). Hierarchical dimensions of leisure stress coping. *Leisure Sciences, 22*, 163-181.

Jenkins, J. & Pigram, J. (2004). *Encyclopedia of leisure and outdoor recreation*. London: Routledge.

Kamlesh, M. L. (2011). *Psychology in physical education and sport*. Charlotte, NC: Pinnacle Technology.

Kelly, J. R. (1972). Work and leisure: A simplified paradigm. *Journal of Leisure Research, 4*(1), 50-62.

Lyubomirsky, S., Sheldon, K. M., & Schkade, D. (2005). Pursuing happiness: The architecture of sustainable change. *Review of General Psychology, 9*, 111-131.

MacNeil, R. D. & Teague, M. L. (1987). *Aging and leisure: Vitality in later life*. Englewood Cliff, NJ: Prentice-Hall, Inc.

Maier, S. F. & Seligman, M. E. (1976). Learned helplessness: Theory and evidence. *Journal of Experimental Psychology, 105*(1), 3-46.

Masten, A. S., Cutuli, J. J., Herbers, J. E., & Reed, M. J. (2009). Chapter 12: Resilience in development. In S. J. Lopez & C. R. Snyder (Eds.) *Oxford handbook of positive psychology* (pp. 117-131). New York: Oxford University Press.

Mayer, J. D. & Salovey, P. (1997). What is emotional intelligence? In P. Salovey & D. Sluyter (Eds.) *Emotional development and emotional intelligence: Implications for educators* (pp. 3-31). New York: Basic Books.

Mayer, J. D., Salovey, P., & Caruso, D. (2000). Chapter 18: Models of emotional intelligence. In R. Sternberg (2000).

Handbook of intelligence (pp. 396-420). Cambridge, UK: Cambridge University Press.

McLeod, S. A. (2008). *Social identity theory*. Retrieved from www.simplypsychology.org/social-identity-theory.html

McLeod, S. A. (2013). *Erik Erikson*. Retrieved from www.simplepsychology.org/Erik-Erikson.html

McLeod, S. A. (2014a). *Carl Rogers*. Retrieved from www.simplypsychology.org/carl-rogers.html

McLeod, S. A. (2014b). *Lev Vygotsky*. Retrieved from www.simplypsychology.org/vygotsky.html

McLeod, S. A. (2015). *Jean Piaget*. Retrieved from www.simplypsychology.org/piaget.html

Mobily, K. E., & Ostiguy, L. J. (2004). *Introduction to therapeutic recreation: U.S. and Canadian perspectives*. State College, PA: Venture.

Moody, H. R. & Sasser, J. R. (2014). *Aging: Concepts and controversies*. New York: Sage Publications.

Mundy, J. (1998). *Leisure education: Theory and practice*. Champaign, IL: Sagamore Publishing.

National Council for Therapeutic Recreation Certification. (2015). *Certification standards part V: NCTRC national job analysis*. Accessed via website https://www.nctrc.org/documents/5JobAnalysis.pdf.

O'Connell, T. S. & Cuthbertson, B. (2009). *Group dynamics in recreation and leisure: Creating conscious groups through an experiential approach*. Champaign, IL: Human Kinetics.

Oxford University Press. (2015). *Competing response theory*. Retrieved from www.oxfordreference.com/view/10.1093/oi/authority.201108 03095628953

Peterson, C. A. & Gunn, S. L. (1985). *Therapeutic recreation program design: Principles and procedures* (2nd ed.). Englewood Cliffs, NJ: Prentice-Hall, Inc.

Peterson, C. & Seligman, M. E. (2004). *Character strengths and virtues: A handbook and classification*. New York: Oxford University Press.

Peterson, C., Maier, S. F., & Seligman, M. E. (1993). *Learned helplessness: A theory for the age of personal control*. New York: Oxford University Press.

Raymore, L. A. (2002). Facilitators to leisure. *Journal of Leisure Research, 34*(1), 37-51.

Ross, J. & Ashton-Shaeffer, C. (2009). Chapter 14: Therapeutic recreation practice models. In N. Stumbo (Ed.) *Professional issues in therapeutic recreation*. Champaign, IL: Sagamore Publishing.

Rowe, J. W. & Kahn, R. L. (1997). Successful aging. *The Gerontologist, 37*(4), 433-440.

Rubin, K. H., Fein, G. G., & Vandenberg, B. (1983). Play. In P. H. Mussen & E. M. Hetherington (Eds.) *Handbook of child psychology* (pp. 693-774). New York: Wiley.

Russell, R. V. (2009). *Pastimes* (4th ed.). Champaign, IL: Sagamore Publishing.

Ryan, R. M. & Deci, E. L. (2000). Self-determination theory and the facilitation of intrinsic motivation, social development, and wellbeing. *American Psychologist, 55*(1), 68-78.

Salovey, P., Mayer, J. D., Caruso, D. & Yoo, S. H (2009). Chapter 22: The positive psychology of emotional intelligence. In S. J. Lopez & C. R. Snyder (Eds.) *Oxford handbook of positive psychology* (2nd ed.) (pp. 237-248). New York: Oxford University Press.

Sander, A., Clark, A., & Pappadis, M. (2010). What is community integration anyway? Defining meaning following traumatic brain injury. *Journal of Head Trauma Rehabilitation, 25*(2), 121-127.

Saracho, O. N. (2013). *An integrated play-based curriculum for early childhood*. Philadelphia: Routledge.

Seligman, M. E. (2011). *Flourish: A visionary new understanding of happiness and wellbeing*. New York: Free Press.

Shaffer, D. (2008). *Social and personality development*. Boston: Cengage Learning.

Shank, J. & Coyle, C. (2002). *Therapeutic recreation in health promotion and rehabilitation*. State College, PA: Venture Publishing.

Sigelman, C. & Rider, E. (2014). *Life span human development*. Boston, MA: Cengage Learning.

Sluss, D. J. (2015). *Supporting play in early childhood* (2nd ed.). Boston, MA: Cengage.

Stebbins, R. A. (1999). Educating for serious leisure: Leisure education in theory and practice. *World Leisure & Recreation, 41*(4), 14-19.

Stebbins, R. A. (2000). *World leisure international position statement on educating for serious leisure*. Retrieved from https://www.worldleisure.org/userfiles/file/seriousleisure.pdf.

Stumbo, N. & Wardlaw, B. (2011). *Facilitation of therapeutic recreation services: An evidence-based and best practice approach to techniques and processes*. State College, PA: Venture Publishing.

Sylvester, C., Voelkl, J. E., & Ellis, G. D. (2001). *Therapeutic recreation programming: Theory and practice*. State College, PA: Venture Publishing.

Tajfel, H. & Turner, J. C. (1979). An integrative theory of intergroup conflict. In W. G. Austin and S. Worchel (Eds.). *The social psychology of intergroup relations*. Monterey, CA: Brooks/Cole.

The Play and Playground Encyclopedia. (2015). *Jean Piaget*. Retrieved from www.playgroundprofessionals.com/encyclopedia/p/jean-piaget.

Tomlin, C. R. (2007). *Play: A historical review*. Accessed via www.earlychildhoodnews.com/earlychildhood/article_print.a spx?ArticleId=618.

Wadsworth, B. J. (2004). *Piaget's theory of cognitive and affective development: Foundations of constructivism* (5th ed.). New York: Pearson.

Widmer, M. A. & Ellis, G. D. (1998). The Aristotelian good life model: Integration of values into therapeutic recreation service delivery. *Therapeutic Recreation Journal, 32*(4), 290-302.

Williams, D. J. (2009). Deviant leisure: Rethinking "the good, the bad, and the ugly." *Leisure Sciences, 31*, 207-213.

Williamson, G. M. & Shaffer, D. R. (2000). Chapter 9: The activity restriction model of depressed affect. In G. M. Williamson, D. R. Shaffer, & P. A. Parmelee (Eds.). *Physical illness and depression in older adults: A handbook of theory, research, and practice* (pp. 173-200). New York: Kluwer Academic /Plenum Publishers.

World Health Organization. (2001). *International classification of functioning, disability, and health*. Geneva, Switzerland: World Health Organization.

Zimmerman, M. A. (2013). Resiliency theory: A strengths-based approach to research and practice for adolescent health. *Health Education and Behavior, 40*(4), 381-383.

II. Techniques and Interventions

11. Activity Pattern Development

Heather R. Porter

The goal of activity pattern development is to modify a client's activity pattern so that it is more healthy and/or therapeutic. Some of the issues involved include understanding the concepts of a leisure repertoire and balanced leisure lifestyle, determining the client's leisure interests, and developing appropriate activity patterns.

Leisure Repertoire vs. Balanced Leisure Lifestyle

The ability to carry out a daily routine (d230 Carrying Out Daily Routine) requires that a client has many different skills and a relatively broad knowledge base of potential actions from which to build a daily routine. If the therapist and client identify a need to increase the number and diversity of leisure activities available to a client, the therapist will want to first help the client identify the activities currently in the client's leisure repertoire (see Interest Exploration below). Mobily, Lemke, and Gisin (1991) define leisure repertoire as the activities that the person feels s/he can do with competence. The authors propose that the more activities the person perceives competence in, the greater the client's ability to adjust to life's challenges.

One of the common terms used in recreational therapy is "balanced leisure lifestyle." A balanced leisure lifestyle is generally considered to be a state in which physical, mental, social, and emotional well-being are all supported by the person's leisure. Edginton et al. (1995) describe the purpose of a balanced leisure lifestyle.

Contemporary society often views leisure as a way of bringing balance into one's life. Leisure is sought not only for the opportunity for relaxation, self-improvement, cultural and family stability and interaction, but also for escape, novelty, complexity, excitement, and fantasy. In many societies, people use leisure as a way of counter-balancing stresses that result from living and working in a technologically oriented, competitive, rapidly changing society that requires attention to a high degree of stimulation in the form of information, media, communications, and human interaction (p. 33).

When the therapist is working on activity pattern development, it is important to make sure that the client has a sufficient leisure repertoire and that the patterns that are being developed allow for balanced leisure.

Indications

Activity pattern development is indicated when life changes, such as injury or disability, occur causing a disruption to the person's ability to engage in leisure activities. It is also indicated when the client's current activity pattern is unhealthy or unbalanced. When it is difficult to see how the current leisure repertoire fills all of the client's leisure needs, the recreational therapist should continue to work with the client to decide if there is a need for activity pattern development.

Recreational therapists who work in day programs or residential settings might analyze each person's activity pattern (or activity patterns of specific units) to ascertain the health of the routine. If concerns are found, the recreational therapist would subsequently evaluate and implement activity changes to optimize the health of the residents.

Contraindications

The extent of client participation in activity pattern development will depend largely on the client's willingness, and extent of investment, to analyze his/her lifestyle. Consequently, leisure education may be required to maximize a client's knowledge and subsequent motivation to evaluate lifestyle choices. Knowledge, however, does not equal action. Making lifestyle changes can be very difficult for some clients, especially those with engrained patterns of behavior. Behaviors, although unhealthy, may yield other desired outcomes, such as emotional escape, which can be difficult to break. (See the Health Behavior Change chapter for more information.)

Developing an activity pattern also requires orientation to time, place, and person; basic and higher-level cognitive skills (e.g., attention, problem solving, planning); knowledge of resources, such as transportation and finances; and the ability to write. Compensatory strategies can, of course, be implemented to minimize challenges and assistance, such as adaptive devices for writing and verbal cues to assist the client in sustaining attention, can be provided by the therapist. Still, a full understanding of the client's ability to actively participate is needed so that engagement is meaningful. For clients who are unable (or minimally able) to participate in activity pattern development, the therapist may seek others, including guardians and family members, who can help.

Protocols and Processes

Interest Exploration

When the therapist is trying to develop appropriate activity patterns, it is important to look at what the client is interested in doing. Even the best program will fail if it doesn't match the client's preferences for leisure. An understanding of a person's leisure repertoire is required prior to developing an activity pattern for a more balanced leisure lifestyle.

There are many different assessment tools that assist the therapist in identifying specific activities or characteristics of activities that appeal to the client. The *Leisure Interest Measure*, the *Activity Card Sort*, and the *Leisure Assessment Inventory* are good measures to consider. The therapist can also opt for a more informal exploration by looking at the client's past interests, future goals, and interests of those who are close to him/her. It is also helpful if the therapist is aware of current activity trends, popular activities in the area, and popular activities by demographics. The more experience a clinician has, the more skilled

s/he becomes at "reading" the characteristics of clients and finding attractive activities for the client. For example, a retired executive with a strong work ethic may gravitate toward more intellectual activities.

However, therapists should also be very careful not to stereotype clients and assume that because of their age or resources that certain activities would not be a consideration. For example, a 75-year-old frail woman may enjoy hiking. The therapist should also remember that recreation is subjective. What is recreation for one person may be work for another. People have different attitudes about tasks like mowing the grass or washing the car. Interest exploration will be a springboard for developing a treatment plan. A treatment plan and functional goals should directly relate to a person's interests.

If a formal assessment tool is used, the name of the tool should be included in your documentation along with the results. The therapist explains the purpose of the assessment and how the information will be used to develop a healthy activity pattern and treatment plan for the client. The ICF can be used to document which aspects of the diagnosis were being treated by developing the plan. For example, a client who is diagnosed with rheumatoid arthritis has mobility deficits. In addition, the assessment notes that the client has not been participating in recreation because she is afraid it will be painful, leading to concerns about cardiovascular issues and overall fitness. Documentation of interest exploration might be documented with a chart note that looks like, "Client seen for assessment of activities that client finds desirable for participation. Post brainstorming, client was able to identify a possible interest in aquatics at the local YMCA. Client and therapist decided that involvement in an aquatic exercise program post d/c would be a good health maintenance activity to help with managing mobility issues (b280 Sensation of Pain, d410 Changing Basic Body Position, d450 Walking) caused by rheumatoid arthritis, as well as help decrease CVA risk (b420 Blood Pressure Functions) improve general fitness (b455 Exercise Tolerance Functions, d570 Looking After One's Health), and provide recreation opportunities (d920 Recreation and Leisure). RT and client to further explore issues related to this task."

Developing Activity Patterns

Developing an activity pattern means creating a coherent, integrated habit of participating in a variety of leisure activities that, as a whole, allow the client to be healthier and happier. One of the therapist's jobs is to help the client develop an activity pattern that is realistic given the circumstances, balanced given the client's needs, and that is enjoyable enough to increase the likelihood that it will become habit.

Once a client determines how s/he currently spends his/her time, s/he can begin to explore modifications to be able to achieve a realistic activity pattern. One way of exploring this is by completing the *Pie of Life* activity (see Appendix). The client may be familiar with the activities in his/her leisure repertoire but may need help from the therapist to broaden his/her options with suggestions of other activities that s/he may find enjoyable, that s/he is likely capable of doing, and that help create a better balance between leisure and other activities.

Activity patterns are developed to encourage health and growth. A realistic, healthy activity pattern can increase the positive outcomes of therapy. There are many ways to design an activity pattern. Most of them involve the therapist working with the client and writing down the plan, allowing the client to work on integrating the activities into his/her normal routine. It should be designed and written in a way that maximizes the client's ability to use it as a recovery and health promotion tool. A general idea of how to put together an activity pattern follows.

The therapist and client begin by making a list of all of the activities that need to fit into the client's daily life. It is helpful to identify and write down broad categories to guide the client in identifying activities prior to making the list (e.g., chores, school, work, recreation, exercise, meals, and therapy). This should include lifestyle changes, which may include items like an altered routine to help the client quit smoking, an exercise program, activity precautions, extra time for preparing healthier meals, and individual quiet time for stress reduction. Next to each activity, the client writes down all of the things that s/he is to remember related to each task, such as "aquatics: three times a week, fill out and send in scholarship application" or "gardening: purchase self-coiling hose, garden in 15-minute increments." This allows the client an opportunity to reflect on his/her lifestyle and the changes to be made. It also gives the therapist an opportunity to evaluate how much the client is able to remember from therapy sessions and how realistic the client is in planning.

If the client's cognitive limitations prevent the client from taking an active role in the development of the list, the therapist puts together the list without the client or develops it with caregivers. Either way, the therapist must discuss the list with the caregivers to promote carryover and follow through.

The client and therapist work from the list with the goal of transferring all of the data into a daily, weekly, or monthly schedule (most typically a week). The schedule resembles an appointment book. Choosing between electronic and paper calendars depends on the preferences of the client; electronic versions have the ability to remind the client about the schedule. The days of the week are listed across the top of the page and underneath each day are half-hour increments (e.g., 8:00, 8:30, 9:00, etc.). The client fills in a time slot with the name of the activity and then draws a line down to the time increment that reflects the end of the activity (e.g., 9:00-9:30 stretching program, 9:30-10:00 shower, 10:00-11:00 dress and breakfast, 11:00-11:15 make brown bag lunch, 11:15 leave for work, and so on).

Some clients find this very frustrating because what they are writing down to happen on a Monday is not necessarily something that will happen every Monday. Clients are told that this is a mock schedule. It is an opportunity to put together a tentative lifestyle plan that allows the client to apply and integrate all of the activities and tasks that are to become part of his/her lifestyle. Clients can use highlighters or different color pens to note activities that will occur regularly on specific days and times. It gives the therapist a clear picture of the client's ability to fully appreciate the role of activity in recovery and health and recall specifics related to each activity. The list of specifics can be long because it includes at least techniques, resources, transportation needs, equipment needs, references, contacts, follow-up responsibilities, techniques utilized, adaptations, any special concerns, precautions and parameters relevant to the activity, and relation of activity to personal health needs. It also provides opportunities to problem solve (e.g., client's medication schedule falls during the YMCA aquatic class) and evaluate his/her ability to incorporate into a comprehensive lifestyle pattern all of the functional skills training, education, counseling, and integration training s/he has received.

If the client is not able to follow through with an activity pattern independently, other people need to be involved. This may include the client's family or caregivers. If the client is going to be discharged to a skilled care facility that employs an activity director, the therapist should call the activity director to discuss activities available, how they relate to the client's interests and needs, and any special accommodations, such as adaptations and cueing, provided permission is granted by the client to do so. A copy of the activity pattern that was developed should be given to the client and family, as well as sent directly to the activity director.

An activity pattern encompasses many different types of activities and may be required for treating aspects of a client's condition described by many different ICF codes including b126 Temperament and Personality Functions, b130 Energy and Drive Functions, b280 Sensation of Pain, b4 Functions of the Cardiovascular, Hematological, Immunological, and Respiratory Systems, b7 Neuromusculoskeletal and Movement-Related Functions, d230 Carrying Out Daily Routine, d240 Handling Stress and Other Psychological Demands, d4 Mobility, d5 Self-Care, d6 Domestic Life, d7 Interpersonal Interactions and Relationships, d8 Major Life Areas, and d9 Community, Social, and Civic Life.

Therapists help clients narrow down what activities to put into an activity pattern by choosing those that are most necessary for health. Having an activity pattern that is realistic and geared toward promoting health and happiness can have a significant impact on preventing illness and secondary complications through its health promotion focus.

Outcomes and Documentation

Recreational therapists document the specific activity pattern issues identified, the method utilized to identify the issues (e.g., standardized measurement tool, clinical interview), methods employed to facilitate change (e.g., discussion, education, counseling, use of particular health behavior change theories, activities), insights gained by the client, barriers to change, facilitators for change, and changes planned or made. Deficits in ICF codes that necessitated activity pattern development should be noted with an explanation of how the new activity pattern will reduce the deficits.

References

Edginton, C., Jordan, D., DeGraaff, D., & Edginton, S. (1995). *Leisure and life satisfaction: Foundational perspectives.* Dubuque, IA: Brown & Benchmark Publishers.
Mobily, K. E., Lemke, J. H., & Gisin, G. J. (1991). The idea of leisure repertoire. *Journal of Applied Gerontology, 10*:208-223.

Appendix: Pie of Life

Objectives

- To help a client identify how s/he spends his/her time.
- To provide the client with a tool to make informed decisions about what to do with his/her time.

Materials

- A piece of paper with each hour of a 24-hour day written down the left column with each hour on its own line. This paper should be labeled "How I spend my day."
- A circle that fills most of an 8½" x 11" piece of paper. The inside of the circle is divided into four equal quarter sections using dotted lines. Each quarter section represents six hours. This second paper can have numerous headings including "REAL" and "IDEAL."
- Something with which to write.
- Colored magic markers.

Procedure

- The client is given two sheets of paper as described in the materials section and writing materials.
- Using the first paper (How I spend my day) the client writes down how each hour is spent. The therapist will need to give clear directions as to whether the client is to record a typical day (not necessarily what really happened on any one day, but what an average day would look like), what happened on a specific day, whether the client should select a specific day that includes time needed for healthcare issues and appointments, and whether the day is a work/school day or not.

- The client breaks down the activities into categories such as sleep, self-care/grooming, work, school, active recreation, reading, transportation, taking care of others, etc. Once the client has a group of activity categories s/he should add up the hours spent in each category.
- The client takes the total hours in each category and transfers this information to the pie chart.
- The six-hour quarters are there just to make it easier for clients to estimate how much of the pie any specific time period represents. For example, if the client spent three hours a day in the car, the client would divide one of the six-hour quarters in half to equal three hours.
- It is helpful if the therapist has pre-determined the activity categories and provides a different color magic marker for each category. That way, if the group compares their pies, each client can judge how much more or less time s/he spends in any one category than others in the group. This can help spur discussions.

Variations

- There are 168 hours in a week. The therapist may want to have a client look at a week as a time unit instead of a day. A week allows a better measurement of how one spends one's time. If a 168-hour time is used, each quarter of the pie represents 42 hours.
- The therapist can use two pies; one for "Real" and one "Ideal"; "While in Rehab" and "Once Discharged"; or "While Using Drugs/Alcohol" and "Not Using."
- The therapist can use different topics besides activities to show in a pie format. For example, Where my money goes; Where my energy goes; What portions of my day are creative? Interesting? Dull? Busy work?

Questions for the Therapist to Ask

After having the client look over his/her own pie and maybe talking about it with the people near him/her:

- Are you comfortable with the relative size of your slices?
- If you want to begin changing the size of any of the slices, what is realistic?
- The changes you have proposed require more/less energy. Is that realistic?

Every time a client decides to spend more time in one activity category, s/he is actively or passively deciding to spend less time in something else:

- When you make a commitment to do something, how often do you stop and ask yourself what you will cut out?
- Is this important to do?
- How would asking yourself this question change your life?

After a client has filled out the "Ideal" pie:

- Do you think that you will usually have enough energy to complete all the hours of activities that you have put down?

Most people find that the majority of their time is spent on work/school, sleep, and caring for self and others, leaving very little time for personal interests or their spouses:

- How important is it for you to increase your time for individual interests or for time with your spouse?
- Many people have a certain image of themselves such as caring mother, athlete, or community activist. What does your pie say about you?
- Does it match your image of yourself, and, if not, why not?

Therapist Notes

- This activity is a good lead in to time management discussions. It also lends itself to discussions about a client's physical needs such as self-care, sleep, and eating. Discussions about obligations and other demands on time are logical with this activity.
- Many people do not understand the difference between a *need* (the client needs something or else his/her health, significant relationships, or life will suffer serious consequences) and a *want* (the client wants something or else s/he will not be as happy, fulfill dreams, etc.). Once a client can be realistic about the difference between needs and wants, prioritization is easier.
- Often people learn better when taught using a multi-sensory approach. Having the client think, write down, color in, discuss, and re-configure is a multi-sensory approach for showing the client how s/he spends his/her time.

12. Adaptive Sports

Neil R. Lundberg and Diane Groff

Sports for people with disabilities have a long and storied history starting as early as the 1870s (Bullock & Mahon, 1997). In the United States wheelchair and other "adapted" sports began as veterans returned from World War II with serious injury (DePauw & Gavron, 2005). In the 1950s the first international competitions began and the first Paralympic games were organized in conjunction with the Olympics held in Rome in 1960 (Bullock & Mahon, 1997).

In addition to these historical markers, sports for people with disabilities continue to be an important and relevant topic. Most recently, the U.S. Government Accountability Office (GAO) (2010) found that public elementary and secondary students with disabilities did not have equal opportunities to engage in extracurricular athletics as required under Section 504 of the Rehabilitation Act of 1973. In response, the GAO clarified for the U.S. Department of Education that schools are responsible to provide separate or equal athletic opportunities for all elementary and secondary students. Furthermore, they identified that college institutions must also provide equal opportunities to participate in sport, including intercollegiate, club, and intramural athletics. The full impact of this ruling has likely not been felt, but it presents a clear legal mandate to increase opportunities for individuals with disabilities to engage in sports while in school (Lakowski & Henkel, 2013).

While the existence of sports for individuals with disabilities has a relatively well-documented history and is at the forefront of current legal movement, the use of sports, particularly adaptive sports, as a therapeutic modality has not been thoroughly acknowledged in the therapeutic recreation and recreational therapy literature. The purpose of this chapter is to provide a starting place, discussing the vast potential for adaptive sports to be utilized as a therapeutic modality to improve the health and well-being of individuals with disabilities and other disabling conditions.

By way of definition, adaptive sports and recreation programs provide opportunities for individuals with disabilities to develop a variety of sports-based skills and compete in sporting events and related activities, essentially achieving the same benefits of participation in sports as individuals without disabilities. The possible benefits include emotional, physical, social, and environmental gains. Adaptive sports can be defined as sports-related activities designed for individuals with disabilities (Martin & Smith, 2001).

Sport is a broad and global term that includes participation in physical activity on various levels under specific standards, rules, or guidelines (Pensgaard & Sorenson, 2002). Levels of sports participation include recreational, competitive, and elite level competition. Participation in recreational sports includes involvement in sports or physical activity for the purposes of health, fun, or socialization. Examples may include spending a weekend skiing during the winter or taking a family bike ride. Competitive sports involve sports participation that is performed to meet certain performance standards with required limitations and imposed conditions. An example of this level of participation would include more formalized community leagues, school, or local competition. The final level of sports participation is considered elite athletic competition. This level of participation includes serious career athletes who participate at regional, national, or international competitions, devoting significant amounts of time, energy, and resources in order to be competitive at the highest levels. It is important to note that adaptive sports participation spans all three levels, and that the benefits gained, and associated problems, are directly related to the level of sports participation (O'Neill & Maguire, 2004; Muraki et al., 2000).

Adaptive sports and recreation activities occur in various settings. Frequently adaptive sports and recreation activities are utilized in a rehabilitation hospital where services are designed to meet the rehabilitative needs of individuals receiving treatment at the hospital. Adaptive sports and recreation activities are also commonly offered through community-based programs or public parks and recreation entities, where individuals with a wide range of disabilities who live in the local community are provided with opportunities to participate in accessible sports and recreation activities. Any combination or variation of the above settings might also be provided.

Regardless of the level of participation or the setting in which adaptive sports and recreation activities are provided, an inherent characteristic of adaptive sports is that they are "adapted," suggesting some level of modification or intentional design in order to create an environment maximizing participation opportunities for an individual with a disability. For example, in the case of skiing, the sport or recreational activity is adapted to include additional equipment options, thereby accommodating individuals with any level of disability. On the other hand, a sport like quad rugby, was not adapted *per se*, but was intentionally designed or created as a competitive contact sport for individuals with quadriplegia. From a recreational therapy standpoint, both of these examples would fit into the definition of adaptive sports and, based on the available evidence, could be utilized for a wide variety of therapeutic purposes including improved physical function or condition, development of social networks, enhancement of self-concept and positive mood states, opportunities for community reintegration, and reduction of disability-related stigma.

Adapting any given sport or recreational activity can be accomplished using the principles provided in the chapter on Activity and Task Analysis. Please refer to that chapter for specific information and principles related to making needed adaptations and modifications to a given sport or recreational activity. For specific recommendations on common equipment or procedural adaptations related to a specific sport, see the resource section of this chapter.

Indications

A significant body of literature supports the benefits of physical activity and sports for individuals of all ages and abilities. The United States Department of Health and Human Services (2005), through the Surgeon General, stated as a national priority having all persons with disabilities "promote their own good health by developing and maintaining healthy lifestyles" (p. 2). Lack of physical activity is a national concern and has been identified as a leading cause of disease in our country. Consistently engaging in physical activities such as adaptive sports can prevent chronic diseases such as diabetes, cancer, hypertension, obesity, depression, cardiovascular disease, and premature death (Warburton, Nicol, & Bredin, 2006). Therefore, facilitating engagement in adaptive sports and recreation is indicated for all persons including individuals with intellectual and developmental disabilities (Wilhite, Biren, & Spencer, 2012), physical and sensory disabilities, and mental and behavioral disabilities (U.S. Department of Health and Human Services, 2005). ICF codes that may indicate a need for adaptive sports can be found in b4 Functions of the Cardiovascular, Hematological, Immunological, and Respiratory Systems.

Adaptive sports can help individuals with physical disabilities increase vitally important flexibility in areas such as the hip flexors, shoulder extensors, knee flexors, and hand flexors (DePauw & Gavron, 2005). Sports can promote endurance in muscles used for ambulation and promote muscular strength in all body functions particularly core muscle groups (Rimmer et al., 2010). Adaptive sports promote muscle coordination that is often negatively impacted by physical disabilities such as ataxia (Groff, Lawrence, & Grivna, 2006; Holland & Steadward, 1990). There are key improvements to cardiovascular health due to engagement in adaptive sports that rely on aerobic conditioning. Positive impacts include improved heart rate, blood pressure, improved oxygen consumption, and blood sugar levels (Santiago, Coyle, & Kinney, 1993; Wilhite et al., 2012). Physical disabilities that indicate a need for adaptive sports can be found in ICF codes b4 Functions of the Cardiovascular, Hematological, Immunological, and Respiratory Systems and d4 Mobility.

Lastly, one should not overlook the vitally important social and emotional benefits of engaging in adaptive sports with other individuals with disabilities and with individuals without disabilities. Particularly for individuals with mental and emotional disabilities such as mild to moderate mental retardation, Down syndrome, or psychiatric disorders, adaptive sports can be an effective context to teach individuals important social and emotional self-management skills (Maiano et al., 2007). The ability to confront things such as one's fears, pressure, winning, losing, interpersonal relationships, and interpersonal disagreements can open vital opportunities for learning life skills. Being a part of a team and working toward group goals can increase opportunities to feel socially connected and bring meaning to life. ICF codes that relate to the social aspects of adaptive sports include d7 Interpersonal Interactions and Relationships and d9 Community, Social, and Civic Life.

Contraindications and Precautions

Participation in adaptive sports is contraindicated for some persons for a variety of reasons. Concerns are similar to sports-related injuries that exist for all people. Individuals should consult with their physician and thoroughly review and monitor any potential physical, emotional, or social complication prior to participation in adaptive sports and physical activity. The National Center on Health, Physical Activity, and Disability (NCHPAD) website (http://nchpad.org) provides a wealth of information on the contraindications of exercise and sports for individuals with a range of disabilities such as cerebral palsy, spinal cord injury, rheumatoid arthritis, Down syndrome, and heart disease. The primary contraindications therapists should be aware of are discussed below.

Engagement in sports can be accompanied by trauma or physical injury to the bones, joints, muscles, head, and skin. Proper equipment, coaching, and supervision are vital components of preventing sports-related physical injury. Environmental hazards such as extreme cold and heat may expose individuals to potential injury. Having a physical disability and using certain medications can impact the body's ability to cool or heat properly. For example, heat may be particularly detrimental to individuals with muscular sclerosis and spinal cord injury. Using wet, cool bandanas or cooling cloths can help an individual cool the body more efficiently. Drinking an adequate amount of water and electrolyte replacement drinks is also vital. Caution should be taken

with some electrolyte replacement drinks that have high sodium levels, which should only be used in endurance-based activities. Otherwise, water is the preferred fluid. Hydration should be particularly monitored in persons who have bladder dysfunction. One of the techniques individuals use to reduce accidents is to limit fluid intake. In this situation caution should be used to increase hydration prior to activity and replace fluids after activity.

Individuals with physical disabilities that involve muscle flexibility and spasticity (such as cerebral palsy, spinal cord injury, or muscular dystrophy) should avoid sitting or lying in one position for extended periods of time and muscle damaging eccentric exercise (such as downhill running). Individuals with disabilities may also fatigue easily, so consideration should also be given to promoting short intervals of participation mixed with rest as needed. To this end, a proper warm-up and cool-down period is vitally important for individuals with disabilities. Some individuals who use wheelchairs are at increased risk of osteoporosis due to the lack of weight-bearing activity in their daily routine. Individuals in this situation should be certain to maintain a healthy, well-balanced diet with adequate calcium and vitamins. They may also benefit from aquatic sports due to the hydrostatic pressure of the water. (See the Aquatic Therapy chapter.) Lastly, individuals who are experiencing some form of acute inflammation to the bone or muscle, as in the case of rheumatoid arthritis, should avoid aggressive stretching or strenuous activity. Gentle stretching and range of motion exercises with the help of a trained staff or family member may be helpful (NCHPAD, 2013). Conversely, individuals with Down syndrome often experience hypermobility and hypertonicity. In these situations taping or braces may be necessary to maintain the proper range of motion during an activity and in some cases contact sports would be contraindicated altogether.

Many individuals with disabilities also experience subtle or more extensive loss of proprioception and feeling in their extremities. For example, as a result of chemotherapy and radiation, many cancer survivors experience loss of sensation in their feet and hands, which can result in increased risk of falls or a weakened grip. Individuals should use caution when walking or running on uneven surfaces, poorly lit areas, or lifting some objects. The aid of visual feedback, such as lifting weights in front of a mirror, can help to offset this hazard.

In the case of individuals with visual impairments, spotting, guiding, or other visual assistance may be required. The therapist, coach, or training partner must be vigilant in identifying hazards that exist and taking action to either remove the threat or verbally inform the individual how to avoid the threat. For example, in a sport such as Goal Ball where players are either blind or required to wear a mask over their eyes, the facilitator must be sure to remove or pad all objects in the playing area and in the surrounding boundary areas prior to the start of play.

Another example of spotting required in the sport of swimming is to have a long stick or pole with a soft object attached to one end (one low cost option is a tennis ball). The facilitator will work with the athlete to identify a distance that they want to be "warned" that they are approaching the wall. When the athlete reaches that distance the facilitator will use the pole to gently tap the athlete on the head or back, warning them that the wall is only a short distance away and they should either reach out to touch the wall of the pool or initiate their flip turn.

Likewise, for individuals with hearing impairments the facilitator should thoroughly discuss potential threats prior to the start of play and discuss plans for how to communicate needs once an activity begins. For example, if an individual with a hearing impairment is engaged in cycling, the use of proper hand signals (e.g., the direction of a turn, slowing, road debris, or stopping) should be used with all participants who are riding.

Lastly, some individuals experience cognitive deficits and memory loss as a result of their disability. This can result in increased risk of injury due to lack of ability to use proper form or remember the proper sequence of events used to perform a sport or exercise. Therapists are encouraged to use verbal, written, and graphic forms of instructions and use frequent reminders on the proper form or ways to use equipment. The use of exercise partners is also encouraged as this facilitates consistent safety monitoring during the activity.

Protocols and Processes

The recommended frequency, duration, and intensity of an adaptive sports and recreation session depends entirely on the intended outcome and the setting in which the protocol is being used. A primary criticism of the therapeutic use of adaptive sports has been the lack of stated goals, objectives, and intended outcomes. For adaptive sports to be an effective therapeutic intervention, regardless of the setting in which they might be used, goals, objectives, and intended outcomes must be established prior to participation. Based on stated goals and objectives, the appropriate frequency and length of sessions can be established.

Goals, objectives, and outcomes of most adaptive sports interventions and activities tend to focus on physical outcomes in the rehabilitation setting and are varied based on individual preference in the community setting. If the focus of adaptive sports participation is in the physical domain the frequency, intensity, and duration of the session should follow recommendations for basic physical exercise or leisure time physical activity. The National Center on Health, Physical Activity, and Disability website provides a wide variety of protocol and process recommendations. Click on the "Articles" tab and then go to the "Disability/Conditions" section.

As one example, individuals who experience a spinal cord injury confront a full range of physical, social, and psychological challenges. In a rehabilitation setting these challenges often coincide with treatment goals designed to improve function and help individuals improve quality of life. Adaptive sports and recreation activities can be used in treatment to teach the individual how to cope with these challenges. Physically, a therapist can use adaptive sports to help individuals strengthen muscles weakened by paralysis. Skill-based activities, such as learning to swing a racket, bounce or shoot a ball, or ride a handcycle address functional deficiencies. The frequency, duration, and intensity of these types of activities should coincide with recommendations for physical activity and exercise for individuals with disabilities, as discussed in http://nchpad.org/14/80/Exercise~Guidelines~for~People~with~Disabilities.

The use of adaptive sports for an individual with a spinal cord injury might also address goals in the social domain. Participation in group- or team-based sports and recreation may allow the individual to meet and socialize with other individuals who are also learning to manage the emotions associated with having recently acquired a disability. It should be noted, however, it is a common recommendation among adaptive sports providers for individuals who have recently acquired a disability to wait one year prior to participating in any high intensity or impact sport. A physician's clearance should be obtained if an individual is interested in participating prior to the one-year stabilization period.

Using sports as a mechanism to provide peer support is a more natural and effective way to offer assistance without relying on a counseling model where individuals meet face to face to discuss issues. Practically speaking, individuals learn vitally important skills and how to adapt techniques and equipment to continue to participate in their favorite pastimes or learn new activities.

Community-based adaptive sports programs tend to be different in their focus and goals when compared to the rehabilitation setting discussed above. The Bridge II Sports program located in Durham, NC, has developed a "Hub Concept" to assist in the development of community-based adaptive sports and physical activity programs for individuals with disabilities (Bedini & Thomas, 2012). Bridge II Sports provides services for children and adults with a wide range of disabilities. They encourage the development of community programs using an integrated "hub" concept where community partners all adhere to one philosophy of operation. Some of the partners are local parks and recreation departments, universities, churches, public and private schools, professional organizations, Veteran's Administration hospitals, and the North Carolina School for the Blind. Bridge II Sports is a non-profit agency that successfully uses this model to offer programs in a wide geographic area including wheelchair basketball, tennis, bocce, sitting volleyball, power and sled hockey, goal ball, yoga, adapted fencing, and golf.

Outcomes and Documentation

The need for participation in physically active recreational activities for all people, with and without disabilities, has become increasingly evident. The hazards of a sedentary lifestyle and the associated complications are increasingly apparent, as the correlation between inactivity and obesity, cardiovascular disease, and other serious health problems has been established. Inactivity for an individual with a disability can be increasingly detrimental as it often

exacerbates the effects of disability (Martin & Smith, 2001) by reducing functioning and life quality. Increased activity, such as that obtained through sports participation, has been shown to decrease risks of cardiovascular disease and reduce hospital visits and admissions in people who use wheelchairs versus those who do not participate in sports (O'Neill & Maguire, 2004). Additional findings have shown that participation is sports activity facilitates the maintenance of good physical condition (b7 Neuromusculoskeletal and Movement-Related Functions), improves upper body strength (b730 Muscle Power Functions), and increases social interactions (d7 Interpersonal Interactions and Relationships) (Tasiemski et al., 2004).

The benefits of participating in adaptive sports are far greater than solely increasing base-line functioning and health-related quality of life. This is due in part to the nature of leisure settings, and more specifically sports participation. Research has demonstrated that leisure contexts are a microcosm of society, reflecting prevailing values, norms, and standards (Devine & Dattilo, 2001). Leisure situations such as adaptive sports not only provide opportunities for self-awareness, freedom, and pleasure, but additionally, they play a role in transcendence of stigma (e4 Attitudes) associated with disability (Brittain, 2004; Devine & Dattilo, 2001; Lundberg et al., 2011).

Sports, specifically, are reflective of society because each time individuals are faced with the challenge of exhibiting their physical skills during any level of sports participation, they are provided direct and immediate positive or negative feedback (Blinde & McClung, 1997; Groff & Kleiber, 2001; Phoenix, 2001). The social nature of sports activity provides individuals with the opportunity to identify with a specific group (Groff & Kleiber, 2001) and develop friendships (Lundberg et al., 2011), which in turn can increases motivation for continual participation (Martin & Smith, 2002). As community reintegration is a key concern in successful rehabilitation, the social nature of sports participation can be an asset for an individual when transitioning from the hospital or rehabilitation center back into the community (O'Neill & Maguire, 2004; Tasiemski et al., 2004). Related ICF codes can be found in d7 Interpersonal Interactions and Relationships and d9 Community, Social, and Civic Life.

From a psychological perspective, sports participation has been shown to reduce depressive mood states and anxiety (b126 Temperament and Personality Functions), while increasing a sense of vigor and vitality (b130 Energy and Drive Functions) (Lundberg, 2010; Muraki et al., 2000). More generally speaking, sports participation for individuals with disabilities improves perceptions regarding quality of life (Groff, Lundberg, & Zabriskie, 2009; O'Neill & Maguire, 2004). Sports provide an overall sense of empowerment: "The goal is to empower the individual through the sports experience by facilitating acquisition of control over personal and environmental resources in order to provide competencies usually limited through disability" (Pensgaard & Sorensen, 2002, p. 51). Sports participation has also been associated with the satisfaction of psychological needs and self-determination (Lundberg, Groff, & Zabriskie, 2010).

The ICF provides a comprehensive framework for organizing outcomes associated with participation in adaptive sports. Designed to measure both the functioning and the disability of an individual, the ICF emphasizes the need to capture an individual's impairments in addition to their strengths and environmental factors that impede or facilitate participation and activity. The following section outlines areas that may be targeted for treatment through participation in adaptive sports.

Body Functions

It is well known that body functions are positively impacted by sports and physical activity. Impairments of body functions that may be improved through adaptive sports include: blood pressure (b420 Blood Pressure Functions), heart rate (b410 Heart Functions), weight maintenance (b530 Weight Maintenance Functions), pain (b280 Sensation of Pain), sleep (b134 Sleep Functions), energy and drive (b130 Energy and Drive Functions), range of motion (b710 Mobility of Joint Functions), muscle tone (b735 Muscle Tone Functions), muscle strength (b730 Muscle Power Functions), and general flexibility (b710 Mobility of Joint Functions). Given that these body functions fall within the scope of various disciplines, recreational therapists might consider collaborating with members of the interdisciplinary teams to further enhance the assessment of body functions that may be positively impacted by adap-

tive sports. Some common assessment methods for measuring body functions include vital signs (blood pressure, heart rate, oxygen saturation level, respiration), body weight, waist circumference, the 0-10 pain scale, client logs (e.g., sleep, energy level, appetite, muscle spasms), goniometer measures for active range of motion, and strength assessment using amount of weight and repetitions and/or the *Manual Muscle Exam*.

In addition to physical skills, adaptive sports can also improve cognitive, psychological, and emotional functions, such as: mood and behavior (b126 Temperament and Personality Functions), energy and drive (b130 Energy and Drive Functions), emotions (b152 Emotional Functions), attention (b140 Attention Functions), cognitive flexibility and other higher-level cognitive skills (b164 Higher-Level Cognitive Functions), confidence (b1266 Confidence), and body image and experience of self (b180 Experience of Self and Time Functions). There are a variety of standardized assessment tools that can be used to measure functions in these areas. Care should be taken to identify reliable and valid assessments tools that are appropriate for the age, gender, and functional level of each participant. A few examples of assessment measures used by recreational therapists include:

Profile of Mood States — Brief (POMS-B): The POMS-B can be used to assess mood states and total mood disturbance (Curren, Andrykowski, & Studts, 1995; McNair & Heuchert, 2005; Shacham, 1983). The POMS-B is a 30-item Likert scale which contains five items for six different mood states including fatigue, vigor, tension, depression, anger, and confusion. Individual items are scored from zero to four with higher scores indicating higher levels of mood state disturbance. A total mood disturbance score or individual-factor mood state scores can be generated and used for comparisons. The total mood disturbance score is obtained by totaling all factors except for vigor, which is subtracted from the other factors to obtain the total score. Internal consistency for each of the six factors shows alpha coefficients ranging from .84 to .95 (McNair & Heuchert, 2005).

Positive and Negative Affect Schedule (PANAS): The PANAS is a 20-item test that is designed to describe different feelings and emotions (e.g., interested, guilty, alert, afraid). Individuals identify from a scale of one (very slightly or not at all) to five (extremely), the extent that they feel that way at the present moment. The individual will derive an overall Positive affect and an overall Negative affect score that ranges from 10 to 50. The reliability of the measure has been established for both constructs of PA (r = .89) and NA (r = .85). Normative data is available for individuals without disabilities (Crawford & Henry, 2004).

STROOP Test: The STROOP test is commonly used as a standard part of neuropsychological tests to assess executive function, reaction time, and information processing and has been validated for use in a vast array of situations (Lezak, Howieson, & Loring, 2004). The test consists of a series of words that are names of colors (red, yellow, blue, green, and orange). To begin the words are printed in black and the individual's simple reaction time is assessed based on how many seconds it takes to read the word. Next, the words appear in colored ink that can either match the word or may be different. For example, Blue may be written in blue ink or the word Blue could appear in yellow ink. The increased amount of time it takes an individual to read the list of words that appear in disharmonious color pairs indicates reaction time, attention, and cognitive flexibility. The test is readily available in on-line or paper versions.

Physical Self-Perception Profile (PSPP): The PSPP measures an individual's perception of physical aspects of the self (Fox & Corbin, 1989). The PSPP uses five subscales to measure physical self-esteem including sports competence, physical condition, bodily attractiveness, physical strength, and overall physical self-worth. The 30-item instrument uses six questions to represent each subscale. Questions are comprised of two general statements (e.g., "Some people feel that they are not very good when it comes to playing sports, BUT, Others feel that they are really good at just about every sport."). Individuals respond to each question by first selecting the general statement which best reflects their beliefs and then indicating if that statement is "Really true for me" or "Sort of true for me."

Activities and Participation

Recreational therapists are probably best trained to facilitate improvements in activities and participation. As mentioned earlier, use of task analysis is central to a comprehensive measurement of activities and participation, and thus recreational therapists

should reply heavily on this skill when measuring potential areas of improvement provided through any given adapted sport. For example, although consistent participation in weight lifting and yoga are both likely to result in improved muscular strength, weight lifting will provide a much different type of strength than will yoga. Weight training, if performed properly, is likely a more effective way to build muscle bulk, and yoga a more effective way to improve muscle tone, endurance, and flexibility. The choice of activity depends on the treatment team's assessment of what the patient needs.

Recreational therapists can use the ICF model to help identify how adaptive sports can improve activities and participation. Learning how to learn skills (d155 Acquiring Skills, d160 Focusing Attention, d175 Solving Problems, d210 Undertaking a Single Task) may be the first objective if the patient has a deficit in skill acquisition. Learning how to ride a bike, water ski, canoe, hike, play bocce, or do T'ai Chi will all result in improvement in sports-specific skills and knowledge (many areas of d4 Mobility and d710 Basic Interpersonal Interactions). These can easily be measured through behavioral objectives, direct observation, interviews, and basic skills assessment tests.

The application of sports-specific knowledge to other areas of life is another potential area of assessment. For example, through sports an individual might improve wheelchair mobility skills (d465 Moving Around Using Equipment) as s/he learns to properly turn, push, and maneuver in the game. These skills can transfer to daily activity and thus be measured through improved mobility skills, especially the ability to navigate a wheelchair in other environments such as home, school, or in the community (d460 Moving Around in Different Locations). There is the potential for adapted sport to influence every area of Activities and Participation in the ICF codes. The proper areas to target are determined by the assessment of the patient and linking the adaptive sports activity to the particular skills needed for the deficit being addressed. For example, a deficit noted in d620 Acquisition of Goods and Services might be addressed by an adaptive sport that included skill training in wheelchair mobility, ability to reach for and carry objects, and assertiveness required to ask teammates for help when required.

Measurement of many of the activity and participation outcomes can be accomplished through a direct review of goals and behavior objectives. Other more standardized measures that have been used by recreational therapists in studies on adaptive sports include:

WHO Quality of Life (WHOQOL-BREF): The WHOQOL-BREF is a generic measurement of quality of life applicable to a wide variety of individuals from differing cultures, living conditions, and health status (WHOQOL Group, 2005). The WHOQOL-BREF contains 26 items categorized into four domains: physical health, psychological health, social relationships, and environment, with two questions that can be analyzed separately focusing on overall quality of life and satisfaction with health. Scores are tabulated on a five-point Likert scale with higher scores indicating higher quality of life. Research has indicated that WHOQOL-BREF scores demonstrate good discriminate, criterion, and content validity; internal consistency; and test-retest reliability (WHOQOL Group, 2005).

Influence on Quality of Life Scale (IQLS): The IQLS was developed in an effort to measure an individual's perception of the influence on their quality of life that resulted from participation in a particular sport, program, or experience (Groff, Zabriskie, & Lundberg, 2009). The IQLS asks respondents to agree or disagree with five statements regarding the influence of adaptive sports on quality of life. Items include the perceived influence of adaptive sports on overall health, quality of life, quality of family life, and quality of social life. Items are scored on a seven-point Likert scale with responses ranging from "Strongly disagree" to "Strongly agree." Total scores for the instrument can range from five to 35 with higher scores indicating that adaptive sports had a more significant impact on perceived quality of life. The IQLS has acceptable internal consistency (0.87).

Athletic Identity Measurement Scale (AIMS): The AIMS is a 10-item instrument that measures athletic identity via three subscales: exclusivity, social identity, and negative affectivity (Brewer, Van Raalte, & Linder, 1993). A seven-point Likert scale is used with responses ranging from "Strongly disagree" to "Strongly agree." Total AIMS scores can range from 10 to 70, with high scores demonstrating strength and exclusivity of identification with the athletic role.

Internal consistency for the overall scale has been reported as 0.93 with test-retest reliability at 0.89. The instrument has been validated for use with athletes with disabilities but caution should be used when interpreting the "social identity" subdomain scores. Score in this domain may be lower for athletes with disabilities compared with normative data for athletes without disabilities (Groff & Zabriskie, 2006).

Perceived Competence Scale (PCS): The PCS is a short four-item questionnaire with individual items ranging from one to seven and the total score ranging from four to 28. Items on the PCS reflect the individual's level of perceived competence in successfully completing an identified behavior. Results have typically indicated a Cronbach's alpha of .80. This scale has been modified to determine an individual's competence in performing sports-related tasks consistent with the program in which s/he participated (Lundberg, Bennett, & Smith, 2011).

Self-Determination in Sport (SDIS): The SDIS is a modified instrument that measures need satisfaction through sports participation (Lundberg, Groff, & Zabriskie, 2010). The SDIS consists of 21 items to be answered on a Likert scale ranging from one, not at all true, to seven, very true. Higher scores represent higher satisfaction of basic psychological needs through sports participation. The SDIS has seven questions relating to autonomy, six questions relating to competence, and eight questions focusing on relatedness. Three items in each subscale are reverse-scored. The subscales can be used separately or totaled to form an overall self-determination score. Testing for internal consistency indicated an alpha coefficient of .86 for the SDIS.

Environmental Factors

Individuals with disabilities face a myriad of barriers that may preclude their participation in physically active lifestyles and adaptive sports (Lollar, 2002). Chief among these barriers are lack of accessible fitness and recreational facilities, presence of architectural barriers in the environment (e150 Design, Construction, and Building Products and Technology of Buildings for Public Use), limited discretionary income due to increased medical expenses and unemployment (e565 Economic Services, Systems, and Policies, e575 General Social Support Services, Systems, and Policies), lack of social support (e3 Support and Relationships), unsupportive public policy (e5 Services, Systems, and Policies), and the presence of societal attitudes and norms (e4 Attitudes) which often discourage them from being active and engaged citizens (Centers for Disease Control and Prevention, 2002). Due to poor community planning, lack of communication and coordination of services, fragmentation of community partners in considering design options, and lack of commitment on the part of decision-makers to create policy that demands activity-friendly environments, communities can contribute to the poor health of individuals with disabilities (Humpel, Owen, & Leslie, 2002; Rimmer, et al., 2004). The ICF model recognizes and values the impact of the environment on health and functioning and thus opens another potential area for assessment when considering adaptive sports.

Recreational therapists can measure the impact of the environment on participation in adaptive sports by conducting an assessment of the accessibility of facilities and services, and by helping to create an infrastructure that supports physically active behavior for individuals with disabilities. Assessing the physical and social environment may appear to be a daunting task, but there are some excellent resources available for recreational therapists. The Robert Woods Johnson Foundation supports research in the area of environmental influence and considers parks and recreation as a vital resource, thus, they have developed several measurements tools available online. These tools include the *Active Neighborhood Checklist*, the *Community Park Audit Tool*, the *Healthy Afterschool Activity and Nutrition Documentation*, and the *Rural Active Living Perceived Environmental Support Scale* (http://activelivingresearch.org/toolsandresources/toolsandmeasures).

Other online assessment resources are available through the North Carolina Office on Disability and Health (www.fpg.unc.edu/projects/north-carolina-office-disability-and-health-ncodh), an organization that promotes the health and wellness of individuals with disabilities across the lifespan. The organization has developed an online publication and assessment tool for professionals interested in accommodating people with disabilities in health and fitness facilities. The guide is an excellent resource for recreational therapists who wish to assess environmental factors related to active lifestyles often associated with participation in adaptive sports (www.fpg.unc.edu/resources/removing-barriers-health-clubs-and-fitness-facilities-guide-accommodating-all-members-incl).

Once a proper assessment of a fitness facility has been conducted, the National Center on Health, Physical Activity, and Disability has an online tool designed to help facilitate the layout of fitness centers to accommodate persons with disabilities interested in adapted fitness and exercise (www.nchpad.org/fitnessCenter/index.html).

Therapists can also use simple measurement counts to determine basic environmental facilitators or barriers in a given community. A tally of the number of accessible trails in a given area or the number of accessible community programs available might give an initial indication of how environmental factors influence participation.

Resources

The following resources give the reader a wide variety of options and ideas when working in the area of adaptive sports. The list, unfortunately, is not all-inclusive, as additional resources continue to become available on a regular basis. This list is only a starting place. In our internet age you will find a wide variety of information by doing a simple search online.

Books

Paciorek, M. J. & Jones, J. A. (2001). *Disability sport and recreation resources* **(3rd ed.). Traverse City, MI: Cooper Publishing Group.**
While there are many valuable books to consider, this one stands out as an indispensable resource. It covers an extensive list of sports with accompanying equipment modifications, various guidelines and recommendations, online resources, organizing bodies, and other valuable information. If you are limited to one source of information on adaptive sports, this book is the right place to start.

DePauw, K. P. & Gavron, S. J. (2005) *Disability sport* **(2nd ed.). Champaign, IL: Human Kinetics.**
This 400-page book provides a comprehensive review of the history and future of disabled sports. A vast array of topics are reviewed including: terminology, sport organization and competitions, international perspectives of sports, coaching principles,

sports medicine, event management, ethical and gender issues, and the future of disabled sports.

Dattilo, J. & McKenney, A. (2011). *Facilitation techniques in therapeutic recreation* (2ⁿᵈ ed.).
This book has two chapters that may be helpful to therapists interested in using adaptive sports and recreation with clients. Broach and Richardson (2011) have elaborated on the "Therapeutic Use of Exercise," and Dattilo, McKenney, and Loy (2011) discuss the "Therapeutic Use of Sports."

Internet Sources

National Center on Health, Physical Activity, and Disability (NCHPAD)
www.nchpad.org.
This is one of the most all-inclusive sites. Information provided on this website covers diverse topics including how to start your own program, the importance of health and nutrition, specific information on disability conditions, information on exercise and fitness, a list of competitive sports, an update on the latest research, video segments, feedback from users, and a wide variety of other helpful information. The range of adaptive sports covered include track and field, sitting volleyball, table tennis, swimming, wheelchair basketball, weight lifting, wheelchair tennis, goal ball, bocce, cycling and hand cycling, rugby, soccer, sledge hockey, alpine skiing, Nordic skiing, wheelchair softball, wheelchair football, power soccer, and golf. In addition, NCHPAD provides a free 14-week web-based, personalized physical activity and nutrition program that individuals with disabilities can sign up for at http://nchpad.org/14weeks/. Populations include individuals with mobility, chronic health, and physical disabilities with the goal of promoting wellness and active lifestyles. Services provided by the free web-based modules include a coach, weekly exercise, physical activity and nutrition tips, weekly recipes, tools to track your progress toward weekly goals, and opportunities to connect with other participants.

Organizations

A wide variety of adaptive sports organizations exist providing programs and other resources locally, nationally, and internationally. It is not feasible to provide an exhaustive sport-by-sport or state-by-state list of resources. Many of these organizations, however, can be found through a simple internet search.

Other organizations offer a wide variety of sports, chapter organizations in various states, and provide nationwide educational or advocacy-related events. While this is not an exhaustive list, start here to look up resources and find adaptive sports and recreation programs in your area.

Access to Recreation
www.accesstr.com/AMAZING/index.asp

Blaze Sports America
www.blazesports.org/

Disabled Sports USA
www.disabledsportsusa.org/

International Paralympic Committee
www.paralympic.org/

National Center on Accessibility
www.ncaonline.org/

Special Olympics International
http://specialolympics.org

U.S. National Sports Center for the Disabled
www.nscd.org/

Wheelchair and Ambulatory Sports USA
www.wasusa.org/

References

Bedini, L. & Thomas, A. (2012). Bridge II Sports: A model of meaningful activity through community-adapted sports. *Therapeutic Recreation Journal, 46*(4), 284-300.

Blinde, E. M. & McClung, L. R. (1997). Enhancing the physical and social self through recreation activity: Accounts of individuals with physical disabilities. *Adapted Physical Activity Quarterly, 14*, 327-344.

Brewer, B., Van Raalte, J., & Linder, D. (1993). Athletic identity: Hercules' muscle or Achilles heel? *International Journal of Sport Psychology, 24*, 237-254.

Brittain, I. (2004). Perceptions of disability and their impact upon involvement in sport for people with disability at all levels. *Journal of Sport & Social Issues, 28*(4), 429-452.

Broach, E. & Richardson, N. (2011). Therapeutic use of exercise. In J. Dattilo & A. McKenney (Eds.). *Facilitation Techniques in Therapeutic Recreation* (pp. 441-487). State College, PA: Venture.

Bullock, C. C. & Mahon, M. J. (1997). *Introduction to recreation services for people with disabilities.* Champaign, IL: Sagamore Publishing.

Centers for Disease Control and Prevention. (2002). Short form of the international physical activity questionnaire. (available at: www.ipaq.ki.se/ipaq.htm).

Crawford, J. R. & Henry, J. D. (2004). The positive and negative affect schedule (PANAS): Construct validity, measurement properties and normative data in a large non-clinical sample. *British Journal of Clinical Psychology, 43*, 245-265.

Curren, S., Andrykowski, M. & Studts, J. (1995). Short form of the profile of mood states (POMS-SF): Psychometric information. *Psychological Assessment, 7*(1), 80-83.

Dattilo, J., McKenney, A., & Loy, D. (2011). Therapeutic use of sport. In J. Dattilo & A. McKenney (Eds.). *Facilitation Techniques in Therapeutic Recreation* (pp. 551-591). State College, PA: Venture.

DePauw, K. P. & Gavron, S. J. (2005) *Disability sport* (2nd ed.). Champaign, IL: Human Kinetics.

Devine, M. A. & Dattilo, J. (2001). Social acceptance and leisure lifestyles of people with disabilities. *Therapeutic Recreation Journal, 34*(4), 306-322.

Fox, K. R. & Corbin, C. B. (1989). The physical self-perception profile: Development and preliminary validation. *Journal of Sport & Exercise Psychology, 11*(4), 408-430.

Groff, D. G. & Kleiber, D. A. (2001). Exploring the identity formation of youth in an adapted sports program. *Therapeutic Recreation Journal, 35*(4)318-332.

Groff, D., Lawrence, E., & Grivna, S. (2006). Effects of a therapeutic recreation intervention using exercise: A case study with a child with cerebral palsy. *Therapeutic Recreation Journal, 25*(4), 269-283.

Groff, D., Lundberg, N., & Zabriskie, R., (2009). Influence of adapted sport on quality of life: Perceptions of athletes with cerebral palsy. *Disability and Rehabilitation, 31*(4), 318-326.

Groff, D. & Zabriskie, R. (2006). An exploratory study of athletic identity among elite alpine skiers with disabilities: Issues of measurement and design. *Journal of Sport Behavior, 29*(2), 1-16.

Groff, D., Zabriskie, R., & Lundberg, N. (2009). Influence of adapted sport on quality of life: Perceptions of athletes with cerebral palsy. *Disability and Rehabilitation, 41*(4), 318-326.

Holland, L. J. & Steadward, R. D. (1990). Effects of resistance in flexibility training and strength, spasticity/muscle tone and range of motion of elite athletes with cerebral palsy. *Palestra,* Summer, 27-31.

Humpel, N., Owen, N., & Leslie, E. (2002). Environmental factors associated with adults' participation in physical activity. *American Journal of Preventive Medicine, 22*(3), 188-199.

Lakowski, T. & Henkel, D. (2013). *New guidance will enhance sports opportunities for students with disabilities inclusive fitness coalition compares impact to title IX* (Retrieved August 18, 2013 at www.nchpad.org/1032/5348/New~Guidance~Will~Enhance~Sports~Opportunities~for~Students~with~Disabilities~Inclusive~Fitness~Coalition~compares~impact~to~Title~IX).

Lezak, M. D., Howieson, D. B., & Loring, D. W. (2004). *Neuropsychological assessment* (4th ed.). New York: Oxford University Press.

Lollar, D. J. (2002, March/April). Public health and disability: Emerging opportunities. *Public Health Reports, 117*, 131-137.

Lundberg, N. (2010). Quality of life and mood state outcomes through participation in adaptive sports for individuals with physical disabilities: A pre-experimental examination. *Annual in Therapeutic Recreation, 19,* 104-112.

Lundberg, N., Bennett, J., & Smith, S. (2011). Adaptive sports participation among veterans returning from combat with acquired disabilities. *Therapeutic Recreation Journal, 45*(2), 105-119.

Lundberg, N., Groff, D., & Zabriskie, R. (2010). Psychological need satisfaction through sports participation among international athletes with cerebral palsy. *Annals of Leisure Research, 13*(1 & 2), 102-115.

Lundberg, N., Taniguchi, S., McCormick, B., & Tibbs, C. (2011). Identity negotiating: Re-defining stigmatized identities through recreational sports participation among individuals with physical disability. *Journal of Leisure Research, 43*(2), 205-225.

Maiano, C., Ninot, G., Morin, J., & Bilard, J. (2007). Effects of sport participation on the basketball skills and physical self of adolescents with conduct disorders. *Adapted Physical Activity Quarterly, 24*, 178-196.

Martin, J. & Smith, K. (2001). Friendship quality in youth disability sport: Perceptions of a best friend. *Adapted Physical Activity Quarterly, 19*, 472-482.

McNair, D. M. & Heuchert, J. P. (2005). *Profile of mood states technical update.* North Tonawanda, NY: Multi-Health Systems Inc.

Muraki, S., Tsunawake, N., Hiramatsu, S., & Yamasaki, M. (2000). The effects of frequency and mode of sports activity on the psychological status in tetraplegics and paraplegics. *Spinal Cord, 38*, 309-314.

O'Neill, S. B. & Maguire, S. (2004). Patient perception of the impact of sporting activity on rehabilitation in a spinal cord injuries unit. *Spinal Cord, 42*, 627-630.

Pensgaard, A. & Sorensen, M. (2002). Empowerment through the sport context: A model to guide research for individuals with disabilities. *Adapted Physical Activity Quarterly, 19*, 48-67.

Rimmer, J. H., Chen, M., McCubbin, J. A., Drum, C., Peterson, J. (2010). Exercise intervention research on persons with disabilities: What we know and where we need to go. *American Journal of Physical Medicine & Rehabilitation, 89*(3), 249-263.

Rimmer, J. H., Riley, B., Wang, E., Rauwroth, A., & Jurkowski, J. (2004). Physical activity participation among persons with disabilities: Barriers and facilitators. *American Journal of Preventative Medicine, 26*(5), 419-425.

Santiago, M. C., Coyle, C. P., & Kinney, M. W. (1993). Aerobic exercise effect on individuals with physical disabilities. *Archives of Physical Medicine and Rehabilitation, 74*(11):1192-1198.

Shacham, S. (1983). A shortened version of the profile of mood states. *Journal of Personality Assessment, 47*(3), 305-306.

Tasiemski, T., Kennedy, P., Gardner, B., & Blaikley, R., (2004). Athletic identity and sports participation in people with spinal cord injury. *Adapted Physical Activity Quarterly, 21*, 364-378.

National Center for Physical Activity, and Disability. (2013). *Recommendations for flexibility and range of motion exercises and rheumatoid arthritis.* http://nchpad.org/112/882/Rheumatoid~Arthritis~and~Exercise#sthash.wSetRpbS.dpufRetrieved August 18, 2013 at http://nchpad.org/112/882/Rheumatoid~Arthritis~and~Exercise. retrieved August 18, 2013.

Phoenix, T. L. (2001). Who am I? Identity formation, youth, and therapeutic recreation. *Therapeutic Recreation Journal, 35*(4), 348-356.

United States Department of Health and Human Services. (2005). *The Surgeon General's call to action to improve the health and wellness of persons with disabilities.* U.S. Department of Health and Human Services, Office of the Surgeon General. Available at: www.surgeongeneral.gov/library/calls/disabilities/calltoaction.pdf.

United States Government Accountability Office. (June 2010). *Students with disabilities: More information and guidance could improve opportunities in physical education and athletics.* No. GAO-10-519, 1, 31. Available at: www.gao.gov/assets/310/305770.pdf.

Warburton, E. R., Nicol, C. W., & Bredin, S. D (2006). Health benefits of physical activity: The evidence. *Canadian Medical Association Journal, 174*(6), 801-809.

WHOQOL Group. (2005). *The World Health Organization Quality of Life instruments: U.S. version WHOQOL-100 and importance items user's manual and interpretation guide.* WA: WHOQOL Group.

Wilhite, B., Biren, G., & Spencer, L. (2012). Fitness intervention for adults with developmental disabilities and their caregivers. *Therapeutic Recreation Journal, 46*(4), 245-267.

13. Adventure Therapy

Elaine M. Hatala

A brief history of the inception and evolution of adventure therapy (AT) provides an important perspective to understand its core values and enormous potential. AT, used as a treatment modality by recreational therapists and other professionals around the world, has its roots in America. The first generation of AT began in the early 20th century when patients with tuberculosis at the state hospital in Manhattan, New York City, were forced to reside in tents on the hospital grounds due to overcrowding. An unforeseen result of this "tent treatment" was that patients showed improved physical and mental health. Similarly, an early 20th century earthquake in San Francisco forced patients to live in tents on hospital grounds and they too showed marked improvement in health and socialization.

Gibson (1979) and White (2012) present extensive histories of AT, tracing the roots of AT from summer camp in the late 1800s to "tent treatment." They discuss observations in the 1930s that camp was an effective therapeutic setting for troubled youth and look at organizations, such as Outward Bound (OB), that took adjudicated and troubled youth into the wilderness for extended periods of time. More recently Project Adventure brought adventure into schools, communities, and corporations.

AT has deep and historic roots in OB. During WW II, Kurt Hahn, an educator from Germany, was hired by a British shipping company to train young sailors who were dying at a higher rate than their older counterparts when their ships were torpedoed. Hahn concluded that the young sailors lacked qualities such as confidence, resilience, problem-solving skills, stamina, and life experiences that their older peers possessed. This observation led to Hahn's development of OB trips that consisted of rigorous 26-day sailing, trekking, rescue training, and service programs to impel young men to develop the qualities they lacked and to recognize their true capabilities. Hahn stressed core values of fitness, initiative and enterprise, memory and imagination, skill and care, self-discipline, and, most importantly, compassion. These are qualities that Hahn believed were missing from the younger generation, largely precipitated by the industrial revolution. Programs were designed to be highly challenging in order to prepare young men for circumstances at sea and in life.

OB expanded into the United States in 1962. Today OB is a worldwide organization that continues to provide extended wilderness courses for at-risk youth and troubled teens as it did in the company's early years. OB also provides courses in the U.S. and worldwide for adults, war veterans (Outward Bound for Veterans, n.d. a), and youth who seek challenge and opportunity to develop the qualities espoused by Kurt Hahn. Prominent adventure-based organizations in the United States such as the National Outdoor Leadership School (NOLS) and Project Adventure are rooted in Outward Bound. Likewise, adventure programming, adventure therapy, wilderness therapy, school-based adventure programs, experience-based training and development, and professional organizations such as the Association for Experiential Education (AEE) all have their roots in Outward Bound.

Adventure Therapy and Wilderness Therapy

AT is an evolving discipline that integrates activities, processes, and practices characteristic of outdoor adventure programming into clinical interventions that may occur indoors or outdoors. There are several terms that practitioners and researchers use interchangeably when referring to AT. As is typical of newer disciplines, a concise definition of AT is evolving. While the interchangeable use of terms and lack of a concise definition does slow the progress of AT, hinder research efforts, and confuse practitioners and clients, the process is typical of a burgeoning field. Recreational therapy, steeped in activity and processing, can play an active role in the evolution of the field and a concise definition of practice.

Therapeutic adventure, adventure-based counseling, experiential therapy, wilderness therapy (WT), and wilderness adventure therapy are common terms found in the literature and used interchangeably with AT. Project Adventure, an organization that has played a pivotal role in the establishment and growth of adventure education and AT in the United States, uses the term adventure-based counseling (ABC) and defines it as "a group counseling model that uses a carefully sequenced and processed series of experiential activities to elicit behavior change. ABC group members share in an engaging, effective, counseling-oriented experience" (Project Adventure, n.d.).

In the RT literature, AT has been described as using outdoor experiential activities to accomplish treatment-related goals (Dattilo, 2000). Elsewhere, AT is defined as "the prescriptive use of adventure experiences provided by mental health professionals, often conducted in natural settings that kinesthetically engage clients on cognitive, affective, and behavioral levels" (Gass, Gillis, & Russell, 2012, p. 1).

Like AT, a clear definition of WT has been difficult to establish. Foundational definitions in the literature are replete with anecdote and early research lacks the methodological rigor required for generalization and replication (Davis-Berman & Berman, 1989). Characteristics of WT include the use of clinical and therapeutic methods in wilderness environments, group therapy, educational and therapeutic sessions, social skills training, and backcountry skill development (Russell & Farnum, 2004). Mental health and substance abuse issues are frequently addressed in WT (Davis-Berman & Berman, 1989).

Though AT and WT are frequently used interchangeably, it is important to make a distinction between AT and WT. While both AT and WT share common roots, philosophies, and practices, in that they both focus on developing trust, cooperation, communication, and problem-solving skills (Bandoroff & Scherer, 1994) they have distinct features.

For the purposes of this chapter three prominent differences will be highlighted.

One distinguishing feature between AT and WT is *the degree to which natural environments are used in the treatment process* (Gass, Gillis, & Russell, 2012). Crisp (1996) describes AT as facility based compared to WT which is wilderness based. Additionally, some components of an AT program (e.g., cooperative activities, trust activities, problem-solving activities, and processing) may routinely be conducted in indoor settings or outdoor settings that are not considered wilderness, while other components (e.g., rock climbing, ropes course) are conducted outdoors (Newes & Bandoroff, 2004). WT programs are residential treatment programs housed in the wilderness. Under the care of mental health professionals 24-hours a day, clients spend an extended time in the wilderness. Greenway (1995) suggests that WT programs should last for a minimum of seven days. In a study of treatment outcomes across eight outdoor behavioral health programs, clients were in treatment for an average of 28 days (Russell, 2001b). Backcountry wilderness is at least two hours away from metropolitan areas (Gass, Gillis, & Russell, 2012).

Another distinguishing feature between AT and WT is the *degree to which adventure experiences are used in an individual's treatment process* (Gass, Gillis, & Russell, 2012). AT is typically considered an adjunct therapy (Clark & Kempler, 1973; Ewert, McCormick, & Voight, 2001; Hatala, 1992; Hyer et al., 1994; Scheinfeld, Rochlen, & Buser, 2011; Wolf & Mehl, 2011) where adventure experiences are one of several different interventions in a treatment process. It is common for AT to be one of several different treatment modalities in an RT program. RTs typically facilitate AT in an hour-long to full-day session format, and in some cases overnight stays in the outdoors. On the other hand, in WT programs adventure activities are primary. Survival skills and the natural consequences of living in nature for an extended period of time are integral to the treatment process.

Finally, *client populations in AT compared to WT programs may differ*. As will be discussed later in this chapter, AT interventions are used across a variety of clinical populations while WT clients are almost exclusively youth with emotional and behavioral problems who were previously in residential treatment centers or counseling settings where their needs were not adequately met (Russell, 2006). Whereas the ages of clients who participate in AT programs vary widely, the age of WT participants is typically 12-17 years old (Russell, 2006). For a more in-depth examination of wilderness therapy refer to Bandoroff and Scherer, (1994), Becker (2010), Davis-Berman and Berman (1989, 1994), Hill (2007), Houston et al. (2010), Russell, (2001a, 2001b, 2006), and Russell, Hendee, and Phillips-Miller (2000).

Outdoor Behavioral Healthcare Programs

Recreational therapists should be aware that in the United States, WT has a growing presence in treatment options for adolescents with persistent behavioral, mental health, and substance abuse problems. This relatively new field of wilderness treatment is referred to as Outdoor Behavior Health (OBH). Since the early days of WT, characterized by lack of standard practice and oversight, the industry has evolved in terms of professionalization and licensure (Russell, 2006). The establishment of the Outdoor Behavioral Healthcare Industry Council (OBHIC) and the National Association of Therapeutic Schools and Programs (NATSP) underscore the increased presence and professionalization of WT in the United States.

The Outdoor Behavioral Healthcare Industry Council was established in 1997 the by a group of OBH organizations to advance the OBH industry through effective treatment and best practices. In 1999 the OBHIC established the Outdoor Behavioral Healthcare Research Cooperative (OBHRC) to conduct comprehensive research of OBH programs in the United States. In 2012 the OBHIC revitalized the Wilderness Therapy Symposium which was first held at Naropa University in 2003 and continued annually until 2010.

The National Association of Therapeutic Schools and Programs (NATSAP) was established in 1999 as a national resource for professionals and programs that provide therapeutic and/or behavioral healthcare services in the United States. Member organizations of NATSAP are required to be licensed by state agencies that oversee therapeutic and/or behavioral health programs for youth, or accredited by national behavioral health accreditation organizations. Additionally, member programs are required to provide

therapeutic services and maintain oversight by a qualified clinician.

Through licensure, clinical oversight, research, integration of evidence-based practices, and professional development, OBH programs have distinguished themselves from other wilderness programs such as Brat Camps and Boot Camps that are portrayed as therapeutic. While popularized in the media, these Brat Camps and Boot Camps have been characterized as militaristic and using harsh and cruel punishment (Gass, Gillis, & Russell, 2012). These programs lack evidence for clinical indication and effectiveness, and do not meet standards of practice established and supported by OBHIC and NATSAP.

Characteristics of Adventure Therapy

Despite what can seem like a multitude of terms and definitions associated with AT, there are several characteristics of AT that are common across settings and populations. In addition to mental health counseling techniques, AT is characterized as

- steeped in experiential and constructivist learning paradigms (Crisp, 1996; Gass, 1993a)
- including challenge, uncertainty, risk, novelty and fun (Haras & Bunting, 2005)
- focusing on group interactions associated with trust, cooperation, communication, and problem solving (Crisp, 1996; Berman & Davis-Berman, 1995; Newes & Bandoroff, 2004; Schoel, Prouty, & Radcliffe, 1988)
- consisting of group development activities that may include activities such as low and high ropes courses (Gillis, Gass, & Russell, 2008)
- having a clearly defined program goal (Ewert, McCormick, & Voight, 2001)
- conducted by qualified facilitators (Gass, 1993a; Gass, Gillis, & Russell, 2012)
- having individual assessments (Ewert et al., 2001; Russell, 2001a)
- establishing individual treatment goals with documented treatment progress and outcomes (Ewert et al., 2001; Russell, 2001a)
- monitoring treatment effectiveness and adjusting treatment to meet the needs of the client (Ewert et al., 2001; Russell, 2001a)
- utilizing cooperative activities as the primary (if not exclusive) genre of activities, where competitive activities are infrequent and competition

between individuals or groups is largely discouraged (Schoel, Prouty, & Radcliffe, 1988)

Benefits of Adventure Therapy

Clients who participate in AT programs have demonstrated improvements and increases in:

- self-concept (Cook, 2008; Jelalian, Sato, & Hart, 2011; Kyriakopoulos, 2011; Wu & Hsieh, 2006).
- relationships and social skills (Glass & Benshoff, 2002; Herbert, 1998; Jelalian et al., 2011; Kyriakopoulos, 2011; Portrie-Bethke, Hill, & Bethke, 2009; Tucker, 2009)
- self-esteem (Herbert, 1998; Lambie et al., 2000; Lemmon, Latourette, & Hauver, 1996; Schell, Cotton, & Luxmoore, 2012; Stevens et al., 2004; Wick, Wick, & Peterson, 1997)
- self-confidence (Clem, Smith, & Richards, 2012; Herskowitz, 1990; Leberman, 2007; Sugerman, 2005)
- self-efficacy (Clem et al., 2012; Tucker, Sugerman, & Zelov, 2013; Wolf & Mehl, 2011)
- locus of control (Hans, 2000; Herbert, 1998; Luckner, 1989; Wolf & Mehl, 2011)
- resilience (Bloemhoff, 2006; Green, Kleiber, & Tarrant, 2000; Lam, Cohen, & Rotter, 2013; Lee, Shek, & Kwong, 2007; SAMHSA, 2012; Walsh & Aubry, 2007; Wynn, Frost, & Pawson, 2012)

Some clients who participated in AT programs showed decreases in symptoms such as:

- anxiety (Hyer et al., 1996; Jelalian et al., 2011; Jorngarden, Mattsson, & von Essen, 2007; Kyriakopoulos, 2011; Santucci, 2013; Wolf & Mehl, 2011)
- depression (Jorngarden et al., 2007; Kyriakopoulos, 2011; Tucker, Javorski, et al., 2013; Wolf & Mehl, 2011)
- post-traumatic symptoms (Attarian & Gault, 1992; Gelkopf et al., 2013; Hyer et al., 1996; Outward Bound, n.d. a; Ragsdale et al., 1996)

Indications

To date, AT is most frequently indicated for adolescents with mental health and substance abuse diagnoses. This reflects the historic roots of AT in camp and Outward Bound programs that served adjudicated youth, at-risk youth, and youth diagnosed with anxiety, depression and substance abuse disorders. AT can be used to treat a large number of

deficits found in ICF codes, such as b126 Temperament and Personality Functions, b130 Energy and Drive Functions, b180 Experience of Self and Time Functions, d175 Solving Problems, d210 Undertaking a Single Task, d3 Communication, and d7 Interpersonal Interactions and Relationships. Other issues related to ICF codes are discussed in the Outcomes section.

The majority of AT research has focused on adolescents 12-18 years old (Gass et al., 2012). Bettmann and Jasperson (2008) note that there is a dearth of research that examines AT with adults. Because the nature and treatment of many conditions vary greatly from childhood and adolescence to adulthood, researchers generally examine the effectiveness and outcomes of AT relative to a specific population. The literature below that indicates AT as an appropriate and effective treatment intervention is organized according to age group and diagnosis or population group.

Children and Adolescents

- depression and anxiety (Autry, 2001; Clark et al., 2004; Cook, 2008; Eikenaes, 2006; Gass, Gillis, & Russell, 2002; Gillis et al., 2008; Harper et al., 2007; Hill, 2007; Lewis, 2013; Russell, 2001b; Schell et al., 2012; Sklar, Anderson, & Autry, 2007; Tucker, Javorski, et al., 2013; Wolf & Mehl, 2011)
- attention deficit/hyperactivity disorder (ADHD) (Bethke, Hill, & Portrie-Bethke, 2009; Fletcher & Hinkle, 2002; Pelham & Fabiano, 2008; Portrie-Bethke et al., 2009)
- sexual offenses (Gillis & Gass, 2010; Lambie et al., 2000; Somervell & Lambie, 2009)
- adjudication (Association for Experiential Education, 2011; Gillis et al., 2008; Jones, Lowe, & Risler, 2004; Leberman, 2007; Russell, Hendee & Phillips-Miller, 2000; SAMHSA, 2012; Walsh & Aubry, 2007)
- substance abuse treatment (note: not wilderness-therapy based) (Bennett, Cardone, & Jarczyk, 1998; Gass & McPhee, 1990; Harper et al., 2007; Hatala, 1992; Lewis, 2013)
- spina bifida (O'Mahar et al., 2010)
- cancer and other serious pediatric illness (Bekesi et al., 2011; Carson & Cook, 2007; Epstein, 2004; Kessell, Resnick, & Blum, 1985; Kinsella et al., 2006; Lee et al., 2007; Martiniuk, 2003;

Smith et al., 1987; Stevens et al., 2004; Torok et al., 2006; Tucker, Sugerman, et al., 2013; Wynn et al., 2012)

- traumatic brain injury (TBI) (Shanahan, McAllister, & Curtin, 2009)
- cognitive impairments (McAvoy, Smith, & Rynders, 2006)
- obesity and weight control (Jelalian et al., 2006; Jelalian et al., 2011; Lloyd-Richardson et al., 2012)
- diabetes (Chadwick & Brown, 1992; Herskowitz, 1990; Hillson, 1984; Kim et al., 2012; McAuliffe-Fogarty, Ramsing, & Hill, 2007; Torok et al., 2006)
- disabilities (Anderson et al., 1997; Bartley, 1997; Brannan et al., 2003; Dillenschneider, 2007; Herbert, 1996, 1998, 2000a, 2000b; Kessell et al., 1985; Tiemens, Beveridge, & Nicholas, 2006)
- substance abuse prevention (Griffin & Botvin, 2010; Harper et al., 2007; SAMHSA, 2013)

Adults and Families

- war veterans and PTSD (Attarian & Gault, 1992; Hyer et al., 1996; Ragsdale et al., 1996)
- mental illness (Chakravorty, Trunnell, & Ellis, 1995; Jerstad & Stelzer, 1973; Kelley & Coursey, 1997; Scheinfeld, Rochlen, & Buser, 2011; Voruganti et al., 2006; Witman & Preskenis, 1996; Wolf & Mehl, 2011)
- adult survivors of breast cancer (Sugerman, 2005)
- traumatic brain injury (TBI) (Lemmon et al., 1996; Thomas, 2004; Walker et al., 2005)
- diabetes (Mancuso & Caruso-Nicoletti, 2003)
- spinal cord and other impairments and disabilities (Bartley, 1997; Beringer, 2004; Hough & Paisley, 2008; Luckner, 1989)
- substance abuse treatment (Bennett et al., 1998; Clem et al., 2012; Gass & McPhee, 1990)
- elderly (Alves & Sugiyama, n.d.; Boyes, 2013)
- marriage and family therapy (Agate & Covey, 2007; Burg, 2001, 2002; Gillis & Gass, 1993; Martiniuk, 2003; Smith et al., 1987)

Contraindications

While there is no research to suggest that AT is contraindicated for any specific diagnostic group or clinical setting, there are several issues that RT

practitioners should consider before conducting AT groups.

Heightened arousal: Adventure activities produce high levels of emotional and cognitive arousal, which can increase perceived risk and improve outcomes (Fletcher & Hinkle, 2002; Gass, 1993a; Kyriakopoulos, 2011). However, the emotional intensity of adventure activities has also been found to provoke dissociative episodes in individuals with multiple personality disorder (Witman & Preskenis, 1996) and trigger acute psychotic symptoms (Wolf & Mehl, 2011). These findings, and findings from Bunting and Gibbons (2001), who found that high ropes course activity elicits more psychosocial stress than physical exertion stress, underscore the need for RTs to conduct thorough assessment and make clinical judgment regarding the use of AT with populations or individuals who may not benefit from heightened arousal;

Medical conditions: Medical conditions such as asthma can be triggered in outdoor settings (Rhee, 2008). AT programs that are not proximal to indoor shelter or that are conducted in remote settings may be contraindicated for some individuals with medical conditions that are triggered or exacerbated by extremely hot or cold weather.

Physical exertion: While most AT activities do not require high levels of physical strength or stamina, the physical demands of being active in the outdoors may be demanding for adults accustomed to a sedentary lifestyle. From 1986-2000, 67% (10) of all sudden deaths on ropes courses were classified as sudden cardiac death; all of these incidents occurred in men 33 to 60 years old (Welch & Ryan, 2002).

Volatile, hostile, or abusive relationships: Since most AT activities rely on social interaction and in some cases close personal contact (e.g., trust activities, low ropes course), some activities may be contraindicated (Burg, 2002) and some individuals or combinations of individuals may be dangerous or disruptive to the group (Creal & Florio, 1993).

Aggressive behavior, crises, and psychiatric emergencies: For off-site AT interventions, therapists must be able to respond to these situations without institutional support (Davis-Berman & Berman, 1994).

Medication: Though not cited in the literature as a contraindication or concern for participation in AT, it is the experience of this author that it may be contraindicated for clients to be outdoors in the sun if their medications produce photoallergies or photo-toxicity. In addition, some states in the United States may require licensure or certification to administer medication. RTs should check with state laws where they practice in order to plan appropriate staffing (e.g., a nurse) for AT sessions that are off site and require the distribution of medication to patients. If staffing arrangements along these lines cannot be met, participation in AT sessions may be contraindicated for some patients.

Protocols

AT sessions or programs can include outdoor adventure activities such as ropes courses, rock climbing, canoeing or kayaking, camping, or backpacking. Because AT is used across a wide range of clinical populations, uses a wide range of activities, and is conducted in indoor and outdoor settings for varying lengths of time, there is no precise established protocol for RTs to follow. In a literature review of how outcomes are achieved in adventure education programs, including AT, McKenzie (2000) found that most models were built on theory, not research. While McKenzie (2000) found that physical environment, use of activities, processing, group, and instructors are all considered to bring about change, he was unable to summarize specific conditions that promote change due to limited research that provided sufficient detail related to processes of change. Crisp (2004) expressed the need for developing evidence-based practices that demonstrate that AT programs are effective, safe, and comparable or even better than other treatment modalities. Tucker and Rheingold (2010) echo concerns expressed by Crisp (2004) and argue that more research is needed to describe intervention protocols and practice models and position AT as a primary intervention. Russell (2006) suggests that more quantitative research needs to be conducted to validate AT interventions.

Processes

AT practice is informed by theories that underlie AT, models put forth in the literature that highlight core components of AT, and by additional AT practices found in the literature. The following highlights three models of core components of AT programs (Crisp, 1996; Gass, 1993a; Tucker, 2009), considerations for AT practice, and information about AT

currently on the National Registry of Evidence-based Programs and Practices.

Models of AT and Adventure Programming

Gass (1993a) proposed that AT programs could be characterized as exhibiting seven characteristics: (1) action-centered therapy; (2) an unfamiliar environment; (3) a climate of change; (4) assessment of capabilities; (5) emphasis on small-group development and a caring community; (6) focus on strengths rather than deficits; and (7) the therapist plays a nontraditional role.

Crisp (1996) examined 14 clinical AT programs that were school, hospital, or wilderness based. Close examination of these programs suggested best practices for using AT with mental health populations. These practices include: assessment and treatment planning, flexibility in interventions to meet client needs, integration of all treatment modalities, monitoring of client outcomes, a theoretical paradigm and therapeutic rationale, therapist skills in individual and group behavior, skills to respond to a broad range of clinical needs and crises in a remote setting, physical and psychological risk management plans, a thorough and practical understanding by the administration and therapist of ethical issues unique to AT, an organizational commitment to program evaluation, and ongoing staff training.

Tucker (2009) proposes that components of AT programs aimed at improving social skills among adolescents include interpersonal learning, social skills development, sequencing, concrete and immediate consequences, problem solving, a novel environment, physical trust, and emotional and physical safety.

Haras and Bunting (2005) proposed that in order to facilitate meaningful ropes course experiences, AT experience should always include challenge, risk, novelty, and fun; the provision of at least two levels of participation (access, order, degree of completion, additional challenge options); challenge by choice; and increased numbers and variety of challenge options that promote purposeful engagement. These strategies were not developed specifically for clinical populations, though they are considerations for RTs to integrate into program planning when using a ropes course as a treatment modality.

These models provide RTs with planning and implementation considerations for effective AT programs. The client population, organizational commitment and resources, therapeutic recreation and AT program goals, individual treatment goals, staff competencies, and access to adventure activities will impact AT models that RTs adopt.

Considerations in AT Sessions

Ethics

For RTs who practice AT there are three primary sources of ethical guidelines. One source is the American Therapeutic Recreation Association (ATRA) Code of Ethics (www.atra-online.com). The other two codes of ethics come from the Association for Experiential Education (www.aee.org) and the AEE Therapeutic Adventure Professional Group (www.tapg.aee.org).

Group Therapy

It is beyond the scope of this chapter to examine theories and practices associated with group counseling. However, because AT relies heavily on processing, RTs who use AT should be familiar with theories and counseling techniques such as cognitive, rational emotive behavioral, reality, behavioral, gestalt, narrative, and constructivism in order to facilitate AT (Fletcher & Hinkle, 2002). Since AT typically is facilitated in groups, RTs who use AT should be skilled at group facilitation. Some RTs may conduct individual AT sessions. In that case, they should be skilled in conducting individual sessions. RTs who use AT with specific clinical populations should have expertise related to that clinical population.

Experiential Learning

AT is steeped in experiential learning. For RTs, it is important to explore and understand theoretical models of experiential learning, given that our profession that is steeped in facilitating learning and functional change through the use of activities, which are a kind of experience. Additionally, an understanding of experiential learning will help the facilitator use a constructivist approach to facilitating AT, an approach embraced by AT practitioners. In constructivism, the learner (client) is invited to construct meaningful learning versus the teacher (therapist) directing all aspects of learning or therapy.

Kurt Lewin, a Gestalt therapist known as the father of social psychology and developer of action research techniques to solve social problems, studied adult learning associated with changes in health-related attitudes and group dynamics. Central to Lewin's (1935) learning theory was the inclusion of concrete experiences and feedback to promote learning. Lewin's action research model, which focuses on problem solving in group situations, continues to be highly influential in AT today, as evidenced by the strong emphasis on group process that is characteristic of the field.

Dewey (1938) developed a theory of learning that, like Lewin, was steeped in experience. Dewey rejected traditional education philosophies that focused on the acquisition of predetermined knowledge. Dewey proposed that the provision of quality educational experiences, learners' observations of their surroundings, and learners' judgments that result in purposeful (versus impulsive) actions were integral components of the learning process. Dewey's seminal *Experience and Education* (1938) continues to inform the field of AT today. Dewey is considered the father of experiential education.

Kolb (1984) popularized Lewin's theory into what is familiarly called the experiential learning cycle. While Lewin and Dewey have a great influence on AT, Kolb's model is the most widely cited today. In his model of experiential learning, Kolb describes four components of learning: concrete experience, observation and reflection, formation of abstract concepts, and testing new ideas or active experimentation in subsequent experiences. Central to learning in Kolb's model, like Lewin's and Dewy's models, is reflection. Guiding reflection and processing experiences with clients are essential elements for RTs to integrate into practice in order to facilitate outcome-based interventions.

Kolb's model is not without its critics and new models of experiential learning are evolving. For example, Jarvis (1995) points out several shortcomings of Kolb's model. One shortcoming Jarvis notes is that the model describes learning in stages, which is too simplistic and does not reflect the reality of how people learn. Additionally, Jarvis (1995) suggests that learning does not always occur through experience. Learning can occur without reflection and learning can occur with reflection. While Jarvis disagrees with some tenets of Kolb's model of experiential learning, he continues to build on Kolb's model to explain the complex nature of learning Jarvis (2004). Other authors (e.g., Cornu, 2005) build on Jarvis's (2004) "work in progress" in order to further examine and understand experiential learning.

Characteristics of AT Experiences

"There is no inherent magic in any specific activities for generating growth" (Allan, McKenna, & Hind, 2012, p. 6). That said, there are several characteristics of AT experiences that are useful for the RT who practices AT to be aware of. The first quality is that the experience is goal-driven (Gass, 1993a; Russell, 2001b). All activities should be identified based on specific client needs and treatment goals. It is both a challenge and hallmark of the RT to facilitate a meaningful experience across multiple individual goals in a group setting. Despite the challenges, it is incumbent on the RT to assess client needs and identify adventure-based activities and settings that will maximize client progress towards achieving predetermined treatment goals. If treatment goals are not being addressed through the activities, then therapy is not being facilitated. Instead, the activities are recreational, and not therapeutic in nature.

In addition to being goal-directed, experiences in an adventure program are proactive in nature. The proactive nature of activities suggests that patients are engaged physically, socially, emotionally, cognitively, and spiritually. Gass, Gillis and Russell (2012, p. 1) refer to this level of engagement as "kinesthetically engaged." Dehn (1995) refers to it as active or creative participation. A proactive approach, where patients are actively engaged in activities (often outdoors) is distinguished from more traditional "talk" or didactic group therapy where discussion is the primary mode of treatment. The proactive nature of AT is facilitated in the context of an ethical and practical practice in AT is known as Challenge by Choice (Rohnke, 1989a; Schoel et al., 1988). Challenge by Choice will be discussed in greater detail later in this chapter.

In *Islands of Healing* (Schoel, Prouty, & Radcliffe, 1988), the first book about adventure-based counseling, the authors emphasized the improvement of self-concept through structured activities that focused on trust building, goal setting, challenge and stress, peak experiences, humor, and problem solving as a goal of adventure-based counseling. In addition to several of these qualities, Butler (1993) added excitement, risk taking, cooperation and competition, communication, physical activity, problem solving and creativity, group and individual skill develop-

ment, and fun as qualities of adventure activities and programs.

Another characteristic of experiential activities that are used in AT is that the activities are prosocial. Prosocial in this context refers to the tradition in AT of facilitating group activities, focusing on positive and productive relationships, and working towards behavior changes that improve interpersonal skills. In their description of the Outward Bound model of adventure programming, Walsh and Golin (1976) asserted that the unique social environment created by participants and leaders was an essential component of the adventure process. It is widely acknowledged that AT programs are group oriented (Gass, 1993b; Nadler & Luckner, 1992; Rohnke, 1989a; Russell & Farnum, 2004; Schoel & Maizell, 2002). For new facilitators, it often takes time to appreciate that AT interventions are a medium to develop prosocial behaviors, not necessarily demonstrate them at early stages of therapy. Often individuals or a group will struggle mightily to learn and demonstrate the knowledge, attitudes, and skills that the activities are designed to promote. A wise supervisor early on in my career as a RT once advised me, "That's why they're here" in response to my frustration that patients were not demonstrating cooperative skills during a session of cooperative activities. This short but powerful statement has proven to be one of the most important and effective tools that I have embraced as an AT facilitator.

The fourth characteristic of experiential activities is that they are sequenced to support mastery and safety (Rohnke et al., 2007; Rohnke, Wall, & Rogers, 2002; Schoel et al., 1988). Group success does not negate failure as a natural component of group dynamics and a valuable window into individual and group behaviors. In fact, attention to failure is central to individual and group growth. Group success in this context means that activities are sequenced so challenges are increased incrementally. Facilitators increase physical, social, emotional, cognitive, and behavioral challenges in a manner that is consistent with flow (Csíkszentmihályi, 1990) so that activities are challenging, but not so challenging across any domain that patients experience anxiety to the extent that they withdraw from activities.

Sequencing activities with regard to safety is paramount in AT. It is vital that participants develop *and demonstrate* knowledge, attitudes, and skills that maximize safety before advancing to activities that have higher levels of inherent risk or that demand higher levels of knowledge, attitudes, skills, and behaviors to participate in the activity safely. Sequencing activities in this manner requires specialized training in adventure-based programming.

Challenge by Choice®

Challenge by Choice (CBC), trademarked by Project Adventure, warrants further discussion because it has substantial ethical and practical impact on AT programming. CBC was briefly mentioned earlier in this chapter in the context of the proactive nature of adventure therapy. CBC was introduced into adventure programming by Project Adventure, one of the first organizations in the United States to provide programming, training, and educational materials to advance and support the development of adventure education in the United States. Project Adventure describes CBC as:

> Recognizing that any activity or goal may pose a different level and type of challenge for each group member and that authentic personal change comes from within, Challenge by Choice creates an environment where participants are asked to search for opportunities to stretch and grow during the experience. The determination of what kind of participation represents an optimal learning opportunity is the responsibility of each group member (Project Adventure, n.d.).

The concept of CBC may be best understood by comparing Project Adventure's definition of CBC to the Outward Bound (OB) paradigm of participation in adventure-based programming. OB embraces a paradigm of "Using unfamiliar settings to impel students into mentally, emotionally, and physically demanding experiences" (Outward Bound, n.d. b). The language and practical ramifications of *impelling* participants to participate in challenging experiences reflects the historic roots and philosophy of OB. This notion positions the leader as the ultimate authority in determining what is challenging to individual participants and diminishes or negates the development of a therapeutic alliance. The development of therapeutic alliance is a primary condition for therapy to occur; therefore the OB model of impelling participants to participate in all aspects of all activities is excluded from AT practice. Minimizing choice, and forcing or

pressuring participants to participate in activities that are innately risky has been strongly rejected by the AT industry and is contraindicated in clinical adventure-based interventions (Russell, 2001b).

It is this author's experience that RTs should consider that types and levels of challenge are highly individual and always legitimate. Challenges may be physical, social, emotional/psychological, cognitive, and/or spiritual in nature and range from minimally challenging to extremely challenging for individuals. The same activity frequently yields different challenges, different combinations of challenge, and different levels of challenge for each member of a group. Trust activities are a good example of activities in which clients may appear to be physically afraid but they are actually more fearful of placing their emotional trust in someone than of being dropped and physically harmed. In group activities, some clients may enjoy or not be distracted by the social nature of an activity and focus on trying to figure out the solution to a team problem-solving challenge. Others in the group may be challenged by the social aspects of the activity to the extent that they do not contribute to the problem-solving aspect of the challenge, or even withdraw. On high ropes course elements (activities) some participants may enjoy the physical challenges of climbing and negotiating elements 25 feet in the air without high levels of fear; other clients may be overcome with fear or anxiety or be preoccupied with their performance in front of peers to the extent that they do not attempt to climb, or withdraw from a high ropes course element because the social and/or emotional experience is too demanding. It is vital for RTs to appreciate and help clients identify and understand their types and levels of challenge versus minimizing or rejecting individuals' apparent and/or expressed challenges.

Risk

There are several considerations concerning risk in AT.

First, not all AT activities are inherently risky (Ewert et al., 2001). There is a wide range of cooperative activities and initiatives (problem-solving activities) associated with AT that are not dangerous by nature.

Second, some AT activities such as ropes courses, rock climbing, and whitewater rafting are inherently risky activities in which serious injury and even death is possible.

Third, in risky activities, real risk is not eliminated; risk is mediated (Lynch & McInnes, 2008). Legal experts support this assertion and advise AT professionals that risk is managed, not eliminated. Clients should not be advised that risk-laden activities are not risky, even in situations where the facilitator is trying to quell fear and anxiety in a supportive manner. Acknowledging the inherently risky nature of many AT activities (e.g., ropes course, rock climbing, backpacking, water-based activity) and managing risk are essential skills for RTs to develop in order to be safe and effective AT facilitators. Complacency is the enemy of effective AT leadership.

Fourth, risk (real and perceived) is important in the therapeutic process because change requires risk (Lynch & McInnes, 2008). Social learning theory (Bandura, 1977) suggests that if individuals take risks in one setting (e.g., AT) they can transfer learning that is achieved in that setting to other (e.g., clinical, "real life") settings. The challenging, highly supportive, and experiential nature of AT is a powerful treatment modality for individuals who are striving to make functional changes that require risk-taking. It is important for RTs to understand the risks and guide clients in taking constructive risks versus destructive risks. RTs must consider that what may be constructive for one client may not be for another. For example, a client may choose to climb an element to challenge himself/herself in order to achieve a personal or treatment goal; this would be considered a constructive challenge. Another client may choose to climb due to perceptions of peer pressure or failure and in doing so disregard personal feelings and choices that would genuinely benefit him/her; this would be considered a destructive risk. When clients disregard personal feelings, goals, or safety parameters, then they are taking destructive risks. Unless clinically indicated, and always if safety is being compromised in any manner, therapists should intervene and, at minimum, discuss and, in some cases, terminate participation in an activity, if destructive choices are being considered or made by a client.

Finally, as in the challenging aspect of AT activities, it is vital for the RT to appreciate and help clients identify and understand their types (physical, social, emotional/psychological, cognitive, spiritual) and levels of risk (minimal to extreme) versus minimizing or rejecting individuals' apparent and/or expressed perceptions of risk. Boyes (2013, p. 648) underscores the personal nature of constructive risk-taking: "Risky activities provide opportunities for individuals to create their own paths and meet self-set personal challenges often against environmental challenges."

Trust

Trust activities in AT are typically characterized as individuals "falling" and "catching" (spotting) one another. These activities serve several purposes in AT. One purpose is to establish emotional and interpersonal trust (Priest, 1998; Rohnke, 1989b; Schoel et al., 1988; Shooter, Paisley, & Sibthorp, 2010). Another purpose of trust activities is for individuals to learn and practice how to protect each other and be protected on activities that require lifting, planned falling, or unexpected falling as occurs on low ropes course activities (Rohnke, 1989b; Rohnke et al., 2007). Other than Rohnke (1989b) and Rohnke and colleagues (2007) there is little in the literature that describes sequences and leadership strategies when leading trust activities. It is the experience of this author that the role of trust activities in establishing genuine trust and safety techniques is frequently minimized by facilitators. This author suggests that an effective trust sequence includes a description for participants concerning the purpose of trust activities (as described above); properly sequenced activities; individuals doing the same trust activity several times with different partners to develop skills in falling and spotting safely; mixing partnerships so males and females, larger and smaller individuals, and individuals with short- or long-term conflicted relationships are paired together in order to prepare the group for the combinations that may occur spontaneously during other activities. Leading trust activities requires specialized training. Facilitators should not lead any trust activities that require falling and catching without proper training.

Facilitation

For the purposes of this discussion, facilitation is defined as "anything and everything you [the facilitator] do before, during, or after the learning experiences to enhance people's reflection, integration, and continuation of lasting change" (Priest, Gass, & Gillis, 2000, p. 19). It is important to operationalize the definition of facilitation here because the term facilitation is frequently used interchangeably in the adventure education and AT literature with processing, debriefing, and reflecting (Seaman & Rheingold, 2013). It is the view of this author that for the RT and AT facilitator, there are many aspects of facilitation. Processing, one component of facilitation, will be examined later in this chapter.

One aspect that is crucial to safe and effective facilitation of AT interventions is the ability to assess a group in order to understand requirements for the design and delivery of the AT intervention. In some cases, assessment impacts facilitation on a macro level and informs the design of an AT program or session. Other times, facilitators have to make more immediate decisions in the moment, on what is considered a micro level. In some circumstances, assessment supports thoughtful planning and delivery strategies; in other circumstances, quick assessment is required to maximize the AT process or ensure the physical and emotional safety of individuals or the group. While examining the many facets of facilitation is beyond the scope of this chapter, two models associated with macro and micro assessment of groups that are most frequently cited in the AT literature and useful facilitation tools unique to AT interventions are briefly described here. An outline of facilitator qualities is also presented to describe areas of expertise that those interested in pursuing AT facilitation should look for in classroom, volunteer, and internship experiences.

One model, developed by Gass and Gillis (1995), uses the acronym CHANGES (Context, Hypotheses, Actions, Novelty, Generate, Evaluation, Solution) as a framework to assess a group on the macro level. By continually considering each aspect of CHANGES, facilitators can make informed decisions that best facilitate functional change among group members. First, facilitators should consider the *Context* of a group. Context refers to characteristics of the group, the facilitator, and the environment. Next, facilitators form tentative *Hypotheses* or assumptions about what they expect from the group based on prior experience with a particular group or similar group. Facilitators then observe *Actions* of group members in order to determine if hypotheses were valid. Based on group actions, a facilitator may have to revise or reject the hypotheses in order to provide an effective intervention. The *Novelty* of adventure activities provides the facilitator with the opportunity to observe spontaneous, therefore true,

core issue behaviors versus behaviors that may be based on individuals' expectations of "socially proper" behaviors. Through observation of group actions, facilitators can *Generate* or identify functional and dysfunctional behaviors and patterns of critical thinking and affect among group members. A positive therapeutic alliance is important in order for the facilitator to perceive patterns accurately. The next step in assessing the group involves the facilitators' *Evaluation* and interpretation of the information they have gathered from the group. The facilitator evaluates which hypotheses are being confirmed or rejected and identifies core issues in the group. Finally, the facilitator identifies and implements *Solutions* to facilitate the group actively working on their issues. The CHANGES model can be a very useful tool in gathering and organizing information about a group in order to inform the diagnosis of a group and the design and delivery of an AT experience.

Another model, developed by Project Adventure, uses the acronym GRABBS (Schoel et al., 1988). GRABBS is an assessment tool that a facilitator can use to scan a group in order to make programmatic decisions in the moment based on client *Goals*; *Readiness* of the group to take physical and psychological risks; *Affect* or mood of the group; presence or lack of supportive and encouraging *Behavior*, *Body strength,* and physical condition of participants; and *Stage* of group development.

Processing

RTs are trained to use activity as a means rather than an end. The purpose is to bring about functional change, not to simply participate in an activity. RTs routinely use reflection and processing as a way for individuals to learn through and draw meaning from activity. Reflection is defined as a post-experience process of reorganizing perceptions, forming new relationships, and influencing future thoughts and actions in order to learn from an experience (Sugerman et al., 2000). As described earlier, Kolb's (1984) experiential learning cycle provides a theoretical rationale for reflection and places reflection in a central role in learning. While there is debate about the precise role of reflection in learning (Cornu, 2005; Jarvis, 2004) there is agreement in the AT field that reflection is an essential component of the AT process (Seaman & Rheingold, 2013).

In its simplest terms, processing can be described as a guided reflection session (Estes, 2008) in a circular discussion group led by a leader who poses questions to the group (Priest & Naismith, 1993). While not all processing techniques include group discussion and circular discussion is not necessarily a given, group discussion in a circle, following an experience, is a typical AT processing technique. Gass (1993a) argues that processing can occur prior to, during, or after the adventure experience. It is the experience of this author that rich processing frequently occurs during adventure experiences and often rich learning opportunities are lost if the facilitator waits until an activity is completed to discuss thoughts, feelings, or actions.

There are many techniques and "generations" of processing AT experiences that position the learner and leader in varying roles of directing learning outcomes. An in-depth discussion is beyond the scope of this chapter, though a brief summary of the generations of processing illustrates different roles the RT takes in guiding learning experiences with clients. The first generation, "letting the experience speak for itself" (Bacon, 1983), is useful when the goal of an experience is fun or recreation; the leader does not guide learning. There are seven additional generations of processing commonly acknowledged in the AT literature. Priest and Gass (1997) and Itin (1995) categorize generations of processing as teacher centered or student centered. The RT can think of the teacher-student roles as therapist-client roles. The second to fourth generations can be considered teacher centered: the leader guides group discussion with questions and provides feedback related to what students are doing well and what they can work on (second generation); the leader asks more questions, provides less feedback, and encourages students to think about and take ownership of their learning (third generation); the leader uses a technique called "front loading" in which the leader "loads" the beginning of the activity with key learning points that the students focus on learning about during the activity (fourth generation). For example, if an RT is working with youth in a substance use rehabilitation setting, the therapist may front-load an activity with a storyline such as, "This is a swamp of addiction. If you step off the mats onto the floor, that represents relapse. At the end of the activity we're going to discuss how you avoided relapse and reasons why you did not avoid relapse during the activity." This technique is considered teacher-centered because the leader decides for the group what is important for them to learn.

The remaining generations of clinical processing techniques (generations five through seven), described by Priest and Gass (1997) and Itin (1995) are used to achieve clinical versus educational goals. They rely more on the use of metaphor, comprehensive needs assessment of clients, and specific client goals. Because these techniques require a high level of facilitation expertise and are clinical in nature, ethical considerations that guide practice are consistent with therapy versus education. The eighth generation of processing is referred to as "self-facilitation" where learners facilitate their own process (Priest, Gass, & Fitzpatrick, 1999). This processing technique has been used with corporate groups versus clinical populations.

It is hopefully clear that RTs should choose processing techniques that match the makeup of a group, the goals of the group, and the level of expertise of the facilitator. While processing techniques vary as described above, Gass (1993a) identifies four primary outcomes that processing activities can be used for: (1) to help individuals focus or increase their awareness on issues prior to an event or the entire experience; (2) to facilitate awareness or promote change while an experience is occurring; (3) to reflect, analyze, describe, or discuss an experience after it is completed; and/or (4) to reinforce perceptions of change and promote integration in participants' lives after the experience is completed.

On a final processing note, the discussion thus far has centered on group discussion where the leader has varying levels of control of the content and direction of reflection. It is the experience of this author that it takes practice to lead group discussions related to thoughts, feelings, and actions that occur during an experience when leaders are preoccupied with leading the activity itself, and processing can be arduous for the leader and the clients.

One processing technique that is gaining popularity is using props to help prompt discussion during processing. Using props relies heavily on metaphor (e.g., symbolism). One example of a processing tool of this type is The Body Parts Debrief, which consists of a small drawstring sack that contains foam items such as an ear, hand, heart, brain, and stomach.

Group members (or the leader if group members cannot or choose not to) assign a quality to each body part that the body part symbolizes. For example, the foam ear may represent something positive that group members heard during the activity; the brain can represent something new that someone learned during the activity; and the hand can represent an instance where someone in the group gave or received help from someone else in the group. The props can be used in many different ways. Individuals can choose a prop, everyone can make a comment using the same prop, and group members can choose props for each other. The types of props that are used and the way they are used are limited only by the creativity of the leader and group members. Kits of themed props can be purchased from companies such as Training Wheels (www.training-wheels.com) or creative RTs can create their own with pictures and everyday items. Props can be a very useful way for leaders and clients to practice reflecting on experiences.

Individuals with Impairments or Disabilities and AT

The Indications section of this chapter demonstrates empirical support for AT being beneficial for persons with an array of impairments, disabilities, and medical conditions. There is, however, little empirical evidence of specific strategies and techniques that are useful. Dillenschneider (2007) makes recommendations that, while they lack empirical support, provide useful insights when individuals with disabilities are members of AT groups: (1) communicate with clients about the fundamental activities and environments they will experience in order to help participants make informed choices about activity participation; (2) always have the person with the impairment assist instructors in understanding his/her actual needs and strengths; (3) commit to possibility thinking and openness to unexpected outcomes; (4) provide appropriate, high quality, and individualized support and adaptation to equipment; and (5) be sure that facilitators have proper training, experience, and make decisions that do no harm. Dillenschneider (2007) also makes recommendations for inclusive practices and equipment adaptations when individuals with disabilities are group members.

Carlson and Cook (2007) describe considerations for working with children with serious medical illness based on Hole in the Wall Gang Camps

founded by Paul Newman in 1988. Children who attend these camps are aged seven to 15 and have serious life-threatening diseases such as cancer, hemophilia, rare blood diseases, sickle cell disease, and immunodeficiencies. Like Dillenschneider (2007), the interventions are not evidence-based but provide some useful insights for RTs who use AT with children with severe medical illness and indicate areas of future research needs.

It is clear from the dearth of research that examines AT practices when AT is used as a treatment intervention for individuals with disabilities, impairments, and serious illness that there is great opportunity and responsibility for RTs to expand this area of research. As individual researchers continue to work towards identifying processes that produce predetermined outcomes, organizations associated with AT are making efforts to advance research in AT. The Association for Experiential Education (AEE) has several groups in the organization that are dedicated to research. AEE's Research and Evaluation in Adventure Programming (REAP) group focuses on researching adventure programming. Since 2007 AEE's Therapeutic Adventure Professional Group (TAPG) has been drafting AT best practices (http://tapg.aee.org/tapg/bestpractices/) and has hosted an annual best practice conference since 2010. The TAPG also sponsors a pre-conference associated with the annual AEE conference in order to discuss and disseminate best practices. Since 2000 the annual AEE conference has hosted a Symposium on Experiential Education Research (SEER). The Outdoor Behavioral Healthcare Research Cooperative (OBHRC) and the American Camping Association (ACA) also support research related to adventure programming and AT.

Professional Preparation

RTs are uniquely prepared to use AT as a treatment intervention. Many of the facilitator competencies outlined by Gass, Gillis, and Russell (2012) are learned and practiced in undergraduate RT programs. It is the experience of this author that students who wish to pursue their senior internship in an AT setting or in a setting that uses AT in an adjunct role are most frequently rejected from these settings due to lack of technical skills. Students interested in AT-focused internships or careers should participate in professional training to develop expertise in activities such as ropes course facilitation, whitewater rafting, backpacking, and wilderness first aid. Leisure participation in these activities provides valuable experience and skill development that may be sufficient for settings that provide additional training or for an entry level or assistant position.

Gass and colleagues (2012) outline 10 areas of competence for AT facilitators. A detailed description of specific skills associated with each competency can be found in Appendix B of *Adventure Therapy: Theory, Research, and Practice* (Gass et al., 2012). This publication is an excellent resource for novice and advanced practitioners of AT. The 10 areas of competence include:

- Technical skills associated with specific adventure activities, risk management, and environmental practices
- Facilitation and processing
- Organizational and administrative skills
- Conceptual knowledge of AT models, practices, philosophies, and applications
- Therapeutic alliance building
- Assessment
- Intervention planning
- Therapeutic monitoring
- Documentation
- Professionalism

SAMHSA National Registry of Evidence-Based Programs and Practices

One program and one practice steeped in AT are currently on the National Registry of Evidence-Based Programs and Practices.

Project Venture: Project Venture is an outdoor experiential youth development program designed primarily for fifth to eighth grade American Indian youth. It aims to develop the social and emotional competence that facilitates youths' resistance to alcohol, tobacco, and other drug use (SAMHSA. 2013).

Behavior Management through Adventure (BMtA): BMtA is a form of outdoor therapy for youth with behavioral, psychological, and learning disabilities; students excluded from school for disciplinary reasons; and juvenile offenders. BMtA incorporates group-based adventure challenges (e.g., ropes courses) and developmental exercises with problem-solving components in an effort to help participants change feelings, thinking, and social behaviors;

reduce dysfunctional behaviors; improve functional life behaviors; and avoid re-arrest (SAMHSA, 2013).

Outcomes and Documentation

The documentation of treatment outcomes is characteristic of AT (Ewert et al., 2001; Russell, 2001b). As can be seen throughout this chapter, there are many outcomes associated with AT. Therefore, there are many measures that are utilized in documenting outcomes. While some commonly used measures are standardized instruments, there are none that are considered standard in the field of AT. Examination of studies that measured AT outcomes portrays a wide use of qualitative research techniques. This section highlights several quantitative measures found in the AT literature that assessed common outcomes of AT.

One common outcome in AT research is self-concept. Cook (2008) and Jelalian and colleagues (2011) used the *Self-Perception Profile for Adolescents* (SPP-A; Harter, 1988) to measure self-concept operationalized as self-worth and self-perception, respectively. Cook (2008) used the measure to identify areas of follow-up questions for semi-structured interviews. In a qualitative study, Kyriakopoulos (2011) measured self-esteem using *Interpretive Phenomenological Analysis* (IPA) to analyze data collected in semi-structured interviews.

Self-esteem has been measured in AT using such scales as the *Rosenberg Self-Esteem Scale* (Rosenberg, 1965). For example, Schell and her team (2012) used the scale to measure self-esteem among young people with mental illness. A meta-analysis of therapeutic camp experiences among children with chronic health conditions identified five additional studies that used the *Rosenberg Self-Esteem Scale* to measure self-esteem (Odar, Canter, & Roberts, 2013). Herbert (1998) used the *Coopersmith Self-Esteem Inventories* (Coopersmith, 1981). NUD*IST 6.0 qualitative software has been used to assist in the analysis of data associated with AT for children with cancer (Stevens et al., 2004).

As described earlier, relationships and social skills (e.g., d7 Interpersonal Interactions and Relationships) are frequently measured as an outcome in AT. The *Social Connectedness Scale — Revised* (Lee, Draper, & Lee, 2001) was used by Schell and colleagues (2012) and Herbert (1998). In her study with colleagues that examined the use of AT in combination with cognitive-behavioral treatment for overweight adolescents, Jelalian et al. (2006) used Harter's (1988) *Self-Perception Profile for Adolescents*. The client self-report and parent assessment versions of the *Youth Outcome Questionnaire* (Burlingame, Wells, & Lambert, 1995) were used by Russell (2001a) in his assessment of treatment outcomes of outdoor behavioral healthcare programs.

Social anxiety (e.g., b126 Temperament and Personality Functions, b152 Emotional Functions, d710 Basic Interpersonal Interactions) was measured by Jelalian and her colleagues (2011) with the *Social Anxiety Scale for Adolescents* (La Greca & Lopez, 1998). The *Depression, Anxiety, and Stress Scales* (DASS), developed by Lovibond and Lovibond (1995) was used by Walker and her team (2005) to measure depression and anxiety among individuals with traumatic brain injury who participated in an AT program. Wolf and Mehl (2011) used the *Beck Depression Inventory* (Beck, Steer, & Brown, 1996) to measure depression among youth who participated in an adjunct therapy AT program in an inpatient treatment program. The *Depression Adjectives Checklist* (DACL) (Lubin, 1965, 1981) was used to measure depression among adults who participated in a ropes course program in a psychiatric hospital (Chakravorty et al., 1995).

Given the preponderance of qualitative studies that measure AT outcomes, it will be useful for researchers to gather quantitative measures of AT outcomes with standardized instruments. This will aid in comparison of interventions across AT studies and across studies that assess interventions other than AT. Mixed methods study designs are also recommended.

AT can be used to work on deficits in several sets of ICF codes. As mentioned earlier, the primary codes that suggest the need for AT are in d7 Interpersonal Interactions and Relationships. It can also be useful for several mental function codes, such as b126 Temperament and Personality Functions, b140 Attention Functions, b147 Psychomotor Functions, and b152 Emotional Functions. Some other ICF codes that might be addressed include b455 Exercise Tolerance Functions, d175 Solving Problems, d210 Undertaking a Single Task, and d3 Communication. While AT may be useful for people who have issues with d4 Mobility and the related Body Function codes, it is probably not a primary means of treating these deficits because it is more centered on the psychosocial aspects of the situation.

Conclusion

Gillis and colleagues (2008) note that one of the challenges of understanding AT is that definitions of AT generally describe *where* AT occurs rather than *what* occurs. While progress has been made in research to elucidate what takes place during AT sessions and programs, there is still work to be done. Future research should continue to examine facilitation, activity choice, processing techniques, and the efficacy of AT with a wider scope of clinical populations and settings. RTs have unique training among professional clinicians, with training in clinical knowledge and skills, process-driven activity leadership, and group facilitation skills. This rich background positions RTs to expand the scope and practice of adventure therapy across a wider scope of clinical populations and settings than is practiced today. Through effective programming and rigorous research, RTs can contribute to the professionalization and evolution of AT, WT, outdoor behavioral healthcare, specialty camps, and many other programs that take children and adults with a wide range of illness, disease, and disability into the outdoors.

While the evidence that supports AT as an effective clinical and community intervention continues to grow, Harper (2010) warns researchers that political and economic forces that drive dominance of randomized controlled trials (RCTs) in determining evidence-based practice may hinder deeper understanding of AT. Harper expresses concerns that RCTs place an overemphasis on demonstrating *that* AT is effective in creating change, but not enough focus on *how* AT creates change. It is incumbent on researchers and practitioners to continue to examine and understand how the unique combination of environment, activities, therapy models, and facilitation techniques that characterize AT create functional change in clients. Gillis (1992) suggests that the types of activities, group size, and qualifications and characteristics of group leaders are important to study. Gillis (1992) also promotes the use of statistical techniques such as regression analysis that can predict those who will benefit the most from AT.

Resources

The Association for Experiential Education (AEE)

www.aee.org

The Association for Experiential Education (AEE) is a nonprofit, professional membership association dedicated to developing and promoting experiential education worldwide.

AEE Therapeutic Adventure Professional Group (TAPG)

http://tapg.aee.org/

The Therapeutic Adventure Professional Group is committed to the development and promotion of adventure-based programming and the principles of experiential education in therapeutic settings.

The Association for Challenge Course Technology (ACCT)

www.acctinfo.org

ACCT is the leading trade association for those working with and on behalf of the challenge course industry.

Outdoor Behavioral Healthcare Industry Council (OBHIC)

www.obhic.com/

OBHIC is an organization of behavioral health providers who are committed to the utilization of outdoor modalities to assist young people and their families to make positive change.

The Outdoor Behavioral Healthcare Research Cooperative (OBHRC)

www.obhrc.org

The purpose of the Outdoor Behavioral Healthcare Research Cooperative is to administer and deliver active, comprehensive research on outdoor behavioral healthcare programs operating in North America.

The National Association of Therapeutic Schools and Programs (NATSAP)

www.natsap.org/

The National Association of Therapeutic Schools and Programs (NATSAP) serves as a national resource for programs and professionals assisting young people beleaguered by emotional and behavioral difficulties.

The Adventure Therapy International Committee (ATIC)

The Adventure Therapy International Committee aims to promote and support professional practice, research, and the development of Adventure Therapy worldwide. ATIC oversees the planning and operation of the International Adventure Therapy Conference (IATC) hosted every three years and publication of proceedings from each conferences. ATIC also provides advocacy and resources to assist in developing national adventure therapy networks.

References

Agate, S. T. & Covey, C. D. (2007). Family camps: An overview of benefits and issues of camps and programs for families. *Journal of Adolescent Psychiatric Clinics of North America, 16*(4), 921-937.

Allan, J. F., McKenna, J., & Hind, K. (2012). Brain resilience: Shedding light into the black box of adventure processes. *Australian Journal of Outdoor Education, 16*(1), 3-14.

Alves, S. & Sugiyama, T. (n.d.). Inclusive design for getting outdoors: Findings for other researchers. Retrieved from www.idgo.ac.uk/useful_resources/for_other_researchers.htm.

Anderson, L., Stuart, J., Schleien, S. J., McAvoy, L., Lais, G., & Seligman, D. (1997). Creating positive change through an integrated outdoor adventure program. *Therapeutic Recreation Journal, 31*(4), 214-229.

Association for Experiential Education. (2011). *Adventure therapy and adjudicated youth.*

Attarian, A. & Gault, L. (1992). Treatment of Vietnam veterans with post-traumatic stress disorder: A model program. *Journal of Physical Education, Recreation & Dance, 63*(4), 56.

Autry, C. E. (2001). Adventure therapy with girls at-risk: Responses to outdoor experiential activities. *Therapeutic Recreation Journal, 35*(4), 289-306.

Bacon, S. B. (1983). *The conscious use of metaphor in Outward Bound.* Denver, CO: Colorado Outward Bound School.

Bandoroff, S. & Scherer, D. (1994). Wilderness family therapy: An innovative treatment approach for problem youth. *Journal of Child and Family Studies, 3*(2), 175-191. doi: 10.1007/bf02234066.

Bandura, A. (1977). *Social learning theory.* Englewood Cliff, NJ: Prentice Hall.

Bartley, N. (1997). Access to success: Team adventure experiences for youth and adults with disabilities. *World Leisure & Recreation, 39*(4), 31-35. doi: 10.1080/10261133.1997.9674087.

Beck, A. T., Steer, R. A., & Brown, G. K. (1996*). Manual for the Beck depression inventory-II.* San Antonio, TX: Psychological Corporation.

Becker, S. P. (2010). Wilderness therapy: Ethical considerations for mental health professionals. *Child and Youth Care Forum, 39*(1), 47-61.

Bekesi, A., Torok, S., Kokonyei, G., Bokretas, I., Szentes, A., Telepoczki, G., & Group, T. E. K. (2011). Health-related quality of life changes of children and adolescents with chronic disease after participation in therapeutic recreation camping program. *Health and Quality of Life Outcomes, 9*(1), 43.

Bennett, L. W., Cardone, S., & Jarczyk, J. (1998). Effects of a therapeutic camping program on addiction recovery: The Algonquin Haymarket Relapse Prevention Program. *Journal of Substance Abuse Treatment, 15*(5), 469-474.

Beringer, A. (2004). Spinal cord injury and outdoor experiences. *International Journal of Rehabilitation Research, 27*(1), 7-15.

Berman, D. & Davis-Berman, J. (1995). Adventure as psychotherapy: A mental health perspective. *Journal of Leisurability, 22*(2), 21-28.

Bethke, J. G., Hill, N. R., & Portrie-Bethke, T. L. (2009). Strength-based mental health counseling for children with ADHD: An integrative model of adventure-based counseling and Adlerian play therapy. *Journal of Mental Health Counseling, 31*, 323-337.

Bettmann, J. E. & Jasperson, R. A. (2008). Adults in wilderness treatment: A unique application of attachment theory and research. *Clinical Social Work Journal, 36*(1), 51-61.

Bloemhoff, H. J. (2006). The effect of an adventure-based recreation programme (ropes course) on the development of resiliency in at-risk adolescent boys confined to a rehabilitation centre. *South African Journal for Research in Sport, Physical Education & Recreation, 28*(1), 1-11.

Boyes, M. (2013). Outdoor adventure and successful ageing. *Ageing & Society, 33*(4), 644-665. doi: 10.1017/s0144686x12000165.

Brannan, S., Fullerton, A., Arick, J. R., Robb, G. M., & Bender, M. (2003). *Including youth with disabilities in outdoor programs: Best practices, outcomes, and resources.* Champaign, IL: Sagamore.

Bunting, C. J. & Gibbons, E. S. (2001). Plasma catecholamine and cardiovascular reactivity during an acute high ropes course event. *International Journal of Psychophysiology, 42*(3), 303-314.

Burg, J. E. (2001). Emerging Issues in therapeutic adventure with families. *Journal of Experiential Education, 24*(3), 118-122.

Burg, J. E. (2002). Crossing the Hot Chocolate River with families. *Journal of Clinical Activities, Assignments & Handouts in Psychotherapy Practice, 2*(3), 13-21. doi: 10.1300/J182v02n03_02.

Burlingame, G., Wells, M. G., & Lambert, M. J. (1995). *The youth outcome questionnaire.* Stevenson, MD: American Professional Credentialing Services.

Butler, S. (1993). The physical education and recreation strand: The history and the future. *Zip Lines, 24*(1), 12-14.

Carson, K. P. & Cook, M. (2007). Challenge by choice: Adventure-based counseling for seriously ill adolescents. *Child and Adolescent Psychiatric Clinics of North America, 16*(4), 909-919. doi: http://dx.doi.org/10.1016/j.chc.2007.05.002.

Chadwick, J. & Brown, K. G. E. (1992). A party of 43 young people with diabetes go skiing. *Diabetic Medicine, 9*(7), 671-673. doi: 10.1111/j.1464-5491.1992.tb01866.x

Chakravorty, D., Trunnell, E. P., & Ellis, G. D. (1995). Ropes course participation and post-activity processing on transient depressed mood of hospitalized adult psychiatric patients. *Therapeutic Recreation Journal, 29*(2), 104-113.

Clark, J. P. & Kempler, H. L. (1973). Therapeutic family camping: A rationale. *The Family Coordinator, 22*(1), 137-142.

Clark, J. P., Marmol, L. M., Cooley, R., & Gathercoal, K. (2004). The effects of wilderness therapy on the clinical concerns (on axes I, II, and IV) of troubled adolescents. *Journal of Experiential Education, 27*(2), 213-232.

Clem, J. M., Smith, T. E., & Richards, K. V. (2012). Effects of a low-element challenge course on abstinence self-efficacy and group cohesion. *Research on Social Work Practice, 22*(2), 151-158. doi: 10.1177/1049731511423672.

Cook, E. C. (2008). Residential wilderness programs: The role of social support in influencing self-evaluations of male adolescents. *Adolescence, 43*(172), 751-774.

Coopersmith, S. (1981). *Self-esteem inventories.* Palo Alto, CA: Consulting Psychologists Press.

Cornu, A. L. (2005). Building on Jarvis: Towards a holistic model of the processes of experimental learning. *Studies in the Education of Adults, 37*(2), 166-181.

Creal, R. S. & Florio, N. (Eds.). (1993). *The family wilderness program: A description of the project and its ethical concerns.* Dubuque, IA: Kendall/Hunt.

Crisp, S. (1996). International models of best practice in wilderness and adventure therapy: Implications for Australia. In W. C. F. F. Report (Ed.). Melbourne, Australia.

Crisp, S. (2004). Envisioning the birth of a profession: A blueprint of evidence-based, ethical, best practice. In S. Bandoroff and S. L. Newes (Eds.), *Coming of age: The evolving field of adventure therapy* (pp. 209-223). Boulder, CO: Association for Experiential Education.

Csíkszentmihályi, M. (1990). *Flow: The psychology of optimal experience.* New York, NY: Harper Perennial.

Dattilo, J. (2000). *Facilitation techniques in therapeutic recreation.* State College, PA: Venture Publishing.

Davis-Berman, J. & Berman, D. (1989). The wilderness therapy program: An empirical study of its effects with adolescents in an outpatient setting. *Journal of Contemporary Psychotherapy, 19*(4), 271-281. doi: 10.1007/bf00946092.

Davis-Berman, J. & Berman, D. (1994). *Wilderness therapy: Foundations, theories and research.* Dubuque, IA: Kendall/Hunt Publishing.

Dehn, D. (1995). *Leisure step up.* Ravensdale, WA: Idyll Arbor.

Dewey, J. (1938). *Experience and education.* New York, NY: Touchstone.

Dillenschneider, C. (2007). Integrating persons with impairments and disabilities into standard outdoor adventure education programs. *Journal of Experiential Education, 30*(1), 70-83.

Eikenaes, I. (2006). Integrated wilderness therapy for avoidant personality disorder. *Nordic Journal of Psychiatry, 60*(4), 275-281. doi: 10.1080/08039480600790093.

Epstein, I. (2004). Adventure therapy: A mental health promotion strategy in pediatric oncology. *J Ped Oncol Nurs, 21*, 103 - 110.

Estes, C. A. (2008). Promoting student-centered learning in experiential education. In K. Warren, D. Mitten, & T. Loeffler (Eds.), *Theory and Practice of Experiential Education.* Boulder, CO: Association for Experiential Education.

Ewert, A. W., McCormick, B. P., & Voight, A. E. (2001). Outdoor experiential therapies: Implications for TR practice. *Therapeutic Recreation Journal, 35*(2), 107-122.

Fletcher, T. B. & Hinkle, J. S. (2002). Adventure based counseling: An innovation in counseling. *Journal of Counseling and Development, 80*(3), 277-285.

Gass, M. A. (1993a). *Adventure therapy: Therapeutic applications of adventure programming.* Dubuque, IA: Kendall/Hunt Publishing Co.

Gass, M. A. (1993b). The evolution of processing adventure therapy experiences. In M. Gass (Ed.), *Adventure therapy: Therapeutic applications of adventure programming* (pp. 219-229). Dubuque, IA: Kendall/Hunt Publishing Co.

Gass, M. A. & Gillis, H. L. L. (1995). CHANGES: An assessment model using adventure experiences. *Journal of Experiential Education, 18*(1), 34-40.

Gass, M. A., Gillis, H. L. L., & Russell, K. C. (2012). *Adventure therapy: Theory, research, and practice.* New York: Taylor & Francis.

Gass, M. A. & McPhee, P. J. (1990). Emerging for recovery: A descriptive analysis of adventure therapy for substance abusers. *Journal of Experiential Education, 13*(2), 29-35. doi: 10.1177/105382599001300206.

Gelkopf, M., Hasson-Ohayon, I., Bikman, M., & Kravetz, S. (2013). Nature adventure rehabilitation for combat-related posttraumatic chronic stress disorder: A randomized control trial. *Psychiatry Research, 209*(3), 485-493, doi: http://dx.doi.org/10.1016/j.psychres.2013.01.026.

Gibson, P. M. (1979). Therapeutic aspects of wilderness programs: A comprehensive literature review. *Therapeutic Recreation Journal, 13*(2), 21-33.

Gillis, H. L. (1992). Therapeutic uses of adventure-challenge-outdoor-wilderness: Theory and research. In K. Henderson (Ed.), *Proceedings of Coalition for Education in the Outdoor*

Symposium. Cortland, NY: Coalition for Education in the Outdoors.

Gillis, H. L. & Gass, M. A. (1993). Bringing adventure into marriage and family therapy: An innovative experiential approach. *Journal of Marital and Family Therapy, 19*(3), 273-286. doi: 10.1111/j.1752-0606.1993.tb00988.x.

Gillis, H. L. & Gass, M. A. (2010). Treating juveniles in a sex offender program using adventure-based programming: A matched group design. *Journal of Child Sexual Abuse, 19*(1), 20-34. doi: 10.1080/10538710903485583.

Gillis, H. L., Gass, M. A., & Russell, K. C. (2008). The effectiveness of project adventure's behavior management programs for male offenders in residential treatment. *Residential Treatment for Children & Youth, 25*(3), 227-247. doi: 10.1080/08865710802429689.

Glass, J. S. & Benshoff, J. M. (2002). Facilitating group cohesion among adolescents through challenge course experiences. *Journal of Experiential Education, 25*(2), 268-277.

Green, G. T., Kleiber, D. A., & Tarrant, M. A. (2000). The effect of an adventure-based recreation program on development of resiliency in low income minority youth. *Journal of Park & Recreation Administration, 18*(3), 76-97.

Greenway, R. (1995). The wilderness effect and ecopsychology. In T. Roszak, M. E. Gomes, & A. D. Kanner (Eds.), *Ecopsychology: Restoring the earth, healing the mind.* Berkeley, CA: Sierra Club.

Griffin, K. W. & Botvin, G. J. (2010). Evidence-based interventions for preventing substance use disorders in adolescents. *Child and Adolescent Psychiatric Clinics of North America, 19*(3), 505-526. doi: http://dx.doi.org/10.1016/j.chc.2010.03.005.

Hans, T. (2000). A meta-analysis of the effects of adventure programming on locus of control. *Journal of Contemporary Psychotherapy, 30*, 33-60.

Haras, K. & Bunting, C. J. (2005). The differences in meaningful involvement opportunities provided by ropes course programs. *Journal of Experiential Education, 27*(3), 297-299.

Harper, N. (2010). Future paradigm or false idol: A cautionary tale of evidence-based practice for adventure education and therapy. *Journal of Experiential Education, 33*(1), 38-55.

Harper, N., Russell, K., Cooley, R., & Cupples, J. (2007). Catherine Freer wilderness therapy expeditions: An exploratory case study of adolescent wilderness therapy, family functioning, and the maintenance of change. *Child and Youth Care Forum, 36*(2-3), 111-129. doi: 10.1007/s10566-007-9035-1.

Harter, S. (1988). *Manual for the self-perception profile for adolescents.* Denver, CO: University of Denver, Department of Psychology.

Hatala, E. (1992). Experiential learning and therapy. Paper presented at the Celebrating Our Tradition, Charting Our Future. Banff, Canada.

Herbert, J. T. (1996). Use of adventure-based counseling programs for persons with disabilities. *Journal of Rehabilitation, 62*(4), 3-9.

Herbert, J. T. (1998). Therapeutic effects of participating in an adventure therapy program. *Rehabilitation Counseling Bulletin, 41*(3), 201.

Herbert, J. T. (2000a). Therapeutic adventure staff attitudes and preferences for working with persons with disabilities. *Therapeutic Recreation Journal, 34*(3), 211-266.

Herbert, J. T. (2000b). Director and staff views on including persons with severe disabilities in therapeutic adventure. *Therapeutic Recreation Journal, 34*(1), 16-32.

Herskowitz, R. D. (1990). Outward Bound, diabetes and motivation: Experiential education in a wilderness setting. *Diabetic Medicine, 7*(7), 633-638. doi: 10.1111/j.1464-5491.1990.tb01463.x.

Hill, N. R. (2007). Wilderness therapy as a treatment modality for at-risk youth: A primer for mental health counselors. *Journal of Mental Health Counseling, 29*, 338-349.

Hillson, R. M. (1984). Diabetes Outward Bound mountain course, Eskdale, Cumbria. *Diabetic Medicine, 1*(1), 59-63. doi: 10.1111/j.1464-5491.1984.tb01925.x.

Hough, M. & Paisley, K. (2008). An empowerment theory approach to adventure programming for adults with disabilities. *Therapeutic Recreation Journal, 42*(2), 89-102.

Houston, P. D., Knabb, J. J., Welsh, R. K., Houskamp, B. M., & Brokaw, D. (2010). Wilderness therapy as a specialized competency. *International Journal of Psychological Studies, 2*(2), 52-64.

Hyer, L., Boyd, S., Scurfield, R., Smith, D., & Burke, J. (1996). Effects of outward bound experiences as an adjunct to inpatient PTSD treatment of war veterans. *Journal of Clinical Psychology, 52*(3), 263-278.

Itin, C. M. (1995). Adventure therapy and the addictive process. *Journal of Leisurability, 22*(2).

Jarvis, P. (1995). *Adult and continuing education. Theory and practice.* London: Routledge.

Jarvis, P. (2004). *Adult and continuing education: Theory and practice* (3rd ed.). London: Routledge.

Jelalian, E., Mehlenbeck, R., Lloyd-Richardson, E. E., Birmaher, V., & Wing, R. R. (2006). "Adventure therapy" combined with cognitive-behavioral treatment for overweight adolescents. *Int J Obes Relat Metab Disord, 30*(1), 31-39.

Jelalian, E., Sato, A., & Hart, C. N. (2011). The effect of group-based weight-control intervention on adolescent psychosocial outcomes: Perceived peer rejection, social anxiety, and self-concept. *Children's Health Care, 40*(3), 197-211. doi: 10.1080/02739615.2011.590391.

Jerstad, L. & Stelzer, J. (1973). Adventure experiences as a treatment for residential mental patients. *Therapeutic Recreation Journal, 7*, 8-11.

Jones, C. D., Lowe, L. A., & Risler, E. A. (2004). The effectiveness of wilderness adventure therapy programs for young people involved in the juvenile justice system. *Residential Treatment for Children & Youth, 22*(2), 53-67. doi: 10.1300/J007v22n02_04.

Jorngarden, A., Mattsson, E., & von Essen, L. (2007). Health-related quality of life, anxiety and depression among adolescents and young adults with cancer. *European Journal of Cancer, 43*, 1952-1958.

Kelley, M. P. & Coursey, R. D. (1997). Therapeutic adventures outdoors: A demonstration of benefits for people with mental illness. *Psychiatric Rehabilitation Journal, 20*(4), 61.

Kessell, M., Resnick, M. D., & Blum, R. W. (1985). Adventure, Etc. — a health-promotion program for chronically ill and disabled youth. *Journal of Adolescent Health Care, 6*(6), 433-438. doi: http://dx.doi.org/10.1016/S0197-0070(85)80048-6.

Kim, T. K., Kang, Y. E., Kim, J. M., Hong, W. J., Kim, K. S., Kim, H. J., … Ku, B. J. (2012). Effects of diabetic camp in type 2 diabetic patients. *Korean J Med, 83*(2), 210-215.

Kinsella, E., Zeltzer, P., Dignan, T., Winter, J., Breatnach, F., & Bouffet, E. (2006). Safety of summer camp for children with chronic and/or life threatening illness. *European Journal of Oncology Nursing, 10*(4), 304-310. doi: http://dx.doi.org/10.1016/j.ejon.2005.12.009.

Kolb, D. A. (1984). *Experiential learning. Experience as the source of learning and development.* Englewood Cliffs, NJ: Prentice-Hall.

Kyriakopoulos, A. (2011). How individuals with self-reported anxiety and depression experienced a combination of individual counselling with an adventurous outdoor experience: A qualitative evaluation. *Counselling & Psychotherapy Research, 11*(2), 120-128. doi: 10.1080/14733145.2010.485696.

La Greca, A. & Lopez, N. (1998). Society anxiety among adolescents: Linkages with peer relations and friendships. *Journal of Abnormal Child Psychology, 26*(2), 83-94.

Lam, C. G., Cohen, K. J., & Rotter, D. L. (2013). Coping needs in adolescents with cancer: A participatory study. *Journal of Adolescent and Young Adult Oncology, 2*(1), 10-16. doi: 10.1089/jayao.2012.0011.

Lambie, I., Hickling, L., Seymour, F., Simmonds, L., Robson, M., & Houlahan, C. (2000). Using wilderness therapy in treating adolescent sexual offenders. *Journal of Sexual Aggression, 5*(2), 99-117. doi: 10.1080/13552600008413302.

Leberman, S. (2007). Voices behind the walls: Female offenders and experiential learning. *Journal of Adventure Education & Outdoor Learning, 7*(2), 113-130. doi: 10.1080/14729670701485832.

Lee, R. M., Draper, M., & Lee, S. (2001). Social connectedness, dysfunctional interpersonal behaviors, and psychological distress: Testing a mediator model. *Journal of Counseling Psychology, 48*(3), 310-318.

Lee, T.-Y., Shek, D. T. L., & Kwong, W.-M. (2007). Chinese approaches to understanding and building resilience in at-risk children and adolescents. *Child and Adolescent Psychiatric Clinics of North America, 16*(2), 377-392. doi: http://dx.doi.org/10.1016/j.chc.2006.12.001.

Lemmon, J., Latourette, D., & Hauver, S. (1996). One year outcome study of Outward Bound experience on the psychosocial functioning of women with mild traumatic brain injury. *Journal of Cognitive Rehabilitation, 14*, 18-23.

Lewin, K. (1935). *A dynamic theory of personality.* New York, NY: McGraw-Hill.

Lewis, S. F. (2013). Examining changes in substance use and conduct problems among treatment-seeking adolescents. *Child & Adolescent Mental Health, 18*(1), 33-38. doi: 10.1111/j.1475-3588.2012.00657.x.

Lloyd-Richardson, E. E., Jelalian, E., Sato, A. F., Hart, C. N., Mehlenbeck, R., & Wing, R. R. (2012). Two-year follow-up of an adolescent behavioral weight control intervention. *Pediatrics, 130*(2), e281-e288. doi: 10.1542/peds.2011-3283.

Lovibond, S. H. & Lovibond, P. F. (1995). *Manual for the depression anxiety stress scales* (2nd ed.). Sydney: UNSW.

Lubin, B. (1965). Adjective checklists for measurement of depression. *Archives of General Psychiatry, 12*, 57-62.

Lubin, B. (1981). *Depression adjective checklist: Professional manual.* Odessa, FL: Psychological Assessment Resources, Inc.

Luckner, J. L. (1989). Altering locus of control of individuals with hearing impairments by outdoor-adventure courses. *Journal of Rehabilitation, 55*(2), 62-67.

Lynch, D. & McInnes, M. (2008). The promise of wilderness therapy. *Journal of Experiential Education, 31*(2), 227-228.

Mancuso, M. & Caruso-Nicoletti, M. (2003). Summer camps and quality of life in children and adolescents with type 1 diabetes. *Acta Biomed Ateneo Parmense, 74*, 35-37.

Martiniuk, A. (2003). Camping programs for children with cancer and their families. *Support Care Cancer, 11*, 749-757.

McAuliffe-Fogarty, A. H., Ramsing, R., & Hill, E. (2007). Medical specialty camps for youth with diabetes. *Child and Adolescent Psychiatric Clinics of North America, 16*(4), 887-908. doi: http://dx.doi.org/10.1016/j.chc.2007.05.006.

McAvoy, L., Smith, J. G., & Rynders, J. E. (2006). Outdoor adventure programming for individuals with cognitive disabilities who present serious accommodation challenges *Therapeutic Recreation Journal, 40*(3), 182-199.

McKenzie, M. D. (2000). How are adventure education program outcomes achieved? A review of the literature. *Australian Journal of Outdoor Education, 5*(1), 19-27.

Nadler, R. S. & Luckner, J. L. (1992). *Processing the adventure experience: Theory and practice.* Dubuque, IA: Kendall/Hunt Publishing.

Newes, S. L. & Bandoroff, S. (2004). What is adventure therapy? In S. L. Newes & S. Bandoroff (Eds.), *Coming of age: The evolving field of adventure therapy* (pp. 1-30). Boulder, CO: Association for Experiential Education.

O'Mahar, K., Holmbeck, G. N., Jandasek, B., & Zukerman, J. (2010). A camp-based intervention targeting independence among individuals with spina bifida. *Journal of Pediatric Psychology, 35*(8), 848-856. doi: 10.1093/jpepsy/jsp125.

Odar, C., Canter, K. S., & Roberts, M. C. (2013). Relationship between camp attendance and self-perceptions in children with chronic health conditions: A meta-analysis. *Journal of Pediatric Psychology, 38*(4), 398-411.

Outward Bound. (n.d. a). Outward Bound for veterans: Reenergizing veterans through adventure and challenge. Retrieved from www.outwardbound.org/veteran-adventures/outward-bound-for-veterans.

Outward Bound. (n.d. b). Outward Bound philosophy. Retrieved from www.outwardbound.org/about-outward-bound/philosophy/

Pelham, W. E. & Fabiano, G. A. (2008). Evidence-based psychosocial treatments for attention-deficit/hyperactivity disorder. *Journal of Clinical Child & Adolescent Psychology, 37*(1), 184-214. doi: 10.1080/15374410701818681.

Portrie-Bethke, T. L., Hill, N. R., & Bethke, J. G. (2009). Strength-based mental health counseling for children with ADHD: An integrative model of adventure-based counseling and Adlerian play therapy. *Journal of Mental Health Counseling, 31*(4), 323-337. doi: 10.1177/08830738050200121301.

Priest, S. (1998). Physical challenge and the development of trust through corporate adventure training. *Journal of Experiential Education, 21*(1), 31-34.

Priest, S. & Gass, M. (1997). *Effective leadership in adventure programming.* Champaign, IL: Human Kinetics.

Priest, S., Gass, M., & Fitzpatrick, K. (1999). Training corporate managers to facilitate: The next generation of facilitating experiential methodologies. *Journal of Experiential Education, 17*(1), 34-39.

Priest, S., Gass, M., & Gillis, H. L. (2000). *The essential elements of facilitation.* Champaign, IL: Human Kinetics.

Priest, S. & Naismith, M. (1993). A model for debriefing experiences. *Journal of Adventure Education & Outdoor Learning, 10*(3), 20-22.

Project Adventure. (n.d.). Glossary of terms. Retrieved from www.pa.org/about-us/glossary-of-terms.

Ragsdale, K., Cox, R., Finn, P., & Eisler, R. (1996). Effectiveness of short-term specialized inpatient treatment for war-related posttraumatic stress disorder: A role for adventure-based counseling and psychodrama. *Journal of Traumatic Stress, 9*(2), 269-283. doi: 10.1007/bf02110660.

Rhee, H. S. M. Y. H. L. (2008). Pearls and pitfalls of community-based group interventions for adolescents: Lessons learned from an adolescent asthma camp study. *Issues in Comprehensive Pediatric Nursing, 31*(3), 122-135. doi: 10.1080/01460860802272888.

Rohnke, K. (1989a). *Cowstails and cobras II.* Dubuque: IA: Kendall Hunt Publishing.

Rohnke, K. (1989b). Silver bullets: *A guide to initiative problems, adventure games, stunts and trust activities.* Dubuque, IA: Kendall/Hunt Publishing Co.

Rohnke, K., Rogers, D., Tait, C. M., & Wall, J. B. (2007). *The complete ropes course manual.* Dubuque, IA: Kendall/Hunt.

Rohnke, K., Wall, J. B., & Rogers, D. (2002). *The complete ropes course manual.* Dubuque, IA: Kendall Hunt Publishing.

Rosenberg, M. (1965). *Society and the adolescent self-image.* Princeton, NJ: Princeton University Press.

Russell, K. (2001a). *Assessment of treatment outcomes in outdoor behavioral healthcare.* Moscow, ID: University of Idaho Wilderness Research Center.

Russell, K. (2001b). What is wilderness therapy? *Journal of Experiential Education, 24*(3), 70.

Russell, K. (2006). Brat camp, boot camp, or...? Exploring wilderness therapy program theory. *Journal of Adventure Education & Outdoor Learning, 6*(1), 51-67.

Russell, K. & Farnum, J. (2004). A concurrent model of the wilderness therapy process. *Journal of Adventure Education and Outdoor Learning, 4*(1), 39-55. doi: 10.1080/14729670485200411.

Russell, K., Hendee, J. C., & Phillips-Miller, D. (2000). How wilderness therapy works: An examination of the wilderness therapy process to treat adolescents with behavioral problems and addictions. Paper presented at the Wilderness Science in a Time of Change, Missoula, MT.

SAMHSA. (2012). Behavior management through adventure. Retrieved from www.nrepp.samhsa.gov/ViewIntervention.aspx?id=260.

SAMHSA. (2013). Evidence-based practices for preventing substance use disorders in adolescents. Retrieved from www.nrepp.samhsa.gov/ViewIntervention.aspx?id=102.

Santucci, L.-M. J. (2013). A randomized controlled trial of the child anxiety multi-day program (CAMP) for separation anxiety disorder. *Child Psychiatry and Human Development, 44*(3), 439-451. doi: 10.1007/s10578-012-0338-6.

Scheinfeld, D. E., Rochlen, A. B., & Buser, S. J. (2011). Adventure therapy: A supplementary group therapy approach for men. *Psychology of Men & Masculinity, 12*(2), 188-194. doi: http://dx.doi.org/10.1037/a0022041.

Schell, L., Cotton, S., & Luxmoore, M. (2012). Outdoor adventure for young people with a mental illness. *Early Intervention in Psychiatry, 6*(4), 407-414. doi: 10.1111/j.1751-7893.2011.00326.x.

Schoel, J. & Maizell, R. (2002). *Exploring islands of healing: New perspectives on adventure based counseling.* Beverly, MA: Project Adventure.

Schoel, J., Prouty, D., & Radcliffe, P. (1988). *Islands of healing: A guide to adventure based counseling.* Hamilton, MA: Project Adventure.

Seaman, J. & Rheingold, A. (2013). Circle talks as situated experiential learning: Context, identity, and knowledgeability in "Learning from Reflection." *Journal of Experiential Education, 36*(2), 155-174. doi: 10.1177/1053825913487887.

Shanahan, L., McAllister, L., & Curtin, M. (2009). Wilderness adventure therapy and cognitive rehabilitation: Joining forces for youth with TBI. *Brain Injury, 23*(13-14), 1054-1064. doi: 10.3109/02699050903421115.

Shooter, W., Paisley, K., & Sibthorp, J. (2010). Trust development in outdoor leadership. *Journal of Experiential Education, 33*(3), 189-207.

Sklar, S. L., Anderson, S. C., & Autry, C. E. (2007). Positive youth development: A wilderness intervention. *Therapeutic Recreation Journal, 41*(3), 223-243.

Smith, K. E., Gotlieb, S., Gurwitch, R. H., & Blotcky, A. D. (1987). Impact of a summer camp experience on daily activity and family interactions among children with cancer. *Journal of Pediatric Psychology, 12*(4), 533-542. doi: 10.1093/jpepsy/12.4.533.

Somervell, J. & Lambie, I. (2009). Wilderness therapy within an adolescent sexual offender treatment programme: A qualitative study. *Journal of Sexual Aggression, 15*(2), 161-177. doi: 10.1080/13552600902823055.

Stevens, B., Kagan, S., Yamada, J., Epstein, I., Beamer, M., Bilodeau, M., & Baruchel, S. (2004). Adventure therapy for adolescents with cancer. *Pediatric Blood & Cancer, 43*(3), 278-284. doi: 10.1002/pbc.20060.

Sugerman, D. (2005). "I am more than my cancer": An exploratory examination of adventure programming and cancer survivors. *Journal of Experiential Education, 28*(1), 72-83. doi: 10.1177/105382590502800108.

Sugerman, D., Doherty, K. L., Garvey, D. E., & Gass, M. A. (2000). *Reflective learning: Theory and practice.* Dubuque, IL: Kendall/Hunt.

Thomas, M. (2004). The Potential Unlimited programme: An outdoor experiential education and group work approach that facilitates adjustment to brain injury. *Brain Injury, 18*(12), 1271-1286. doi: 10.1080/02699050410001698776.

Tiemens, K., Beveridge, H. L., & Nicholas, D. B. (2006). A therapeutic camp weekend for adolescents with craniofacial differences. *The Cleft Palate-Craniofacial Journal, 43*(1), 44-46. doi: 10.1597/04-124r.1.

Torok, S., Kokonyei, G., Karolyi, L., Ittzes, A., & Tomcsanyi, T. (2006). Outcome effectiveness of therapeutic recreation camping program for adolescents living with cancer and diabetes. *J Adolescent Health, 39*, 445- 447.

Tucker, A. R. (2009). Adventure-based group therapy to promote social skills in adolescents. *Social Work with Groups, 32*(4), 315-329. doi: 10.1080/01609510902874594.

Tucker, A. R. & Rheingold, A. (2010). Enhancing fidelity in adventure education and adventure therapy. *Journal of Experiential Education, 33*(1), 258-273.

Tucker, A. R., Javorski, S., Tracy, J., & Beale, B. (2013). The use of adventure therapy in community-based mental health: Decreases in problem severity among youth clients. *Child and Youth Care Forum, 42*(2), 155-179.

Tucker, A. R., Sugerman, D., & Zelov, R. (2013). On belay: Providing connection, support, and empowerment to children who have a parent with cancer. *Journal of Experiential Education, 36*(2), 93-105. doi: 10.1177/1053825913487889.

Voruganti, L. N. P., Whatham, J., Bard, E., Parker, G., Babbey, C., Ryan, J. ... & MacCrimmon, D. J. (2006). Going beyond: An adventure- and recreation-based group intervention promotes well-being and weight loss in schizophrenia. *Canadian Journal of Psychiatry, 51*(9), 575-580.

Walker, A. J., Onus, M., Doyle, M., Clare, J., & McCarthy, K. (2005). Cognitive rehabilitation after severe traumatic brain injury: A pilot programme of goal planning and outdoor adventure course participation. *Brain Injury, 19*(14), 1237-1241. doi: 10.1080/02699050500309411.

Walsh, J. & Aubry, P. (2007). Behavior management through adventure. *Reclaiming Children and Youth, 16*(1), 36-39.

Walsh, V. & Golin, G. L. (1976). *The exploration of the Outward Bound process.* Denver, CO: Outward Bound School.

Welch, T. R. & Ryan, R. (2002). Sudden unexpected death on challenge courses. *Wilderness & Environmental Medicine, 13*(2), 140-142. doi: http://dx.doi.org/10.1580/1080-6032(2002)013[0140:SUDOCC]2.0.CO;2.

White, W. (2012). A history of adventure therapy. In M. Gass, H. L. L. Gillis, & K. C. Russel (Eds.) *Adventure therapy: Theory, research, and practice.* New York, NY: Routledge.

Wick, D. T., Wick, J. K., & Peterson, N. (1997). Improving self-esteem with Adlerian adventure therapy. *Professional School Counseling, 1*(1), 53-56.

Witman, J. P. & Preskenis, K. (1996). Adventure programming with an individual who has multiple personality disorder: A case history. *Therapeutic Recreation Journal, 30*(4), 289-296.

Wolf, M. & Mehl, K. (2011). Experiential learning in psychotherapy: Ropes course exposures as an adjunct to inpatient treatment. *Clinical Psychology & Psychotherapy, 18*(1), 60-74. doi: 10.1002/cpp.692.

Wu, C.-C. & Hsieh, C.-M. (2006). The effects of a leisure education programme on the self concepts and life effectiveness of at-risk youth in Taiwan. *World Leisure Journal, 48*(2), 54-60. doi: 10.1080/04419057.2006.9674444.

Wynn, B., Frost, A., & Pawson, P. (2012). Adventure therapy proves successful for adolescent survivors of childhood cancers: Wilderness journeys for teenage cancer survivors are helping address many of their long-term health issues. *Nursing New Zealand, 18*, 28-30.

14. Anger Management

Alexis McKenney

Although anger is a normal, healthy emotion, it is also one that can escalate into feelings that range from aggression to rage (Spielberger, 1991). It typically manifests itself through behavioral symptoms, such as grinding teeth or raised voices, and physiological symptoms, such as tensed muscles or perspiration (Novaco, 1975). Anger is a natural response to a situation when a person feels threatened or unfairly treated (Reilly et al., 2002), but the expression of anger can become problematic if it is expressed inappropriately or experienced for intensive and extended periods of time (Hagiliassis et al., 2005). Anger, furthermore, is often an antecedent to physical or passive aggression (Hagiliassis et al., 2005) and may involve violent actions directed towards a target with an aim to destroy or injure that target (Lochman & Lenhart, 1993). According to the World Health Organization, there are three types of violence: self-directed, interpersonal, and collective. In self-directed violence the victim and perpetrator are the same individual. Interpersonal violence involves violent behaviors between individuals. Collective violence is defined as acts performed by a group for social, political, or economic reasons.

According to Porter and burlingame (2006), "When handled in a positive manner (e.g., talking out the problem, going for a walk to calm down), it can move people toward a positive result (e.g., solve a problem, learn something new)" (p. 492). A common approach to providing anger management programs that focus on teaching people to handle anger appropriately is through the use of cognitive-behavioral strategies. Cognitive behavioral therapy (CBT) is a primary orientation of psychotherapy. This form of treatment is unique in that it is derived from the behavioral and cognitive models of behavior (Roth & Fonagy, 2005). In other words, the model recognizes the importance of an individual's cognitive experi-

ences while preserving the best of clinical behavioral interventions. The behavioral model is based on the argument that behavior is determined by external events (Good & Brophy, 1990), and the cognitive model is centered on how an individual cognitively processes a situation (Beck, 1995). Cognitive-behavioral interventions center on a person's cognitive deficiency relative to maturity, complexity, expression of emotions, and distorted thinking that could lead to false assumptions and related reactions (Sofronoff et al., 2007). According to Ekman (2003), these interventions align with current theoretical models on human emotions: As one becomes more aware of his/her emotional state, s/he becomes more sensitive to how other people are feeling. Because dysfunctional thinking is central to negative behaviors and emotions, cognitive-behavioral interventions are used to change the manner in which a person conceptualizes situations.

This chapter provides a summary of how a cognitive-behavioral-based anger management program can serve as a recreational therapy protocol. Indications, contraindications, a description of the protocol, and resources are provided.

Causes of Anger

To be able to address anger and/or aggression, the recreational therapist, along with the interdisciplinary treatment team, work to identify the cause of the anger experienced by the participant. According to Porter and burlingame (2006), failing to address anger might hinder a participant's progress. "For example, a client may be so angry at his current situation that it impedes his ability to concentrate and learn new skills. It may also affect his social relationships with others and his ability to problem solve for barriers (because 'life just stinks and I'm too angry to deal with it'). Anger can also lead to adjustment problems (e.g., depression, anxiety, inability to work with caregivers)" (Porter & burlingame, 2006, p. 492).

Examples of causes of anger include those related to medical illness, such as brain tumors or other cancers, influenza, encephalitis, multiple sclerosis, substance-induced mood disorder, and bipolar disorder. Anger can also arise because of task-related anxiety that is more than a participant can cope with or an inability to express needs, for example as a result of a speech impairment or poor communication ability. Behaving in a negative manner with the goal of receiving attention or other reinforcers, and as a way to escape or avoid a situation because of feeling vulnerable, may also be seen as an expression of anger.

A participant might also demonstrate aggression as a side effect of medication (Porter & burlingame, 2006). Examples of such medications include "neurological medications, nonsteroidal anti-inflammatory drugs, anticancer medications, anesthetic medications, antibiotic medications, penicillin, procaine, heavy metals and toxins such as organic tin (which can cause unprovoked rage attacks), amphetamines, bromides, cocaine, corticosteroids, levodopa, MAOI, tricyclic antidepressants, methylphenidate, over-the-counter stimulants and appetite suppressants, vitamin deficiencies, excess of fat-soluble vitamins, phenobarbital, anticonvulsant medication, and methamphetamines" (Porter & burlingame, 2006, p. 492).

Golant and Crane (1987) noted that individuals are not born with a natural understanding of how to control and cope with anger and associated feelings of aggression and violence. They argued that it must be learned. Anger is a common emotion, but if it is expressed inappropriately or experienced for an extended period of time, it can become problematic (Hagiliassis et al., 2005). This is evidenced by a high number of clinical referrals to behavioral health services. Lipman and Offord (2006) contended that anger-driven aggression and violence is, perhaps, the most common reason for referrals of children and adolescents to clinical behavioral health services, and accounts for more than one-third of referrals to outpatient services.

Indications

According to Porter and burlingame (2006), "Any medical condition that affects the brain may

cause anger" (p. 492). Examples of illnesses or disabilities that are documented as affecting emotions include traumatic brain injury (TBI), cerebrovascular accident, multiple sclerosis, behavior disorders, developmental disabilities, learning disabilities, and substance-induced mood disorders. Strategies for teaching individuals anger coping strategies depend on the problems the individual is experiencing specific to their illnesses. For example, an individual who has sustained a TBI might experience impairments in social and/or behavioral functioning (Campbell, 2000) that might include verbal and/or physical aggression (Kim et al., 2007).

Cognitive behavioral interventions are commonly used to teach anger coping skills to children and adolescents with behavior disorders; however, research has shown that such strategies can also be helpful in treating individuals with TBI. In a study that included 28 participants (M = 26, F = 2), Medd and Tate (2000) examined the effects of an anger-management program over six one-hour sessions. Participants in the treatment group were guided through a process that began with learning principles of brain injury and how anger problems can result, to practicing strategies, such as relaxation, self-talk, and time-out procedures. Using the *State-Trait Anger Expression Inventory* (STAXI) (Spielberger, 1988), participants in the treatment group demonstrated improvements from pre-test to post-test and again two months after completing the program.

ICF codes that may indicate the need for anger management training include b126 Temperament and Personality Functions, b130 Energy and Drive Functions, b152 Emotional Functions, b164 Higher-Level Cognitive Functions, d2 General Tasks and Demands, especially d240 Handling Stress and Other Psychological Demands, and d7 Interpersonal Interactions and Relationships. Deficits in d3 Communication, d6 Domestic Life, d8 Major Life Areas, and d9 Community, Social, and Civic Life should be evaluated to see if they have an anger management component. More details on specific scoring of the intervention related to the ICF are discussed in the Outcomes section.

Contraindications

How to cope with and control anger often requires the development of anger coping strategies taught through a planned process (Golant & Crane,

1987). This is particularly true for individuals who have sustained a TBI, for they often experience feelings of frustration, anxiety, and stress in addition to feelings of anger (Denmark & Gemeinhardt, 2002). When stress and anxiety levels limit a participant's success in the anger management program, the facilitation of stress management techniques, such as progressive relaxation and yoga, might be considered. Progressive relaxation involves the use of techniques that help participants to relax or reduce physical tension through a process of tensing and releasing each of the 16 muscle groups (Bernstein & Borkovec, 1973; Lucic et al., 1991). Yoga focuses on the mind, body, and spirit (Smith, 1986) and focuses on five points, each of which is designed to address needs specific to the individual (Angus, 1989).

Protocols

For the purpose of this chapter, several programs and ideas are described. The main emphasis is on the Anger Coping Program (ACP) (Gongora, McKenney, & Godinez, 2006). Other ideas include the ZIPPER Strategy and "In Control." McKenney and Dattilo (2011) looked at average time frames from select anger management programs designed for working with children and adolescents with behavior disorders and/or learning disabilities (Cobb et al., 2005; Etscheidt, 1991; Hagiliassis et al., 2005; Willner et al., 2002). They found that programs are most effective when planned for 12 to 18 sessions, one hour per session.

Prior to starting any program, assessment data are collected. Gongora, McKenney, and Godinez (2006) recommend that recreational therapists use two assessment tools: the *Functional Independence Measure*™ (FIM™) (Guide for the Uniform Data Set for Medical Rehabilitation, 1997), and the *Functional Assessment Measure*™ (FAM™) (Hall, 1997) to score participants' overall levels of functioning. Each member of the treatment team should be responsible for administering discipline-specific components of the assessment. The FIM™ assessment involves categorizing results on a seven-point rating scale that ranges from "complete independence" to "total assist" and measures independent functioning in self-care, transfers, communication, locomotion, and social cognition (Center for Outcome Measurement in Brain Injury, n.d.). The FAM™, similarly, involves a seven-point rating scale that involves categorizing

patient functioning levels from "independence" to "complete dependence" (Hall, 1997). Examples of items assessed include community access, communication, attention and concentration, and psychosocial adjustment. Additionally, the *Comprehensive Evaluation in Recreational Therapy — Psych/Behavioral Revised* (Parker et al., 1998) can be used to measure the participants' abilities to function in an RT treatment group.

Gongora, McKenney, and Godinez (2006) additionally recommended that a leisure-related assessment specific to RT services be administered to determine participants' past and present leisure interests. Two examples of leisure-related assessments include the *Leisurescope Plus* or *Teen Leisurescope Plus* (Schenk, 1998) and the *Leisure and Recreation Involvement* assessment tool (Ragheb, 2002).

Anger Coping Program (ACP)

The ACP includes eight, one-hour sessions designed for individuals who have sustained a traumatic brain injury (TBI). Although this program is described as it is used with individuals who have sustained a TBI, the steps (identifying and coping with anger, discussing assertive behavior, modeling assertive behavior, role-playing assertive behavior, and processing feelings) can be used with other populations, such as youth with behavior disorders or who are at risk.

Once assessment data are collected, the planning phase begins. It is at this time that goals are formulated and strategies are determined. The implementation phase involves the actual delivery of the ACP. Sessions are designed to teach participants anger coping skills, reinforce what was learned in prior sessions, and help them prepare for the next ACP session. The order of sessions should include identifying anger, reacting to anger, the boiling point, coping with stress and anger, discussing assertiveness, modeling assertiveness, role-playing, and processing feelings. Descriptions of each session follow. The ACP can be delivered to participants individually or in a group.

Identifying anger: During the first session, activities are implemented to help participants increase their awareness of what makes them angry. Participants are asked to define anger, identify stressors they experience in their daily lives, and categorize stressors into levels of anger. The recreational therapist explains how anger is used as a means of responding to stressors and is expressed through verbal or physical aggression. Participants are then asked to identify situations that cause them to experience anger and categorize these situations into ones that irritate them, make them angry, and/or cause them to respond aggressively. See Table 7 for an example of what the categories might look like.

Table 7: Example of Self-Reported Reactions to Anger-Producing Situations

Irritated

Anger producing situations

- Other people's lack of compassion and consideration
- Other people's lack of awareness of the diagnosis
- Inability to contribute to daily family activities
- Overprotective mother
- Anybody driving fast
- Difficulty driving at night
- People not living up to their word
- Other people behaving irresponsibly

Reaction to situation
A little irritated; accepts situation

Mad

Anger producing situations

- Over stimulation
- Lack of involvement and consistency from father in relationship
- Lack of understanding from father in reference to diagnosis
- Lack of commitment and support from father
- Frustration with trying to reintegrate into the community
- Awareness of deficits as they emerged
- Memory problems

Reaction to situation
Upset; reacts verbally

Explosive

Anger producing situations

- Inability to be flexible with unexpected changes
- Multi-tasking and over-stimulation

- Brother not helping around the house with chores

Reaction to situation
Very angry; reacts physically

Gongora, McKenney, and Godinez (2006)

Reacting to anger: Participants are next asked to recall the last time they felt angry, what it felt like both emotionally and physically, and identify corresponding bodily reactions. This is done to help participants identify their bodily reactions to anger, which helps them to become aware of their physiological signs of anger escalation. The recreational therapist, furthermore, explains that as a result of an escalation in feelings of anger, bodily reactions occur that individuals might not notice. These reactions occur when the nervous system and muscles prepare for an "attack" that might manifest physically or verbally.

The boiling point: During the third session, participants are asked to draw comparisons of anger to temperatures measured on a thermometer. The recreational therapist explains that when situations arise that elicit anger, a person's emotional temperature increases. A picture of a thermometer is provided to help participants visualize their individual "boiling point" and to better understand what triggers their anger at different times during the day or week.

Coping with stress and anger: Next, participants are provided with information that guides them in learning how to identify the "fight or flight" response to anger. The purpose of this session is to help participants understand means for confronting emotions. In particular, they learn to identify strategies that help them to cope with stress. For example, participants might be asked to imagine that they are in the woods when they see a bear that they believe is going to attack them. The recreational therapist provides suggestions for coping with the stress of such a confrontation, attempting to injure or kill the bear, diverting the bear's attention by tossing something distracting (e.g., food) toward the bear, or avoiding the bear by running away. The example of the confrontation with the bear is described as a metaphor for other potential stressors or anger producing situations.

Discussing assertiveness: The fifth session centers on teaching participants how to respond to anger-provoking situations in an assertive manner.

Assertiveness involves employing a direct and honest approach to expressing thoughts and feelings. Gongora, McKenney, and Godinez (2006) argue that when an individual is assertive, s/he is confidently demonstrating respect for the rights of other people while assuring that the individual's own needs and rights are respected. The person speaks clearly at appropriate times and confidently expresses his/her needs, opinions, thoughts, and feelings, such as during situations that cause the person to experience anger. A person who assertively verbalizes feelings without becoming aggressive is demonstrating the capacity to properly channel anger. Alternatively, a person who responds passively is demonstrating fear and is less likely to appropriately express feelings.

Modeling assertive behavior: Next, the recreational therapist models ways to appropriately express feelings of anger in a manner that helps participants develop the ability to apply coping strategies in a variety of environments. For example, the recreational therapist might model different verbal and physical reactions that participants could use when they feel threatened. To illustrate this strategy, the recreational therapist might model leaving a potentially threatening situation by showing how to turn and walk away after someone makes a disparaging comment.

Role-playing assertive behavior: During the seventh session, the recreational therapist organizes role-play activities that parallel situations participants have confronted in the past or might confront in the future. Before each role-play activity is initiated, participants decide how they should react in that particular situation. These activities should be designed to help them express their feelings in an assertive manner. At the close of this session, the authors recommended that recreational therapists provide participants with notebooks to document anger-provoking situations that they confront each day. Participants are asked to use the notebooks for the remainder of the program and to continue to use them after the program ends. Participants are asked to be ready to discuss one of their entries while participating in the last session.

Processing feelings: The last session involves discussing anger-provoking situations that participants wrote about in their notebooks. To provide guidance, participants are asked to describe one positive result of the confrontational situation, how

they handled the situation, and what they might do in the future to handle the confrontational situation differently.

At the close of the ACP, a systematic process of gathering and analyzing information to assess quality, effectiveness, and/or outcomes should be conducted (Peterson & Stumbo, 2000). A formative evaluation of participants' responses during the ACP sessions that involves conducting ongoing observations of participants' behaviors, along with interviews conducted by the recreational therapist, is recommended. In addition, Gongora, McKenney, and Godinez (2006) recommended that recreational therapists complete evaluations to determine if they had attained goals set prior to the implementation of the ACP.

ZIPPER Strategy

Wilkening and Gazitt, (1991) developed the ZIPPER Strategy. ZIPPER is a mnemonic (Zip your mouth, Identify the problem, Pause, Put yourself in charge, Explore choices, and Reset) that was created to help participants remember how to respond when confronted with an anger-provoking situation. Exercises include: (1) getting started, (2) introducing ZIPPER, (3) promoting cognitive modeling, (4) practicing with help, (5) practicing self-instruction, (6) fading self-instruction, and (7) committing to using the strategy.

Getting started involves conducting interviews with participants to determine types of situations that might provoke them to respond aggressively. For example, a question might be, "Can you remember a time that you were so angry that you felt like hitting someone or something?" Introducing ZIPPER involves using cue cards and picture prompts that outlines what each letter represents: Z — Zip your mouth, I — Identify the problem, P — Pause, P — Put yourself in control, E — Explore other solutions, and R — Reset.

To promote cognitive modeling, the recreational therapist uses a "thinking aloud" procedure to demonstrate how to use verbal and physical cues. It is recommended that recreational therapists choose a scenario that the participant identified as aggression producing. To practice with help, the recreational therapist uses scenarios based on situations identified by participants while providing verbal cues as the participant models a physical response. The ZIPPER steps are reviewed then spoken out loud while participants show the recreational therapist physical cues that they were taught. Participants then demonstrate the strategy with prompts provided only as needed. Fading occurs as participants whisper verbal cues while modeling physical cues. Practice sessions then allow them to think through the steps by themselves. To reinforce participation beyond the group, the recreational therapist might ask them to consider good things they think will happen if they use the ZIPPER strategy at home or in school (Wilkening & Gazitt, 1991).

In Control

The In Control program involves ten weekly, 30-minute skill-building sessions (Kellner, 2008). Similar to the ZIPPER Strategy, the In Control program uses a cognitive-behavioral intervention to teach participants skills for reducing aggressive behavior while developing prosocial behavior skills. Participants learn to identify anger triggers, degree of anger arousal, how to use a log to record instances, and how to use techniques for deescalating. Central to the program is the use of the anger log sheets. Included on the sheets are spaces for participants to identify the causes of anger, an appraisal of the degree of their anger from not angry to extremely angry, a plan for how they will deal with a similar anger inducing occurrence, and an overall evaluation of how they feel they handled themselves. Skill acquisition occurs through a series of sessions that include discussions, modeling, and role-play activities. After the conclusion of the program, "booster sessions" are conducted during which anger logs are monitored and opportunities for skill strengthening are offered.

Individualized Plans

Anger triggers and reactions vary greatly between individuals (Ekman, 2003). Because of the great differences, there is sometimes a need to develop a plan specific to an individual. Porter and burlingame (2006) offer the following suggestions for recreational therapists in developing individualized anger management plans.

First, because learning how to manage anger requires being able to identify the cause of the anger, it is important for participants to be able to identify anger "triggers." For example, an adolescent partici-

pant feels angry because his mother asks him to do something when he is busy doing something else.

Second, the recreational therapist should assist participants to critically evaluate identified triggers and identify corresponding distorted thinking patterns. For example, the recreational therapist might assist a participant in evaluating whether he, indeed, "knows" the he cannot do something that he used to do. Similarly, it is important for participants to be aware of internal and external warning signs such as, clenched fists and perspiration. This sets the stage for teaching participants appropriate coping strategies. For example, counting backwards from 10 or physical and/or relaxation exercises.

Finally, participants sometimes demonstrate anger in a manner that is considered unacceptable to their families or cultures. Consequently, the recreational therapist should assist participants in understanding that anger is a natural emotion and that it is important to develop the coping strategies necessary to express the anger effectively while keeping it from manifesting itself in a way that is harmful to the person feeling the anger or to others.

Outcomes and Documentation

The ICF does not include anger specifically. The manifestations of anger can be documented using several ICF codes. If anger is a result of a medical condition, it could by scored using the appropriate subcodes in b126 Temperament and Personality Functions, b130 Energy and Drive Functions, and b152 Emotional Functions. The same codes could be used with stress-related anger, which should also be documented with b164 Higher-Level Cognitive Functions, d2 General Tasks and Demands, and d240 Handling Stress and Other Psychological Demands.

The consequences of anger generally show up in d7 Interpersonal Interactions and Relationships, but they may affect many parts of the Activities and Participation codes, such as d3 Communication, d6 Domestic Life, d8 Major Life Areas, and d9 Community, Social, and Civic Life. When scoring the ICF make a notation to the right of the scoring area about anger, aggression, irritability, or rage. Recreational therapists teaching clients anger management and coping skills should document the intervention by using the codes noted in the client assessments. Because anger can be a pervasive problem for clients, the recreational therapist should be sure to note all of the ICF codes that the intervention will improve.

Outside of the ICF, anger management skills can be measured and documented in other ways. For example, behavioral observations (Lochman & Curry, 1986), tracking of acting-out behaviors (Feindler et al., 1986), self-reported levels of anger (Hagiliassis et al., 2005), and summative evaluations (Gongora, McKenney, & Godinez, 2006). Specifically, anger can be measured and documented by assessing the following areas, as outlined by Porter and burlingame (2006):

- Frequency of angry verbalizations or gestures during a specific time frame
- Identification of current and resolved causes of anger
- Identification and use of anger coping skills
- Documentation of clients' comments specific to anger

Resources

The Louis de la Parte Florida Mental Health Institute

http://home.fmhi.usf.edu/.
Offers a curriculum for teaching children and adolescents appropriate ways to express anger.

National Institute of Mental Health

www.nimh.nih.gov/nimhhome/index.cfm
Public Information and Communications Branch

The Center for Mental Health Services, U.S. Department of Health and Human Services

http://mentalhealth.samhsa.gov/cmhs/
Provides information and services designed to help improve and increase the quality and range of treatment and support services to individuals experiencing mental health problems.

References

Angus, S. F. (1989). Three approaches to stress management for children. *Elementary School Guidance and Counseling, 23,* 228-233.

Beck, J. S. (1995). *Cognitive therapy: Basics and beyond.* New York: Guilford Press.

Bernstein, D. A. & Borkovec, T. D. (1973). *Progressive relaxation training: A manual for the helping professions.* Champaign, IL: Research Press.

Campbell, M. (2000). *Rehabilitation for therapeutic brain injury: Physical therapy practice in context.* Churchill Livingston, NY: Harcourt Publisher Limited.

Cobb, B., Sample, P., Alwell, M., & Johns, N. (2005). *The effects of cognitive behavioral interventions on dropout for youth with disabilities.* Paper presented at 2004 Annual Council for Exceptional Children Conference. New Orleans, LA.

Center for Outcome Measurement in Brain Injury. (n.d.). FAM syllabus. Retrieved from http://tbims.org/combi/FAM/famsyl.html.

Denmark, J. & Gemeinhardt, M. (2002). Anger and its management for survivors of acquired brain injury. *Brain Injury, 16,* 91-108.

Ekman, P. (2003). *Emotions revealed: Recognizing faces and feelings to improve communication and emotional life.* New York: Times Books.

Etscheidt, S. (1991). Reducing aggressive behavior and improving self-concept: A cognitive-behavioral training program for behaviorally disordered adolescents. *Behavioral Disorders, 16,* 107-115.

Feindler, E. L., Ecton, R. B., Kingsley, D., & Dubey, D. R. (1986). Group anger control training for institutionalized psychiatric male adolescents. *Behavior Therapy, 17,* 109-123.

Golant, M. & Crane, B. (1987). *Sometimes it's o.k. to be angry!* New York: Tom Doherty Associates.

Gongora, E., McKenney, A., & Godinez, C. (2006). A multidisciplinary approach to teaching anger coping after sustaining a traumatic brain injury: A case report. *Therapeutic Recreation Journal, 39,* 229-240.

Good, T. L. & Brophy, J. E. (1990). *Educational psychology. A realistic approach.* White Plains, NY: Longman.

Hagiliassis, N., Gulbenkoglu, H., DiMarco, M., Young, S., & Hudson, A. (2005). The anger management project: A group intervention for anger in people with physical and multiple disabilities. *Journal of Intellectual & Developmental Disability, 30,* 86-96.

Hall, K. M. (1997). The functional assessment measure (FAM). *Journal of Rehabilitation Outcomes, 1*(3), 63-65.

Kellner, N. H. (2008). Anger management effects on middle school students with emotional/behavioral disorders: Anger log use, aggressive and prosocial behavior. *Child and Family Behavior Therapy, 30,* 215-230.

Kim, E., Lauterback, E., Reeve, A., Arciniegas, D., Coburn, K., Mendez, M., Rummans, T., & Coffey, E. (2007). Neuropsychiatric complications of traumatic brain injury: A critical review of the literature. *Journal of Neuropsychiatry & Clinical Neurosciences, 19,* 106-127.

Lipman, E. L. & Offord, M. H. (2006). Conduct disorder in girls. In S. Roman & M. Seeman (Eds.), *Women's mental health: A life cycle approach* (pp. 93-107). Philadelphia: Lippincott, Williams & Wilkins.

Lochman, J. E. & Curry, J. F. (1986). Effects of social problem-solving training and self-instruction training with aggressive boys. *Journal of Clinical Child Psychology, 15,* 159-164.

Lochman, J. E. & Lenhart, L. A. (1993). Anger coping intervention for aggressive children: Conceptual models for outcome effects. *Clinical Psychology Review, 13,* 785-805.

Lucic, K. S., Steffen, J. J., Harrigan, J. A., & Stuebing, R. C. (1991). Progressive relaxation training: Muscle contraction before relaxation? *Behavior Therapy, 22,* 249-256.

McKenney, A. & Dattilo, J. (2011). Anger management. In J. Dattilo & A. McKenney, *Facilitation techniques in therapeutic recreation* (pp. 43-68). State College, PA: Venture.

Medd, J. & Tate, R. L. (2000). Evaluation of an anger management therapy programme following acquired brain injury: A preliminary study. *Neuropsychological Rehabilitation, 10*(2), 185-201.

Novaco, R. W. (1975). *Anger control: The development and evaluation of an experimental treatment.* Lexington, MA: D.C. Heath and Company.

Parker, R. A., Ellison, C. H., Kirby, T. F., & Short, M. J. (1998). Comprehensive Evaluation in Recreational Therapy — Psych/Behavioral Revised. Enumclaw, WA: Idyll Arbor.

Peterson, C. A. & Stumbo, N. J. (2000). *Therapeutic recreation design: Principles and procedures* (3rd ed.). Boston: Allyn & Bacon.

Porter, H. R. & burlingame, j. (2006). *Recreational therapy handbook of practice: ICF-based diagnosis and treatment,* Enumclaw, WA: Idyll Arbor.

Ragheb, M. (2002). *Assessment of leisure and recreation involvement (LRI).* Ravensdale, WA: Idyll Arbor.

Reilly, P. M., Shopshire, M. S. Durazzo, T. C., & Campbell, T. A. (2002). *Anger management for substance abuse and mental health patients: A cognitive behavioral therapy manual and participant workbook.* Rockville, MD: National Clearinghouse for Alcohol and Drug Information.

Roth, A. & Fonagy, P. (2005). *What works for whom? A critical review of psychotherapy research* (2nd ed.). New York: Guilford.

Schenk, C. (1998). *Leisurescope plus.* Enumclaw, WA: Idyll Arbor.

Smith, H. (1986). *The religions of man.* New York: Harper & Row.

Sofronoff, K., Attwood, T., Hinton, S., & Levin, I. (2007). A randomized controlled trial of a cognitive behavioural intervention for anger management in children diagnosed with Asperger syndrome. *Journal of Autism and Developmental Disorders, 37,* 1203-1214.

Spielberger C. D. (1988). *Manual for the state-trait anger expression inventory* (STAXI). Odessa, FL: Psychological Assessment Resources.

Spielberger, C. D. (1991). *State-trait anger expression inventory: Revised research edition professional manual.* Odessa, FL: Psychological Assessment Resources.

Wilkening, P. & Gazitt, N. (1991). *The ZIPPER strategy.* Unpublished manuscript, University of Florida, Department of Special Education, Gainesville, FL.

Willner, P., Jones, J., Tams, R., & Green, G. (2002). A randomized controlled trial of the efficacy of a cognitive-behavioral anger management group for clients with learning disabilities. *Journal of Applied Research in Intellectual Disabilities, 15,* 224-235.

World Health Organization. (n.d.). *Definition and typology of violence.* Retrieved July 31, 2008, from www.who.int/violenceprevention/approach/definition/en/index.html.

15. Animal Assisted Therapy

Daniel D. Ferguson

For many years the term "Pet Therapy" was used to describe the use of animals for deriving a therapeutic benefit. Pet therapy was talked about jokingly, much like people joke about "retail therapy" today. Through the years an evolution occurred in the label for the use of animals in therapeutic settings as practitioners tried to legitimize the use of dogs, cats, and other animals as treatment. It was called pet-facilitated therapy, pet-assisted therapy, pet-oriented child psychotherapy, animal-facilitated therapy, and animal visitation (Connor & Miller, 2000).

As positive anecdotal evidence piled up, physicians, nurses, psychotherapists, occupational therapists, and recreational therapists began to take the link between animals, treatment, recovery, and humans more seriously (Martin & Farnum, 2002; Velde, Cipriani, & Fisher, 2005). The relationship between humans and animals became known as the "human-animal bond" and it is inseparable from Animal Assisted Therapy (AAT) as it is now called (RHMSS Pty Ltd, 2003). Furthermore, a healthy respect developed for AAT as investigators began to collect empirical evidence concluding that there are positive outcomes to be derived from a planned, therapeutic involvement of various animals with children, adolescents, adults, and the elderly (RHMSS Pty Ltd, 2003; Adams, 2009). Recognition and respect for the human-animal bond is taken seriously now as researchers from various disciplines are exploring the use of animals to facilitate therapeutic outcomes. This research is encouraging but it will be years before the impact of human-animal interactions on human development, health, and behavior will be fully known (Esposito et al., 2011). There is a great need for well-designed studies to supplement the many case studies and anecdotal reports already in the literature (Marr et al., 2000).

The research that has been done ranges widely from qualitative studies to experimental designs. Researchers have explored the use of animals with various client groups including children (Martin & Farnum, 2002; Sobo, Eng, & Kassity-Krich, 2006), adolescents with behavior problems (Adams, 2009), cardiac rehabilitation clients (Cole et al., 2007), geriatric clients (Nordgren & Engström, 2012; Filan & Jones, 2006), individuals with aphasia (Macauley, 2006), and others. In some cases, the results have been positive and encouraging, but in many cases the results have been inconclusive for methodological reasons, small sample size, lack of controls, or statistically insignificant results.

There are few specific protocols describing how to use animals for treatment purposes and, as Banks and Banks (2002) point out, most of the published results of AAT are anecdotal. For this reason it is important to recognize that what is often referred to as AAT may, in reality, just be Animal Assisted Activities (AAA). Animal assisted activities have been defined as "goal directed activities that improve a client's quality of life through the use of the human-animal bond. They are not guided by a professional or necessarily evaluated" (RHMSS Pty Ltd, 2003, p. 3). AAA can include nearly any activity involving the use of animals such as a pet visitation program in a long-term care facility, a class of children making a trip to the zoo or aquarium, or a group home of intellectually impaired clients making a trip to a farm or county fair to see, touch, and experience the animals. While such activities may elicit a positive emotional reaction or recall a memory from the past, these activities are recreational in nature as opposed to therapeutic in nature. Recreational therapists must keep in mind that as Beck and Karcher (1984) were quoted in Rowan and Thayer (2000, p. 419), "It should not be concluded that any event that is enjoyed by the patients is a kind of therapy."

Animal Assisted Therapy Defined

AAT is specifically designed to elicit a desired response and has been defined by several authors in a similar manner. Barba (1995) states that AAT "is an interdisciplinary treatment involving nursing, medicine, psychology, social work, and occupational, physical, and recreational therapy" (p. 91). She further states that AAT is "a therapeutic intervention that brings animals together with persons with physical and/or emotional needs as a way of meeting those needs." Chandler (2012) says, "AAT is a therapeutic modality with goals that are consistent with all of the basic counseling theoretical orientations. It is considered an adjunct to therapy in that it encourages and facilitates client motivation and participation, enhances the client-therapist relationship, stimulates client focus and attention to task, and reinforces positive clinical change" (p. 166). Connor and Miller (2000) go beyond Chandler by saying "AAT is a scheduled intervention designed to improve a patient's cognitive or physical functioning with specific short- and long-term goals. It is generally done by a skilled practitioner, and the patient/animal interaction is usually one-on-one. Animal-assisted therapy uses specially trained therapy animals, not the patient's own pet" (p. 20).

Perhaps the best definition of AAT is provided by the Delta Society (2000), which is now called Pet Partners. For more than two decades, they have defined AAT in Standards of Practice for Animal-Assisted Activities and Therapy as

> AAT is a goal-directed intervention in which an animal that meets specific criteria is an integral part of the treatment process. AAT is directed and/or delivered by a health/human service professional with specialized expertise, and within the scope of practice of his/her profession. AAT is designed to promote improvement in human physical, social, emotional, and/or cognitive functioning [cognitive functioning refers to thinking and intellectual skills]. AAT is provided in a variety of settings and may be group or individual in nature. This process is documented and evaluated (p. 9).

There are four key differences between this definition of AAT and those presented earlier. These differences help to separate AAT from AAA and justify AAT as a recreational therapy intervention. The first key difference is that AAT "is an integral part of the treatment process," which suggests that goals are formally established and are incorporated into the client's treatment plan. The second difference is that "AAT is directed and/or delivered by a health/human service professional with specialized expertise." For example, a certified therapeutic recreation specialist might recruit an animal therapy team from Pet Partners or Therapy Dogs International and assign them to specific clients with specific treatment goals. The third key difference is that AAT falls "within the scope of practice of the human service professional's position." There can be little argument that AAT falls within the scope of practice of recreational therapy. The final key difference is that "the process is documented and evaluated." The outcome is measured and recorded as part of the daily responsibility of a recreational therapist.

A clear differentiation between AAT and AAA is critical because as Richeson and McCullough (2002) inform us, "animal-assisted therapy has been identified as one of the modalities in which CTRSs are expected to have a demonstrated competency" (p. 25).

To illustrate this point, an example is given of an adult female with a brain injury who presents with a partial hemiparesis of the left side and signs of neglect of the left arm. After assessing the degree of the problem and incorporating a treatment goal into the client treatment plan, the therapist decides to work on range of motion, strength, and dexterity by inviting a Pet Partners animal therapy team to visit the client three times a week to help relieve the left-side neglect. While interacting with a small dog, the therapist directs the client to use her left arm to open a food container to give the dog a treat, to unlock and lock the carrying cage for the dog repeatedly while using the left hand, to reach to pet the dog, and other activities that motivate the client while forcing her to use her left hand. All of this is aimed at accomplishing a specific treatment goal and would be considered AAT as opposed to having a pleasant visit with a cute, well-behaved, affectionate dog every other day, which would be an Animal Assisted Activity.

The account above is but one example of how animals can be used for therapy and not just for activity. More examples of evidence-based benefits of AAT as shown in the literature are listed below. Each listing includes the symptoms that were improved, the ICF codes to use when documenting the symptoms, and the authors who reported the result.

Aphasia: Increased spontaneous social interaction — d7 Interpersonal Interactions and Relationships, d9205 Socializing (Macauley, 2006).

Autism: Much greater use of language when engaged with animals, increased social interaction — d3 Communication and d7 Interpersonal Interactions and Relationships (Sams, Fortney, &Willenbring, 2006).

Coronary issues: Lowered heart rates — b4100 Heart Rate, lowered blood pressure — b4200 Increased Blood Pressure, and decreased state anxiety — b126 Temperament and Personality Functions (Friedman et al., 1980; Cole et al., 2007).

Depression (mild): Decreased depression using dolphins — b126 Temperament and Personality Functions and b130 Energy and Drive Functions (Antonioli & Reveley, 2003).

Developmental disability: Improved playful moods — b126 Temperament and Personality Functions, d710 Basic Interpersonal Interactions, d720 Complex Interpersonal Interactions, and d9200 Play (Martin & Farnum, 2002).

Older adults in residential care: Reduced behavioral and psychological symptoms of dementia — b117 Intellectual Functions, b126 Temperament and Personality Functions, b144 Memory Functions, and other b1 Mental Functions (Nordgren & Engström, 2012; Filan & Llewellyn-Jones, 2006); improved systolic and diastolic blood pressure — b420 Blood Pressure Functions (Stasi et al., 2004 in Morrison, 2007); decreased agitation and increased spontaneous social behavior — b126 Temperament and Personality Functions and d7 Interpersonal Interactions and Relationships (Richeson, 2003); walking further with a dog than walking alone — b455 Exercise Tolerance Functions, d450 Walking, and d460 Moving Around in Different Locations (Herbert & Greene, 2001 in Velde et al., 2005); improved *Mini-Mental State Examination* after caring for an animal — b114 Orientation Functions (Colombo et al., 2006).

Older adults in residential care with a history of pet ownership: Decreased loneliness — b126 Temperament and Personality Functions, d720 Complex Interpersonal Interactions, d730 - d779 Particular Interpersonal Relationships, and d9 Community, Social, and Civic Life (Banks & Banks, 2002).

Pediatric cardiology: Decreased stress and increased morale — b126 Temperament and Personality Functions and d240 Handling Stress and Other Psychological Demands (Wu et al., 2002 in Morrison, 2007).

Pediatric surgery with 5-18 year old patients: Decreased pain perception post-surgery — b280 Sensation of Pain (Sobo, Eng, & Kassity-Krich, 2006).

It can be seen that the research articles on AAT have focused on just a few of the many disability groups that recreational therapists serve. AAT has been tried in many treatment settings and with varying populations from pediatrics to geriatrics, from physical rehabilitation to adolescent treatment, and from developmental disability to mental health. However, most of the published literature is either anecdotal or provides too little information to report the findings with confidence. For this reason these articles were not cited above. Anecdotal benefits of AAT that are worthy of consideration for program development and future investigation are listed below.

Physical Benefits

- Lowered blood pressure and increased skin temperature (Friedman et al., 1980).
- Decreased preoperative anxiety (Connor & Miller, 2000; Velde et al., 2005).
- Decreased fear and anxiety in psychiatric clients (Velde et al., 2005).
- Increased range of motion (Velde et al., 2005).
- Improved sensory modulation and sensory interpretation (Velde et al., 2005).
- Increased tolerance for physical activity with pain present (Sobo et al., 2006).
- Improved sitting balance and strength (RHMSS Pty Ltd, 2003; All et al., 1999).
- Improved posture (Heimlich, 2001; All et al., 1999).

Mental and Psychological Benefits

- Increased attention skills such as paying attention and staying on task (Delta Society, 2000).
- Developed leisure and recreation skills (Delta Society, 2000; Quinlan, n.d.).
- Increased self-esteem (Delta Society, 2000).
- Reduced loneliness (Banks & Banks, 2002; Connor & Miller, 2000).
- Increased feelings of safety (Velde et al., 2005).
- Decreased irritability in psychiatric clients (Sobo et al., 2006).
- Increased alertness and cognitive ability with chronic mental illness (Velde et al., 2005).
- Brightening of the day for hospice clients (Velde et al., 2005).
- Increased emotional support for pediatric clients (Zissleman et al., 1996).

Educational Benefits

- Increased vocabulary (Delta Society, 2000; Sams et al., 2006).
- Aided in long-term or short-term memory (Banks & Banks, 2002; Quinlan, n.d.).
- Improved knowledge of concepts, such as size, color, etc. (Quinlan, n.d.).
- Increased reminiscence in older adults when animals are present (Velde et al., 2005).

Motivational Benefits

- Increased speech motivation (Sams et al., 2006; Macauley, 2006).
- Increased motivation to attend group treatment sessions when an animal would be there (Velde et al., 2005).
- Improved willingness to be involved in group activity when an animal is present (Quinlan, n.d.).
- Improved interactions with others (Macauley, 2006).
- Improved willingness to be involved in long-term treatment (Quinlan, n.d.).
- Increased motivation to walk for older adults when a dog is involved (Herbert & Greene, 2001).
- Increased motivation to persevere in HIV/AIDS clients who have pets (Velde et al., 2005).

Indications

The evidence base is not extensive, but AAT has been used with many populations and may be an effective treatment in a variety of situations for which it is not yet proven. AAT has been shown to be an effective intervention with several disability groups and is positively indicated with:

- Pediatric and adult cardiac rehabilitation clients (Cole et al., 2007; Friedman et al., 1980; Wu et al., 2002).
- Clients with high levels of pain (Sobo et al., 2006).
- Older adults with dementia (Filan & Llewellyn-Jones, 2006; Nordgren & Engström, 2012).
- Individuals with autism to improve speech or socialization (Sams et al., 2006).
- Individuals with aphasia to improve communication (Macauley, 2006).

Contraindications

Morrison (2007) conducted an extensive review of the literature on AAT. Her conclusion was that while there are many indications for the use of what she called Animal-Assisted Interventions, there are few contraindications. Yet it would be irresponsible to establish any AAT program without considering the guidelines that have been published by Pet Partners (Delta Society, 2005). The following conditions or circumstances would contraindicate the use of AAT.

- Client is allergic to animals or pet dander.
- Client is afraid of an animal.
- Client has expressed or demonstrated disinterest in the AAT program.
- Client has a history of animal abuse or is unable to treat an animal appropriately.
- Caution should be exercised with children who have witnessed or experienced abuse.
- There is a danger to the client of infection or other negative impact on their medical condition, such as a client who is immunocompromised, has open sores, etc.
- There is danger of injury to either the animal or the client resulting from mishandling or abuse.

Protocols

Choice of Animal

Both farm and domestic animals have been used in AAT programs. Some of these include rabbits, guinea pigs, llamas, dolphins, and even fish aquariums. House cats have also been used but the most common animals for AAT programs are dogs of various breeds (Delta Society, 2000). There is no research to indicate that any one breed is preferred over another, but there are some obvious considerations in choosing appropriate animals for specific client. For example some breeds tend to be nervous or frisky and might not be well suited to older adults or physically weak clients. Other breeds tend to be docile or affectionate and probably better suited for older adults or clients who are physically weak. Some breeds have a coarse coat that is not enjoyable to pet, while other breeds are silky like a greyhound or fluffy like a poodle and tactilely stimulating for those being visited. The energy level of the animal must also be matched to the energy level of the person. Energetic dogs should not be matched with a person with low energy or confined to a bed (Therapy Dogs International, 2008). Animals must feel comfortable being touched. Their behavior must also be predictable and reliable in any situation, as therapy animals must be able to cope with stressful situations and be controllable at all times to insure client safety (Delta Society, 2005).

A therapist should give more than casual consideration to the animal of choice for clients. It should not be assumed that "any dog will do" or any animal can be a therapy animal. An animal that is a fantastic match for one client may not be an appropriate match for another. By the same token it should not be assumed that every client is well suited to an animal therapy intervention.

Length and Frequency of AAT Sessions

Evidence indicates that individual AAT sessions with a dog can be successful when they last in the range of 12 to 30 minutes (Cole et al., 2007). The frequency of AAT sessions vary, however Banks and Banks (2002) found no significant difference in benefit to an older adult population between one and three visitations per week.

Facilitator Qualifications

The animals used in AAT may be owned by the facility or brought into the facility by staff, volunteers, or animal therapy organizations. The individuals who provide AAT and their animals are a team. Together they work to produce a therapeutic effect. For this to happen the staff member or volunteer should be trained in AAT and the animal should be a Certified Pet Partner or tested and certified by Therapy Dogs International so the therapeutic impact will be maximized (Connor & Miller, 2000).

Structure of AAT Sessions

When structuring AAT sessions, the therapist should consider the items below:

Screen animals carefully and match them to clients and treatment goals so each AAT session has a specific purpose.

The animal owner should be briefed as to the purpose of the AAT session and how both the animal and the owner should interact with the client to achieve treatment goals.

The AAT session may be overseen by the therapist or the therapist may be directly involved in the AAT session, depending upon the goals of the session.

During the AAT session, clients may be involved with the animal in a variety of ways to address treatment goals. Such activities might include talking to the animal, petting it, holding it, walking with it, giving commands to do tricks, reminiscing about animals they have had, giving treats to the animal, or other activities deemed to be appropriate to client treatment goals and the abilities of the animal and/or its handler.

Outcomes from the AAT session should either be observed by or reported to the therapist and recorded in the client chart.

Establishing and Implementing an AAT Program

Assuming that the therapist does not have a trained animal of his/her own to use for AAT, or that s/he wishes to establish an ongoing program with multiple animals, the following process for developing an outcome-oriented procedure should be used:

Step 1: Identify and recruit qualified Pet Partners through the Pet Partners online directory or through the Therapy Dogs International online directory. Only certified animals should be used because owners are trained to facilitate therapeutic sessions and animals are tested for behavior in many problematic situations they may encounter with clients.

Step 2: Recruited animals and handlers should visit the facility to meet the therapist, tour the facility, and get a feel for the clients, the level of activity at the facility, the objectives of the program, and an understanding of how the Pet Partner Team (PPT) might be most useful. The therapist will also gain a sense of how to best use the PPT to facilitate treatment.

Step 3: A visitation schedule for the PPT should be established for regular therapeutic sessions.

Step 4: As clients are admitted and discharged on an irregular basis, the PPT should have a brief meeting with the therapist at the beginning of each visit to learn which clients they should visit and what the treatment objectives for the day might be. Best use of the animal can also be discussed to maximize outcomes (e.g., walking the dog, giving treats, etc.). The team can then either proceed on their own to facilitate the sessions or conduct the sessions with the therapist.

Step 5: At the conclusion of the AAT session, the outcomes are discussed with the therapist and charted by the therapist in the client record.

Outcomes and Documentation

Through empirical research AAT has yielded positive outcomes for clients from pediatrics to geriatrics and across diagnostic groups from cardiology to aphasia, to autism and developmental disability, to depression and surgery. Because AAT has been a useful intervention strategy in so many different settings and with so many different diagnostic groups, it makes good sense to use ICF codes to further advance our understanding of the relationship of interactions between humans and animals and application to clinical treatment. The ICF codes listed earlier provide a snapshot of some of the codes that can be applied when documenting treatment. This will provide another avenue to replicate outcomes that have already been seen through the systematic bringing together of clients and animals.

Careful examination of the places where success of AAT has been documented shows several commonalities between the client types and the outcomes produced. For example, animals promote spontaneous socialization in older adults, individuals with aphasia, and individuals with autism (b126 Temperament and Personality Functions, d7 Interpersonal Interactions and Relationships). Likewise animal visitation has helped improve blood pressure in individual with cardiac conditions and older adults (b420 Blood Pressure Functions). When these common outcomes occur, one begins to think that the same results could be obtained with other types of clients and it becomes possible to set up an experiment using the ICF codes to develop treatment goals, monitor progress, and document change in the client chart or record.

The ICF codes are extremely comprehensive and there is barely an aspect of physical, mental, intellectual, emotional, or daily life function that is not included among the code numbers. Deficits in many of the codes in b1 Mental Functions, b280 Sensation of Pain, b4 Functions of the Cardiovascular, Hematological, Immunological, and Respiratory Systems, and b7 Neuromusculoskeletal and Movement-Related Functions can be addressed with AAT interventions. Similarly, documented deficits in d3 Communication, d4 Mobility, d7 Interpersonal Interactions and Relationships, and d9 Community, Social, and Civic Life may be treated with appropriate AAT techniques.

Here is a simple example with at least five ICF codes that could be worked on and progress documented from a single AAT session of taking a dog for a walk around the hospital: b130 Energy and Drive Functions (dogs provide motivation to get exercise), b455 Exercise Tolerance Functions (walking improves fitness), d450 Walking (people walk farther with a dog), d460 Moving Around in Different Locations (going in areas that may be more challenging, such as outside), d710 Basic Interpersonal Interactions, d720 Complex Interpersonal Interactions, and d750 Informal Social Relationships (forming relationships with the dog and handler). To be effective the therapist has to incorporate a set of measurable treatment goals for each ICF target into the client treatment plan. Then, following an AAT session the success of that treatment activity has to be recorded in the client chart.

Resources

Care should be taken when developing an AAT program. It is highly recommended that certified therapy animals and handlers be used. There are two organizations that certify therapy teams. They are Pet Partners (formerly Delta Society) and Therapy Dogs International. Both of these organizations have certified trainers that extensively train and test the animals and handlers to be sure that clients will have a safe and pleasant experience in every situation.

Pet Partners

www.petpartners.org

At the Pet Partners website there is an excellent description of how to establish and AAA or AAT program that adheres to the Pet Partners Scope of Practice and Code of Ethics. There is also information about how to become a Registered Pet Partners Facility. More information about all of their services and programs can be found at Pet Partners, 875 124th Ave NE #101, Bellevue, WA 98005, USA. 425-679-5500. E-mail info@petpartners.org.

Therapy Dogs International (TDI)

www.tdi-dog.org

Therapy Dogs International is a volunteer organization dedicated to regulating, testing, and registering therapy dogs and their volunteer handlers for the purpose of visiting nursing homes, hospitals, other institutions, and wherever else therapy dogs are needed. They have almost 25,000 certified dog/handler teams that provide free visits to facilities. All teams have been heavily tested and the health of the dogs is constantly monitored for safety. More information about TDI and its programs can be obtained from their website. To learn more about how to arrange for visits or to access the dog/handler directory TDI can be contacted at their mailing address: 88 Bartley Road, Flanders, NJ 07836; by telephone at 973-252-9800; by fax at 973-252-7171; or by e-mail: tdi@gti.net.

Animal Behavior Institute (ABI)

www.animaledu.com/Programs/AnimalAssistedTherapy.aspx

The Animal Behavior Institute (ABI) in Durham, North Carolina is an organization that provides online training for therapists and other professionals who wish to use their own animals in an AAT program. Their catalog of courses includes education in general animal behavior and the human-animal bond, animal training, feline, canine, and equine behavior, and activities. There is also a course titled Behavior and Training of Marine Mammals. In addition to online coursework ABI requires 40 hours of relevant, hands-

on experience as an employee, intern, or volunteer at an approved institution chosen by the student. The mailing address for ABI is Animal Behavior Institute, Inc., 4711 Hope Valley Road, Suite 4F-332, Durham, NC 27707. 866-755-0448, support@animaledu.com.

References

Adams, N. (2009). Animal assisted interventions for adolescents with emotional and behavioural problems: A review of selected literature. (Unpublished paper for Postgraduate Diploma of Psychology), Monash University, Melbourne, Australia.

All, A. C., Loving, G. L., & Crane, L. L. (1999). Animals, horseback riding, and implication for rehabilitation therapy. *Journal of Rehabilitation 65*(3) 49-57.

Animal Behavior Institute, Inc. (ABI). (2011). Animal assisted therapy 15 credits/30 CEUs. Retrieved from www.animaledu.com/student/Programs.aspx.

Antonioli, C. & Reveley, M. A. (2005). Randomized controlled trial of animal facilitated therapy with dolphins in the treatment of depression. *BMJ. 331*, 1231-1234.

Banks, M. A. & Banks, W. A. (2002). The effects of animal-assisted therapy on loneliness in an elderly population in long term care facilities. *Journals of Gerontology: Medical Sciences. 57A*(7), M428-32. Retrieved from http://search.proquest.com/docview/208635810?accountid=13211.

Barba, B. E. (1995). The positive influence of animals: Animal assisted therapy in acute care. *Clinical Nurse Specialist, 9*(4), 91-95.

Beck, A. & Karcher, A. (1984). A new look at pet facilitated therapy. *Journal of the American Veterinary Medicine Association, 184*, 414-421.

Chandler, C. K. (2012). *Animal assisted therapy in counseling* (2nd ed.). New York, NY: Routledge.

Cole, K. M., Gawlinski, A., Steers, N., & Kotlerman, J. (2007). Animal assisted therapy in patients hospitalized with heart failure. *American Journal of Critical Care, 16*, 575-585.

Colombo, G., Dello-Buno, M., Smania, K., Raviola, R., & DeLeo, D. (2006). Pet therapy and institutionalized elderly: A study of 144 cognitively unimpaired subjects. *Archives of Gerontology and Geriatrics, 42*, 207-216.

Connor, K. & Miller, J. (2000). Animal-assisted therapy: An in-depth look. *Dimensions of Critical Care Nursing, 19*(3), 20-26.

Delta Society. (2000). *The pet partners team training course manual: A Delta Society program for animal-assisted activities and therapy*. Renton, WA: Delta Society.

Delta Society. (2005). *Introduction to animal assisted activities and therapies*. Renton, WA: Delta Society.

Esposito, L., McCune, S., Griffin, J. A., & Maholmes, V. (2011). Directions in human-animal interaction research: Child development, health, and therapeutic interventions. *Child Development Perspectives, 5*, 205-211. DOI: 10.1111/j.1750-8606.2011.00175.x

Filan, S. L. & Llewellyn-Jones R. H. (2006). Animal-assisted therapy for dementia: A review of the literature. *International Psychogeriatrics, 18*, 597-611. doi:10.1017/S1041610206003322.

Friedman, E., Katcher, A. H., Lynch, J. J., & Thomas, S. A. (1980). Animal companions and one year survival of patients after discharge from a coronary care unit. *Public Health Report, 95*, 307-312.

Heimlich, K. (2001). Animal-assisted therapy and the severely disabled child: A quantitative study. *Journal of Rehabilitation, 67*(4), 48-54.

Herbert, J. D. & Greene, C. (2001). Effect of preference on distance walked by assisted living residents. *Physical and Occupational Therapy in Geriatrics, 19*, 1-15.

Lange, A. M., Cox, J. A., Bernert, D. J., & Jenkins, C. D. (2006). Is counseling going to the dogs? An exploratory study related to the inclusion of an animal in group counseling with adolescents. *Journal of Creativity in Mental Health, 2*(2), 17-31.

Macauley, B. L. (2006). Animal assisted therapy for persons with aphasia: A pilot study. *Journal of Rehabilitation Research and Development, 43*, 357-366.

Marr, C. A., French, L., Thompson, D., Drum, L., Greening, G., Mormon, J., & Hughes, C. (2000). Animal-assisted therapy in psychiatric rehabilitation. *Anthrozoos, 13*(1), 43-47.

Martin, F. & Farnum, J. (2002). Animal-assisted therapy for children with pervasive developmental disorder. *Western Journal of Nursing Research, 24*, 657-670.

Morrison, M. L. (2007). Health benefits of animal-assisted interventions. *Complimentary Health Practice Review, 12*(1), 51-62.

Nordgren, L. & Engström, G. (2012). Effects of animal-assisted therapy on behavioral and psychological symptoms of dementia: A case report. *American Journal of Alzheimer's Disease and Other Dementias. 27*. 625-632.

Pet Partners. (2012). Animal-assisted therapy (AAT). Retrieved from www.deltasociety.org/page.aspx?pid=320.

Pet Partners. (2012). Developing a visiting animal program. Retrieved from www.petpartners.org/page.aspx?pid=271.

Quinlan, S. (n.d.). Animal assisted therapy: Therapeutic interventions in working with children who have a diagnosis of selective autism and autism disorder. Unpublished paper retrieved from Google Scholar at http://scholar.google.com/scholar?q=Stephen+Quinlan+AND+Selective+Mutism&btnG=&hl=en&as_sdt=0%2C5.

RHMSS Pty Ltd. (2003). *Animal assisted therapy and young people: A review of selected literature*. Melbourne, AU: Menzies Inc.

Richeson, N. E. (2003). Effects of animal-assisted therapy on agitated behaviors and social interactions of older adults with dementia. *American Journal of Alzheimer's Disease & Other Dementias, 18*, 353-358.

Richeson, N. E. & McCullough, W. T. (2002). An evidence based animal-assisted therapy protocol and flow sheet for the geriatric recreation therapy practice. *American Journal of Recreation Therapy, 1*(1), 25-29.

Rowan, A. & Thayer, I. (2000). Forward. In A. Fine (Ed.) *Handbook on animal assisted therapy: Theoretical foundations and guidelines for practice*. San Diego, CA: Academic Press.

Sams, M. J., Fortney, E. V., & Willenbring, S. (2006). Occupational therapy incorporating animals for children with autism: A pilot investigation. *American Occupational Therapy Association, 60*, 268-274.

Sobo, E. J., Eng, B., & Kassity-Krich, N. (2006). Canine visitation (pet) therapy. *Journal of Holistic Nursing, 24* (1), 51-57.

Stasi, M. F., Amati, D., Costa, C., Resta, D., Senepa, G., Scarafioti, C., & Motosachi, M. (2004). Pet therapy: A trial for institutionalized frail elderly patients. *Archives of Gerontology and Geriatrics, 9*, 407-412.

Therapy Dogs International. (2008). Therapy dogs international (TDI) testing requirements. Retrieved from www.tdi-dog.org/images/TestingBrochure.pdf.

Velde, B. P., Cipriani, J., & Fisher, G. (2005). Resident and therapist views of animal-assisted therapy: Implications for occupational therapy practice. *Australian Occupational Therapy Journal 52*, 43-50.

Wu, A. S., Niedra, R., Pendergast, L., & McCrindle, B. W. (2002). Acceptability and impact of pet visitation on a pediatric cardiology inpatient unit. *Journal of Pediatric Nursing, 17*, 354-362.

Zissleman, M. H., Rovner, B. W., Shmuely, Y., & Ferrie, P. (1996). A pet therapy intervention with geriatric psychiatry inpatients. *American Journal of Occupational Therapy, 50*(1), 47-51.

16. Aquatic Therapy

Ellen Broach

Aquatic therapy (AT) includes passive or active techniques for rehabilitation/habilitation of health conditions using water as the therapeutic medium. Recreational therapists can use AT to promote health and well-being of clients while facilitating independence or interdependence in water activity (Broach & Dattilo, 2011).

There is a difference between aquatic therapy and adapted aquatics, which teaches swimming and skills. While AT may use adapted aquatics as a facilitation technique, AT is a specialized area of skilled practice that is implemented to improve or maintain function (Broach & Dattilo, 2011). Therefore, the recreational therapist using AT must have knowledge of and skills in intervention strategies that produce specialized outcomes. This knowledge includes indications, contraindications, precautions, and protocols that involve aquatic principles of hydrodynamics and thermodynamics, as well as methods of practice.

Indications

The buoyancy, support, accommodating resistance, and other unique properties of the aquatic environment enhance interventions for clients across the age span with musculoskeletal, neuromuscular, cardiopulmonary, and psychological diseases, disorders, or conditions. Aquatic therapy interventions are designed to improve or maintain functions that can include balance, motor coordination, oral-facial control, postural stabilization, respiration and vital capacity, muscle strength and endurance, range of motion, gait, weight bearing, proprioception, circulation, edema reduction, relaxation, self-esteem, mood, skill, and life activity level (Broach & Dattilo, 2011; Vargas, 2004). AT is also indicated for clients with goals that include reduction in pain, muscle fatigue, spasticity, depression, and anxiety. Some specific examples of clients who might be appropriate for AT are individuals who have difficulty with land exercise, have chronic pain, have low endurance, are obese, or are athletes.

Contraindications and Precautions

A recreational therapist conducting AT must be aware of contraindications and precautions associated with water activity in general and those pertaining to specific impairments. The therapist must also understand the pathology of the impairment and be prepared to apply appropriate AT principles. General contraindications identified by Broach and Dattilo (2011) include:

- skin infections
- open wounds
- vomiting
- recent bowel incontinence
- diseases transmissible by water
- hepatitis-A
- open tracheotomies that are not healed
- uncontrolled seizures

Precautions require the therapist to closely monitor clients. Therapists must monitor individuals with intravenous sites, ostomies, central line catheters, bowel incontinence, epilepsy, unstable blood pressure, decreased vital capacity, weakness, fear, impulsivity, swallowing issues, recent radiation, body temperature regulation issues, eardrum perforation, no cough reflex, and clients who use psychotropic drugs. Because of the various client precautions in an aquatic environment, the therapist must consider waterproof dressings, water temperature, humidity, water quality, noise, accessibility, anxiety, movement restrictions, and immersion times (Sova, 2004).

Principles

Using AT, the recreational therapist applies the principles of hydrodynamics and thermodynamics to meet treatment goals. Hydrodynamics involves a complex interrelationship of the physical properties of the water and the principles that affect movement in the water. Aquatic interventions rely on the properties of the water to provide an environment that is more beneficial than land-based treatments for many individuals (Broach & Dattilo, 1996). Thermodynamics involves the exchange of work and heat between systems. Water temperature has an effect on a body and, therefore, performance in the aquatic environment. In pools, water temperature can affect the physiological and psychological success of a session. While research specific to AT interventions is still sparse, AT has a wealth of basic science research related to the effects of immersion and properties of the water as a foundation. This significant research is an outcome of studies that used water immersion to examine the cardiopulmonary responses to changes in blood volume and weightlessness associated with preparing individuals for spaceflight (Becker, 2011). Knowledge of the properties of water and the consequent evidence of effects of immersion and movement in the water are important for the recreational therapist to understand to provide appropriate techniques and justification for interventions. The profound biologic effects of water immersion can be used to address a variety of client issues. For example, the effects of immersion result in physiological changes with implications to the following body systems (Becker, 2009):

- circulatory (improved stroke volume, lower heart rate, decrease in blood pressure)
- pulmonary system (increased pulmonary blood flow with a reduction in vital capacity due to increased thoracic blood volume which increases work of breathing)
- musculoskeletal (increased blood supply to muscles and skin, improved oxygen delivery to the muscles, reduction in edema, increased muscle relaxation in warm water)
- renal (diuretic effect)
- nervous system (relaxation, mood effect)

The effects of immersion on body systems are linked to buoyancy, hydrostatic pressure, viscosity, centers of gravity and buoyancy, temperature, and autonomic nervous system changes. These will be described next.

Buoyancy

Buoyancy is known as Archimedes' principle (Giancoli, 1985). When an object is immersed in water, it experiences an upward thrust that is equal to its weight resulting in less gravitational pull on the body. As gravity decreases, weight bearing will also decrease. When considering buoyancy, the therapist must understand relative density. The relative density (specific gravity) of water is 1.0. Relative density of a human body fluctuates slightly above or below 1.0 (Koury, 1996). Individuals with low body fat percentages (greater lean body mass) often find it difficult to float because their body mass is slightly greater than 1.0. Individuals with more flaccidity will find it easier to float because fat has a specific gravity lower than 1.0. In other words, if a person's body weighs more than the amount of water it displaces, that individual may have difficulty floating. This relative density of a human body also increases with spasticity and tenseness (Bloomfield, Fricker, & Fitch, 1992). Buoyancy results in decreased weight bearing with partial off-loading when standing in the water (Harrison & Bulstrode, 1992). For example, a person who is standing still in the water is typically 10% of their weight at neck depth, 25% at chest depth, and 50% at waist depth (Becker, 2011).

Implications: Buoyancy allows a reduction in joint compression forces during a client's water activity allowing for improved movement with less pain and increased ease of handling for the therapist (Broach & Dattilo, 2011). The recreational therapist can use buoyancy to assist or resist a movement for range of motion, weight bearing, gait, and strengthening activities.

Hydrostatic Pressure

According to Pascal's Law, when a body is immersed in the water there is hydrostatic pressure exerted by the fluid that varies with depth of immersion and density of the fluid (salt water is denser than fresh water) (Becker, 2009). This pressure is equal around a body at a given depth while it increases with the depth of the water. Becker added that a person immersed to a depth of 48 inches is subjected to a force equal to 88.9 mmHg. This is slightly greater than typical diastolic blood pressure. When a person is standing at neck level, the pressure is twice as high as that experienced when standing at hip level with the pressure being greater on the lower extremities. Vital capacity (VC) decreases about 10% when immersed to the neck and the work of breathing increases about 60% (Arborelius et al., 1972). This VC reduction is due to increased thoracic blood volume and hydrostatic forces countering inspiration.

Implications: Clinical implications of hydrostatic pressure are numerous. First, the heart works more efficiently in deep water. Because of hydrostatic pressure, venous blood return to the heart is enhanced, improving circulation while decreasing the heart rate during exercise (Starling's Law) (Garbielsen et al., 2000). Second, hydrostatic pressure is the force that aids resolution of edema of the extremities and greater oxygen delivery to the muscles. This improved blood supply in warm water also aids muscle relaxation. Third, when immersed at shoulder level the pressure will assist vital capacity while resisting inspiratory capacity resulting in strengthening of the diaphragm (Vargas, 2004). This is also a precaution because some clients with compromised vital capacity will feel the effects when breathing against the pressure of the water. Fourth, the sensory input that occurs with the equal pressure around a body may decrease tactile defensiveness and be an indication for individuals with sensory deficits. Finally, with immersion to the neck, sodium excretion increases up to 10 times the normal rate, leading to a diuretic effect. Therefore, individuals who are immersed in the water should drink fluids and empty leg bags (when appropriate) prior to entering water (Broach & Dattilo, 2011).

Viscosity

Viscosity is the resistance that occurs between molecules of a liquid. It affects the body as it moves through the water. Water acts to resist movement as molecules are attracted to each other (cohesion) and to the body in the water (adhesion) (Becker, 2011). When a body or limb moves through the water there is resistance produced by friction. This friction is greater in front of the moving body than behind. Also, as the body moves faster through the water, it experiences greater resistance, but that resistance drops to zero almost immediately when a movement stops (Poyhonen et al., 2000).

Implications: Because of viscosity, when a client in the water feels pain and stops movement, the force drops abruptly allowing an enhanced control of strengthening activities within the clients' comfort level (Becker, 2009). In addition, the viscosity principle is useful for balance and strength training. Finally, the increased resistance allows for greater response time to maintain balance resulting in less fear of falling in the water than on land. This decrease in fear can result in less tense movement, improved relaxation, and a reduction in pain (Broach & Dattilo, 1996, 2011).

Center of Gravity and Buoyancy

The center of buoyancy is generally located around mid-chest while the center of gravity is located around the pelvis. When these two centers are in alignment, the body is in a state of equilibrium in the water. According to Bougier's theorem, a person's state of equilibrium will determine their stability in the water (Becker, 2011).

Implications: The center of buoyancy and gravity concept explains the stability of clients with disabilities in the water. Spasticity, flaccidity, or loss of limbs affects the alignment of a body. Therefore, in a supine position in the water, clients who have limitations from a disability will roll towards the side with greater tone or spasticity until the center of buoyancy and gravity are aligned. Because of the shift in the alignment of one or both centers, a person with a flaccid limb will roll away from the affected side. Therefore, the therapist should understand how the head, upper extremities, and lower extremities in relation to the trunk or affected limb can affect position. This can be addressed as the therapist works in the mental adjustment phase of the Halliwick technique described below.

Temperature

The temperature of water can affect treatment outcomes. The rate of heat gain or loss is 25 times greater in water than on land. Warm water affects circulation due to the dilation of blood vessels, which in turn improves skin condition, enhances relaxation, and decreases pain (Becker, 2011; Vargas, 2004). When warm blood reaches the muscles, there is an increase in muscle temperature causing less muscle stress and enhanced movement. Typical therapy pools operate in the range of 90° to 94°F (32.2° to 34.4°C) permitting immersion without chilling or overheating. However, water can be used therapeutically over a wider range of temperatures. After a review of the research, Becker and Cole (2011) stated that many studies showed positive effects in water temperatures in the range of 80° to 87°F (26.7° to 30.6°C). The current consensus of the rehab community is that pools with warmer temperatures may be more effective for rehabilitation.

Implications: For session content, water temperature should be considered because of physiological changes that occur to the body. It is difficult to have the ideal temperature for every client. The therapist may have to consider warm attire for some clients to help retain body heat in a cooler pool or lower the intensity of programming in warmer pools. While the ideal temperature is 92°F (33.3°C) for most clients (Sova, 2004), warmer water (94°-96°F; 34.4°-35.5°C) should be used for passive treatments and moderate water (86°-90°F) can include more active programs. Clients with multiple sclerosis, cardiac issues, prenatal women, and clients who are obese may overheat in warmer water with active treatment. Clients with arthritis, fibromyalgia, pain, and some children could become chilled in cooler water and experience an exacerbation of tone, pain, or joint issues (Sova, 2004).

Autonomic Nervous System Changes

Research strongly indicates that aquatic immersion can result in mood changes. Parasympathetic nervous system (PNS) activity becomes more prevalent than sympathetic nervous system (SNS) activity (Becker, 2011). The parasympathetic and sympathetic nervous systems are part of the autonomic nervous system. The SNS action mobilizes the body's resources under stress by inducing "fight-or-flight" responses. The PNS generally works to promote maintenance of the body at rest. While the functions of both systems are complicated, the description above is a common rule of thumb (Broach & McKenney, 2012). Becker cites various studies that yield findings specific to improved mood states and increases in plasma dopamine levels from warm water immersion or water exercise. Plasma dopamine levels correlate positively with mood state (Becker, 2011). Similarly, Becker found that both anxiety and depression are reduced after water- and land-based exercise. Becker contends that the important

outcomes associated with mental health benefits of immersion need further study; however, the effect produced does have important implications for positive emotions from aquatic immersion.

Aquatic Intervention Studies

Research related to the effectiveness of aquatic interventions indicates that AT can be used by recreational therapists to promote functional improvement while facilitating independence or interdependence in water activity. Most of the studies have examined the effects of swimming and exercise rather than specific AT techniques (Becker, 2011; Broach & Dattilo, 2011). Physical outcomes from aquatic activity include decreases in pain (Cantarero-Villanueva et al., 2012; Guillemin et al., 1994; Hauser et al., 2010; Langridge & Phillips, 1988; Templeton, Booth, & O'Kelly, 1996; Woods, 1989) bone loss (Tsukahara et al., 1994; Benedict & Freeman, 1993), fatigue (Broach et al., 1998; Hauser et al., 2010), and limb edema (Tidhar and Katz-Leurer, 2009). The physical outcomes also include increases in motor performance (Broach & Dattilo; 2001; Broach et al., 1998), strength (Broach & Dattilo, 2003; Gehlsen, Grigsby, & Winant, 1984), endurance (Broach, Groff, & Dattilo, 1997; Burke & Keenan, 1984; Edlund et al., 1986; Routi, Troup, & Berger, 1994; Wright & Cowden, 1986), fitness (Wang et al., 2007), and pulmonary function (Bar-Or & Inbar, 1992; Getz, Hutzler, & Vermeer, 2006; Haung et al., 1989; Ide, Belini, & Caromano, 2005).

Psychological implications included improved body image (Benedict & Freeman, 1993; Smith & Michel, 2006) enhanced mood (Berger & Owen, 1992; Berger, Owen, & Man, 1993; Hauser et al., 2010), and decreased anxiety (Parker & Smith, 2003). Finally, studies indicated leisure and life activity benefits through adherence to aquatic activity (Beaudouin & Keller, 1994) as well as improved communication skills (Bumin et al., 2003), social function (Getz et al., 2006), self-esteem (Peganoff, 1984), decreased dependence on pain medications (Guillemin et al., 1994), improved quality of life (Fernandez-Lao et al., 2012; Hauser et al., 2010), and less time out of school for medical reasons (Haung et al., 1989).

Processes

A number of factors must be considered when *active* (e.g. Halliwick, active exercise) or *passive* (e.g. Watsu, passive Bad-Ragaz) treatment is given. First, session length will vary from 15 minutes to one hour depending on the endurance of the client. Second, when considering aquatic therapy, an understanding of the differences between land and water movement is essential. Often the same exercises used on land will work different muscle groups when used in the water. Thus, different outcomes will be achieved. Third, regardless of the AT intervention used, it is important to include the analysis of mental adjustment followed by techniques to improve the client's comfort in the water (Broach & Dattilo, 2011). AT is enhanced when the client understands how to use the properties of water to maintain balance and improve function. Mental adjustment strategies are described in the Halliwick Concept description.

General principles for *active* aquatic therapy involve a task-oriented approach with an emphasis placed on using functional positions, functional activities, problem solving, and challenges that equal a client's skill level. These task-type training approach principles described by Morris (2004) require the client and therapist to:

- Work in the shallowest water tolerated.
- Use activities as a whole that are similar to the land function to be improved.
- Systematically remove external stabilization (e.g., progress from your support, to the client using the pool edge, to a floating barbell, to no support).
- Use sitting or standing positions as much as possible while promoting balance and postural stability (e.g., putting ball in basket).
- Use functional activities that require quick reciprocal movement with sudden movement changes (e.g., move legs as if bicycling while floating, or high stepping in place).
- Use active movement problem solving to increase likelihood of learning by allowing clients to critique performance and provide solutions to their movement activity (e.g. How can I achieve this movement safely?).
- Increase the challenge as skill level increases (e.g., throwing a ball at different speeds, distances, and positions).

Broach and Dattilo (2011) added that clients should progress from the slower, less water-resisted movements to faster movements where resistance is increased. Also, the use of swimming naturally incorporates functional movements and should be utilized as a part of treatment when appropriate.

Protocols

While there are many interventions used in AT, the following includes a brief description of some of the common techniques that recreational therapists use in AT practice including the Halliwick Concept, Watsu, Ai Chi, Back Hab, Bad Ragaz, Aquatic PNF, Sensory Integration, and Swimming.

Halliwick Concept

The Halliwick Concept was developed by James McMillan in 1949 in London, England, as a swimming instruction method for children with cerebral palsy. Using the principles of hydrodynamics described above, the method is designed to assist an individual in progressions that lead to swimming. The concept is used as a clinical approach for appropriate clients of all ages. It provides treatment applications from balance control to swimming. The Halliwick method provides clients with the opportunity to understand how their body works in the water while meeting goals. It involves body function and activity and participation domains of the ICF. The Halliwick process revolves around theories of motor control, balance control, and the neurodevelopmental stages of growth. No flotation devices are used during instruction since the purpose is to teach a client how their body works in the water, leading to independence. The theory is that floatation adjusts the client's buoyancy to an unnatural state, resulting in having to re-teach any movements learned when the floatation is removed. Because this technique was originally developed for children, there are numerous games documented for the Halliwick progressions (Campion, 1985). The Halliwick concept consists of four phases of instruction that include mental adjustment, balance control, inhibition, and facilitation.

Mental adjustment: While described as part of the Halliwick concept, mental adjustment and disengagement strategies that emphasize client comfort and safety in the water should be used as part of most AT treatments. As the client becomes more comfortable, s/he will be able to progress to the other phases of Halliwick and AT in general. Most of the activities in this phase are performed vertically, which is the most comfortable position for the client in the water. Mental adjustment involves maintaining balance in a vertical position, breath control, and activities with gradual disengagement from the therapist or other sources of stability. While vertical, the therapist helps the client through a variety of movement patterns to experience buoyancy and resistance, which helps the client learn to use his/her head and trunk for control and balance. Disengagement is an ongoing process in every phase of Halliwick. Disengagement involves withdrawing support to increase the challenge, which is the basis of motor learning (Lambeck & Gamper, 2011). Disengagement strategies can include changes in placement of hand supports, depth of the water, and turbulence. Therapeutic objectives for mental adjustment can be oral facial control (e.g., lip closure, vocalization, breathing through nose, diaphragm contraction), head and trunk control that works on normalizing tone, and righting reactions. This phase also helps clients understand the effects of water while the therapist works on activities such as walking, squatting, turning around, and reaching (Vargas, 2004). Finally, understanding the concept that one cannot sink (upthrust) is fundamental to safety and comfort in the water. Many are afraid to go under the water. With simple activities a client is able to understand that they will generally float to the top after submersion (Lambeck & Gamper, 2011).

Balance control: Balance control involves the use of arms and/or legs to restore balance and postural control in the water and increases the clients understanding of the concept of upthrust (floating). Sagittal rotation, transverse rotation (vertical to horizontal rotation), longitudinal rotation (vertical rotation around a horizontal axis), and combined rotations are taught (Lambeck & Gamper, 2011).

Sagittal rotation is required for movements such as walking sideways and changing directions. These movements are facilitated in both upright and supine positions such as lateral flexion of the trunk or swimming a crawl stroke. It usually involves reaching the arm and looking at the hand.

Lambeck and Gamper explain that transverse rotations involve moving from a vertical position to a supine or prone position. It could even involve a sitting to standing movement. Therapeutic applications could include head control and trunk strength.

Longitudinal rotation occurs around the midline of the body. While the goal is to rotate in supine it can begin in an upright position while passing an object in a circle or turning around while walking. The client rotates by using the head to look in the direction of the roll and by crossing the midline of the body with the arm and leg. Ultimately, the goal is a 360° roll (Lambeck & Gamper, 2011). The therapeutic aspect of this rotation could include facilitating the head and trunk righting reactions, trunk strength necessary for walking, decreasing tone in the trunk, and/or swimming.

Combined rotation includes the transverse and longitudinal together. This is a more complicated move that can help a client regain balance in a vertical and supine position. Teaching a client how to fall and stand up again is an important safety skill that involves combined rotations. The client learns that the head controls movement in the water. The therapist usually begins teaching a vertical to horizontal to vertical rotation followed by a 360° lateral rotation of the entire body and then combined rotations. This activity is first practiced with support but gradually contact is reduced as the client acquires the skill.

Inhibition and facilitation: Inhibition involves holding a desired position in the water while the therapist challenges balance and stability by using turbulence or altering the center of buoyancy. Inhibition can be used to improve stability through isometric activity in addition to being an important skill for facilitation. This can occur while a participant is standing, squatting, or in a supine position. Facilitation is the ability to create a controlled movement through the water, such as swimming.

Overall, clinical objectives of the Halliwick method include but are not limited to: improved strength, motor control of trunk and extremities, improved circulation, improved breathing patterns, improved static and dynamic balance, improved gait pattern, improved postural tone, and independent swimming (Broach & Dattilo, 2011; Lambeck & Gamper, 2011; Vargas, 2004).

Watsu

Watsu, developed by Harold Dull in the 1980s, is a passive technique that incorporates shiatsu with stretches that are performed at the water's surface. The primary objective is to allow the body to drift into a state of relaxation, which in turn affects flexibility (Schoedinger, 2011). The client is held or cradled by the therapist at the surface of the water throughout the varied movement sequences. The therapist learns a variety of moves in Watsu to address the client's needs. When considering Watsu, a number of practice principles are observed. Schoedinger cited the following.

- The optimal water temperature is 90° to 92°F (32.2° to 33.3°C).
- The ideal depth for effective Watsu is three to four feet.
- The client's cervical region must be supported at all times.
- The client's face and nose must be kept above water at all times.
- The pool environment should be calm.
- The practitioner must thoroughly explain to the client the process and outcomes.
- Certain movements may be contraindicated for certain orthopedic clients.
- Before a session the therapist needs to explain the technique and goals to the clients.
- Clients are instructed to notify the therapist immediately if a movement causes discomfort or motion sickness.

Watsu influences both the neuromuscular and musculoskeletal systems. Faull's (2005) research indicates that Watsu helps clients to experience movements with less pain and greater freedom of mobility. Other research found Watsu helpful in controlling spasticity and improving ambulatory function (Chon, Oh, & Shim, 2008). Additional effects may include improved circulation, flexibility, postural alignment, sleep patterns, and quieting of the sympathetic nervous system (Schoedinger, 2011). Vargas (2004) contends that Watsu can result in a decrease in edema, tension, muscle spasms, fatigue, and muscle tone from stimulating the vestibular system and immersion in warm water.

Ai Chi

Ai Chi, developed by Jun Konno, is a total body strengthening and relaxation exercise progression (Sova & Konno, 2003). It combines T'ai Chi and Qi Gong concepts and is performed standing in shoulder-depth warm water using a combination of deep breathing and slow, broad movements of the arms, legs, and torso. The Ai Chi progression moves from simple breathing to the incorporation of upper-extremity movements, trunk movements, lower-extremity movements, and finally total body involvement. Ai Chi is designed to affect oxygen and caloric consumption through correct form and positioning in the water to improve relaxation, range of motion, and core stability. One study was found pertaining to Ai Chi combined with the Halliwick (Noh et al., 2008). These researchers found that postural balance and knee flexor strength were improved after Ai Chi and Halliwick interventions.

BackHab

BackHab is a form of active aquatic therapy based on a walking program in the pool using a variety of strides and stretching exercises to increase overall fitness, to eliminate low-back and hamstring inflexibility, to improve postural alignment, and to strengthen the abdominals (Sova, 2004).

Bad Ragaz

Bad Ragaz involves proprioceptive neuromuscular facilitation concepts. This technique uses flotation devices that allow three-dimensional access to the patient who is in a horizontal position (Meno, 2000). Bad Ragaz involves movement patterns that can involve a client's lower extremity, trunk, and/or upper extremity. The patterns are passive with the therapist moving the client or command movement where the therapist instructs the client to perform specific movement patterns. These command patterns can be isometric (client holds a position while being moved), isotonic (movement is assisted or resisted by the therapist), or isokinetic (client controls the resistance by speed of movement). Meno (2000), a CTRS, details the protocol and patterns that are most commonly used in aquatic rehabilitation. The recommended water depth for effective application of Bad Ragaz is three to four feet with the water level between the T8 and T11 vertebrae for the best stability for the therapist. Indications for this treatment include clients who have pain with movement, decreased range of motion, increased tone, muscle imbalance and weakness, decreased coordination, proprioceptive deficits, sensory deficits, restricted weight bearing, or back problems.

Aquatic Proprioceptive Neuromuscular Facilitation

Aquatic PNF is a form of active aquatic therapy modeled after the principles and movement patterns of Proprioceptive Neuromuscular Facilitation (PNF). PNF describes the methods used to promote or hasten the response of the neuromuscular mechanisms through stimulation of proprioceptors (Morris, 2004). Aquatic PNF can be provided in either a hands-on or a hands-off manner by the provider. The client is verbally, visually, and/or tactilely instructed in a series of functional, spiral, and diagonal mass movement patterns while standing, sitting, or lying in the water (Jamison & Ogden, 1994).

Sensory Integration

Recreational therapists can use movement in the water to facilitate sensory integration. The method, described by Broach and Dattilo (2011), is characterized by an informal but carefully planned progression of activities that result in successful movement experiences to meet a participant's functional objectives. As sensory integration is facilitated, participants develop body awareness (including image and functions), spatial awareness (including laterality and directionality, such as right, left, up, down, forward, backward, sideways), levels (high, medium, low), relationships (over, under, in, out, around, together, beside), experience with central part movements (bending, stretching, twisting, pushing, pulling, kicking), and, finally, practice with locomotor movements (walking, running, jumping, hopping, climbing). According to Buis and Schane (1980), the objectives of sensory integration may embody improvements associated with vestibular (balance, equilibrium, and posture), proprioceptive (body position processing), tactile (sense of touch for motor planning), auditory (interpret sounds), and bilateral (using both sides of the body simultaneously and crossing midline) integration.

Swimming

Most of the efficacy research in the aquatic literature describes outcomes using swimming and vertical exercise. This is logical since swimming can play an important role in improving strength, range of motion, and endurance while facilitating normal patterns of movement (Broach & Dattilo, 2011). Swimming involves all muscle groups while having the added benefit of encouraging independence and reintegration. When using swimming, Broach and Dattilo emphasize that the therapist should pay attention to body mechanics and any movements that might be contraindicated for some clients. While swimming is a useful method of AT, teaching swimming using methods such as the Halliwick Concept can also assist in achieving treatment goals.

Assessment, Outcomes, and Documentation

Once the therapist has completed the assessment of the client, the goals have been established, and the plan designed, the next step is to introduce the client to the water. Specific interventions of aquatic therapy are usually based on a land assessment; however, when in the water the recreational therapist must consider the effects of water on movement (Broach & Dattilo, 2011).

In general, before an AT intervention, the recreational therapist will acquire the client's medical diagnosis, medical history, chief complaints (e.g., impairments, activity, participation, and environmental factors), community support, client goals, and physician goals. The assessment and goals may include land-based information on impairments that may be retrieved from the medical history such as the client's current status. Other AT assessment and goal areas may involve ratings of physical, psychosocial, cognitive, and activity level functioning. Personal, societal, or healthcare system goals may also be included such as drug use, number of times restrained, re-admissions to the hospital, general community activity level, school attendance, and community re-integration. The following list shows common preliminary aquatic assessment areas and related ICF codes.

- *Affect*: b126 Temperament and Personality Functions, b152 Emotional Functions
- *Ambulation*: d450 Walking
- *Anxiety*: b152 Emotional Functions
- *Arousal*: b110 Consciousness Functions, b130 Energy and Drive Functions, b140 Attention Functions
- *Attending to task*: b140 Attention Functions, d160 Focusing Attention
- *Balance*: b755 Involuntary Movement Reaction Functions, d410 Changing Basic Body Position, d415 Maintaining a Body Position

- *Coordination and motor control*: b760 Control of Voluntary Movement Functions, d4 Mobility
- *Endurance*: b455 Exercise Tolerance Functions, b740 Muscle Endurance Functions
- *Fatigue*: b455 Exercise Tolerance Functions
- *Following direction*: d210 Undertaking a Single Task, d155 Acquiring Skills
- *Gait*: b770 Gait Pattern Functions, d450 Walking
- *Leisure skill level*: d920 Recreation and Leisure, d155 Acquiring Skills
- *Mood*: b126 Temperament and Personality Functions, b152 Emotional Functions
- *Oral facial control*: b760 Control of Voluntary Movement Functions, d335 Producing Nonverbal Messages
- *Other functional activities*: Choose appropriate ICF codes
- *Pain*: b280 Sensation of Pain
- *Performing tasks*: d210 Undertaking a Single Task, d220 Undertaking Multiple Tasks
- *Posture*: d410 Changing Basic Body Position, d415 Maintaining a Body Position
- *Proprioception*: b260 Proprioceptive Function
- *Range of motion*: b710 Mobility of Joint Functions, b735 Muscle Tone Functions
- *Self-esteem*: b126 Temperament and Personality Functions
- *Self-initiation*: b130 Energy and Drive Functions, d220 Undertaking Multiple Tasks
- *Sensation*: b2 Sensory Functions and Pain, b780 Sensations Related to Muscles and Movement Functions
- *Sleep*: b134 Sleep Functions
- *Social skills*: b126 Temperament and Personality Functions, b152 Emotional Functions, d7 Interpersonal Interactions and Relationships, d910 Community Life, d920 Recreation and Leisure
- *Spasticity*: b735 Muscle Tone Functions
- *Stair climbing*: d4551 Climbing
- *Strength*: b730 Muscle Power Functions
- *Transfer status*: d420 Transferring Oneself
- *Vital capacity*: b430 Hematological System Functions, b455 Exercise Tolerance Functions
- *Weight-bearing status*: b715 Stability of Joint Functions, b7603 Supportive Functions of Arm or Leg

After land-based strengths and needs are determined, a water-based assessment is conducted. The list below shows some of the ICF codes that can be used to document specific deficits.

- *Arousal level*: b110 Consciousness Functions, b130 Energy and Drive Functions, b140 Attention Functions
- *Attending*: b140 Attention Functions, d160 Focusing Attention
- *Balance* (static, dynamic, and challenged): b235 Vestibular Functions, b755 Involuntary Movement Reaction Functions
- *Buoyancy*: d4554 Swimming
- *Comfort in the water*: d4554 Swimming
- *Following direction*: d210 Undertaking a Single Task, d155 Acquiring Skills
- *Gait*: b770 Gait Pattern Functions, d450 Walking
- *Perceived exertion*: b455 Exercise Tolerance Functions, b740 Muscle Endurance Functions
- *Range of motion*: b710 Mobility of Joint Functions, b735 Muscle Tone Functions
- *Repetitions*: d135 Rehearsing, d210 Undertaking a Single Task
- *Safety awareness and performance*: d570 Looking After One's Health
- *Sitting tolerance*: d4153 Maintaining a Sitting Position
- *Stair performance*: d4551 Climbing
- *Standing tolerance* (how long the client can stand and level of weight bearing): d4104 Standing, d4106 Shifting the Body's Center of Gravity, d415 Maintaining a Body Position
- *Swimming ability*: d4554 Swimming
- *Time the client tolerated activity*: b140 Attention Functions, b455 Exercise Tolerance Functions, d210 Undertaking a Single Task, d220 Undertaking Multiple Tasks

The plan of care based on the assessment should include the specific AT strategies to be implemented such as: Bad Ragaz (relaxation, trunk stabilization, upper extremity PNF, lower extremity PNF), Halliwick (mental adjustment, balance, inhibition, facilitation, skill development), Watsu (stretching, relaxation), swimming (strength, endurance, range of motion, proprioception, skill development), sensory integration (balance, coordination, tactile defensiveness), Aquatic PNF (functional movement patterns),

Ai Chi (relaxation, range of motion, mobility), family training, community resources, community evaluation, and other areas according to specific client needs. The type of equipment to be utilized should also be included in the plan of care (Vargas, 2004), such as ankle floats, aqua dumbbells, buoyant collar, blow toys, floatation jacket, floatation belt, fins, kick board, noodle, resistance paddles, snorkel/mask, weights _____ lbs, and other equipment. When documenting a client's session in aquatic therapy, the recreational therapist should note the length of treatment, water temperature, water depths, exercises, progressions in exercises, improvements in participant's condition, and activity level, as well as any effects or other activities related to the goals.

Resources

National Parkinson's Foundation

www.parkinsonswny.com/Aquatic-Handbook.pdf
Provides a free "Parkinson's Disease Aquatic Exercise" manual.

The following organizations offer certifications or training related to Aquatic Therapy.

Aquatic Therapy and Rehabilitation Institute

www.atri.org
Aquatic Therapy Certification, Ai Chi, Aqua Stretch, Back Hab.

Arthritis Foundation

www.arthritis.org
Arthritis Aquatic Exercise Certification.

Aquatic Exercise Association

www.aeawave.com
AEA Aquatic Fitness Professional Certification.

International Halliwick Association

halliwick.org
Halliwick Certifications.

National Multiple Sclerosis Society

www.nationalmssociety.org
Multiple Sclerosis Aquatic Exercise Certification.

Worldwide Aquatic Bodywork Association (WABA)

www.watsu.com and www.minakshiwatsu.com
Watsu certifications.

References

Arborelius, M., Balldin, U., Lila, B., & Lundgren, C. C. (1972). Regional lung function in man during immersion and with the head above water. *Aerospace Medicine, 7,* 701-707.

Bar-Or, O. & Inbar, O. (1992). Swimming and asthma: Benefits and deleterious effects. *Sports Medicine, 14,* 397-405.

Bloomfield, J., Fricker, P. A., & Fitch, D. (1992). *Textbook of science and medicine in sport.* Champaign, IL: Human Kinetics.

Beaudouin, M. & Keller, J. (1994). Aquatic solutions: A continuum of services for individuals with physical disabilities in the community. *Therapeutic Recreation Journal, 28,* 193-202.

Becker, B. E. (1997). Aquatic physics. In R. Routi, D. Morris, & A. J. Cole. (Eds.), *Aquatic rehabilitation* (pp. 15-23). Philadelphia, PA: Raven Publishers.

Becker, B. E. (2009). Aquatic therapy: Scientific foundations and clinical rehabilitation applications. *Physical Medicine and Rehabilitation, 1,* 859-872.

Becker, B. E. (2011). Biophysiologic aspects of hydrotherapy. In B. E. Becker & A. Cole (Eds.). *Comprehensive Aquatic Therapy* (3rd ed.) (pp. 23-76). Pullman, WA: Washington State University.

Becker, B. E. & Cole, A. J. (2011). *Comprehensive aquatic therapy* (3rd ed.). Pullman, WA: Washington State University Press.

Benedict, A. & Freeman, R. (1993). The effect of aquatic exercise on aged persons' bone density, body image and morale. *Activities, Adaptation & Aging, 17,* 67-85.

Berger, B. & Owen, D. (1992). Mood alteration with yoga and swimming: Aerobic exercise may not be necessary. *Perceptual and Motor Skills, 75,* 1331-1343.

Berger, B., Owen, D., & Man, F. (1993). A brief review of the literature and examination of the acute mood benefits of exercise in Czechoslovakian and United States swimmers. *International Journal of Sport Psychology, 24,* 130-150.

Bloomfield, J., Fricker, P., & Fitch, K. (1992). *Textbook of science and medicine in sport.* Champaign IL: Human Kinetics Books.

Broach, E. & Dattilo, J. (1996). Aquatic therapy: A viable therapeutic recreation option. *Therapeutic Recreation Journal 30,* 213-239.

Broach, E. & Dattilo, J. (2001). Effects of aquatic therapy on adults with multiple sclerosis. *Therapeutic Recreation Journal, 35,* 141-154.

Broach, E. & Dattilo, J. (2003). The effect of aquatic therapy on strength of adults with multiple sclerosis. *Therapeutic Recreation Journal, 37,* 224-239.

Broach, E. & Dattilo, J. (2011). Aquatic Therapy. In J. Dattilo & A. McKenney (Eds.). *Facilitation techniques in therapeutic recreation* (2nd ed.) (pp. 69-106). State College, PA: Venture.

Broach, E., Dattilo, J., & McKenney, L. (2007). The effects of aquatic therapy on perceived enjoyment or fun experiences of participants with MS. *Therapeutic Recreation Journal, 27,* 179-200.

Broach, E., Groff, D., & Dattilo, J. (1997). The effects of swimming therapy on individuals with spinal cord injury. *Therapeutic Recreation Journal, 21,* 159-172.

Broach, E., Groff, D., Dattilo, J., Yaffe, R., & Gast, D. (1998). The effects of aquatic therapy on the physical behavior of people with Multiple Sclerosis. *ATRA Annual.*

Broach, E. & McKenney, A. (2012). Social fun and enjoyment: Viable outcomes in aquatics for individuals with disabilities. *International Journal of Aquatic Research and Education, 6,* 171-187.

Bumin, G., Uyanik, M., Yilmaz, I., Kayihan, H., & Topcu, M. (2003). Hydrotherapy for Rett syndrome. *Journal of Rehabilitation Medicine, 35,* 44-45.

Buis, J. M. & Schane, C. S. (1980). Movement exploration as a technique for teaching pre-swimming skills to students with developmental delays. *Practical Pointers, 4*(8), 1-110.

Burke, E. J. & Keenan, M. D. (1984). Energy cost, heart rate, and perceived exertion during the elementary backstroke. *The Physician and Sports Medicine, 12*(12), 75-79.

Campion, M. R. (1985). *Hydrotherapy in pediatrics.* Oxford, United Kingdom: Heinemann Medical Books.

Campion, M. R. (1990). *Adult hydrotherapy.* Oxford, United Kingdom: Heinemann Medical Books.

Cantarero-Villanueva, I., Fernandez-Lao, C., Fernandez-de-las-Penas, C., Lopez-Barajas, I. B., Del-Moral, Avila, R., Isabel de la Llave-Rincon, A., Arroyo-Morales, M. (2012). Effectiveness of water physical therapy on pain, pressure pain sensitivity, and myofascial trigger points in breast cancer survivors: A randomized, control clinical trial. *Pain Medicine, 13*, 1509-1519.

Chon, S. C., Oh, D. W., & Shim, J. H. (2009). Watsu approach for improving spasticity and ambulatory function in hemiparetic patients with stroke. *Physiotherapy Research International, 2*, 128-136.

Edlund, L. D., French, R. W., Herbst, J. J., Ruttenberg, H. D., Ruhling, R. O., & Adams, T. D. (1986). Effects of a swimming program on children with cystic fibrosis. *American Journal of Diseases in Children, 140,* 80-83.

Faull, K. (2005). A pilot study of the comparative effectiveness of two water-based treatments for fibromyalgia syndrome: Watsu and Aix massage. *Journal of Bodywork and Movement Therapies, 9*, 202-210.

Fernandez-Lao, C., Vantarero-Villanueva, I., Ariza-Garcia, A., Cortney, C., Fernandez-de-la-Penas, C. & Morales, M. (2012). Water versus land-based multimodal exercise program effects on body composition in breast cancer survivors: a controlled clinical trial. Support Care Cancer, DOI 1-.1007/s00520-012-1549-x.

Garbielsen, A., Sorensen, V., Pump, B., et al., (2000). Cardiovascular and neuroendocrine responses to water immersion in compensated heart failure. *American Journal of Physiology: Heart and Circulatory Physiology. 279*(4), 1931-1940.

Gehlsen, G., Grigsby, S., & Winant, D. (1984). Effects on an aquatic fitness program on the muscular strength and endurance of participants with multiple sclerosis. *Physical Therapy, 64,* 653-657.

Getz, M., Hutzler, Y., & Vermeer, A. (2006). Effects of aquatic interventions in children with neuromotor impairments: A systematic review of the literature. *Clinical Rehabilitation, 20,* 927-936.

Giancoli, D. C. (1985). *Physics: Principles with applications* (2nd ed.). Englewood Cliffs, NJ: Prentice Hall.

Guillemin, F., Constant, F., Collin, J. F., & Boulange, M. (1994). Short- and long-term effect of spa therapy in chronic low back pain. *British Journal of Rheumatology, 33,* 148-151.

Harrison, R. A. & Bulstrode, S (1992). Loading of the lower limb when walking partially immersed. *Physiotherapy, 78,* 165.

Haung, S., Veiga, R., Sila, U., Reed, E., & Hines, S., (1989). The effect of swimming in asthmatic children: Participants in a swimming program in the city of Baltimore. *Journal of Asthma, 26,* 117-121.

Hauser, W., Klose, P., Langhorst, J., Moradi, B., Steinbach, M., Schiltenwolf, M., & Busch, A. (2010), Efficacy of different types of aerobic exercise in fibromyalgia syndrome: A systematic review and meta-analysis of randomized controlled trials. *Arthritis Research & Therapy, 12*:R79, retrieved from www.biomedcentral.com/content/pdf/ar3002.pdf.

Ide, M. R, Belini, M A., & Caromano, F. A. (2005). Effects of an aquatic versus non-aquatic respiratory exercise program on the respiratory muscle strength in healthy aged persons. *Clinics, 60*, 151-158.

Jamison, L. & Ogden, D. (1994). *Aquatic therapy: Using PNF patterns.* San Antonio, TX: Therapy Skill Builders.

Koury, J. M. (1996). *Aquatic therapy programming: Guidelines for orthopedic rehabilitation.* Champaign, IL: Human Kinetics.

Lambeck, J. & Gamper, U. (2011). The Halliwick concept. In B. E. Becker & A. Cole (Eds.) *Comprehensive Aquatic Therapy* (3rd ed.) (pp. 77-108). Pullman, WA: Washington State University.

Langridge, J. C. & Phillips, D. (1988). Group hydrotherapy exercises for chronic back pain sufferers. *Physiotherapy, 74,* 269-273.

Meno, J. (2000). *Bad Ragaz Ring Method. An introduction. A visual instructional manual for aquatic therapists.* Jackson, WY: Therapeutic Aquatics Inc.

Morris, D. M. (2004). Aquatic rehabilitation for the treatment of neurologic disorders. In Cole, A., J. & Becker, B. E. (Eds.) *Comprehensive aquatic therapy* (2nd ed.) (pp. 151-176). Philadelphia, PA: Butterworth Heinemann.

Noh, D. K., Lim, J., Shin, H., & Paik, N. (2008). The effect of aquatic therapy on postural balance and muscle strength in stroke survivors: A randomized controlled pilot. *Clinical Rehabilitation, 22,* 966-976.

Parker, K. M. & Smith, S. A. (2003). Aquatic aerobic exercise as a means of stress reduction during pregnancy. *Journal of Perinatal Education, 12,* 6-17.

Peganoff, S. A. (1984). The use of aquatics with cerebral palsied adolescents. *The American Journal of Occupational Therapy, 38,* 469-473.

Poyhonen, T., Keskinen, K. L., Hautala, A., & Malkia, E. (2000). Determination of hydrodynamic drag forces and drag coefficients on human leg/foot model during knee exercise. *Clinical Biomechanics, 4,* 256-260.

Routi, R. G., Troup, J. T., & Berger, R. A. (1994). The effects of nonswimming water exercises on older adults. *Journal of Sports Physical Therapy, 19,* 96-103.

Schoedinger, P. (2011). Watsu. In B. E. Becker & A. Cole (Eds.) *Comprehensive aquatic therapy* (3rd ed.) (pp. 137-154). Pullman, WA: Washington State University.

Skinner, A. T. & Thomson, A. M. (Eds.). (1989). *Duffield's exercise in the water* (3rd ed.). Philadelphia, PA: Bailliere Tindall.

Smith, S. A., & Michel Y. (2006). A pilot study on the effects of aquatic exercises on discomforts of pregnancy. *Journal of Obstetric, Gynecologic, & Neonatal Nursing, 35,* 315-323.

Sova, R. (2004). *Introduction to aquatic therapy.* Port Washington, WI: DSL, Ltd.

Sova, R. & Konno, J. (2003). *Ai Chi balance, harmony and healing.* Port Washington, WI: DSL, Ltd.

Templeton, M. S., Booth, D. L., O'Kelly, W. D. (1996). Effects of aquatic therapy on joint flexibility and functional ability in subjects with rheumatic disease. *Journal of Orthopedic Sports Physical Therapy, 23,* 376-381.

Tidhar, D. & Katz-Leurer, M. (2009). Aqua lymphatic therapy in women who suffer from breast cancer treatment-related lymphedema: A randomized controlled study. Support Care Cancer. DOI 10.1007/sf00520-009-0669-4.

Tsukahara, N., Toda, A., Goto, J., & Ezawa, I. (1994). Cross-sectional and longitudinal studies on the effect of water exercise in controlling bone loss in Japanese postmenopausal women. *Journal of Nutrition and Science Vitaminology, 40,* 37-47.

Vargas, L. G. (2004). *Aquatic therapy: Interventions and applications.* Ravensdale, WA: Idyll Arbor.

Wang, T. J., Belza, B., Thompson, F. E., Whitney, J. D., & Bennett, K. (2007). Effects of aquatic exercise on flexibility, strength and aerobic fitness in adults with osteoarthritis of the hip or knee. *Journal of Advanced Nursing 57,* 141-152.

Woods, D. A. (1989). Rehabilitation aquatics for low back injury: Functional gains or pain reduction? *Clinical Kinesiology, 43,* 96-103.

Wright, J. & Cowden, J. E. (1986). Changes in self-concept and cardiovascular endurance of mentally retarded youths in a Special Olympics swim training program. *Adapted Physical Activity Quarterly, 3,* 177-183.

17. Assertiveness Training

Gena Bell Vargas

Assertiveness training (AT) is a behavioral training method that involves teaching clients when and how to refuse requests and how to make sure their rights are being respected while respecting the rights of others. The term was first coined by a psychotherapist in 1958 who suggested AT as a means to reciprocally inhibit anxiety (Wolpe, 1958). AT experienced a lot of popularity starting in the late 1960s into the late 1980s (Ruben & Ruben, 1989). At this point it was noted that while some success had been documented, often results were very mixed. These mixed results were reportedly caused by a "diffusion of the brand." From the training of the facilitators to the way in which assertiveness itself was defined, everything about AT programs varied greatly (Ruben & Ruben, 1989). Evidence-based practice as to the effectiveness of AT was lacking at this point. As a result, potential clients were missing out on many possible benefits. Since that time techniques have become more refined and consistent, as is reflected in this chapter.

To begin, behaviors are a product of personality and environment. Thus, some people are already assertive. People who tend to be more reserved are sometimes seen as non-assertive or passive, while people who are too outspoken are seen as aggressive. In addition, some people are seen as displaying a combination of these behaviors (passive-aggressive). Each of these types of people would benefit from AT. The following list further expands upon the different characteristics of each of these personality types, as well as the feelings associated with them (modified from Moles, 2003).

Passive

- Indirect, anxious, inhibited.
- Avoids addressing issues with others.

- Says "yes" when they would prefer to say "no."
- Difficulty advocating for self (speaking up for their rights).
- For some, anger builds and can result in aggression, depression, physical symptoms such as aches, pains, and stomach issues, or anxiety.
- May cause those on the receiving end of the behavior to respond by taking advantage or ignoring.

Aggressive

- Threatening, attacks others.
- Bossy, dominating, loud, and sarcastic.
- External locus of control (blames others, will not accept responsibility).
- Behavior does not result in the respect of others.
- May cause those on the receiving end of the behavior to respond by feeling hurt, humiliated, threatened, and possibly to act angrily or vengefully.

Passive-Aggressive

- Does not address problems directly.
- Indirectly works to retaliate in an anonymous way.
- Because problems are not directly addressed, this behavior generally results in dissatisfaction, as the person's needs are not being met.

Assertive

- Confident, clear, honest, autonomous.
- Addresses problems directly by seeking out compromises.
- Says "No" when necessary.
- Advocates for self and others.
- Has needs met without hurting others.

Indications

AT is indicated when passive, aggressive or passive-aggressive behavior is exhibited with resultant negative consequences. This may be seen in, among other indicators, difficulties forming and maintaining relationships or conveying needs and thoughts. It is important to note, however, that behavior can vary in different situations and with new life experiences. Therefore, therapists must be observant. For example, an individual who recently sustained a spinal cord injury may have been very assertive prior to the injury, yet finds himself being passive in community settings after the injury due to psychosocial adjustment issues. Other possible causes of dysfunctional communication include personal (e.g., learned behavior, beliefs, values, personality) and environmental (e.g., situation, setting, relationship) factors. When working with individuals who have disabilities, AT can be a vital tool in teaching clients how to be their own best advocate in attaining wants, needs, and personal rights. For example, the Substance Abuse and Mental Health Services Administration (SAMSHA, 2002) has a program called "Speaking Out" designed to assist individuals with mental illness to improve their ability to advocate for themselves by working on their assertiveness skills.

Additional indications for AT will vary by population. For example, individuals with intellectual disabilities may have behaviors that are perceived as challenging by others. AT has been shown to improve such behaviors (Hassiotis & Hall, 2008). Individuals in physical rehabilitation settings who have sustained a spinal cord injury or traumatic brain injury can also benefit from developing or strengthening assertiveness skills, as such skills can improve ability to adapt to life changes (Dorstyn, Mathias, & Denson, 2011; Gongora, McKenney, & Godinez, 2005).

In general, the following populations have been shown to experience a range of benefits from assertiveness training including improved social skills, decreased social anxiety, improved self-esteem, and improved mood:

- Individuals with a mental illness (Douglas, 1980; Lin et al., 2008; Park et al., 2011; Weinhardt et al., 1998; Seo, Ahn, Byun, & Kim, 2007).
- Individuals with intellectual disabilities (Hassiotis & Hall, 2008; Laxton, Gray, & Watts, 1997; McGillicuddy & Blane, 1999; Nezu, Nezu, & Arean, 1991).

- Individuals with post-traumatic stress disorder (Cloitre, 2013).
- Individuals at risk for diabetes (CDC, 2013a).
- Adults and adolescents with visual impairments (Hersen et al., 1995; Kim, 2003).
- Older adults with hearing loss (Ryan, Anas, & Friedman, 2006).
- Older adult residents of nursing homes experiencing depression (Segal, 2005).
- Older adults with chronic pain (Andersson et al., 2012).
- Children who have run away (Rotheram-Borus et al., 1991).
- Rural adolescents at risk of abusing alcohol (Goldberg-Lillehoj, Spoth, & Trudeau, 2005).
- Students at risk of bullying (Crothers & Kolbert, 2004).
- Women at risk of violent attack (Brecklin & Ullman, 2005).
- People who have experienced a traumatic brain injury (TBI) (Gongora et al., 2005).
- People who have experienced a spinal cord injury (SCI) (Dorstyn et al., 2011).
- Caregivers for persons who have experienced a stroke (van den Heuvel, 2000).

ICF codes that may indicate a need for assertiveness training include these codes and their subcodes: b126 Temperament and Personality Functions, b152 Emotional Functions, b280 Sensation of Pain, d240 Handling Stress and Other Psychological Demands, d3 Communication, d550 Eating, d570 Looking After One's Health, d630 Preparing Meals, and d7 Interpersonal Interactions and Relationships. The relationship between ICF codes and other measures of the client's need for assertiveness training is discussed in the Outcomes section.

Contraindications

There are no contraindications in the literature for AT. As with any treatment, however, it is important to consider all aspects of a person (including readiness and interest) before determining treatment. For example, if a potential client is assessed and found to be highly delusional and/or paranoid and has a strong, unfounded belief that others are mistreating him/her, AT would most likely not be appropriate. Likewise, a client who is in the acute stage of rehabilitation might not be ready to learn about AT due to increased focus on other recovery issues (Stumbo & Caldwell, 2002).

Protocols and Processes

Given the variety of populations in which AT is used, a wide variety of protocols and processes are utilized. Recreational therapists can seek out professional textbooks (e.g. Hutchins, 2011), specific workbooks (e.g., Bunnell, 2004; Gingerich & Mueser, 2005; Moles, 2003) or journal articles on AT as they relate to the specific setting and population served. Protocols vary in length from a single session to a multi-week program. The content (processes) also varies depending on the specific needs of the individual or group. Common themes across protocols and programs are

- General education on assertiveness
- Identification of client's personal tendencies
- Education on "I" messages
- How to come to a compromise
- How to make and refuse requests
- Planning appropriate assertive responses to anticipated life situations
- Practicing assertiveness skills via relevant techniques, including role-play, writing, visualization, etc.

The manner in which AT is administered can also vary. It may be part of a larger, more ambitious protocol, paired or imbedded in other technique-specific programs and protocols, or delivered as a sole intervention. A sampling of such programs and protocols are provided below.

AT in Larger Protocols

Assertiveness is often included as one piece of a larger protocol. For example, the CDC "Street Smart" program has eight 1.5-2 hour group sessions over the course of six weeks designed to reduce risky sexual behaviors of runaway youth. It integrates principles of assertiveness throughout the program.

In addition, AT has been recognized to be a valuable component in cognitive behavioral therapy, anger management, and social skills training:

AT in cognitive behavioral therapy (CBT): Andersson and colleagues (2012) conducted a controlled pilot trial of 21 older adults with chronic pain. In the study, participants engaged in six CBT group treatment sessions focusing on applied relaxation.

The program also included problem solving, assertiveness, communication strategies, sleep management, and relapse prevention. Findings indicated positive changes in pain, mood, anxiety, and quality of life. In another study, a meta-analysis was conducted on the efficacy of CBT for psychological adjustment in adults with spinal cord injury (Dorstyn, Mathias, & Denson, 2011). A total of 10 studies were identified. Findings indicated that CBT was effective in improving assertiveness, coping, self-efficacy, depression, and quality of life. As a final example, Hassiotis and Hall (2004) conducted a meta-analysis to investigate the effectiveness of CBT on outwardly directed aggressive behavior by individuals with intellectual disabilities. The authors identified three studies, of which only two provided data appropriate for analysis. Findings indicated that direct interventions based on CBT methods (modified relaxation, assertiveness training with problem solving, and anger management) appear to reduce outwardly directed aggressive behavior that can cause social exclusion.

AT in anger management: Although assertiveness is frequently included when teaching anger management in the clinical setting as it is seen as a healthy way to respond to negative situations, there is a lack of research on its efficacy. One example in recreational therapy literature describes a case study in which it was included as a portion of an anger coping program developed to assist individuals with traumatic brain injury respond more effectively to their anger (Gongora et al., 2005). The program utilized a CBT framework and was carried out with one participant across eight sessions, 45 minutes in length, delivered three times a week. Assertiveness was focused on in session five (discussing assertive reactions), session six (modeling assertive behavior), and session seven (role-playing assertive behavior). The researchers observed improvements in the participant's social interactions, which were seen as helpful in future transitions to work and social environments after discharge.

AT in social skills training: Assertiveness has also been included as part of social skills training (SST). In one instance, a research team compared a virtual reality (VR) application to traditional role-playing to see which was more likely to improve social skills in individuals with schizophrenia (Park et al., 2011). Those in the study participated in 10 semi-weekly sessions, of which three sessions focused on AT (making a demand, rejecting a demand, and making a compromise). The researcher-developed VR program allowed participants to practice their assertiveness skills in a virtual environment, interacting with simulations of people as opposed to actual people. It was shown to be more effective in improving assertiveness and conversational skills than the traditional role-playing program. This is of particular interest to recreational therapists working with participants that might prefer a different approach to SST if they are hesitant to or have difficulty interacting with peers (Park et al., 2011).

AT Only Application

In addition to AT as a component of a larger protocol, as previously described, AT might be a sole intervention. For example, a study performed by Glueckauf and Quittner (1992) focused solely on AT. They developed an 11-week AT program with the hopes of making improvements in the self-efficacy and interpersonal skills in 34 adults without cognitive impairment who utilized wheelchairs at least 50% of the time. The sessions were 2½ hours long and met once a week. Nine of the sessions were in a group with the other participants, and the other two sessions were in a small group consisting of one other participant and the therapist to allow participants to practice application skills. Group sessions consisted of:

- Discussion of outside assignments or "homework" regarding learning and/or practicing assertiveness skills learned in the prior session.
- Didactic educational presentations by the therapist on assertiveness using audiovisual methods and modeling of skills.
- Discussion on, and practicing of, new assertiveness skills via role-playing.
- Introduction to the new outside assignment for the following week, generally composed of practicing communication skills and reading from an assigned book.

Participants completed a pretest at the beginning of the study, a posttest immediately after, and were contacted for follow-up six months after the conclusion of the training. Results showed participants increased how frequently they responded to situations assertively, and decreased how frequently they responded to situations passively.

In another study by Lin and colleagues (2008), AT was utilized to increase self-esteem and decrease social anxiety in 68 inpatients with depression, anxiety, or adjustment disorders. The study consisted of two-hour AT sessions twice a week for four consecutive weeks. Sessions covered the following topics:

- Education on assertiveness and the related behaviors.
- Education on basic personal rights.
- Practicing listening skills and how to question others.
- Education on self-esteem and its relation to assertiveness.
- How to withstand criticism and express dissatisfaction.
- How to refuse requests and make definitive requests.
- Verbal and non-verbal assertive techniques.
- How to give and receive praise.
- Education on empathy.

Participants completed a pretest at the beginning of the study, a posttest immediately after, and completed surveys one month after the conclusion of the training. Results showed an increase in assertiveness skills and decrease in social anxiety. A significant increase of self-esteem was not shown.

AT through Vicarious Learning

As is often the case, vicarious learning is an effective method for teaching AT. The therapist should strive to always be an example of how to interact assertively with peers and participants. Techniques that have been discussed should be demonstrated in all interactions. This also helps to improve the overall milieu as staff and participants come to treat each person with whom they interact with respect and honesty.

Outcomes and Documentation

Possible outcomes of AT-specific programs and programs that integrate AT include improvements in the following areas found as deficits during the assessment process:

- Assertiveness (b126 Temperament and Personality Functions) (Lin et al., 2008; Weinhardt et al., 1998).

- Social anxiety (b152 Emotional Functions, d240 Handling Stress and Other Psychological Demands, d710 Basic Interpersonal Interactions) (Lin et al., 2008).
- Conversational skills (d3 Communication, d710 Basic Interpersonal Interactions) (Park et al., 2011).
- Self-esteem or self-worth (b126 Temperament and Personality Functions) (Seo et al., 2007).
- Socialization (d7 Interpersonal Interactions and Relationships) (Gongora et al., 2005).
- Eating habits (d550 Eating, d570 Looking After One's Health, d630 Preparing Meals) (Gongora et al., 2005).
- Pain tolerance (b280 Sensation of Pain, d570 Looking After One's Health, d7 Interpersonal Interactions and Relationships, and other ICF codes affected by pain issues) (Andersson et al., 2012).
- Mood (b126 Temperament and Personality Functions, b130 Energy and Drive Functions) (Hassiotis & Hall, 2008).
- Self-efficacy (b126 Temperament and Personality Functions, d710 Basic Interpersonal Interactions) (Glueckauf & Quittner, 1992).
- Interpersonal skills (d7 Interpersonal Interactions and Relationships) (Glueckauf & Quittner, 1992).
- Quality of life (usually a client's self-assessment that can include all of the areas described above) (Hassiotis & Hall, 2008).

Recreational therapists who provide AT should consider the use of the following measures:

The Wolpe-Lazarus Assertiveness Scale (WLAS): This is one of the earliest self-report scales on assertiveness (Wolpe & Lazarus, 1966) and is still in use. It consists of 30 items rated as yes/no or true/false. Responding "yes" or "true" results in one point towards an overall score. The higher the score, the more assertive a person is said to be. It has been tested and found to produce reliable and consistent results (Hersen et al., 1979).

The Rathus Assertiveness Schedule: Published in 1973, this schedule employs 30 items to measure degree of assertiveness, 17 of which are reversed (Rathus, 1973). The intent was for it to be used to establish a baseline measurement in clients prior to receiving AT. It is self-report and each item is given a rating ranging from +3 to -3 based on how much the clients agree that the item is one of their characteristics. Adding all of the responses together gives the total score. Some items were based on previous scales (Wolpe & Lazarus, 1966). The schedule was tested and shown to be reliable and valid.

The Galassi College Self-Expression Scale — A Measure of Assertiveness: This measure was published by Galassi and colleagues (1974). The scale looks at three dimensions of assertiveness (positive assertiveness, negative assertiveness, and self-denial), as measured in multiple relational contexts (peers, family, strangers, authority figures, etc.). The scale provides an overall score where higher scores indicate more assertiveness. Only college students were utilized in developing the scale and, thus, it would be most accurate when measuring assertiveness in similar young adults.

The Gambrill Assertion Inventory: In 1975, Gambrill and Richey published a self-report inventory of assertion containing 40 items. They had observed a need for such an inventory in clinical settings (as well as for research) to detect a client's current assertiveness. The inventory is based on the concept that a person's behavior type can be determined by evaluating the person's level of anxiety in and likelihood to respond to various possible situations. Responding to the survey consists of rating each of the 40 items twice. First, each item is reviewed and rated by the individual on a scale of one to five as to how anxious or discomforting the situation would be. Second, each item is again reviewed (while covering the first rating) and rated on a scale of one to five as to how likely the individual is to display the behavior in question. Finally, the individual is asked to go back and circle the situations they would like to handle more assertively. After analysis, the client is classified into one of four profiles (see below). In testing the inventory, the authors found results to be reliable and valid for undergraduate students, as well as women seeking assertiveness training.

- *Doesn't care*: discomfort low, response probability low
- *Assertive*: discomfort low, response probability high
- *Unassertive*: discomfort high, response probability low
- *Anxious-performer*: discomfort high, response probability high

The Bakker Assertiveness-Aggressiveness Inventory: This 36-item measure, completed by self-report, was developed in order to separately measure defensive and initiating behaviors (Bakker et al., 1978). The authors viewed the then current operationalization of assertiveness to be murky at best, mostly due to there being two undifferentiated elements — assertiveness and aggressiveness. Thus, the 36-item measure has two 18-item subscales. One measures likelihood of an assertive response, the other measures likelihood of aggressive behavior. The inventory was found to produce valid and reliable results.

As the number of assertion inventories grew, a set of authors decided to conduct a factor analysis to review current inventories and determine the direction of future efforts (Henderson & Furnham, 1983). Results showed that the inventories reviewed (the Wolpe-Lazarus Assertion Inventory, the Rathus Assertiveness Schedule, the Galassi College Self Expression Scale, the Gambrill Assertion Inventory, and the Bakker Assertiveness-Aggressiveness Inventory) were able to account for a minority of the variance, which highlighted the multidimensional nature of assertiveness. The inventories acknowledged this characteristic, however, each only provided a global score. The authors recommended that future efforts focus on separating the items by dimension and attributing a different score to each (Henderson & Furnham, 1983). Two scales have been developed in response to this:

The Scale for Interpersonal Behavior (SIB): Arrindell and Van der Ende first published this scale in 1985. Developed in the Netherlands, the scale has since been tested and proved reliable with psychiatric and non-psychiatric participants in Europe and the United States (Arrindell & van der Ende, 1985; Arrindell et al., 1988, 1999, 2001, 2005). The 50-item scale was developed on the premise that past scales did not utilize systematic research to determine validity and or cross-sample generalizability. The development of the SIB supported the validity of four factors when measuring assertiveness: display of negative feelings (negative assertion), expression of and dealing with personal limitations, initiating assertiveness and praising others, and the ability to deal with compliments or praise of others (positive assertion). This has proven to be a more accurate representation of the multidimensional nature of assertiveness. The factors are represented as subscales in

the SIB having a range of eight to fifteen questions for each. A "general assertiveness" score can be determined by summing all of the subscales. However, this can be seen as oversimplifying the results (Arrindell et al., 1999).

Adaptive and Aggressive Assertiveness Scales (AAA-S): This 19-item instrument combines two scales — one to measure adaptive assertiveness, and the other to measure aggressive assertiveness (Thompson & Berenbaum, 2011). The authors saw a need for these to be distinguished, as certain aspects of assertiveness and aggressiveness have previously been confounded, in that behaviors interpreted by some to be assertive can also be seen by others to be aggressive. In testing the scale, the authors utilized a clinical sample as well as a student sample. Their results were shown to have good validity and psychometric properties.

Resources

The following is a list of books and training guides that are helpful resources on AT for therapists and consumers. Many include protocols, activities, and worksheets.

- *Coping Skills Groups* (Gingerich & Mueser, 2005)
- *Strategies for Anger Management* (Moles, 2003)
- *Strategies Using Art for Self-Reflection* (Bunnell, 2004)
- *Speaking Out for Yourself: A Self-Help Guide* (SAMSHA, 2002)
- *Street Smart: Reducing HIV Risk among Runaway and Homeless Youth* (CDC, 2013b)
- *Clinical Skills: Skill Training in Affect and Interpersonal Regulation (STAIR)* (Cloitre, 2013)
- *Assertiveness: Practical Skills for Positive Communication* (Hermes, 1998)
- *The Assertiveness Workbook* (Paterson, 2000)

Organization

National Alliance on Mental Illness (NAMI)
www.nami.org/

References

Andersson, G., Johansson, C., Nordlander, A., Asmundson, G. (2012). Chronic pain in older adults: A controlled pilot trial of a brief cognitive-behavioural group treatment. *Behavioural and Cognitive Psychotherapy, 40*(2), 239-244.

Arrindell, W. A., Akkerman, A., van der Ende, J., Schreurs, P. J. G., Brugman, A., Stewart, R., & Sanderman, R. (2005).

Normative studies with the Scale for Interpersonal Behaviour (SIB): III. Psychiatric inpatients. *Personality and Individual Differences, 38*(4), 941–952.

Arrindell, W. A., Bridges, K. R., van der Ende, J., St. Lawrence, J. S., Gray-Shellberg, L., Harnish, R., Rogers, R., & Sanderman, R. (2001). Normative studies with the Scale for Interpersonal Behaviour (SIB): II. U.S. students. *Behaviour Research and Therapy, 39*(12), 1461–1479.

Arrindell, W. A., Ende, J. van der, Sanderman, R., Oosterhof, L., Stewart, R., & Lingsma, M. M. (1999). Normative studies with the Scale for Interpersonal Behaviour (SIB): I. Nonpsychiatric social skills trainees. *Personality and Individual Differences, 27*(3), 417–431.

Arrindell, W. A., Sanderman, R., Van der Molen, H., Van der Ende, J., & Mersch, P.-P. (1988). The structure of assertiveness: A confirmatory approach. *Behaviour Research and Therapy, 26*(4), 337–339.

Arrindell, W. A. & van der Ende, J. (1985). Cross-sample invariance of the structure of self-reported distress and difficulty in assertiveness. *Advances in Behaviour Research and Therapy, 7*(4), 205–243.

Bakker, C., Bakker-Rabdau, M., & Breit, S. (1978). The Measurement of Assertiveness and Aggressiveness. *Journal of Personality Assessment, 42*(3), 277–284.

Brecklin, L. & Ullman, S. (2005). Self-defense or assertiveness training and women's responses to sexual attacks. *Journal of Interpersonal Violence, 20*(6), 738-762.

Bunnell, L. (2004). *Strategies using art for self-reflection.* Wilkes-Barre, PA: Wellness Reproductions and Publishing.

Centers for Disease Control (CDC). (2013a). *Lifestyle coach facilitation guide: Post-core.* Atlanta, GA: Centers for Disease Control and Prevention.

Centers for Disease Control (CDC). (2013b). *Street smart: Reducing HIV risk among runaway and homeless youth* (DHHS Publication No. CS210399U). Atlanta, GA: Centers for Disease Control and Prevention.

Cloitre, M. (2013, August 30). *Clinical Skills: Skill Training in Affect and Interpersonal Regulation (STAIR).* Retrieved from www.ptsd.va.gov/professional/continuing_ed/ ClinSkills/STAIR_online_training.asp.

Crothers, L. & Kolbert, J. (2004). Comparing middle school teachers' and students' views on bullying and anti-bullying interventions. *Journal of School Violence, 3*(1), 17-32.

Dorstyn, D., Mathias, J., & Denson, L. (2011). Efficacy of cognitive behavior therapy for the management of psychological outcomes following spinal cord injury: A meta-analysis. *Journal of Health Psychology, 16*(2), 374-391.

Douglas, R. (1980). Assertiveness training for emotionally disturbed clients. *Journal of Rehabilitation, 46*(1), 46-47.

Galassi, J., Delo, J., Galassi, M., & Bastien, S. (1974). The college self-expression scale: A measure of assertiveness. *Behavior Therapy, 5*(2), 165-171.

Gambrill, E. & Richey, C. (1975). An assertion inventory for use in assessment and research. *Behavior Therapy, 6*(4), 550-561.

Gingerich, S. & Mueser, K. (2005). *Coping skills group: A session-by-session guide.* Wilkes-Barre, PA: Wellness Reproductions and Publishing.

Glueckauf, R. & Quittner, A. (1992). Assertiveness training for disabled adults in wheelchairs: Self-report, role-play, and activity pattern outcomes. *Journal of Consulting and Clinical Psychology, 60*(3), 419-425.

Goldberg-Lillehoj, C., Spoth, R., & Trudeau, L. (2005). Assertiveness among young rural adolescents: Relationship to alcohol use. *Journal of Child & Adolescent Substance Abuse, 14*(3), 39-68.

Gongora, E. L., McKenney, A., & Godinez, C. (2005). A multidisciplinary approach to teaching anger coping after sustaining a traumatic brain injury: A case report. *Therapeutic Recreation Journal, 39*(3), 229-240.

Hassiotis, A. & Hall, I. (2008). Behavioural and cognitive-behavioural interventions for outwardly-directed aggressive behaviour in people with learning disabilities. *Cochrane Database of Systematic Reviews 2008, Issue 3.*

Henderson, M. & Furnham, A. (1983). Dimensions of assertiveness: Factor analysis of five assertion inventories. *Journal of Behavior Therapy and Experimental Psychiatry, Volume 14*(3), 223-231.

Hermes, S. (1998). *Assertiveness: Practical skills for positive communication.* Center City, MN: Hazelden.

Hersen, M., Bellack, A., Turner, S., Williams, M., Harper, K., & Watts, J. (1979). Psychometric properties of the Wolpe-Lazarus assertiveness scale. *Behaviour Research and Therapy, 17*(1), 63–69.

Hersen, M., Kabacoff, R., Van Hasselt, V., Null, J., Ryan, C., Melton, M., & Segal, D. (1995). Assertiveness, depression, and social support in visually impaired adults. *Journal of Visual Impairment and Blindness, 89*(6), 524-531.

Hutchins, D. (2011). Assertiveness Training. In N. Stumbo, & B. Wardlaw (Ed.), *Facilitation of therapeutic recreation services: An evidence-based and best practice approach to techniques and processes* (pp. 237-245). State College, Pa: Venture Pub.

Kim, Y. (2003). The effects of assertiveness training on enhancing the social skills of adolescents with visual impairments. *Journal of Visual Impairments & Blindness, 97*(5), 285-298.

Laxton, M., Gray, C., & Watts, S. (1997). Teaching assertiveness skills to people with learning disabilities: A brief report of a training programme. *Journal of Intellectual Disabilities, 1*(2), 71-76.

Lin, Y., Wu, M, Yang, C., Chen, T., Hsu, C., Chang, Y., et al. (2008). Evaluation of assertiveness training for psychiatric patients. *Journal of Clinical Nursing, 17*(21), 2875-2883.

McGillicuddy, N. & Blane, H. (1999). Substance use in individuals with mental retardation. *Addictive Behaviors, 24*(6), 869-878.

Moles, K. (2003). *Strategies for anger management.* Wilkes-Barre, PA: Wellness Reproductions and Publishing.

Nezu, C., Nezu, A., & Arean, P. (1991). Assertiveness and problem-solving training for mildly mentally retarded persons with dual diagnoses. *Research in Developmental Disabilities, 12*(4), 371-386.

Park, K., Ku, J., Choi, S., Jang, H., Park, J., Kim, S., Kim, J. (2011). A virtual reality application in role-plays of social skills training for schizophrenia: A randomized, controlled trial. *Psychiatry Research, 189*(2), 166-172.

Paterson, R. (2000). *The assertiveness workbook.* Oakland, CA: New Harbinger.

Rathus, S. A. (1973). A 30-item schedule for assessing assertive behavior. *Behavior Therapy, 4*(3), 398–406.

Rotheram-Borus, M., Koopman, C., Haignere, C., & Davies, M. (1991). Reducing HIV sexual risk behaviors among runaway adolescents. *Journal of the American Medical Association, 266*(9), 1237-1241.

Ruben, D. & Ruben, M. (1989). Why assertiveness training programs fail. *Small Group Behavior, 20*(3), 367-380.

Ryan, E., Anas, A., & Friedman, D. (2006). Evaluations of older adult assertiveness in problematic clinical encounters. *Journal of Language and Social Psychology, 25*(2), 129-145.

Substance Abuse and Mental Health Services Administration (SAMHSA) (2002). *Speaking out for yourself: A self-help guide.* (DHHS Publication No. SMA-3719). Rockville, MD.

Segal, D. (2005). Relationships of assertiveness, depression, and social support among nursing home residents. *Behavior Modification, 29*(4), 689-695.

Seo, J.-M., Ahn, S., Byun, E.-K., & Kim, C.-K. (2007). Social skills training as nursing intervention to improve the social skills and self-esteem of inpatients with chronic schizophrenia. *Archives of Psychiatric Nursing, 21*(6), 317–326.

Stumbo, N. & Caldwell, L. (2002). Leisure education and learning theory, *ADOZ: Boletin del Centro de Docmentacion en Ocio, 23* (Spanish version pp. 29-35; English version pp. 35-40).

Thompson, R. J. & Berenbaum, H. (2011). Adaptive and aggressive assertiveness scales (AAA-S). *Journal of Psychopathology and Behavioral Assessment, 33*(3), 323–334.

van den Heuvel, E., de Witte, L., Nooyen-Haazen, I., Sanderman, R., & Meyboom-de Jong, B. (2000). Short-term effects of a group support program and an individual support program for caregivers of stroke patients. *Patient Education and Counseling, 40*(2), 109-120.

Weinhardt, L., Carey, M., Carey, K., & Verdecias, R. (1998). Increasing assertiveness skills to reduce HIV risk among women living with a severe and persistent mental illness. *Journal of Consulting and Clinical Psychology, 66*(4), 680-684.

Wolpe, J. (1958). *Psychotherapy by reciprocal inhibition.* Stanford, CA: Stanford University Press.

Wolpe, J. & Lazarus, A. (1966). *Behavior therapy techniques.* New York, NY: Pergamon.

18. Balance Training

Heather R. Porter

Balance (also referred to as postural control) is a dynamic process in which the body maintains its center of gravity over its base of support so it can hold a position against gravity, whether in a static (stationary) or dynamic (moving) state (Rose, 2010; O'Sullivan & Schmitz, 2007). For example, when skiing, the skier tries to keep his/her weight balanced over the center of the skis in such a manner that gravity does not cause a fall. The center of gravity for a typical skier versus a skier who has an above the knee amputation is different and requires different positions and strategies to keep from falling. (One of the strategies for skiers who have had amputations is to use ski poles with short skis on the end of the pole instead of a spike and basket.)

There are a number of important concepts associated with a client's ability to maintain balance during activities. The recreational therapist begins to address balance as s/he expands the client's movements and actions beyond the basic skills and equipment taught by physical therapy (PT) and occupational therapy (OT). For example, PT and OT may have prescribed a walker and reacher for the client to use after discharge. However, the client has always been an avid gardener and these two pieces of equipment do not allow the client to continue to garden. It is the recreational therapist's task to determine further adapted equipment and transfer procedures that allow the client to garden again and address balance issues in the activity.

In addition to addressing balance skills in specific activities, recreational therapists might also facilitate specific balance training sessions or classes for those who are at risk of falling. For example, older adults are at a higher risk of falls due to the deterioration of key sensory systems that are involved in balance. According to Rogers (2012), visual acuity, depth perception, peripheral field and sensitivity to

low spatial frequencies (requiring more contrast to detect spatial differences) decrease with age. At approximately age 40, vestibular neurons begin to decrease in size resulting in various impairments, including dizziness. Skin sensitivity decreases with age. Decreased input from tactile, pressure, and vibration receptors make it difficult to walk, stand, and detect heel-to-toe body weight shifts needed to maintain balance. To compensate for these losses, the therapist must have a solid understanding of balance in different positions and using different adapted equipment.

Basic concepts related to balance include the following (Rose, 2003; O'Sullivan & Schmitz, 2007; Finlayson, 2013).

Postural Orientation

Good posture is the positioning of the body so that the client is able to complete activities with the least amount of internal energy and the least amount of wear and tear on the body. It's the ability to maintain normal alignment relationships among body segments and between the body and the environment. Maintaining postural orientation requires active muscle effort. In a quiet standing position, the line of gravity passes in front of the ankle and knee joints, slightly behind the hip joints, and in front of the thoracic and neck segments, with the calf muscles and hip and trunk extensors holding the body in an upright position. In a seated position, ears are aligned with the center of the hips and knees are aligned with the ankles.

Postural Control and Stability

Anticipatory postural control: Anticipatory postural control refers to learned actions that a client makes to ensure that his/her postural balance remains stable even when the environment changes. A client is able to increase functional balance through instruction and practice. For example, a recreational therapist, working with a client who uses a wheelchair, teaches how to balance on the back two wheels of the wheelchair in anticipation of using this skill to drop down from a curb that has no curb cut. Another example is teaching a client how to balance with both crutches in one hand while opening a door. Anticipated postural control is always a planned action.

Reactive postural control: Reactive postural control is a quick action that must be taken to maintain postural balance in response to an unexpected challenge in the environment. One example of reactive postural control is when a client grabs onto the stair railing to break the forward fall when his foot does not quite clear the step. Another example is when a client puts his hands on the seat in front of him to stop forward movement when the city bus on which he is riding makes a sudden stop. Reactive postural control is a reaction to an event and not a planned action.

Dynamic postural control (also referred to as dynamic balance): Dynamic balance is the ability to maintain stability and orientation with the center of mass over the base of support when the body is in motion (e.g., standing and throwing a baseball). Dynamic balance is often described by the client's body position (e.g., dynamic standing balance, dynamic sitting balance), as well as the extent of the challenge and support. The extent of the challenge is described as being within min ranges, mod ranges, or max ranges. Min ranges refers to movements that are closest (most proximal) to the body, such as standing at a table and assembling a wood project that is immediately in front of the client. Mod ranges are movements of full extension, such as standing at a table and assembling a wood project where project pieces are at arm's length on the table. Max ranges are movements past full extension, such as standing at a table and assembling a wood project where the project pieces are across the other side of the table, requiring the client to bend at the hips in order to further extend his/her reach. Dynamic balance is also described by support provided, including type of support (e.g., with unilateral upper extremity support, such as supporting one's balance with one hand on the table top; with an adaptive device, such as a single point cane), support strategy utilized (e.g.,

using hip strategy), or the absence of a particular support (e.g., unsupported). See Postural Responses and Control in the Protocols and Processes section below

Postural stability control (also referred to a static balance): Static balance is the ability to maintain stability and orientation with the center of mass over the base of support with the body at rest (no motion, stationary; such as sitting still or standing still).

Stability Limits

Stability limits are the greatest distance in any direction the client is able to (or feels comfortable to) move without changing his/her base of support, while still maintaining balance. Stability limits tend to shrink as an individual ages or develops sensory losses. Stability limits are part of engaging in many activities such as preparing a meal, gardening, arts and crafts, and sports. Even playing bingo (leaning forward to mark a number on the bingo sheet) involves a client consciously or unconsciously moving within stability limits. Just as with range of motion, stability limits shrink with inactivity. Engaging in regular activity that moves a person safely to the edges of his/her stability should be a daily occurrence. Just like cardiovascular endurance, stability limits are maintained or increased only through regular and ongoing activity.

Sway Envelope

Sway envelope is the common range of movement that an individual stays within during activity without changing his/her base of support. It is not unusual for people to have a smaller sway envelope than their stability limits. Sway envelopes are often "lopsided" as individuals lose function, favor one side due to pain, or lose function through neurological or musculoskeletal degeneration. For clients who seldom venture outside of their sway envelope or have a restricted sway envelope, the therapist will want to ensure that activities are offered that help "exercise" the stability limits beyond the sway envelope. For clients who have impairments that often cause them to venture outside of their sway envelope and outside their stability limits, balance safety should be taught.

Balance

The skill of balance requires the integration of multiple body systems and a full understanding of each system is needed in order to identify, and subsequently address, the underlying causes of balance dysfunction. Each is described below (Rose, 2010; Gillen, 2011; Rogers, 2012):

Visual system: The visual system provides a visual layout of the environment, and one's position related to environmental objects, allowing for safe navigation (e.g., anticipation of environmental challenges, obstacle avoidance).

Somatosensory system: The somatosensory system perceives touch, pressure, pain, temperature, position, movement, and vibration that arise from receptors in the skin, muscles, and joints. This information helps a person to know his/her body position. For example, feeling the pressure on the bottom of the foot when stepping forward tells the person that s/he has made full contact with the ground. Likewise, if the client feels that s/he has not made full contact with the ground surface (e.g., foot is half on the curb and half off the curb), the body would then react to the signal of questionable support through reactive or planned postural control (e.g., swinging arms to the front or side to maintain center of gravity or readjusting footing). If the somatosensory system is impaired, and information is not effectively sent from the proprioceptors in the muscles and joints, then reactive and planned postural control responses might not be signaled and subsequently performed, thus increasing the risk of falling. It is also important to note that this system is more challenged when the visual system is impaired or absent in a dark environment or because of visual impairment.

Vestibular system: The vestibular system is housed in the inner ear and is activated when the head is moved. It aids in determining head position and head motion in space relative to gravity.

Motor system: The integration of the visual, somatosensory, and vestibular information results in the development of a sensory strategy. A sensory strategy activates the motor system response (referred to as a sensory-motor interaction). The specific motor response will vary depending upon the sensory information received (e.g., stiffening muscles, coordinating muscles). Specific muscle response synergies are activated leading to a pattern of movement triggered through a single neural command. The sensory-motor interaction continues as the challenge is negotiated. This is referred to as the perception-action cycle. In addition to the motor system response, the health of the motor system (e.g., strength, flexibility, coordination, endurance) also plays a role in balance.

Cognitive system: The cognitive system also plays a role in the motor response. For example, the processing speed of incoming stimuli can slow the timing and reduce the accuracy of the motor response. Memory of how best to respond to the challenge and attention skills (sustained, divided, shifting) can influence the motor response performed. Intelligence can influence the person's ability to anticipate and subsequently adapt to environmental challenges.

Nervous system: The cerebellum receives information from various structures and sends out information to control smooth, coordinated movement, including appropriate timing, muscle tone, and synergy of muscle groups. An indication of dysfunction in the cerebellum includes ataxia, unsteady gait, and visual disturbance. The basal ganglia influence the sequencing of automatic postural reactions. Indications of dysfunction in the basal ganglia include rigidity, bradykinesia, akinesia, tremors (resting or intention), chorea, and athetosis. The brain stem integrates vestibular input and initiates compensatory eye movements. An indication of dysfunction in the brain stem includes dysfunctional compensatory eye movements and vestibular dysfunction.

Indications

Balance training is indicated when the person has balance deficits, a history of falls, a particular impairment in one or more of the systems involved in balance, or a particular condition that increases the risk of falls (e.g., Parkinson's, multiple sclerosis, stroke, joint replacement, amputation). Balance training is also indicated to maintain and strengthen balance-related body systems in older adults, as balance-related body systems deteriorate due to the normal aging process. Individuals who do not present with balance deficits, or who are not identified as being a falls risk, may additionally require balance training due to psychological-emotional factors. For example, Miller and Deathe (2011) measured balance confidence and social activity in 65 individuals with a lower extremity amputation at the time of discharge from an inpatient rehabilitation facility, and then again at a three-month follow-up. They found that balance confidence at the three-month follow-up remained low despite improvements in walking ability, and that the balance confidence scores predicted three-month social activity scores. The authors recommended that therapists augment traditional balance training to include strategies based on Bandura's Social Cognitive Learning Theory to build confidence and subsequently improve social activity engagement.

The primary ICF code that indicates a need for balance training is b755 Involuntary Movement Reaction Functions. Other ICF codes that influence balance include b156 Perceptual Functions, b160 Thought Functions, b210 Seeing Functions, b235 Vestibular Functions, b715 Stability of Joint Functions, b730 Muscle Power Functions, b735 Muscle Tone Functions, b765 Involuntary Movement Functions, b770 Gait Pattern Functions, and d4 Mobility.

Contraindications

When engaging a client in balance training there is increased risk of falling. Consequently, all precautions must be taken to prevent or minimize falls. This includes beginning with simple tasks and progressing to more complex tasks as the client improves, removing unnecessary environmental challenges that are not the focus of treatment, and using fall prevention devices as appropriate or needed, such as ambulatory aids, gait belts, or physical assistance from the therapist.

Protocols and Processes

A balance assessment is conducted which includes (1) a clinical interview to ascertain information about activities that are important and meaningful to the client, along with information about the client's perception of abilities and challenges, (2) observation of the client performing meaningful activities to determine if the client's self-perceptions are congruent with the therapist's observations and to observe patterns of dysfunction that could be helpful in determining underlying causes of balance problems, (3) direct requests, such as asking the client to perform specific balance tasks (e.g., tandem walking), and (4) utilization of standardized measurement tools. Standardized measurement tools for considera-

tion are discussed below. Go to www.rehabmeasures.org for more information about each tool. Many of them are copyright free and available on the website.

Berg Balance Scale: A 14-item tool that measures balance in older adults and subsequently categorizes the individual into low, medium, or high fall risk.

Functional Gait Assessment: A 10-item tool that measures postural stability during various walking tasks.

Dynamic Gait Index: An eight-item tool that measures the person's ability to modify balance while walking in the presence of external demands.

Four Step Square Test: A simple four step square design placed on the ground to test dynamic balance by testing the ability to step over objects forward, sideways, and backwards.

Activities-Specific Balance Confidence Scale: A 16-item self-report measure in which clients rate their balance confidence in performing various ambulatory activities without falling or experiencing a sense of unsteadiness.

Functional Reach Test: A simple task that measures the maximum distance a client can reach while standing in a fixed position.

Community Balance and Mobility Scale: The client is asked to perform a total of 13 tasks that are commonly encountered in community environments to detect high-level balance and mobility deficits.

Tinetti Performance Oriented Mobility Assessment: A 16-item tool used to screen older adults for gait and balance impairments and subsequently categorize the individual into low, medium, or high falls risk.

Dizziness Handicap Inventory: A 25-item tool designed to evaluate the self-perceived handicapping effects imposed by dizziness.

Motion Sensitivity Quotient Test: A 16-item tool that requires quick changes to head or body positions to measure motion-provoked dizziness.

Mini Balance Evaluation Systems Test: A 14-item tool that measures six different balance control systems so that specific rehabilitation approaches can be designed for different balance deficits.

The Vestibular Activities and Participation Measure: A 34-item self-report questionnaire to assess the extent of activity limitations and participation restrictions created by vestibular disorders (based on the ICF).

Romberg Test: Assesses static standing balance by asking the client to stand on a hard floor surface without shoes, feet together, eyes closed, with arms at his/her sides. If the client is unable to hold the posture, it is considered a positive Romberg test and the amount of time the client is able to hold this position is recorded. Observation times are usually about 30 seconds.

ICF Components

The recreational therapist should record observations about the client with the appropriate ICF codes. The Body Functions code usually associated with balance concerns is b755 Involuntary Movement Reaction Functions. There may also be aspects that contribute to balance problems, such as b156 Perceptual Functions (especially b1561 Visual Perception), b160 Thought Functions, b210 Seeing Functions, b235 Vestibular Functions, b715 Stability of Joint Functions, b730 Muscle Power Functions, b735 Muscle Tone Functions, b765 Involuntary Movement Functions, and b770 Gait Pattern Functions. In the Activities and Participation codes, the primary deficits will be recorded in aspects of d4 Mobility. Balance issues can also restrict the client from participating in many other activities. Some examples include d230 Carrying Out Daily Routine, d5 Self-Care, d6 Domestic Life, and d920 Recreation and Leisure. If the client says that balance problems are keeping him/her from a particular activity that s/he wants to pursue, the appropriate ICF code should be noted as part of the assessment. The ICF codes, as part of the results of the assessment process, should be used to decide which components and which techniques will be used in treatment.

Balance Training Components

Depending upon the underlying causes of the balance deficits, the therapist will determine if balance training should focus on remediation, compensation, or a combination of both. Typical components of balance training include (O'Sullivan & Schmitz, 2007, p 498):

- Static postural control, biomechanical alignment, and symmetrical weight distribution.

- Dynamic postural control including musculoskeletal responses necessary for movement and balance.
- Adaptation of balance skills for varying tasks and environmental conditions.
- Sensory function including sensory integration and sensory compensation.
- Safety awareness and compensatory strategies for effective fall prevention.

Balance Training Techniques

The type of facility that the recreational therapist is working in and the make-up of its team members, will determine the responsibilities for working on specific interventions related to improving balance. When clients are medically cleared to participate in activities, ensure that the activities offered have a variety of movements helping maintain or improve posture and stability. Activities utilized in balance training must also be important and meaningful to the client to maximize skill transfer, foster motivation for engagement, and contribute to functional abilities in the specific task, all contributing to quality of life. Utilizing the specific activities desired by the client will also allow for the opportunity to identify and address activity-specific needs and concerns that have the potential to influence success in activity engagement. The types of movements the therapist will want to include are (Rose, 2003):

- Moving from different positions back to good standing posture. (Also, practice this with eyes closed.) For clients with significant limitations, lateral weight shifts in different directions may be a good place to begin. For clients with greater skill, leaning over and reaching for something on the ground and then returning to a good postural position may be appropriate.
- Moving from different positions (forward to backward and diagonal forward to backward) to reach a balanced seated position. (Also, practice this with eyes closed.)
- Maintaining balance while slowly raising each arm over the head, one at a time and together. If possible, the arm should be relatively straight and the elbow should be above the client's ear. Not only does this movement help with range of motion and stability, but it also helps expand the lungs and increases lung capacity.

- Moving the arms in an "airplane" movement. In an airplane movement the arms are stretched horizontally out to the client's side with palms down. As one arm is raised the other one drops as if the two arms together make up the wings of an airplane. (Also, practice this with eyes closed.)
- Turning the head and shoulders in a slow, lateral trunk rotation while the hips remain in the same place. This is the movement made when you look behind you as you are driving to see if anything is in the way of your backing up.
- Alternatively lifting one foot off the ground, then the other while standing and while seated. The therapist must ensure that the client is safe during these activities, spotting the client and ready to stop any fall. An intermediate step may be just lifting either the heel or the toe off the ground while leaving part of the foot still on the ground. For clients with less stability, seated "marches" or single leg raises may be appropriate.

Except for the first exercise, all of the exercises can be done in a sitting or standing position. The sitting position may be on a stool, but it is often better to use a balance ball. Balance balls are rubber balls of various sizes that are strong enough for clients to sit on for balance training. The therapist must use the right size ball for the client. The size of ball used is based on the client's standing height. Rose (2003, p. 95) provides the following rule of thumb for selecting ball sizes based on the height of the client.

Below 5' 5"	45 cm ball
5' 5" to 5' 8"	55 cm ball
5' 9" to 6' 3"	65 cm ball
6' 4" to 6' 9"	75 cm ball
6' 10" and taller	85 cm ball

During balance training, activities are chosen based on impaired systems and specific activities that are challenging for the client (e.g., engaging in postures such as bending or tandem walking, quickly scanning for items in a store). The activities are then gradually made more difficult by controlling the conditions in which the activities are performed, including the type of surface (smooth, uneven, tile, carpet, grass, cobble stones), types of items (size, weight), body position (sitting, standing, squatting, bending), balance range challenges (min, mod, max ranges), level of physical support provided by the therapist (max, mod, min support), type of support devices utilized (ambulation device, object in the environment), and complexity of tasks. A possible range of task difficulties looks like this: standing and holding an item, standing and placing an item at different heights, walking in challenging environments such as dimly lit or crowded areas, walking and carrying an item, walking and carrying an item while transitioning from one flooring surface to another, walking and carrying an item while paying attention to external stimuli such as a conversation, walking and carrying an item while overcoming environmental challenges, walking and carrying an item while overcoming environmental challenges and scanning store shelves for particular items — requiring head movements.

Engaging the client in general exercise programs can also be helpful to enhance strength, endurance, and flexibility. Therapists might also use standardized equipment to challenge balance further during activities such as the use of a rocker board, foam rolls, or bubble domes. When working on balance, therapists need to additionally consider the impact of medical issues (e.g., low blood pressure, medication), cognitive impairments, and psychological-emotional issues (e.g., balance confidence, self-efficacy, learned helplessness) and alter interventions accordingly.

Strategies for controlling balance (which are also practiced as part of balance training) include (Rose, 2010; Gillen, 2011; DeLisa, 2005):

Corrective Responses

Ankle strategy/response: The upper and lower body move in the same direction (as a single entity) while the individual rocks on his/her ankle joint to maintain balance. The muscles surrounding the ankle joint are small, therefore this strategy is used when standing upright or swaying ever so slightly (a minimal challenge, e.g., recovering from a small push or nudge, small sways while waiting in line at a store). This strategy can be challenging if there is limited ankle range of motion or strength, an unstable flooring surface with a surface that isn't firm or broad, and/or impaired sensation in the feet.

Hip strategy/response: The upper and lower body move in different directions while the individual activates the large hip muscles (e.g., leaning forward or sideways) to more quickly restore the center of mass. The hip muscles are stronger than the ankle muscles and are therefore better able to recover balance when postural alignment is moderately challenged (e.g., a large push, standing on a small beam). This strategy can be challenging if there is limited hip range of motion or strength.

Stiffening strategy/response: Contraction of all muscles in the ankle, knee, and hip joints, as well as the muscles of the back and neck. This type of response is commonly evoked with a vibration challenge.

Counterbalance strategy/response: Movement of the arm in front of the body to minimize the center of gravity shift from the center to the limits of the stability.

Protective Responses

Step strategy/response: When the center of mass is displaced beyond a person's limit of stability or the speed of sway is so fast that the hip strategy is ineffective, the person needs to establish a new base of support by stepping one or more steps in the direction of the loss of balance. This strategy can be challenging if there is inadequate lower body range of motion, strength, or power. Slowed central processing speed may also impact the person's ability to quickly initiate the steps.

Grabbing external support response: Reaching for and grabbing an external support such as a railing, pole, piece of furniture, etc.

Rescue response with support by outstretched arm to minimize impact of fall and break the fall: Putting arms out in front of the body to help decrease the impact or extent of a fall. For example, landing on hands or forearms prevents the head from hitting the ground.

Outcomes and Documentation

Recreational therapists document the specific balance impairments observed along with related criteria. The information reported includes time, support, device, assistance, position, balance range, surface, strategies utilized, type and amount of cueing, and characteristics of items such as size and weight. Examples of documented baselines include:

- Engages in dynamic standing balance in mod ranges with minimum assistance.
- Able to maintain unsupported static sitting balance for 10 minutes.

- Employs hip strategy to maintain balance with minimal verbal cues.
- Ambulates approximately 120 feet on outdoor uneven surfaces with a single point cane with contact guard secondary to occasional episodes of loss of balance.
- Reports experiencing vertigo two times during 10-minute visual scanning activity.

If the therapist used a standardized assessment tool during the initial assessment, the tool is re-administered to assess changes. Changes in ICF codes noted during the assessment process should also be documented.

Resources

Go4Life from the National Institute on Aging
http://go4life.nia.nih.gov
An exercise and physical activity campaign that provides a variety of resources (e.g., booklets, videos, tip sheets).

Preventing Falls: How to develop a community-based fall prevention programs for older adults.
www.cdc.gov/homeandrecreationalsafety/images/cdc_guide-a.pdf
A free 100-page resource book developed by the National Center for Injury Prevention and Control.

Rehabilitation Measures Database
www.rehabmeasures.org
An online database with rehabilitation measures and other measurement-related information including webinars.

Fallproof! A comprehensive balance and mobility training program.
The book contains an excellent set of exercise protocols that can be used by a recreational therapist (Rose, 2010).

Workout to Go
www.nia.nih.gov/sites/default/files/workout_to_go.pdf
A free 24-page exercise booklet for older adults developed by the National Institute on Aging at the National Institutes of Health. It contains strengthening, balance, and flexibility exercises.

References

DeLisa, J. A. (2005). *Physical medicine and rehabilitation: Principles and practice* (4th ed.). Philadelphia PA: Lippincott Williams & Wilkins.

Finlayson, M. (2013). *Multiple sclerosis: From impairment to participation*. New York, NY: CRC Press.

Gillen, G. (2011). *Stroke rehabilitation: A function-based approach*. St. Louis, Missouri: Elsevier.

Miller, W. C. & Deathe, A. B. (2011). The influence of balance confidence on social activity after discharge from prosthetic rehabilitation for first lower limb amputation. *Prosthetics and Orthotics International, 35*(4), 379-385.

O'Sullivan, S. B. & Schmitz, T. J. (2007). *Physical rehabilitation* (5th ed.). Philadelphia, PA: F. A. Davis Company.

Rogers, M. E. (2012). Balance and falls preventions. Retrieved from www.acsm.org/access-public-information/articles/2012/01/10/balance-and-fall-prevention.

Rose, D. (2003). *Fallproof!: A comprehensive balance and mobility training program*. Champaign, IL: Human Kinetics.

Rose, D. (2010). *Fallproof!: A comprehensive balance and mobility training program*. Champaign, IL: Human Kinetics.

19. Behavior Strategies and Interventions

Kari Kensinger

Behavior can be defined as any action or reaction that is observable and measurable. When a person's behavior is harmful or disruptive to his/her self, peers, or the community, that behavior might need to be changed, altered, or prevented. Traditionally concepts such as behavior modification and behavior management have been used by professionals in education, healthcare, and human services. More recently the concepts of functional behavioral assessment and applied behavioral analysis have gained in popularity. All of these concepts use similar strategies and interventions based on behavioral principles; therefore this chapter will broadly refer to behavioral strategies and interventions.

Recreational therapists can use behavioral strategies and interventions in almost any setting and with almost any diagnostic group since the clientele seen by recreational therapists exhibit a myriad of behaviors. For example:

- A nursing home resident with dementia may wander when bored.
- A client with a spinal cord injury in a rehabilitation hospital may abuse alcohol when depressed.
- A child with autism in a school setting might become physically aggressive when frustrated.
- A client with depression in a behavioral health setting might eat too much when under stress.
- An adolescent in a correctional facility might steal for attention.

In each of these scenarios, behavioral techniques can be utilized at any point along the continuum of care, including assessment, treatment, education, and participation. During assessment the therapist observes the frequency, intensity, and duration of behaviors across time, people, and environment. Baseline data can be collected and effective techniques can be identified. Preferred activities can be identified and later used as reinforcers. During treatment, positive reinforcement, negative reinforcement, or punishment can be used to change or alter behavior. During education, prompts, cues, and reinforcement schedules can be used to help teach new skills or behaviors. During participation, generalization can occur or the environment can be altered or modified.

In order for behavioral strategies and interventions to be successful in the practice of recreational therapy, the recreational therapist must understand the principles of behaviorism. Behaviorism is one paradigm that can be used to explain human behaviors. There are many ways to conceptualize behaviors.

The *biological viewpoint* looks at the actions of clients by evaluating physiological changes occurring in the body as the antecedents and the consequences. People who use the biological viewpoint may examine pharmacological or surgical means of altering behaviors. Recreational therapists do not prescribe medications; therefore recreational therapists would not be associated with the antecedents of biological actions. Recreational therapists may, however, see the consequences from the pharmacological methods and, therefore, should have knowledge of pharmaceuticals to be able to communicate with other healthcare providers.

Other therapists may believe in a *psychoanalytic approach* to behavior. This approach looks first at the consequences and the behaviors and then seeks to explore causes in the subconscious. As recreational therapists, we might see coping mechanisms and behaviors that can be attributed to the subconscious, but recreational therapists are not trained at analyzing or altering the subconscious.

A *humanistic approach* to understanding behaviors involves a client analyzing his/her own behavior while a therapist asks the client processing questions and offers the client resources for personal growth and development. An example might be if a student asks a professor a question and the professor responds, "What do you think the answer is?" This approach is commonly used by recreational therapists in behavioral health settings when teaching anger management or coping skills.

The *cognitive-behavioral approach* involves looking at how thoughts cause behaviors and how feelings are the reactions to behaviors. Some recreational therapists who use this approach believe that we cannot change our feelings but can change our thoughts and our behaviors. Recreational therapists might help clients recognize and be aware of feelings via some emotional intelligence activities, but would predominantly address changing thoughts to subsequently change behaviors. See the Cognitive Behavioral Counseling chapter for more information.

The final approach to looking at behaviors is called the *behavioral approach*, which is considered to be a temporal approach, meaning there are a beginning, middle, and end (Havens, 1987). The behavioral approach is based on the belief that behaviors are learned and therefore can be altered, shaped, or enforced. Almost every group of clients a recreational therapist works with exhibits behaviors and, if a recreational therapist is called to alter, shape, or enforce behaviors during education, treatment, or participation, the approaches that are based on behaviorism might be helpful. Therefore, this chapter will focus on the principles of behaviorism.

The basic premise behind behaviorism is that for every behavior there is an antecedent and consequence. An antecedent, which is often called a trigger, is the condition that occurs before a behavior is exhibited. Some examples of common antecedents for negative behaviors include task difficulty, boredom, time of day, social interaction, negative consequence, weather, illness, sensory overload, hunger, and noise. The therapist can help control these antecedents by altering environmental concerns (e.g., time of day, room temperature, distraction) or therapist behavior (e.g., commands, directions, attitude, and rules).

The term consequence is used to describe the outcome of the behavior. Consequences can be positive or negative (e.g., attention or avoidance; reward or punishment). Collectively, the antecedent,

behavior, and consequence determine the function of the behavior. Some functions of behavior might be to obtain attention, obtain sensory stimulation, obtain an object or a desired activity, escape a demand or request, escape an activity, or escape a social interaction.

Using a behavioral approach in recreational therapy practice involves manipulating the antecedent or consequence in order to bring about the desired behaviors of clients.

The theories of classical conditioning (Pavlov, 1927) and operant conditioning (Thorndike, 1901; Skinner, n.d.) illustrate some of the ways a therapist can shape a client's behavior. At the foundation of both forms of conditioning are the phenomena of stimulus and response. In classical conditioning the client will associate negative or positive feelings with a given experience. The stimulus in classical conditioning is the experience. The response in classical conditioning is the feeling that results from the client's behavior. Some examples in recreational therapy might be swimming eliciting feelings of joy, relaxation from listening to music, or frustration from knitting.

According to Pavlov, there is evidence that therapists can manipulate an experience to bring about positive or negative results. This is why techniques such as aversion therapy and systematic desensitization work.

Similarly, operant conditioning involves the utilization of both a stimulus and a response. In operant conditioning, the therapist can influence the stimulus and response via the use of positive or negative reinforcement. According to Dattilo and Murphy (1987) "positive reinforcement is the presentation or delivery of a consequence that makes a behavior occur more often in the future" (p. 11). They define "negative reinforcement" as the process that "increases the strength of the behavior by removing or postponing an aversive antecedent contingent on the occurrence of the behavior" (p. 63). Anything can be a reinforcer, but some of the most common types of reinforcement include food, toys, favorite activities, money, hugs, praise, and recognition. In order for a reinforcement to be effective, the method and intensity of the reinforcers should be varied. If the same reinforcer is used all of the time, a client can get bored and the unique properties of that reinforcer diminish. The frequency of reinforcement also should vary according to the situation. It is recommended that continuous reinforcement, providing a reinforcer each time a behavior is exhibited, be used when teaching a new skill. Intermittent reinforcement, providing reinforcement occasionally when a behavior is demonstrated, is most typically used to maintain a behavior.

Indications

According to Schloss and Smith (1998) behavioral strategies and interventions associated with the principles of behaviorism can help people: pay attention, volunteer responses, and make and keep friends. They also suggest that that these principles can help decrease or eliminate behaviors such as swearing, fighting, and destroying property. Clients who have these issues are prime candidates for behavioral strategies.

Weiss (1990) suggests asking the following questions to determine whether a behavior should be changed.

- Is the individual's behavior currently or potentially dangerous?
- Does behavior interfere with the individual's ability to learn essential skills?
- Does the behavior limit the individual's ability to participate in other activities?
- Does the behavior limit integration into the community?
- As a result of this behavior, is the individual more dependent on other people?
- Is medication or another restrictive measure necessary to manage the behavior?
- Do other people agree that this behavior should be changed?

Chandler and Dahlquist (2002) similarly suggest asking the following questions:

- Does this behavior interfere with the individual's learning?
- Does this behavior interfere with other's learning?
- Does the behavior interfere with or impede social relationships?
- Does the behavior have a negative impact on self-esteem?
- Is the behavior harmful or dangerous to the individual?

- Is the behavior harmful or dangerous to other individuals?
- Does the behavior occur frequently or infrequently?
- Is the behavior age-appropriate?

The ICF does not have a code that states behavioral strategies are required. The therapist needs to look at codes that have been cited and ask the questions discussed in this section to decide if the code is a candidate for behavioral strategies. There are some codes which clearly outline behaviors that can be modified with these strategies, such as d710 Basic Interpersonal Interactions. Deficits in other codes, such as b140 Attention Functions, b152 Emotional Functions, b455 Exercise Tolerance Functions, d1 Learning and Applying Knowledge, d2 General Tasks and Demands, d5 Self-Care, d7 Interpersonal Interactions and Relationships, and d8 Major Life Areas may be improved with behavioral strategies depending on the underlying cause of the deficit. The general rule is that deficits can be treated with behavioral strategies when they are caused by client behaviors that can be changed.

Contraindications

According to Schloss and Smith (1998) the reputation of "behavior modification" has been tarnished by misuse and misunderstanding. They report that there have been incident reports where individuals "have been at risk for or have actually experienced neglect or injury as the result" of misuse of a specific strategy such as time out (p. 1). According to Schloss and Smith some common problems that can arise when using behavioral strategies include:

- Inconsistent uses across therapists, teachers, and family members.
- Behavioral change that can be seen as a violation of an individual's "free will."
- Abuse and neglect if practitioners do not adequately assess client needs, assess risks, and monitor progress.
- Behavior changes for the practitioner's convenience, not in the person's best interest.
- Concerns about cultural insensitivity caused by the language used in behavioral literature such as "control, reinforcement, and punishment … [which is] seen as coercive and controlling"

(Axelrod, 1992, p. 31, as cited by Schloss & Smith, 1998).

- Lack of generalization because there is improper planning and follow-through maintenance.

Protocols

As with any recreational therapy program, the assessment, planning, implementation, and evaluation (APIE) process should be followed. Applied Behavioral Analysis (ABA) is the systematic use of the principles of behaviorism and therefore utilizes similar processes. At the heart of ABA is systematic data collection. Functional Behavioral Assessment and Behavior Intervention Plans are two terms identified in the Individuals with Disabilities Education Act. While these concepts are designed to be used with school-aged children, similar concepts are discussed throughout the literature in the field of recreational therapy and are applicable to other settings. Consequently, the Functional Behavioral Assessment and Behavior Intervention Plan will be discussed in this chapter. Behavioral interventions are often researched using single-subject design. Progress and effectiveness of the interventions are determined from base-line data. Thus assessment is the foundation of both recreational therapy (Stumbo & Peterson, 2006; Austin, 2009) and applied behavioral analysis (Schloss & Smith, 1998; Chandler & Dahlquist, 2002; Zirpoli, 2008).

Assessment

According to Reed and Azulay (2011), "functional behavioral assessment is a system of data collection of the environmental events both preceding and following a target behavior in an effort to understand the communicative intent" (p. 13). They suggest three approaches: indirect assessment, direct observation, and functional analysis.

Indirect assessment is used to gather background information about the client. This information does not come from direct face-to-face contact or observation with the client but rather relies on second-hand information. Some common methods of indirect assessment include record reviews or behavioral interviews with caregivers.

Direct observation is also referred to as behavioral observation and is the most common form of assessment utilized for gathering and monitoring behaviors. Tarbox, Najdowski, and Lanagan (2011)

describe the following steps associated with behavioral observation and assessment.

- Define a target behavior.
- Choose a method of measurement.
- Collect baseline data.
- Collect treatment data.
- Make data-based decisions.
- Consider collecting inter-observer agreement (IOA) data where multiple therapists or staff members collect the same data.

The method of measurement can be one or more of the following techniques

Frequency: The number of times a behavior occurs.

Rate: The number of times a behavior occurs divided by the amount of time the client is observed.

Duration: The amount of time a behavior occurs.

Latency: The length of time it takes a client to respond to a command. For example if the recreational therapist asks a client to "sit at the table," it may take five minutes before the client actually sits.

Percent correct: Looks at the number of behaviors performed correctly divided by the number of attempts.

The amount of sampling is usually one of these three possibilities.

Partial-interval: Looks at five minutes of a 20-minute session to see what behaviors occur.

Whole-interval: Examines behaviors for the full 20 minutes that a session occurs.

Momentary time sampling: Looks at behavior at a particular time. It might be quite often or less frequently, such as one time per week.

According to Chandler and Dahlquist (2002) functional assessments provide answers to the question, "Why does challenging behavior occur?" without falsely blaming the behavior on the "student, other individuals, or family and home situations" (p. 24). They suggest that functional assessments are based on four assumptions (Chandler & Dahlquist, 2002, p 25):

- Challenging behavior and appropriate behavior are supported by the current environment.
- Behavior serves a function.
- Challenging behavior can be changed using positive interventions that address the function of the behavior.

- Functional assessment should be a team-based process.

Other forms of assessment that can be used for behavioral techniques are stimulus preference assessments that assess client-preferred activities and items that can be used for reinforcement (Tiger & Kliebert, 2011), intervention integrity assessments that assess how well an intervention is being implemented (DiGennaro Reed, & Codding, 2011), skills assessments that determine the extent to which a client can perform a skill (Rue, 2011), and outcome assessments that determine if a client meets his or her goals (Wilczynski, 2011). burlingame and Blaschko (2010) provide examples of how all of these assessments are used in the field of recreational therapy.

Once the therapists, family members, and others who have contact with the client identify the antecedents, behavior, consequence, and function of challenging behaviors, a Behavior Intervention Plan is developed. This plan identifies two types of intervention strategies based on either the antecedent and setting or the consequence. Behavioral Intervention Plans are individualized and are different according to setting and client needs. Some specific techniques that can be part of this plan can found in the Processes section of this chapter.

Processes

Several techniques and strategies, including the use of positive behavioral support, can be used by a recreational therapist before, during, and after a behavior occurs to alter an individual's behavior. The term positive behavioral support (sometimes referred to as an antecedent approach) is used to describe the "use of positive reinforcement strategies as the principal method of changing behaviors" (Zirpoli, 2008, p. 303). Examples of such techniques and strategies that a recreational therapist might utilize in a behavior plan are provided below.

Strategies to be Used before an Activity

Strategies that can be used before an activity start with assessing the client ahead of time to make sure activities will be appropriate for the client's skill level. The recreational therapist should also establish rules and routines prior to starting any program. The rules include establishing physical boundaries and defining expectations about appropriate client behavior.

The therapist may want to establish a system-wide behavioral plan, which may include token economies — reinforcement schedules for an entire community. In a token economy all clients in the program might receive a sticker for helping others, sharing, and/or taking turns. There should also be systematic policies and procedures for de-escalation, punishment, suspension, and expulsion. For example, all corrective action must require a verbal warning or written warning, prior to suspension. If a client has been suspended three times, they might be expelled.

Before the activity the recreational therapist should educate clients about the system policies and procedures. It is often a good idea to have clients and perhaps caregivers sign behavioral contracts prior to participation to indicate that they understand the expectations.

Strategies to be Used during the Activity

Activities should be kept as simple or complex as is appropriate for the therapy objectives. Some ideas for keeping activities simple include hiding supplies that could become distracting, tempting, or misused; keeping clients busy by having a plan, a schedule, and back-up activities; and minimizing noise and distractions.

During an activity, recreational therapists can use a variety of behavioral strategies to alter or manage a client's behavior. These strategies can be classified as teaching strategies or facilitation strategies. Teaching strategies are used to teach new skills or behaviors, while facilitation strategies help manage behaviors. Some teaching strategies are described below.

Discrete trials: A systematic way of introducing new knowledge and skills to a client. In this process, the therapist uses a stimulus or a specific phrase such as "Do this." and then demonstrates an action that the therapist would like the client to replicate. In the beginning of this process the therapist gives the client reinforcement for every correct response. After the client masters the first skill, a second skill is introduced in the same way. Once the client understands two skills, the therapist will alternate between the two skills in order to make sure the client understands the skill instead of merely the command.

Shaping: A technique often used in the discrete trial format when a client might not be able to master a skill. In this case, a task analysis is performed and the client is rewarded using a reinforcement schedule until s/he masters each task or skill. For example, if the skill the therapist is teaching is dribbling and the client holds the ball, any time the client bounces the ball s/he may be rewarded.

Chaining: A technique often used to teach a concept. In chaining each step is identified and the client is asked to complete the first step before advancing to the second step. After each step is completed, the client is rewarded until mastery occurs.

Reverse chaining: Used when the therapist teaches the last step first. For example, when teaching a client how to do a nine-piece puzzle, the therapist may start by leaving eight pieces assembled. The therapist would then ask the client to "do puzzle" and reward the client with a reinforcer each time the client completes the puzzle correctly. After the client demonstrates mastery with that step, the therapist would remove two puzzle pieces. This process would continue until the client can successfully do a nine-piece puzzle at a level that fulfills the goal independently.

The ultimate goal of teaching behaviors is that the behavior will be generalized across different settings and with different people and that the behavior would be maintained after the client leaves the training program. In order to enhance generalization, there needs to be consistency of the behavioral strategies and expectations among therapists, teachers, and parents in different settings such as hospital, school, home, and community. An activity is likely to be maintained if the client sees benefits to the behavior after the therapist instructs the client in the appropriate behavior. Therefore, intermittent or occasional reinforcement is recommended.

Prompting and cueing are two terms used to describe the methods that a therapist can use to offer assistance and guidance to clients. According to Zirpoli (2008) the word cueing is used to describe verbal guidance. Prompts describe physical guidance. Zirpoli also suggests that prompting is the more global concept and can be used to describe both forms of guidance or, in other words, actions performed by the therapist to help clients understand a command. There are several methods of prompting which include:

- *Verbal prompts*: More specific verbal commands.
- *Gestural prompts*: Pointing to what needs to be done.

- *Modeling prompts*: The therapist demonstrates what the client needs to do.
- *Physical prompts*: Hand-over-hand assistance whereby the therapist physically helps the client perform the task.

When prompting, the therapist will want to utilize the least restrictive method. Therefore, the therapist starts with verbal prompts and progressively goes to more direct methods if the client needs more assistance. As the client becomes independent, the prompts should be faded so the client can perform the task as independently as possible.

Once the client has learned what is expected of him/her and how to meet those expectations, the therapist can use facilitation techniques to create an environment that can help the client succeed. The following techniques might be helpful:

Catch clients behaving positively. By recognizing the good the clients do, attention-seeking clients will receive more attention from behaving instead of misbehaving.

Enforce rules consistently. Therapists need to enforce rules among all clients fairly so that expectations are clear.

Pick your battles. Determine what behaviors really need to be altered and focus on one at a time. If a client swears and hits others, focus on the behavior that is inflicting the most harm (in this case, hitting).

Follow through with consequences. If a therapist says s/he is going to put a client in time-out, remove a barrier, or use a recovery room, the therapist must follow through or the client will push the boundaries.

Model behaviors. Therapists should model the behaviors they expect of the clients.

Interrupt the behavior chain. Therapists should monitor the activities of their clients and be physically present to stop behaviors that might be developing (called proximity control).

Use punishment as a last resort. Therapists need to be familiar with principles of de-escalation, time-out, restraints, and recovery. De-escalation is a preventative measure used to prevent more serious behavioral consequences. Time out, restraints, and recovery can all be part of the punishment process. Punishment is dangerous in that it can lead to physical, psychological, and emotional abuse. It can be avoided if the therapist is familiar with sound behavioral strategies.

Zirpoli (2008) uses the term behavior reduction strategies "to identify procedures that, when implemented immediately after a target behavior, reduce the future probability of the target behavior recurring" (p 381). There are many ways that a therapist can react to behaviors. For positive behaviors these include:

Positive reinforcement: Providing a satisfying consequence.

Negative reinforcement: Removal or avoidance of a consequence which a client dislikes.

Differential reinforcement: Using alternative consequences for participating in activities that are incompatible with the challenging behavior, are an alternative to a challenging behavior, cause the challenging behaviors to occur at a lower-rate, or lead to omission of challenging behavior.

For targeted negative behaviors, the therapist may use these strategies:

Punishment: Decreasing behavior through an unpleasant consequence.

Extinction: Withholding reinforcement for a behavior. This might also be considered as ignoring a behavior.

Response cost: Involves taking away a reinforcer.

Time-out: Removing individuals from a reinforcing environment. Prior to utilizing time-out, consider the potential side effect of neglect that may occur and what material the client might be missing out on. According to Lavay, French, and Henderson (2006), there are four types of time-out:

- *Observational*: The client watches but does not participate.
- *Exclusion*: The client is removed from the environment where s/he cannot see the activity.
- *Seclusion*: The client leaves the setting of the activity.
- *Self time-out*: The client removes himself/herself from the activity to cool-off.

Verbal reprimands: The therapist talks to the client about his/her inappropriate behavior and why it is inappropriate.

Corporal punishment: This involves "using physical force with the intention of causing pain, but not injury, for the purpose of correction or behavior control" (Lavay, French, & Henderson, 2006, p 102.). Corporal punishment is illegal in several states and is considered physical abuse. Therapists should avoid using this practice.

Physical restraint: Physical restraint, such as a small child restraint or team supine restraint, might be used to stop a violent individual from hurting himself/herself or others. Since this technique involves a therapist physically interacting with a client, it too is regulated and may be illegal in many states. Therapists who use this technique should be trained to do so by their employer. Information on common restraint training programs can be found in the Resources section of this chapter. The programs train therapists and educators to use restraints as a last resort after other de-escalation principles have not worked.

Outcomes and Documentation

By using behavioral strategies before, during, and after a behavior, the therapist should be able to alter, change, and treat the challenging and problem behaviors exhibited by clients. Yet, unless there is documentation, a therapist cannot demonstrate the effectiveness of the strategies used. Behavioral strategies follow a systemic process where assessment, actions, and evaluation are documented consistently. The targeted behaviors identified by the therapist and each behavioral objective should be documented. Behavioral checklists such as those included in the Appendix are the most common form of documentation.

When using the ICF as a basis for making treatment decisions, the therapist scores the ICF codes selected for treatment using behavioral strategies. Improvements in the codes demonstrate the effectiveness of treatment. Looking at all the techniques that were used to treat each particular code suggests how much of the improvement is caused by each of the strategies.

Resources

Applied Behavioral Analysis International
http://ebpsig.org
Contains a special interest section related to evidence-based practice on Applied Behavioral Analysis and numerous articles supporting its practice.

The National Professional Development Center for Autism Spectrum Disorders
http://autismpdc.fpg.unc.edu/content/briefs

Identifies 24 evidence-based practices that can be used to identify behavior interventions that will work with this population.

American Therapeutic Recreation Association

Dementia Practice Guideline for Recreational Therapy: Treatment of Disturbing Behaviors by Buettner and Fitzsimmons (2003) outlines evidence-based practices that recreational therapy uses to reduce challenging behaviors of individuals with dementia.

Behavior Analyst Certification Board (BACB)

www.bacb.com/

The BACB offers certification in applied behavioral analysis. Recreational therapists who work in settings where behavioral goals are common may be interested in seeking this certification.

Physical Restraining Training Programs

Crisis Prevention Institute

www.crisisprevention.com/Resources/Knowledge-Base/Physical-Intervention-Training

SafeGuards

http://safeguards-training.net/TCI-SystemOverview.aspx

The Mandt System

www.mandtsystem.com/

Appendix: Sample Documentation Tracking Problem Behaviors

In the first column, the therapist identifies any problem behaviors exhibited by a client (e.g., wandering, verbal aggression, physical aggression). The therapist then uses the same unit of measurement that s/he used for the assessment. Data is collected each time the client is seen by the therapist. The number of occurrences or percentage of occurrences of the behavior is reported.

Client Goal: Joe will reduce negative self-talk during recreational therapy groups.

Baseline Summary: On average Joes makes 3 negative statements about himself during each therapy session. Therapist sees Joe 3x per day 5 days a week.

Objective 1: After 2 weeks, Joe will make less than 3 negative statements about self per day.

Interventions:

- Reinforcement (praise or edibles) for positive self-talk.
- Prompting after the first negative statement.
- Redirective statement affirming positive behavioral traits.

Client: Joe
Week of observation: Week 1
Behavior being measured: Negative Self-Talk

	Mon	Tues	Wed	Thu	Fri
Activity 1	6	6	8	2	4
Activity 2	2	3	3	3	3
Activity 3	4	3	2	1	0

References

Austin, D. R. (2009). *Therapeutic recreation: Processes and techniques* (6th ed.). Champaign, IL: Sagamore Publishing.

Axelrod, S. (1992). Disseminating an effective educational technology. *Journal of Applied Behavioral Analysis, 25*, 31-35.

Buettner, L. & Fitzsimmons, S. (2003). *Dementia practice guidelines for recreational therapy: Treatment of disturbing behaviors*. Alexandria, VA: American Therapeutic Recreational Association.

burlingame, j. & Blaschko, T. (2010*). Assessment tools for recreation therapy and related fields* (4th ed.). Ravensdale, WA: Idyll Arbor, Inc.

Chandler, L. K. & Dahlquist, C. M. (2002). *Functional assessment: Strategies to prevent and remediate challenging behaviors in school settings*. Upper Saddle River, NJ: Pearson.

Dattilo J. & Murphy W. (1987). *Behavior modification in therapeutic recreation*. State College, PA: Venture.

DiGennaro Reed, F. D. & Codding, R. S. (2011). Intervention integrity assessment. In J. K. Luiselli (Ed.) *Teaching and behavior support for children and adults with autism spectrum disorder: A practitioner's guide* (pp. 38-47). New York: Oxford University Press.

Havens, L. (1987). *Approaches to the mind: Movement of the psychiatric schools from sects toward science*. Cambridge, MA: Harvard University Press.

Lavay, B. W., French, R., & Henderson, H. L. (2006). *Positive behavior management in physical activity settings* (2nd ed.). Champaign, IL: Human Kinetics.

Luiselli, J. K. (2011). *Teaching and behavior support for children and adults with autism spectrum disorder: A practitioner's guide*. New York: Oxford University Press.

Pavlov, I. (1927). *Conditioned reflexes: An investigation of the physiological activity of the cerebral cortex*. Retrieved from http://psychclassics.yorku.ca/Pavlov/.

Reed, D. D. & Azulay, R. L. (2011). Functional behavioral assessment (FBA). In J. K. Luiselli (Ed.) *Teaching and behavior support for children and adults with autism spectrum disorder: A practitioner's guide* (pp. 13-21). New York: Oxford University Press.

Rue, H. C. (2011). Skills assessment. In J. K. Luiselli (Ed.) *Teaching and behavior support for children and adults with autism spectrum disorder: A practitioner's guide* (pp. 48-54). New York: Oxford University Press.

Schloss, P. & Smith, M. A. (1998). *Applied behavior analysis in the classroom* (2nd ed.). Needham Heights, MA: Allyn & Bacon.

Skinner, B. F. (n.d.). A brief survey of operant conditioning. Retrieved from www.bfskinner.org/brief_survey.html.

Stumbo, N. J., & Peterson, C. A. (2009). *Therapeutic recreation program design: Principles and procedures* (5th ed.). San Francisco: Pearson Benjamin Cummings.

Tarbox, J. L., Najdowski, A. C., & Lanagan, T. M. (2011). Behavioral observation and measurement. In J. K. Luiselli (Ed.) *Teaching and behavior support for children and adults with autism spectrum disorder: A practitioner's guide* (pp. 5-12). New York: Oxford University Press.

Thorndike, E. L. (1901). Animal intelligence: An experimental study of the associative processes in animals. *Psychological Review Monograph Supplement, 2*, 1-109.

Tiger, J. H. & Kliebert, M. L. (2011). Stimulus preference assessment. In J. K. Luiselli (Ed.) *Teaching and behavior support for children and adults with autism spectrum disorder: A practitioner's guide* (pp. 30-37). New York: Oxford University Press.

Weiss, N. (1990). Positive behavioral programs. In J. F. Gardner & M. S. Chapman (Eds.). *Programming issues in developmental disabilities*. Baltimore: Paul H. Brooks.

Wilczynski, S. M. (2011). Outcome assessment. In J. K. Luiselli (Ed.) *Teaching and behavior support for children and adults with autism spectrum disorder: A practitioner's guide* (pp. 5-12). New York: Oxford University Press.

Zirpoli, T. J. (2008). *Behavior management: Applications for teachers*. Upper Saddle River, NJ: Pearson.

20. Bibliotherapy

Erin K. Moore

Jack and Ronan (2008) and McCulliss (2012) describe the changing perception and use of the term bibliotherapy over time. Historically, bibliotherapy was an adjunctive therapy used by physicians working with the mental health population. In the 19th and early 20th centuries bibliotherapy referred to recommended literature (both fiction and non-fiction) and use of libraries in institutions. Although librarians continued to be involved in the field of bibliotherapy, by mid-20th century additional professionals such as psychologists, therapists, social workers, and educators had also begun to use bibliotherapy with different populations. As the practice of bibliotherapy expanded, additional terms were developed (Jack & Ronan, 2008; McCulliss, 2012; Moore & Coyle, 2007).

Clinical bibliotherapy refers to literature used for clients with emotional or behavioral problems for the purpose of meeting therapeutic goals. *Developmental bibliotherapy* refers to literature used to maintain well-being. It is also called self-help bibliotherapy. *Interactive bibliotherapy* refers to a technique in which a therapist facilitates a discussion or reflection following review of a written work.

The National Federation for Biblio/Poetry Therapy refers to bibliotherapy as "all forms of the interactive use of literature and/or writing to promote growth and healing," such as poetry therapy, journal therapy, bibliotherapy, biblio/poetry therapy, and poetry/journal therapy (National Foundation for Biblio/Poetry Therapy, 2013). The diversity within the field of bibliotherapy makes it a modality that can be utilized by recreational therapists in different settings to accomplish goals. This chapter will focus on three bibliotherapy interventions that can be utilized in practice: interactive bibliotherapy, self-help bibliotherapy, and writing.

Indications

Jack and Ronan (2008) identify divorce, alcohol or chemical dependency, abuse, fear, grief, anxiety, tension relief, and social-emotional skills as appropriate reasons for using bibliotherapy. Additionally, Hevey, Wilczkiewicz, and Horgan (2012) suggest that clients with Type D personality (negative affect and emotional suppression) might benefit from expressive writing interventions. Although bibliotherapy is most indicated for mental health populations, it can also be used with non-mental health populations for the reasons listed above. Indications for the specific types of bibliotherapy reviewed in this chapter are as follows:

Interactive bibliotherapy was noted to have positive research outcomes for clients with anxiety, depression, and schizophrenia (Santacruz, Méndez, & Sánchez-Meca, 2006; Shechtman & Nir-Shfrir, 2008; Moore & Coyle, 2007; Wang, 2007).

Self-help bibliotherapy research documents effectiveness with anxiety, depression, post-traumatic stress, headaches and migraines, drinking, insomnia, bulimia, and sexual dysfunction (Apodaca et al., 2007; Febbraro, 2005; Floyd et al., 2006; Jernelöv et al., 2012; Jones, 2002; McCulliss, 2012; Morgan & Jorm, 2008; Reeves, 2010).

Writing research identified effective outcomes for both physical illnesses (arthritis, asthma, irritable bowel syndrome, myocardial infarction, insomnia, and breast cancer) and mental health (Fair et al., 2012; Gillispie, 2003; Halpert, Rybin, & Doros, 2010; Hevey, Wilczkiewicz, and Horgan, 2012; Lowe, 2006; Mooney, Espie, & Broomfield, 2009; Moore & Coyle, 2007; Mosher et al., 2012; Pennebaker & Evans, 2014; Smyth, Hockemeyer, & Tulloch, 2008).

While recreational therapists often utilize a strength-based approach to treatment planning, there is limited exploration in the research as to whether or not bibliotherapy is indicated specifically for clients who have identified leisure interests in literature or creative outlets. Although Gillispie (2003) utilized this approach and reported positive outcomes in his single case study, there is limited generalizability.

ICF codes that suggest considering bibliotherapy include b126 Temperament and Personality Functions, b130 Energy and Drive Functions, b134 Sleep Functions, b140 Attention Functions, b152 Emotional Functions, b160 Thought Functions, b180 Experience of Self and Time Functions, b435 Immunological System Functions, d240 Handling Stress and Other Psychological Demands, d3 Communication, d570 Looking After One's Health, and d7 Interpersonal Interactions and Relationships. More details on the relationship between specific codes and types of bibliotherapy are presented in the Outcomes section.

Contraindications

Due to the extent of emotions that can be involved with bibliotherapy, this intervention is contraindicated for clients with post-traumatic stress disorder who are unable to demonstrate competence in coping skills. Bibliotherapy is also contraindicated for those who have limited literacy skills. Although Sagan (2007) did report on a case study in which creative writing was beneficial for one client with low literacy levels and chronic mental illness, improvements were noted after a three-year period of working with the client. While some recreational therapists may have the opportunity to develop interventions of similar length, bibliotherapy is not recommended for settings that are unable to facilitate this level of involvement with clients who have low literacy. Although bibliotherapy has been recommended for many different populations, recreational therapists should always consider individual client assessments when choosing types of bibliotherapy interventions to make sure they are appropriate.

Protocols

Since there are many styles of bibliotherapy interventions, there is not one specific protocol identified in evidence-based research. Further research comparisons are needed to evaluate frequencies and methodology for structuring sessions. Research does indicate that interventions occurring over multiple sessions have increased effectiveness, as evidenced by increased statistical significance and greater retention of outcomes at subsequent follow up. Recreational therapists interested in using bibliotherapy should consider becoming credentialed in its use (Chamberlain, Heaps, & Robert, 2008; Brewster, 2008; Fanner & Urquhart, 2008). Organizations that provide instruction and credentialing are listed in Resources.

Processes

Interactive Bibliotherapy

While suggested for use with groups, interactive bibliotherapy can be utilized for one-on-one sessions as well. Sessions are often 45 minutes to an hour in length. While each individual session is an independent intervention, research findings also demonstrate outcomes from multiple-session interventions. The process of interactive bibliotherapy originally described by Arleen McCarty Hynes and Mary Hynes-Berry consists of four stages: recognition, examination, juxtaposition, and application to self (McCulliss, 2012). A condensed process described by Kay Adams included only three stages: recognition, examination, and self-reflection (Moore & Coyle, 2007). Although the number of stages differs, the protocol for implementation is similar.

Interactive bibliotherapy begins by reading a written work (poetry, short story, literature, etc.). Usually this written work will be read once more to assist with clarity and reflection, often with the therapist or client reading it out loud. Following the initial introduction to the work, the therapist facilitates examining the content by asking questions such as, "What do you notice?" and asking if certain parts of the written work stand out. This interactive discussion is followed by questions such as "What can you relate to?" and "What did you learn?" These questions help facilitate a time of self-reflection and comparison of reactions among group members.

Selecting a work: Since interactive bibliotherapy begins with a written work, it is important for the therapist to carefully select an appropriate written work as a starting point, reviewing the entire work prior to utilizing it with clients. Considerations include topic, length, structure, and style. One form of bibliotherapy conducive to achieving healthcare goals is poetry therapy (Rojcewicz, 1999), but even this requires consideration of which poem. A decision about a poem involves a choice between different structural options (e.g., alphapoem, cinquain, free verse, haiku, renku, spoken word) and themes (e.g., anger management, leisure education, overcoming grief). Additional considerations include age-appropriateness, literacy level based on vocabulary and grammar, and cultural preferences

To assist with the selection process, recreational therapists should become familiar with available resources and utilize evidence-based practice to inform decision-making.

Facilitating self-reflection: Interactive bibliotherapy sometimes utilizes a task to facilitate additional self-reflection. Although most often writing is utilized (e.g., free writing, story writing, poetry), research also identified other creative tasks such as art (drawing and collages), music, movement, and different games to reinforce the message of the written work (Briggs & Pehrsson, 2008; Fair et al., 2012; Heath et al., 2011; Pennebaker & Evans, 2014; Santacruz et al., 2006). While it may be useful for all ages to have a task-based reflection component, it appears most indicated for children and adolescents.

Self-Help Bibliotherapy

The process of self-help bibliotherapy is usually initiated by a physician or therapist who recommends review of a written work (e.g., literature, non-fiction book, cognitive behavioral workbook) as a component of treatment. Typically it is utilized as an adjunct to group or individual psychotherapy sessions. The client is assigned a reading that is then processed in a discussion during subsequent sessions with the therapist. For example, a recreational therapist working with a client on leisure education might recommend a book on coping skills to expand the client's understanding of the role of leisure. While Morgan and Jorm (2008) identified two books (*Feeling Good* by Burns, 2008, and *Control Your Depression* by Lewinsohn, Munoz, Youngren, and Zeiss, 1978) with beneficial outcomes during clinical trials with depression, there is little evidenced-based research that evaluates the clinical effectiveness of specific literature. Instead, there are a variety of resources that recommend books for self-help bibliotherapy based upon the suggestions of practicing

clinicians including the Department of Veterans Affairs: Bibliotherapy Resource Guide, Bibliotherapy Education Project, and Books on Prescription. These programs are described in the Resources section.

The process of self-help bibliotherapy relies extensively on client participation in their treatment during unstructured time. To improve effectiveness, the recreational therapist should be able to identify components of independence and self-motivation at the time of client assessment. The time frame of this style of bibliotherapy is determined both by frequency of sessions with the therapist and by the length of assigned written work. Some research studies involved a four- to eight-week intervention independent of therapist involvement, but noted increased statistical outcomes when supportive telephone calls were offered for clients during those weeks (Febbraro, 2005; Jernelöv et al., 2012). This suggests that the recreational therapist can have an important role in the process of self-help bibliotherapy.

Writing

There are many styles of writing such as expressive writing, journaling, free writing, and creative writing. Expressive writing refers to disclosures about specific emotional experiences or traumas. Journaling refers to the written description of personal feelings or experiences. Free writing refers to a technique in which clients write for a specified time period without regard for grammar or spelling. Creative writing refers to the development of fiction and non-fiction writing, such as short stories, life stories, autobiographies, newsletters, poetry, playwriting, etc. Writing can also be utilized as a task during the reflection component of interactive bibliotherapy.

Facilitating writing: Writing can be utilized in interventions with individuals or groups, and usually consists of twenty minutes of writing followed by sharing and processing with the therapist. Although there are few evidence-based protocols, many research studies involved writing for three or more sessions over a time frame of several weeks. James Pennebaker in Pennebaker and Evans (2014) describes the methodology which produced the first experimental proof that expressive writing produced positive health results as four 20-minute sessions on four consecutive days. Writing can also be assigned as an intervention to be completed independently and later shared with the recreational therapist. For example, one recreational therapist provided a notebook and writing assignments to a client for several weeks in order to develop journaling as a coping skill (Gillispie, 2003).

Each writing session begins with the recreational therapist providing instructions appropriate to the selected writing style. For expressive writing, the therapist will direct the client to write about a traumatic emotional experience (e.g., reactions to diagnosis or illness) without regard to spelling and grammar. For clients who have not used writing before or who are looking to enhance creativity, starting points can be utilized to promote involvement in writing:

- Music or art as inspiration (e.g., song, still life, photo, picture).
- Pre-recorded poetry or written work as inspiration.
- Start phrase or word bank or quotes to be included.
- Fill-in-the blank poetry or story structure.
- Assigned task or topic (e.g., newsletter, autobiography, playwriting, or letter writing).

For collaborative group story writing or poetry, the therapist can utilize clipboards and white boards as resources and instruct each group member to provide one line at a time. This process might be utilized to support communication and concentration goals.

Sharing writing: The writing component of the session is often followed by a sharing component, especially in group therapy with clients who have mental health conditions. Sharing can consist of a time period in which participants read aloud what they have written. Sharing can also consist of a discussion that reflects on the completed writings or benefits of writing. For interventions completed independently, the therapist can organize poetry slams or open mic sessions to provide a sharing opportunity. Additional variations of sharing include publication of finished works in a facility newsletter or displaying them on a bulletin board. These variations can be utilized to support self-esteem and socialization outcomes. Some researchers utilized independently completed internet-based expressive writing interventions and still noted beneficial outcomes even without a sharing component (Penne-

baker & Evans, 2014). Some authors argue strongly that sharing may be inappropriate and that forcing a client to share should never be done. Therapy occurs because of the writing. Forcing a client to reveal what s/he has written has the effect of convincing the client to not write anything meaningful because forced sharing can be harmful emotionally and potentially in other ways (Pennebaker & Evans, 2014).

Outcomes and Documentation

One difficulty of evaluating evidence-based research on bibliotherapy is the diversity in the field of bibliotherapy itself. Bibliotherapy research not only incorporates different styles (e.g., interactive bibliotherapy, self-help bibliotherapy, and writing), but also different outcome measures and treatment designs that make it difficult to generalize results. While practitioners have been asserting the benefits of bibliotherapy for the last century, there is still a limited evidence base. Despite efforts in the profession to advocate for assessment and documentation of outcomes (McCarty Hynes, 1988), current research often involves case studies or qualitative investigations with limited systematic approaches or quantitative analyses. Documentation of outcomes varied, but often involved statistical analysis of pre-post test scales. None of the articles referred to ICF coding.

Interactive Bibliotherapy

Many research outcomes for interactive bibliotherapy were improvements on assessments of mental health symptomatology. Moore and Coyle (2007) reviewed research on implementation of poetry therapy interventions with behavioral health clients and identified several qualitative and quantitative outcomes: enhanced ratings of affect, acceptance, and creativity; increased social interaction and unity (b126 Temperament and Personality Functions, d7 Interpersonal Interactions and Relationships); increased communication and language expression (d3 Communication); improved concentration (b140 Attention Functions, b160 Thought Functions); and improved self-concept (b126 Temperament and Personality Functions, b180 Experience of Self and Time Functions). Additional research determined outcomes of:

- Greater affective exploration, less resistance, and decreased use of simple responses during bibliotherapy sessions for clients with anxiety and depression (b126 Temperament and Personality Functions, b130 Energy and Drive Functions) (Shechtman & Nir-Shfrir, 2008).

- Decrease in fearful behavior for children with darkness phobia following intervention (b126 Temperament and Personality Functions, b134 Sleep Functions) (Santacruz et al., 2006).

- Reduction in depression symptoms (according to the *Hamilton Depression Scale*), and improvement in problem solving (according to the *Coping Methods Inventory*) and social support (according to *Social Support Rating Scale*) for clients with depression (b126 Temperament and Personality Functions, d240 Handling Stress and Other Psychological Demands, d7 Interpersonal Interactions and Relationships) (Wang, 2011).

Self-Help Bibliotherapy

Although many research studies explored the plausibility of self-help bibliotherapy as a cost-effective treatment, current research outcomes appear to promote self-help bibliotherapy as a supplement to therapy rather than a replacement. Several research studies identify mental health benefits of self-help bibliotherapy, often via use of cognitive behavioral bibliotherapy interventions:

- Reduction on quantitative measures of anxiety, depression, stress, and panic attacks (b126 Temperament and Personality Functions, b152 Emotional Functions, d240 Handling Stress and Other Psychological Demands) (Febbraro, 2005; Floyd et al., 2006; Jones, 2002; Reeves, 2010).

- Improved measures of self-concept and internal locus of control with inmates in a correctional setting (b126 Temperament and Personality Functions, b180 Experience of Self and Time Functions, d940 Human Rights) (Kohutek, 1983).

- Qualitative outcomes of increased self-expression for children with short stature or diabetes using fiction stories (b126 Temperament and Personality Functions, d710 Basic Interpersonal Interactions) (Amer, 1999).

Other research studies alluded to the physical benefits of self-help bibliotherapy:

- Improvement in sleep onset latency for people with insomnia (b134 Sleep Functions) (Jernelöv et al., 2012).

- Decrease in harmful alcohol use and possible trending pattern of seeking further treatment (d570 Looking After One's Health) (Apodaca & Miller, 2003; Apodaca et al., 2007).

- Improved immune system function (increase in saliva antibodies that protect against infection) (b435 Immunological System Functions) following positive poetry intervention (Lowe, 2006).

While self-help bibliotherapy did produce positive outcomes following interventions for both physical and mental health, some research studies documented that outcomes were not maintained after extended follow up (Floyd et al., 2006; Kohutek, 1983). Further research could explore the possibilities of extending protocol time to include additional maintenance or increased therapeutic support.

Writing

Frisina, Borod, and Lepore (2004) suggest from their meta-analysis that expressive writing does improve health outcomes and indicate that it is more effective on physical rather than psychological health outcomes. However, this statement has limited generalizability as their meta-analysis only included nine research studies. Some research studies refer to the benefits of expressive writing on physical health:

- Improved physical wellness (as evidenced by decrease in health center visits and assessed stress levels) for healthy participants (d240 Handling Stress and Other Psychological Demands, d570 Looking After One's Health) (Lowe, 2006).

- Reduced symptoms (according to illness ratings scales) for people with arthritis, asthma, and irritable bowel syndrome (use ICF codes specific to the diagnoses, possibly including d570 Looking After One's Health) (Lowe, 2006; Halpert et al., 2010).

- Improvements on the *Health-Related Quality of Life* scale for people who had recently had a myocardial infarction (use ICF codes specific to the diagnoses, possibly including d570 Looking After One's Health) (Hevey et al., 2012).

- Decrease in pre-sleep cognitive arousal for people with insomnia (b134 Sleep Functions) (Mooney, Espie, & Broomfield, 2009).

Although a study of expressive writing for clients with cancer resulted in no statistically significant outcomes, the authors attributed the lack of results to poor adherence among participants and limitations of the research design (Bruera et al., 2008).

Additional research supports the benefits of writing on mental health outcomes, specifically on mood and self-esteem (b126 Temperament and Personality Functions, b152 Emotional Functions). In a case study of expressive writing with one client with anxiety, depression, and post-traumatic stress, Smyth and Helm (2003) note qualitative outcomes of: improved mood and sleep, decreased anxiety, improved coherence of written expression, and decreased physical symptoms. They also provide qualitative outcomes of increased optimism and ability to sustain a job at six-month follow-up. Further research identifies mental health benefits of:

- Qualitative increase in self-efficacy and self-esteem for adolescents utilizing the Writing for Resilience to Increase Self-Esteem (WRITE) program (b126 Temperament and Personality Functions) (Chandler, 1999).
- Qualitative outcomes of improved confidence (b1266 Confidence), communication skills (d3 Communication), improved self-expression and writing skills (d170 Writing), and increased support network (d7 Interpersonal Interactions and Relationships, e3 Support and Relationships) for adolescents perinatally infected with HIV (Fair et al., 2012).
- Quantitative outcomes of reduction in tension and anger (using the *Profile of Mood States* scale) and improvements in post-traumatic growth for people with post-traumatic stress (b152 Emotional Functions) (Smyth et al., 2008).
- Decrease in aggression according to qualitative teacher ratings for adolescents living in high-violence urban neighborhoods (b152 Emotional Functions, d240 Handling Stress and Other Psychological Demands) (Kliewer et al., 2011).
- Increased utilization of mental health services for breast cancer patients (d570 Looking After One's Health) (Mosher et al., 2012).

Limitations of Research

While research has identified different outcomes and goals of bibliotherapy, sometimes the question remains: What component makes bibliotherapy work? The evidence base of all three methods (interactive bibliotherapy, self-help bibliotherapy, and writing) has questionable validity due to research limitations and confounding variables. For example, group interactive bibliotherapy outcomes may be confounded by benefits derived merely from the structure of group therapy. Also, quantitative scales can provide documentation of the efficacy of self-help bibliotherapy, but research does not usually analyze the role of the literature in achieving outcomes by studying the increased knowledge related to the implementation of skills. Although writing may produce a decrease in stress outcome measures, it is difficult to identify whether these are attributed to self-expression or reorganization and reframing of emotional stories (Smyth & Helm, 2003). Preliminary work by Pennebaker suggests that the reorganization and reframing are the key elements (Pennebaker & Evans, 2014).

Deborah Dysart-Gale (2008) suggests that quantitative research and evidence-based medicine practices do not effectively evaluate bibliotherapy. She proposes that the practice of comparing large numbers of clients utilizing pre-post tests ignores some of the subjective responses and emotional engagement, as well as the fact that different readers may react differently to assigned texts. Dysart-Gale recommends additional qualitative research to analyze both specific texts and the reactions of clients.

Resources

Bibliotherapy Education Project
dev3.ehs.cmich.edu/index.php
EHS and the Kromer Instructional Materials Education Center
Central Michigan University
Mount Pleasant, Michigan, 48859
This online resource provides information on a variety of books for the recreational therapist to evaluate their potential for use in bibliotherapy interventions. There is an advanced search option, allowing the therapist to refine the search by age group, subject, etc. Reviews are submitted by practitioners, evaluated using the Bibliotherapy Evaluation Tool.

Books on Prescription (BOP)

www.booksonprescription.org.uk/

A program in Great Britain. The organization provides a list of books related to a variety of health conditions. Access to the literature is facilitated by select libraries. Physicians prescribe these books as self-help bibliotherapy treatment.

Center for Journal Therapy

www.journaltherapy.com

3798 Marshall St., Suite #5

Wheat Ridge, CO 80033

This organization provides resources, credentialing, and training in journal therapy.

Department of Veterans Affairs: Bibliotherapy Resource Guide

www.mirecc.va.gov/docs/VA_Bibliotherapy_Resource_Guide.pdf

Mental Illness Research

Education and Clinical Centers Office of Mental Health Services

VA Central Office

810 Vermont Avenue NW

Washington, DC 20420

This guide provides information about bibliotherapy resources that can serve as supplements to treatment. It categorizes resources according to different mental health diagnoses.

National Association for Poetry Therapy

www.poetrytherapy.org

256 McCaslin Blvd. #100

Louisville, CO 80027

This membership organization has information on educational opportunities and poetry resources. They have several publications available for purchase.

National Federation for Biblio/Poetry Therapy

www.nfbpt.com

1625 Mid Valley Dr. #1, Suite 126

Steamboat Springs, CO 80487

This organization provides information on credentialing requirements, the field of biblio/poetry therapy, and a list of resources. It offers three credentialing options: certified applied poetry facilitator (CAPF), certified poetry therapist (CPT), or registered poetry therapist (PTR).

***Therapeutic Value of Creative Writing* by Paul M. Spicer**

www.venturepublish.com

Available from Venture Publishing, Inc.

1999 Cato Ave.

State College, PA 16801

This workbook provides an introduction to the healing value of creative writing as well as exercises to develop writing skills.

References

Amer, K. (1999). Bibliotherapy: Using fiction to help children in two populations discuss feelings. *Pediatric Nursing, 25,* 91-95.

Apodaca, T. R., Miller, W. R., Schermer, C. R., & Amrhein, P. C. (2007). A pilot study of bibliotherapy to reduce alcohol problems among patients in a hospital trauma center. *Journal of Addictions Nursing, 18,* 167-173.

Apodaca, T. R. & Miller, W. R. (2003). A meta-analysis of the effectiveness of bibliotherapy for alcohol problems. *Journal of Clinical Psychology, 59,* 289-304.

Brewster, L., (2008). Medicine for the soul: Bibliotherapy. *Aplis, 21*(3), 115-119.

Briggs, C. A. & Pehrsson, D. E. (2008). Use of bibliotherapy in the treatment of grief and loss: A guide to current counseling practices. *Adultspan Journal, 7*(1), 32-42.

Bruera, E., Willey, J., Cohen, M., & Palmer, J. L. (2008). Expressive writing in patients receiving palliative care: A feasibility study. *Journal of Palliative Medicine, 11*(1), 15-19.

Burns, D. (2008). *Feeling Good: The New Mood Therapy.* New York: Harper.

Chamberlain, D., Heaps, D. & Robert, I. (2008). Bibliotherapy and information prescriptions: a summary of the published evidence-base and recommendations from past and ongoing Books on Prescription projects. *Journal of Psychiatric and Mental Health Nursing, 15,* 24-36.

Chandler, G. E. (1999). A creative writing program to enhance self-esteem and self-efficacy in adolescents. *Journal of Child and Adolescent Psychiatric Nursing, 12*(3), 70-78.

Dysart-Gale, D. (2008). Lost in translation: Bibliotherapy and evidence-based medicine. *Journal of Medical Humanities, 29,* 33-43.

Fair, C. D., Connor, L., Albright, J., Wise, E., Jones, K. (2012). "I'm positive, I have something to say": Assessing the impact of a creative writing group for adolescents living with HIV. *The Arts in Psychotherapy, 39,* 383-389.

Fanner, D. & Urquhart, C. (2008). Bibliotherapy for mental health service users part 1: A systematic review. *Health Information and Libraries Journal, 25,* 237-252.

Febbraro, G. A. R. (2005). An investigation into the effectiveness of bibliotherapy and minimal contact interventions in the treatment of panic attacks. *Journal of Clinical Psychology, 61*(6), 763-779.

Floyd, M., Rohen, N., Shackelford, J. A. M., Hubbard, K. L., Parnell, M. B., Scogin, F., & Coates, A. (2006). Two-year follow-up of bibliotherapy and individual cognitive therapy for depressed older adults. *Behavior Modification, 30*(3), 281-294.

Frisina, P. G., Borod, J. C., & Lepore, S. J. (2004). A meta-analysis of the effects of written emotional disclosure on the health outcomes of clinical populations. *Journal of Nervous & Mental Disease, 192*(9), 629-634.

Gillispie, C. (2003). A case report illustrating the use of creative writing as a therapeutic recreation intervention in a dual-diagnosis residential treatment center. *Therapeutic Recreation Journal, 37*(4), 339-348.

Halpert, A., Rybin, D., & Doros, G. (2010). Expressive writing is a promising therapeutic modality for the management of IBS:

A pilot study. *The American Journal of Gastroenterology, 105,* 2440-2448.

Heath, M. A., Moulton, E., Dyches, T. T., Prater, M. A., & Brown, A. (2011). Strengthening elementary school bully prevention with bibliotherapy. *Communiqué, 39*(8), 12-14.

Hevey, D., Wilczkiewicz, E., & Horgan, J. H. (2012). Type D moderates the effects of expressive writing on health-related quality of life (HRQOL) following myocardial infarction (MI). *The Irish Journal of Psychology, 33,* 107-114.

Jack, S. J. & Ronan, K. R. (2008). Bibliotherapy: Practice and research. *School Psychology International, 29*(2), 161-182.

Jernelöv, S., Lekander, M., Blom, K., Rydh, S., Ljótsson, B., Axelsson, J. & Kaldo, V. (2012). Efficacy of a behavioral self-help treatment with or without therapist guidance for co-morbid and primary insomnia — a randomized controlled trial. *Biomed Central Psychiatry, 12,* 1471-1484.

Jones, F. A. (2002). The role of bibliotherapy in health anxiety: An experimental study. *British Journal of Community Nursing, 7,* 498-503.

Kliewer, W., Lepore, S. J., Farrell, A. D., Allison, K. W., Meyer, A. L., Sullivan, T. N., & Greene, A. Y. (2011). A school-based expressive writing intervention for at-risk urban adolescents' aggressive behavior and emotional lability. *Journal of Clinical Child & Adolescent Psychology, 40*(5), 693-705.

Kohutek, K. J. (1983). Bibliotherapy within a correctional setting. *Journal of Clinical Psychology, 39*(6), 920-924.

Lewinsohn, P., Munoz, R., Youngren, M. A., & Zeiss, A. (1978). *Control your depression.* New York: Prentice Hall.

Lowe, G. (2006). Health-related effects of creative and expressive writing. *Health Education, 106,* 60-70.

McCarty Hynes, A. (1988). Some considerations concerning assessment in poetry therapy and interactive bibliotherapy. *The Arts in Psychotherapy, 15,* 55-62.

McCulliss, D. (2012). Bibliotherapy: Historical and research perspectives. *Journal of Poetry Therapy: The Interdisciplinary Journal of Practice, Theory, Research and Education, 25*(1), 23-38.

Mooney, P., Espie, C. A., & Broomfield, N. M. (2009). An experimental assessment of a Pennebaker writing intervention in primary insomnia. *Behavioral Sleep Medicine, 7*(2), 99-105.

Moore, E. K. & Coyle, C. (2007). Using poetry in therapeutic recreation interventions with a focus on applications in behavioral healthcare. *American Journal of Recreation Therapy, 6*(3), 35-47.

Morgan, A. J. & Jorm, A. F. (2008). Self-help interventions for depressive disorders and depressive symptoms: A systematic review. *Annals of General Psychiatry, 7,* 13.

Mosher, C. E., DuHamel, K. N., Lam, J., Dickler, M., Li, Y., Massie, M. J., & Norton, L., (2012). Randomised trial of expressive writing for distressed metastatic breast cancer patients. *Psychology & Health, 27,* 88-100.

National Foundation for Biblio/Poetry Therapy. Retrieved January 13, 2013, from www.nfbpt.com/about.html.

Pennebaker, J. & Evans, J. (2014). *Expressive writing: Words that heal.* Enumclaw, WA: Idyll Arbor.

Reeves, T. (2010). A controlled study of assisted bibliotherapy: An assisted self-help treatment for mild to moderate stress and anxiety. *Journal of Psychiatric and Mental Health Nursing, 17,* 184-190.

Rojcewicz, S. (1999). Medicine and poetry: The state of the art of poetry therapy. *International Journal of Arts Medicine, 6*(2), 4-9.

Sagan, O. (2007). An interplay of learning, creativity and narrative biography in a mental health setting: Bertie's story. *Journal of Social Work Practice, 21*(3), 311-321.

Santacruz, I., Méndez, F. J., & Sánchez-Meca, J. (2006). Play therapy applied by parents for children with darkness phobia: Comparison of two programmes. *Child & Family Behavior Therapy, 28*(1), 19-35.

Shechtman, Z. & Nir-Shfrir, R. (2008). The effect of affective bibliotherapy on clients' functioning in group therapy. *International Journal of Group Psychotherapy, 58*(1), 103-117.

Smyth, J. & Helm, R. (2003). Focused expressive writing as self-help for stress and trauma. *Journal of Clinical Psychology: In Session: Psychotherapy in Practice, 59*(2), 227-235.

Smyth, J. M., Hockemeyer, J. R., & Tulloch, H. (2008). Expressive writing and post-traumatic stress disorder: Effects on trauma symptoms, mood states, and cortisol reactivity. *British Journal of Health Psychology, 13,* 85-93.

Van Emmerik, A. A. P., Reijntjes, A., Kamphuis, J. H. (2013). Writing therapy for posttraumatic stress: A meta-analysis. *Psychotherapy and Psychosomatics, 82,* 82-88.

Wang, Y. (2011). Bibliotherapy for Chinese patients with depression in rehabilitation. In L. L'Abate, *Mental illnesses — understanding, prediction and control.* (pp. 407-422). Rijeka, Croatia: Intech.

21. Cognitive Behavioral Counseling

Cynthia Carruthers and Colleen Deyell Hood

Cognitive-behavioral therapies and related counseling techniques have gone through an evolution (Kellogg & Young, 2008; Reinecke & Freeman, 2005). The first wave of cognitive behavioral therapy (CBT) was behavior therapy with a focus on changing directly observable (overt) maladaptive behaviors (Spiegler, 2010). The second wave was cognitive therapy with a focus on changing cognitions (covert or private behaviors) (Spiegler, 2010). Currently most therapists who practice behavioral or cognitive therapies have fully integrated these approaches into a multimodal cognitive-behavioral approach (Lebow, 2008). The third wave of CBT is mindfulness-based cognitive-behavioral therapies (Kingdon & Dimech, 2008; McCracken, 2011) that apply mindfulness principles to the alleviation of distress and the cultivation of well-being. Cognitive-behavior therapeutic interventions have received wide empirical support in controlled trials with a diverse variety of populations (Hofmann et al., 2012).

Indications

Cognitive behavioral therapy does not represent a singular approach, but rather a body of strategies and interventions that help individuals take constructive action in their lives (Mayer & Van Acker, 2009). Cognitive behavioral counseling techniques have been used traditionally with individuals who are attempting to reduce the emotional distress in their lives, such as anxiety, depression, and anger, as well as maladaptive or problematic behaviors (Mayer & Van Acker, 2009; Radnitz, 2000). More recently, cognitive behavioral techniques are being used with individuals who wish to develop their full potential as human beings and create a meaningful life (Luoma, Hayes, & Walser, 2007; Spiegler & Guevremont, 2010). The specific techniques used are determined by the clients' assessed needs, strengths, and goals

(Mayer & Van Acker, 2009) and are monitored and modified as required during therapy based on their effectiveness (Lambert, 2010; Spiegler & Guevremont, 2010).

Contraindications

Cognitive behavioral counseling techniques have been used effectively with a wide variety of populations (Antony, Ledley, & Heimberg, 2005; Hofmann et al., 2012; Radnitz, 2000). The cognitive behavior techniques chosen for therapy should be selected and modified based on the functional level of the clients served, the complexity of the emotional or behavioral challenge, the availability of the resources and supports needed to be successful, and clients' monitored responses to the interventions and therapeutic alliance (Spiegler & Guevremont, 2010; Wampold, 2010).

Protocols and Processes
Outcomes and Documentation

This section will describe three types of cognitive behavioral counseling: behavior therapy, cognitive therapy, and mindfulness-based cognitive-behavioral therapy.

Behavior Therapy

Traditional behavior therapy applies learning theory to the understanding and modification of maladaptive behaviors (Naugle & O'Donohue, 1998; Zinbarg & Griffith, 2008). Behavior therapy is based on the premise that psychological distress is a result of learned behaviors. If new, more adaptive behaviors are learned and adopted successfully, the distress will abate (Zinbarg & Griffith, 2008). Dealing with the problematic behaviors directly is viewed as the fastest approach to problem resolution (Drummond & Kennedy, 2007).

Traditional behavior therapy identifies the problematic behaviors, as well as the antecedents and consequences of those behaviors, specifically and objectively (Drummond & Kennedy, 2007). Therapy is targeted at directly changing the current factors that "predispose, trigger, strengthen, or maintain" the maladaptive behaviors (Antony & Roemer, 2005, p. 182). Strategies include stimulus control, reinforcement, punishment, exposure, modeling, and skills training, which may include communication, anger management, relaxation, problem solving, and other cognitive skills, as required (Spiegler, 2008). Additionally, learning adaptive behaviors prior to the development of maladaptive behaviors is an important aspect of primary prevention (Naugle & O'Donohue, 1998). Although some authors (Antony & Roemer, 2005) suggest contemporary behavior therapy does not represent a singular approach to treatment, but is, instead, an amalgamation of evidence-based strategies found useful for a variety of clinical populations, other authors argue that behavior therapists should be well grounded in learning theory in order to skillfully address complex client behaviors (Naugle & O'Donohue, 1998).

Behavioral Activation Therapy (BAT) is one contemporary form of behavioral therapy that reflects many traditional strategies. BAT was originally used effectively in the treatment of depression (Sturmey, 2009), but there is growing evidence that it is helpful with a variety of populations (Busch et al., 2010). Depression is characterized by sad mood, feelings of hopelessness, isolation, loss of interest in previously enjoyable experiences, and avoidance of distressing or challenging experiences (Kanter et al., 2008). As individuals withdraw increasingly from positive engagement with their lives, the frequency and intensity of the positive reinforcement they experience diminishes, creating a downward spiral into depression (Kanter et al., 2008). The focus of behavior activation is to systematically help clients build positively reinforcing activities back into their lives, resulting in the elevation of moods, thoughts, and quality of life (Busch et al., 2010; Hopko, Bell, et al., 2008). In BAT, clients begin by self-monitoring current activities as a base-line measure and make a plan to reduce the current reinforcers of depression (Hopko, Armento, et al., 2005). Therapists then guide

clients in the identification of immediately pleasurable activities, as well as activities that would contribute to their future quality of life in a variety of life domains (Hopko, Bell, et al., 2008). Through this process, clients create a hierarchy of 15 activities ranked from easiest to most difficult to accomplish. Using a master activity log and daily behavioral checklist, the client works progressively through the accomplishment of the identified activities (Hopko, Armento, et al., 2005). In the early stages of the process, it is extremely important that the client identifies readily achievable activities that are immediately reinforcing in order to keep the client's behavior activated (Kanter et al., 2008). The therapist monitors the clients' progress and provides the psychological education necessary for successful engagement in the activities, as well as helping clients overcome avoidance and solve problems with enacting the plan (Martell, Dimidjian, & Herman-Dunn, 2010).

The Transtheoretical Model of Behavior Change (TTM), also known as the Transtheoretical Change Model (TCM) and Stage of Change Model (Prochaska & DiClemente, 1982), provides a helpful framework for understanding and supporting client behavior change that falls within the cognitive behavioral perspective. The TTM was originally developed to describe the experiences of individuals who are drug and alcohol dependent. It was developed to support efforts towards recovery (Prochaska & DiClemente, 1982) but has also been used to describe efforts toward behavior change in areas other than addiction, including physical activity (Fetherman, Hakim, & Sanko, 2011), and health related behaviors (Andrews, Gomez, & Saldana, 2008; Arden & Armitage, 2008). Prochaska and DiClemente (1982) suggested that people progress through various stages as they begin to contemplate behavior change. Intervention strategies must recognize the stages and support movement through the stages to the point where the person is willing to act towards a desired goal. The five stages of change identified by Prochaska and DiClemente are precontemplation, contemplation, preparation, action, and maintenance. In the precontemplation stage, the individual is not considering the possibility of change and does not believe that the current behavior is a problem. In the contemplation stage, the individual is beginning to recognize that the behavior may be causing a problem but is ambivalent about making any changes, still perceiving significant reasons to continue the behavior. In the preparation stage, the individual has an intention to change in the immediate future and has a plan in mind for the change. In the action stage, the individual is actively taking action towards the desired behavior change. Finally, in the maintenance stage, the person is striving to maintain and integrate the new behavior into a habitual pattern of action. The TTM assumes that "as people progress through these stages, they will experience normal fluctuations in ambivalence, problem recognition, and willingness to take action" (Levensky et al., 2007, p. 52). Therapeutic interventions must address these issues if clients are to be successful in initiating and maintaining behavior change.

Motivational Interviewing (Miller & Rollnick, 2002) is a clinical method that is based on the TTM to support individuals in exploring and resolving their ambivalence about behavioral change. It is a directive, client-centered approach that uses a supportive, non-judgmental therapeutic alliance to facilitate the exploration of motives for change, readiness for change, ambivalence about change, and confidence levels for change. The primary belief associated with Motivational Interviewing is that trying to convince individuals to make necessary behavior changes increases resistance and arguments. The most effective way to support change is to elicit the arguments for change from the individuals themselves. As Levensky et al. (2007) stated, "Motivational interviewing is not a 'fixing method' in which the provider says 'I have what you need,' but rather an 'evocative method' in which the provider says 'You have what you need'" (p. 52). The four key principles that underlie the practice of Motivational Interviewing are "(a) roll with resistance to avoid fruitless argumentation; (b) ask open-ended questions to explore the client's ambivalence about change; (c) use affirming statements to selectively reinforce change-supporting arguments; and (d) support client's autonomy and self-efficacy" (Leffingwell et al., 2007, p. 31). The primary therapist skills associated with Motivational Interviewing are the ability to convey empathy and understanding; active, reflective listening; asking change-oriented questions; and the ability to listen for and focus on change statement arising from the clients themselves. Motivational

Interviewing has been used with success in a variety of settings, including clinical, community, and public health, and with a variety of clients seeking change (Dunn, DeRoo, & Rivera, 2001; Hettema, Steele, & Miller, 2005; Knight et al., 2006). As a result, it has a great deal of applicability to the breadth of recreational therapy practice.

The majority of studies on the efficacy of recreational therapy have examined the impact of behavioral interventions. Studies have examined the impact of recreational therapy behavioral interventions on a variety of client outcomes. The following list describes the effect seen with ICF codes that might have been seen in the diagnosis assessment to justify treatment with behavioral interventions. The positive results of behavioral interventions include goal setting on physical activity level (b455 Exercise Tolerance Functions, d570 Looking After One's Health) (Farhney et al., 2010), visual activity schedules on independent transitioning (d910 Community Life) (Whatley, Gast, & Hammond, 2009), anger management intervention for anger control (b126 Temperament and Personality Functions, b130 Energy and Drive Functions, d710 Basic Interpersonal Interactions) (Marcus & Mattiko, 2007), camp experiences to support autonomy of self-management (d5 Self-Care) (Hill & Sibthorp, 2006), social skills program on social competence (d7 Interpersonal Interactions and Relationships) (Rothwell, Piatt, & Mattingly, 2006), music instruction on identity reconstruction (b126 Temperament and Personality Functions, b180 Experience of Self and Time Functions) (Montgomery, Booth, & Hutchinson, 2009), as well as leisure education on social knowledge for youth with cognitive disabilities (d155 Acquiring Skills, d710 Basic Interpersonal Interactions, d9 Community, Social, and Civic Life) (Cory, Dattilo, & Williams, 2006), community reintegration (d910 Community Life) (Ryan et al., 2008), and quality of life (Nour et al., 2002). To date, however, there are no studies examining the use and impact of Motivational Interviewing in recreational therapy practice. Although the preponderance of recreational therapy research has examined behavioral interventions, there is great need for additional recreational therapy research (Stumbo & Pegg, 2010).

Cognitive Therapy

Cognitive therapy is based on the premise that maladaptive cognition creates psychological distress and maladaptive behaviors. It asserts that if new logical, rational cognitions are learned and applied successfully, the distress and maladaptive behaviors will abate (Spiegler & Guevremont, 2010). Faulty cognitions are distorted beliefs about oneself or the world that shape the clients' anticipation and interpretation of internal and external events. There are many types of cognitive distortions, including absolute (dichotomous) thinking, overgeneralization, emotional reasoning, personalization, and catastrophizing. If these are unexamined, they can become deeply engrained, rigid schemas through which the world is processed (Kellogg & Young, 2008). Cognitive therapy focuses on changing the content of thought to produce client change (Hofmann et al., 2012). In cognitive therapy, clients are taught how to monitor their thoughts, identify and challenge maladaptive thoughts, and replace maladaptive thoughts with more adaptive thoughts (Spiegler, 2010). Homework is an important aspect of cognitive therapy and serves as a context in which to practice and monitor the effectiveness of the clients' cognitive restructuring skills in the context of their daily lives (Kellogg & Young, 2008).

The two most common cognitive restructuring approaches are Ellis' Rational Emotive Behavior Therapy and Beck's Cognitive Behavioral Therapy (Beck, 2011; Ellis & Ellis, 2011; Spiegler, 2010).

In Rational Emotive Therapy, clients learn about the relationship among activating events, rational and irrational beliefs, and their resultant consequences for feelings and behaviors, as well as how to effectively identify, monitor, actively dispute, and replace their irrational beliefs (Archer & McCarthy, 2007). In sessions, therapists actively challenge clients' irrational beliefs and clients practice the skills (Spiegler, 2010).

Although Beck's Cognitive Behavioral Therapy also questions irrational beliefs, it uses a slightly different approach that focuses on empirically testing the accuracy of the actual content of the belief (Archer & McCarthy, 2007). The therapeutic relationship is collaborative, and the therapist and client act as co-investigators to examine the validity of clients' automatic beliefs using a wide variety of techniques, such as examining evidence, defining terms, testing thoughts, and evaluating thought logic (Kellogg & Young, 2008). Thoughts that are deemed irrational and maladaptive are then replaced with more adaptive, flexible thoughts, resulting in more adaptive thoughts, schemas, and behaviors (Archer & McCarthy, 2007).

As mentioned earlier, the cognitive and behavior therapies have been largely integrated into CBT (Spiegel, 2010). One example of this integrated CBT is coping skills therapy (Spiegler, 2010). The first stage of coping skills therapy is to develop a thorough base-line assessment of the presenting problems and coping deficits, including behavioral, cognitive, emotional, and environmental components (Ronen, 2007). Then the therapist and client identify target behaviors and goals, as well as the cognitive and behavioral skills necessary for successful coping, implement the plan through coping skills acquisition, practice and complete homework in the clients' natural environment, and monitor goal attainment (Ronen, 2007, Spiegler, 2010). Given the importance of measurable outcomes in both behavior therapy and cognitive therapy, it is not surprising that outcome assessment is a core tenet of CBT (Kellogg & Young, 2008). CBT is a therapist-directed but collaborative process that serves as the foundation for many of the brief therapies (Antony & Roemer, 2005; Feltham & Dryden, 2006).

CBT has been suggested as an important theoretical framework for the development and implementation of recreational therapy services. It has been argued that an important focus of recreational therapy services should be helping clients acquire coping skills, the cognitive and behavior skills necessary to respond effectively to the evolving challenges of life (d2 General Tasks and Demands) (Hood & Carruthers, 2002). More recently, it has been suggested the focus of recreational therapy should be helping clients acquire the cognitive and behavioral capacities and resources necessary to thrive, not only survive (d3 Communication, d6 Domestic Life, d7 Interpersonal Interactions and Relationships, d9 Community, Social, and Civic Life) (Carruthers & Hood, 2004; McCormick & Iwasaki, 2008). Although less prevalent than studies of behavior interventions, the recreational therapy literature contains some examples of CBT interventions. Studies have examined the impact of recreational therapy CBT interventions on a variety of client outcomes, such as leisure education on ability to change negative thoughts and cope effectively (d240 Handling Stress and Other Psychological Demands) (Carruthers, 1995), attribution retraining on personal control and stability attributions (b126 Temperament and Personality Functions, d710 Basic Interpersonal Interactions) (Dieser & Ruddell, 2002), and rational emotive recreation therapy on irrational beliefs (b160 Thought Functions) (Lundberg et al., 2006).

Mindfulness-Based Cognitive Behavioral Therapy

Mindfulness-based cognitive behavioral therapies incorporate many of the same principles and techniques of the first two waves of cognitive behavioral therapies with some important differences (Spiegler, 2010). First, the focus of the therapy is not the amelioration of emotional and behavioral problems. Instead the focus is on helping clients take action to create a life based on what is most meaningful and important to them (Spiegel, 2010). Second, rather than challenging the content of thoughts or avoiding emotional distress, clients learn to become mindfully aware and accepting of these internal experiences as a normal part of life, neither getting caught up in them nor avoiding them, while simultaneously taking mindful action in a valued direction (Borkovec & Sharpless, 2004; Germer, 2009).

Often, people avoid situations that generate uncomfortable thoughts and emotions, even though engaging in those experiences will bring them closer to what they most value in life. They may attempt to suppress negative internal events, such as thoughts, feelings, memories, and physical sensations, with the unintended consequence of no longer feeling engaged or present for their lives (Luoma, Hayes, & Walser, 2006). Mindfulness is the awareness that emerges through paying attention, purposefully and nonjudgmentally, to the unfolding of experience, moment by moment (Kabat-Zinn, 2003). It allows individuals to disengage from automatic thoughts and habitual, maladaptive behavior patterns (Brown & Ryan, 2003). Mindfulness contributes to a more flexible, autonomous, responsive engagement in one's life (McCracken, 2011).

One example of mindfulness-based cognitive behavioral therapy is Hayes and colleagues (2004) Acceptance and Commitment Therapy (ACT). Through the therapeutic process, clients look at distressing internal experiences with the goal of understanding the relationship between the avoidance of these experiences and difficulties in creating a joyful and meaningful life. Clients develop and practice mindfulness skills, identify and prioritize their life values, establish goals and specific action items that reflect their values, make a commitment to their goals, and identify potential barriers and strategies to navigate setbacks (Luoma, Hayes, & Walser, 2006). Throughout the process, clients are encouraged to stay in the moment and defuse from their thoughts, accept their emotions and present reality, and continuously return to committed action in pursuit of their valued lives (Wilson & Defrene, 2008). Therapists flexibly, compassionately, and authentically respond to the needs, motivations, experiences, and situations of clients, modeling acceptance of challenging content and respecting clients' ability to change (McCracken, 2010). Motivational Interviewing and Acceptance and Commitment Therapy (ACT) share many similarities in technique, therapeutic stance, behavioral goals, and concepts. Methods from Motivational Interviewing can be integrated easily into the practice of ACT (Gillanders, 2011).

Although Carruthers and Hood (2011) articulated the important role of mindfulness-based cognitive behavioral therapy in recreational therapy practice, there are few empirical studies supporting its efficacy. Examples of studies that have been reported include the use of yoga and guided imagery on pain and anxiety reduction (b280 Sensation of Pain, d240 Handling Stress and Other Psychological Demands) (Bonadies, 2004, 2009), mindfulness-based biofeedback on heart rate coherence (b410 Heart Functions) and quality of life (Groff et al., 2010), and mindfulness-based stress reduction on coping, depression, and anxiety (b126 Temperament and Personality Functions, b130 Energy and Drive Functions, b152 Emotional Functions, d240 Handling Stress and Other Psychological Demands) (Van Puymbroeck & Hsieh, 2010). Much more efficacy research on comprehensive mindfulness-based cognitive behavioral recreational therapy interventions is needed (Carruthers & Hood, 2011).

References

Andrews, A, Gomez, J, & Saldana, C (2008). Challenges and applications of the transtheoretical model in patients with diabetes mellitus. *Disease Management and Health Outcomes, 16*, 31-47.

Antony, M., Ledley, D., & Heimberg, R. (Eds.) (2005). *Improving outcomes and preventing relapse in cognitive-behavioral therapy*. New York: Guilford Press.

Antony, M. & Romer, L. (2005). Behavior therapy. In A. Gurman & S. Messer (Eds.), *Essential psychotherapies: Theory and practice* (2ⁿᵈ ed.) (pp. 182-223). New York: Guilford Press.

Archer, J. & McCarthy, C. (2007). *Theories of counseling and psychotherapy: Contemporary applications.* Upper Saddle River, NJ: Pearson Education.

Arden, M. A. & Armitage, C. J. (2008). Predicting and explaining transtheoretical model stage transitions in relation to condom-carrying behavior. *British Journal of Health Psychology, 13,* 719-735.

Beck, J. (2011). *Cognitive behavior therapy: Basics and beyond* (2ⁿᵈ ed.). New York: Guilford Press.

Bonadies, V. (2009). Guided imagery as a therapeutic recreation modality to reduce pain and anxiety. *Therapeutic Recreation Journal, 43,* 43-55.

Bonadies, V. (2004). A yoga therapy program for AIDS-related pain and anxiety: Implications for therapeutic recreation. *Therapeutic Recreation Journal, 38,* 148-166.

Borkovec, T. & Sharpless, B. (2004). Generalized anxiety disorder: Bringing cognitive-behavioral therapy into the valued present. In S. Hayes, V. Follette, & M. Linehan (Eds.), *Mindfulness and acceptance: Expanding the cognitive-behavioral tradition* (pp. 209-242). New York: Guilford Press.

Brown, K. & Ryan, R. (2003). The benefits of being present: Mindfulness and its role in psychological well-being. *Personality and Social Psychology, 84,* 822-848.

Busch, A., Uebelacker, Z., & Miller, I. (2010). Measuring homework completion in behavioral activation. *Behavior Modification, 34,* 310-329.

Carruthers, C. (1995). Model leisure education program for people with addictions. *The Counselor, 13,* 35-39.

Carruthers, C. & Hood, C. (2004). The power of the positive: Leisure and well-being. *Therapeutic Recreation Journal, 38,* 225-245.

Carruthers, C. & Hood, C. (2011). Mindfulness and well-being: Implications for therapeutic recreation practice. *Therapeutic Recreation Journal, 45,* 171-189.

Cory, L., Dattilo, J., & Williams, R. (2006). Effects of a leisure education program on social knowledge and skills of youth with cognitive disabilities. *Therapeutic Recreation Journal, 40,* 144-164.

Dieser, R. & Ruddell, E. (2002). Effects of attribution retraining during therapeutic recreation on attributions and explanatory styles of adolescents with depression. *Therapeutic Recreation Journal, 36,* 35-47.

Drummond, L. & Kennedy, B. (2007). Behavioral psychotherapy. In S. Bloch (Ed.). *An introduction to the psychotherapies* (4ᵗʰ ed.) (pp. 167-196). New York: Oxford University Press.

Dunn, C., DeRoo, L., & Rivera, F. P. (2001). The use of brief interventions adapted from motivational interviewing across behavioral domains: A systematic review. *Addiction, 96,* 1725-1742.

Ellis, A. & Ellis, D. J. (2011). *Rational emotive behavior therapy* (3ʳᵈ ed.). Arlington, VA: Amer Psychological Assn.

Farhney, S., Kelley, C., Dattilo, J., Rusch, F. (2010). Effects of goal setting on activity level of senior exercisers with osteoarthritis residing in the community. *Therapeutic Recreation Journal, 44,* 87-102.

Feltham, C. & Dryden, W. (2006). *Brief counseling: A practical, integrative approach* (2ⁿᵈ ed.). Berkshire, England: Open University Press.

Fetherman, D. L., Hakim, R. M., & Sanko, J. P. (2011). A pilot study of the application of the transtheoretical model during strength training in older women. *Journal of Women and Aging, 23,* 58-76.

Germer, C. (2009). *The mindful path to self-compassion: Freeing yourself from destructive thoughts and emotions*. New York, NY: Guilford Press.

Gillanders, D. (2011). Acceptance and Commitment Therapy and Motivational Interviewing for health behavior change. In L. McCracken (Ed.), *Mindfulness and acceptance in behavioral medicine: Current theory and practice.* (pp. 217-242). Oakland, CA: New Harbinger Publications.

Groff, D., Battaglini, C., Sipe, C., Peppercorn, J., Anderson, M., & Hackney, A. (2010). "Finding a new normal": Using recreation therapy to improve the well-being of women with breast cancer. *Annual in Therapeutic Recreation, 18,* 40-52.

Hayes, S., Strosahl, K., Bunting, K., Twohig, M., & Wilson, K. (2004). What is Acceptance and Commitment Therapy? In S. Hayes & K. Strosahl (Eds.). *A practical guide to Acceptance and Commitment Therapy* (pp. 3-29). New York: Springer.

Hettema, J., Steele, J., & Miller, W. R. (2005). Motivational interviewing. *Annual Review of Clinical Psychology, 1,* 91-111.

Hill, E. & Sibthorp, J. (2006). Autonomy support at diabetes camp: A self-determination theory approach to therapeutic recreation. *Therapeutic Recreation Journal, 40,* 107-125.

Hofmann, S., Asnaani, A., Vonk, I., Sawyer, A., & Fang, A. (2012). The efficacy of cognitive behavioral therapy: A review of meta-analyses. *Cognitive Therapy and Research, 36,* 427-440.

Hollan, S. & Beck, A. (2004). Cognitive and cognitive behavioral therapies. In M. Lambert (Ed.), *Bergin and Garfield's Handbook of psychotherapy and behavior change* (5ᵗʰ ed.) (pp. 447-492). New York: John Wiley and Sons.

Hood, C. & Carruthers, C. (2002). Coping skills theory as an underlying framework for therapeutic recreation services. *Therapeutic Recreation Journal, 36,* 137-153.

Hopko, D., Armento, M., Hunt, M., Bell, J., & Lejuez, C. (2005). Behavior therapy for depressed cancer patients in primary care. *Psychotherapy: Theory, Research, Practice, Training, 42,* 236-243.

Hopko, D., Bell, J., Armento, M., Robertson, S., Mullane, C., Wolf, J., & Lejuez, C. (2008). Cognitive-behavior therapy for depressed cancer patients in a medical care setting. *Behavior Therapy, 39,* 126-136.

Kabat-Zinn, J. (2003). Mindfulness-based interventions in context: Past, present, and future. *Clinical Psychology: Science and Practice, 10,* 144-156.

Kanter, J., Manos, R., Busch, A., & Rusch, L. (2008). Making behavioral activation more behavioral. *Behavior Modification, 32,* 780-803.

Kellogg, S. & Young, J. (2008). Cognitive therapy. In J. Lebow (Ed.), *Twenty-first century psychotherapies* (pp. 43-79). Hoboken, NJ: John Wiley & Sons.

Kingdon, D. & Dimech, A. (2008). Cognitive and behavioral therapies: The state of the art. *Psychiatry, 7,* 217-220.

Knight, K. M., McGowan, L., Dickens, C., & Bundy, C. (2006). A systematic review of motivational interviewing in physical health care settings. *British Journal of Health Psychology, 11,* 319-332.

Lambert, M. (2010). Yes, it is time for clinicians to routinely monitor treatment outcome. In B. Duncan, S. Miller, B. Wampold, & M. Hubble (Eds.). *The heart and soul of change* (2ⁿᵈ ed.) (pp. 239-266). Washington, DC: American Psychological Association.

Lebow, J. (2008). Introduction. In J. Lebow (Ed.), *Twenty-first century psychotherapies* (pp. 1-7). Hoboken, NJ: John Wiley & Sons.

Leffingwell, T. R., Neumann, C. A., Babitzke, A. C., Leedy, M. J., & Walters, S. T. (2007). Social psychological and motivational interviewing: A review of relevant principles and recommendations for research and practice. *Behavioral and Cognitive Psychotherapy, 35,* 31-45.

Levensky, E. R., Forcehimes, A., O'Donohue, W. T., & Beitz, K. (2007). Motivational interviewing: An evidence-based approach to counseling helps patients follow treatment recommendations. *American Journal of Nursing, 107*(10), 50-58.

Lundberg, N., Widmer, M., McCormick, B., & Ward, W. (2005/2006). Rational emotive recreation therapy: Using adventure and recreation in reducing irrational beliefs among adolescent males with behavior disorders. *Annual in Therapeutic Recreation, 14,* 59-69.

Luoma, J., Hayes, S., & Walser, R. (2007). *Learning ACT: An Acceptance and Commitment Therapy skills-training manual for therapists.* Oakland, CA: New Harbinger.

Marcus, D. & Mattiko, M. (2007). An anger management program for children with attention deficit, hyperactivity disorder. *Therapeutic Recreation Journal, 41,* 16-28.

Martell, C., Dimidjian, S., & Herman-Dunn, R. (2010). *Behavioral activation for depression: A clinician's guide.* New York: Guilford Press.

Mayer, M. & Van Acker, R. (2009). Historical roots, theoretical and applied developments, and critical issues in cognitive-behavior modification. In M. Mayer, R. Van Acker, J. Lochman, & F. Greham (Eds.), *Cognitive-behavioral interventions for emotional and behavioral disorders: School-based practice.* New York: Guilford Press.

McCormick, B. & Iwasaki, Y. (2008). Mental health and transcending life challenges: The role of therapeutic recreation services. *Therapeutic Recreation Journal, 42,* 5-23.

McCracken, L. (2011). History, context, and new developments in behavioral medicine. In L. McCracken (Ed.), *Mindfulness and acceptance in behavioral medicine: Current theory and practice.* (pp. 3-30). Oakland, CA: New Harbinger Publications.

Miller, W. R. & Rollnick, S. (Eds.) (2002). *Motivational interviewing: Preparing people for change* (2nd ed.). New York: Guilford Press.

Montgomery, E., Booth, R., & Hutchinson, S. (2009). From a focus on function to rediscovering the self: A case report of an individual with post-stroke depression. *Therapeutic Recreation Journal, 43,* 25-41.

Naugle, A. & O'Donohue, W. (1998). The future directions of behavior therapy: Some applied implications of contemporary learning research. In W. Donohue (Ed.), *Learning and behavior therapy* (pp. 545-558). Boston: Allyn & Bacon.

Nour, K., Desrosiers, Gauthier, P., & Carbonneau, H. (2002). Impact of a home leisure educational program for older adults who have had a stroke. *Therapeutic Recreation Journal, 36,* 48-64.

Prochaska, J. O. & DiClemente, C. C. (1982). Transtheoretical therapy: Toward a more integrative model of change. *Psychotherapy, 19*(3), 279-288.

Radnitz, C. (Ed.) (2000). *Cognitive-behavioral therapy for persons with disabilities.* Northvale, NJ: Jason Aronson Inc.

Reinecke, M. & Freeman, A. (2005). Cognitive therapy. In A. Gurman & S. Messer (Eds.), *Essential psychotherapies: Theory and Practice* (2nd ed.) (pp. 182-223). New York: Guilford Press.

Ronen, T. (2007). Clinical social work and its commonalities with cognitive behavior therapy. In T. Ronen & A. Freeman (Eds.), *Cognitive behavior therapy in clinical social work practice* (pp. 3-24). New York: Springer Publishing.

Rothwell, E., Piatt, J., & Mattingly, K. (2006). Social competence: Evaluation of an outpatient recreation therapy treatment program for children with behavioral disorders. *Therapeutic Recreation Journal, 40,* 241-254.

Ryan, C., Stiell, K., Gailey, G., & Makinen, J. (2008). Evaluating a family centered approach to leisure education and community reintegration following a stroke. *Therapeutic Recreation Journal, 42,* 119-131.

Spiegler, M. (2008). Behavior therapy I: Cognitive-behavioral therapy. In J. Frew & M. Spiegler (Eds.), *Contemporary psychotherapies for a diverse world* (pp. 275-319). Boston: Houghton Mifflin.

Spiegler, M. & Guevremont, D. (2010). *Contemporary behavior therapy* (5th ed.). Belmont, CA: Wadsworth.

Stumbo, N. & Pegg, S. (2010). Outcome and evidence-based practice: Moving forward. *Annual in Therapeutic Recreation, 18,* 12-23.

Sturmey, P. (2009). Behavioral activation is an evidence-based treatment for depression. *Behavior Modification, 33,* 818-829.

Van Puymbroeck, M. & Hsieh, P. (2010). The influence of mindfulness-based stress reduction and walking on the psychological well-being of female informal caregivers: A pilot study. *American Journal of Recreation Therapy, 9,* 15-25.

Wampold, B. (2010). The research evidence for the common factors models: A historically situated perspective. In B. Duncan, S. Miller, B. Wampold, & M. Hubble (Eds.). *The heart and soul of change* (2nd ed.) (pp. 49-82). Washington, DC: American Psychological Association.

Whatley, A., Gast, D., & Hammond, D. (2009). Visual activity schedules: Teaching independent transitioning during recreation and leisure. *Therapeutic Recreation Journal, 43,* 27-42.

Wilson, K. & Defrene, T. (2008). *Mindfulness for two: An Acceptance and Commitment Therapy approach to mindfulness in psychotherapy.* Oakland, CA: New Harbinger Publications.

Zinbarg, R. & Griffith, J. (2008). Behavior therapy. In J. Lebow (Ed.), *Twenty-first century psychotherapies* (pp. 8-42). Hoboken, NJ: John Wiley & Sons.

22. Cognitive Retraining and Rehabilitation

Heather R. Porter

As the saying goes, "use it or lose it." This holds true not only for physical skills such as muscle strength, but also for cognitive skills such as memory. The brain needs continuous challenges to develop, strengthen, and shed neural pathways. Brain development is not a one-time event. The brain continually changes its structure to meet the demands placed upon it.

The specific process involved in challenging the brain after injury is called cognitive rehabilitation. Cognitive rehabilitation is an "umbrella term for a group of interventions that are used to support or ameliorate cognitive impairments, as well as the changes that occur in everyday functioning as a result of these impairments" (Koehler, Wilhelm, & Shoulson, 2011, p. 86). Interventions employed may target a specific impairment (e.g., memory deficits) or address multiple impairments (e.g., memory, self-awareness, and attention), but either way, the interventions are individually tailored to meet the needs of each client (Koehler et al., 2011).

Due to the diversity of interventions and the various ways interventions are combined and modified to meet the needs of the individual client, there is a lack of a unified theoretical framework for defining and quantifying cognitive rehabilitation treatments, making it particularly challenging to evaluate their effectiveness (Koehler et al., 2011). However, it is important to note that "limited evidence regarding the effectiveness of cognitive rehabilitation therapy does not indicate that the effectiveness of cognitive rehabilitation therapy treatments are 'limited'; the limitations of the evidence do not rule out meaningful benefit" (Koehler et al., 2011, p. 257).

Cognitive rehabilitation is used by many different disciplines, including recreational, physical, occupational, and speech therapy, to promote neuroplasticity. It is commonly used after brain damage (e.g., stroke, traumatic brain injury, multiple sclerosis) to recover lost cognitive skills, throughout a progressive neurological disease (e.g., Alzheimer's disease, multiple sclerosis) to help promote maintenance of current cognitive skills, and to promote developmental growth of cognitive skills related to intellectual disability. Therapists use a variety of approaches to promote cognitive abilities. They are best understood by dividing them into two types of interventions. The first is called restoration or development where the focus is on recovery of lost skills, the development of skills, or the refinement and maintenance of skills. The second is compensation where the focus is on adaptations and modification to compensate for cognitive dysfunction (Riccio, 2007). Both are explained in more detail in the Protocols and Processes section.

Indications

Cognitive rehabilitation is implemented when cognitive impairments are present and when the client could benefit from skill restoration or compensatory management to optimize recovery, functioning, health, and quality of life. ICF codes directly tied to cognitive function can be found in b1 Mental Functions, s110 Structure of Brain, and d1 Learning and Applying Knowledge. Specific skills that show deficits may be found in many other areas of the ICF codes. Some examples include d2 General Tasks and Demands, d3 Communication, d7 Interpersonal Interactions and Relationships, and d8 Major Life Areas.

Contraindications

Current literature indicates that potential adverse outcomes and risk for harm associated with cognitive rehabilitation are rare, although more research is needed for confirmation, as this has not been addressed regularly in the literature (Koehler et al., 2011).

Protocols and Processes

Prior to implementing cognitive rehabilitation interventions, it is important for the therapist to recognize that cognitive processes (and recovery in general) are impacted by multiple factors and that addressing only cognitive processes might not yield optimal outcomes. Factors that impact recovery, in addition to cognitive impairments, include, but are not limited to, physical impairments (e.g., fatigue, pain, poor sleep), psychological impairments (anger, irritability, anxiety, depression, stress), and a lack of ability to carry out important activities in the physical and social environment. There may also be issues with community participation, educational attainment, employment status, family or caregiver health, quality of life and well-being, role in the home, family functioning, social support, transportation access, behavioral problems, comorbid conditions, and quality of care (Koehler et al., 2011).

Restoration and Development Approach

Cognitive rehabilitation, although appearing easy in application, requires the clinician to integrate a variety of approaches and to continually modify the task, the environment, and the therapeutic input. The therapist needs to maintain a balance between tolerated, guided challenges and detrimental frustration of the client, all the while tracking the client's performance and reaction to the challenge. The steps to implement this process are described below.

Step 1: Identify the skills in a functional task and determine a baseline of functioning

Restoring and developing cognitive skills begins by identifying the specific cognitive skills that need to be addressed and evaluating the client's current functional status. For example, if the client needs to address sequencing, short-term memory, and problem solving, the therapist might find the following functional status: Client requires moderate verbal cues to sequence five steps involved in staining a wood project; client is able to recall three of six grocery items after a five-minute delay; client requires minimal multi-modal cues to problem solve for issues related to using public transportation. Notice that the tasks in the examples are all functional tasks (wood-

working, grocery shopping, public transportation). Generalizing cognitive skills from one task to another is a separate and distinct cognitive process and it can be very difficult for some clients to do, especially those who have had a brain injury. Therefore, it is recommended that the therapist address the specific deficit in a functional task that will be both familiar to the client and also part of the client's lifestyle after therapy.

The therapist should also continue to use the same functional task throughout the course of cognitive rehabilitation as much as possible. For example, if the therapist is using the task of repotting a plant to address the skill of sequencing and the client becomes proficient with the task, the therapist would then need to increase the complexity of the task to further challenge the client (e.g., tending a flower garden). When tasks are changed, the therapist still must be attentive to choosing a task that is going to be part of the client's activity pattern after discharge. In the literature, it has been argued that activities that are "within a familiar environment, or deal with personally important tasks, are likely to enhance motivation for treatment, improve self-awareness of strengths and weaknesses, and ensure that the strategies learned are applicable to the patient's personal situation" (Koehler et al., 2011, p. 83).

Step 2: Once a baseline for a deficit skill in a functional task has been determined, the therapist implements various strategies to develop the skill. Below is a list of basic strategies utilized in interventions.

Manipulate the environment. The therapist begins by treating the client in a quiet, non-distracting environment and gradually increases the complexity of the environment. The environment can be manipulated by increasing or decreasing the number of supplies, the type and degree of distractions (e.g., people, pictures on the wall, a ringing telephone, an open door to a busy hallway), and paying special consideration to the type of environment chosen (e.g., non-threatening, exciting, calming) and the emotional reaction of the client to the environment. Clients do not all perceive an environment the same way. For example, one client may enjoy the peacefulness of a private therapy room while another client may become anxious in such a setting. A quiet, non-distracting environment can enhance a client's attention and concentration on the skill being addressed, thus maximizing neuroplasticity. However this type of environment is not always found in the real world. Therefore, the therapist begins with a quiet, non-distracting environment with the goal of increasing the complexity of the environment to match the client's anticipated real-life setting or to reach a level of functioning that can be reasonably accommodated.

Graduated stepping: Graduated stepping refers to small and progressive changes in the challenges presented to the client. The therapist can either increase or decrease the steps presented as long as they reflect a positive change (e.g., gradually decrease the verbal cues given to the client, gradually increase the complexity of the task). Negative stepping is not desirable, yet it is necessary at times (e.g., increasing the verbal cues given to the client, decreasing the complexity of the task) if the task presented is too difficult or there is a negative change in the status of the client. The goal is to increase the skill set of the client through cognitive retraining. Therefore, the therapist wants to always present a challenge slightly above the client's current level of cognitive functioning. Examples of what a therapist can change include the amount of cueing provided, the type of assistance provided (e.g., decrease from a hand-over-hand assist to a verbal cue, decrease from moderate gestural cues to minimal gestural cues), the complexity of the activity (e.g., increase from a two-step activity to a three-step activity, increase from solving familiar problems to solving moderately familiar problems), and the environment (e.g., increase from a non-distracting environment to a minimally distracting environment).

Cueing: The therapist provides the client with a variety of cues to help the client complete the task without the therapist doing the task for the client. Cues can include verbal cues, tactile cues, demonstrative cues, auditory cues, gestural cues, and/or visual cues. Cueing helps the client figure out the task. It does not give the client the answer (e.g., "What do we need next?" "It is on your right side" "It begins with the letter 's'." "You use it to scoop up soil.", "What do we have to do before we put in the seed?"). Cues without answers are important to facilitate neuroplasticity as it challenges the brain to reorganize. Cueing is given in a graduated fashion and may need to be altered depending on the environment. For example, a client may require minimal verbal cues in a moderately distracting clinic (capac-

ity qualifier in the ICF) and when in the community require moderate verbal cues (performance qualifier in the ICF).

Reinforced practice: This refers to the need to practice the skill repetitively and consistently for facilitation of learning. The same skill is practiced at each therapy session with the client using the same activity. The skill does not need to be practiced for the duration of each session, thus hindering your ability to address other issues with the client, but it should be practiced for a specific duration in the treatment session. For example, if you are addressing problem solving for familiar tasks, ask the client one or two problem-solving questions at the beginning of each therapy session. It is also important to be consistent in the approach taken with the client (cueing, level of assistance, task, environment), especially if the entire treatment team is focusing on the same skill. For example, if a client lacks insight about his impairments, the team may agree to jointly address this issue by tying a laminated list of the client's five prominent impairments onto the side of her wheelchair and asking the client at the beginning of each therapy session to name the five impairments without looking at the list. If deficits were missed, the client is asked to refer to the list to identify deficits she didn't name. The results could be recorded on a traveling documentation sheet on the back of the client's wheelchair.

Compensation Approach

The compensation approach is used when there is not enough time to gradually increase the client's cognitive skills to achieve skill independence in the anticipated real-life environment or the client is not able to fully recover some cognitive skills, resulting in the need to adapt for the cognitive deficit. This approach can be detrimental to the client in the long run if the activities are not also structured in a manner that promotes continued recovery of function. Brain function can be recovered over long periods of time, including after discharge from an inpatient rehabilitation facility. A compensation approach, while it can slow down the recovery process, may be required for two primary reasons:

Safety: Without compensatory strategies the client has a high risk of harm to self or others, for example, without a curtain hung in front of the main house door, the client would wander outside.

Activity participation restrictions: Without compensatory strategies, the client's activity involvement would be restricted impacting physical and emotional health, functioning, independence, or productivity. For example, without a beeping watch that reminds the client to go outside to wait for the bus, the client would miss the school bus.

Recreational therapists understand the value of participating in leisure and recreation experiences for the pleasure they bring. Designing activities that require the assistance of another person, a special environment that is not typical of a real-life setting, and challenges that can be frustrating all limit the benefits of participation. Consequently, therapists often seek to balance both recovery and compensation. Therapists do this by (1) teaching the client's caregiver how to continue to facilitate improvement with activities after discharge (recovery approach) and (2) teaching the client and caregiver how to adapt the activity so that the client can participate in the activity with the greatest level of independence and pleasure (compensation approach).

Choosing Interventions

The majority of literature surrounding the use of cognitive rehabilitation relates to the treatment of brain injury. The Cognitive Rehabilitation Task Force of the Brain Injury Interdisciplinary Special Interest Group (BI-ISIG) of the American Congress of Rehabilitation Medicine (ACRM) conducted several systematic reviews of the literature related to cognitive rehabilitation and recommend the following treatment approaches and strategies based on the evidence, as well as clinical experience (Haskins, 2012). Those who practice in the cognitive rehabilitation field should read this reference for more detailed information. To determine the course of treatment, the BI-ISIG recommends that therapists use the following decision tree:

1. If a client is not aware of his/her deficits, use techniques to increase awareness.

2. If the client achieves (or already has) awareness of deficits, AND...

a. the client is able to use an external strategy and has a mild to moderate brain injury, then internal strategies (as able) and/or external strategies (with assistance, as needed) should be used.

b. the client is able to use an external strategy and has a severe brain injury, then specific ap-

proaches (errorless learning, spaced retrieval, chaining) and/or external strategies with cueing and assistance should be used.

c. the client is UNABLE to use an external strategy (despite the level of brain injury impairment), then task-specific approaches (errorless learning, spaced retrieval, chaining) should be used.

The decision tree leads the therapist to identify the best types of strategies for intervention based on the client's level of self-awareness and extent of brain injury. Although not meant to be an exhaustive review, Haskins (2012) provides therapists with more detailed instructions on how to apply each of the interventions in the decision tree based on available evidence, as reviewed below.

Self-Awareness

To improve awareness of deficits in general, it is recommended that therapists point out the concern or deficit; provide information about the condition through information, discussion, or formal materials such as handouts and videos; provide psychoeducation about brain injury; and explain and normalize common symptoms related to brain injury to increase self-identification and relateableness (e.g., "I don't have a memory impairment, but I do forget where I have to go sometimes"). If the client still doesn't have insight, the therapist should identify evidence that highlights the problem and pose a non-confrontational question such as "I wonder if you are having trouble with your memory or if something else is really causing the problem." The therapist and client can then explore the issue together. The therapist should be aware of remarks such as "I don't remember it because it is not important to me." The therapist then continues to track problems and successes and share these routinely with the client to help raise awareness, not highlight failures. Other techniques to help improve awareness, related to the underlying cause, include:

Neurocognitive causes: Provide awareness that deficits can be caused by damage to the right hemisphere, right or left parietal regions, the frontal lobe, or diffuse brain injury. Parietal lesions however, most often yield insight problems. For example, damage to the left parietal lobe can result in aphasia and damage to the right parietal lobe can cause left neglect, both of which are impairments related to difficulty perceiving and recognizing impairments. The problem results from an underlying inability to generalize. The ability to generalize means that the person is able to recognize a mistake, make the connection that the mistake indicates impairment, and that the impairment can impact everyday tasks. If a client has difficulty with awareness due to neurocognitive causes, then the therapist should (1) build a therapeutic relationship with the client and validate any frustration or distress, (2) select the key tasks and environments where awareness behaviors are most important, (3) provide clear feedback and structured opportunities to help the client evaluate his/her performance, discover errors, and compensate for deficits, (4) focus on habit formation through repetition and procedural or implicit learning, (5) train for generalization, but be realistic and understand the client's limitations in this area, and (6) consider group therapy, family education, and environmental supports to provide external compensation.

Psychological causes: Recognizing that one has a cognitive impairment can result in emotionally painful thoughts leading to the development of denial. It could be related to a personality trait (denial and repression as a defense mechanism) or not having worked through the normal grief process (which includes acceptance and adjustment). If a client has difficulty with awareness due to psychological causes, then the therapist should (1) build a therapeutic relationship with the client and validate any frustration or distress (a strong therapeutic relationship is a foundation to work collaboratively on self-image, coping strategies, and acceptance); (2) avoid direct confrontation and education; (3) foster hope for continued recovery to facilitate adjustment; (4) use non-confrontational approaches to teach adaptive coping strategies, such as relaxation techniques, before attempting to change any maladaptive strategies that may be protecting the client from emotional distress; (5) enhance perceived control over the therapy process by presenting choices; (6) use psychotherapy and adjustment counseling techniques to help to re-establish a sense of self and self-mastery by exploring the subjective meaning of loss and to acknowledge grief; (7) consider family therapy to help the client adjust to new roles, discuss expectations, and identify and establish external supports to maximize generalization of learned strategies to real-world environments; and (8) promote and reinforce acceptance of change, and gradually develop modified goals for the future. Care needs to be taken

because there can be feelings of vulnerability when awareness of an impairment begins to emerge. Subtle feedback or comments can easily be perceived by the client as being confrontational or insensitive.

Social-environmental causes: Unawareness of deficits may stem from a variety of social-environmental causes including a general lack of information about brain injury and functional impairments, not having been told about the impairments, not having had an opportunity to engage in tasks that demonstrate the existence of impairments, family members minimizing the client's cognitive deficits (for various reasons) and increasing focus on physical impairments, being inadvertently encouraged or reinforced by well-intentioned family members to deny the existence of problems, being fearful of disclosing cognitive challenges due to uncertainty of how the information will be used, and/or cultural issues impacting the understanding of the assessment or rehabilitation process. If a client has difficulty with awareness due to social-environmental causes then the therapist should (1) clarify the rationale for the assessment, help the client identify concerns, and provide education; (2) consider the timing of the intervention and the need for safe and supportive opportunities to observe post-injury changes; (3) educate significant others on how to provide appropriate feedback and support; (4) connect family members to support or education groups to provide a positive social context and normalize their experiences; (5) seek advice from a cultural liaison office or other professional and speak to the family and friends of the individual to develop a shared understanding; and (6) provide psychoeducation about brain injury and rehabilitation to clarify misinformation and misunderstandings, answer questions, validate experiences, and explain cognitive deficits common to brain injury. Education can help clarify the unusual behaviors observed by family. However, it may not be helpful if the family is defensive.

Internal Strategies

Internal strategies teach clients how to cue themselves to use an image, word, or action sequence as a trigger to take the appropriate steps to address a task or problem at hand. Examples of internal strategies include:

Problem-solving strategies: These are strategies that are used to help clients improve self-awareness, identify problems, and implement solutions. The client is trained to use a particular strategy consistently whenever a problem is encountered. Strategies typically begin with the use of an external strategy (e.g., a list of steps to follow), which is gradually faded away so that it becomes an internal strategy (self-talk). Strategies can vary from simple (e.g., the three-step process of Stop, Think, Plan as done in Goal Management Training; the four-step process of Goal, Plan, Do, Review in the Goal-Plan-Do-Review procedure) to more complex. In general, it is recommended that steps move along a continuum of *awareness* (recognizing there is a problem, deciding on its relevance, defining the problem), *anticipation/planning* (such as, deciding what information is needed to make a decision, listing possible solutions to the problem, identifying pros and cons, choosing the best option, identifying and learning the steps involved related to the option), *execution/self-monitoring* (e.g., executing the solution in an effective manner while monitoring progress in following the identified solution), and *self-evaluation* (e.g., exploring the effectiveness of the solution).

Self-instructional strategies: Self-instructional strategies (also referred to as metacognitive strategies) aim to increase the client's awareness of, and control over, behavior. It's the process of thinking about thinking. Strategies usually begin with the use of external strategies (e.g., a written list) while fostering the use of internal strategies, with the goal of then eliminating the external strategies and solely using the internal strategy. The task is broken down into simple steps, and written down if needed. The client is instructed to say the steps out loud when performing the task, while receiving any needed assistance from the therapist (e.g., cueing, modeling, picture cards). Once the client demonstrates success without assistance from the therapist or use of external strategies, such as picture cards or a list, the therapist then instructs the client to whisper the steps out loud as s/he completes the task (faded verbalization). Once the client is successful with this step, the client is then instructed to say the steps in his/her head rather than out loud (inner speech), thus moving from the use of external strategies such as picture cards or lists to the use of an internal strategy such as inner speech.

Internal memory strategies: This includes the use of mental processes to cue memory. Some internal memory strategies include:

- *Chunking or grouping*: Provides a way of organizing information to be recalled, such as putting things into categories (e.g., organizing a grocery list by types of items needed). The information doesn't have to be in a written format. For example, the client might remember that she needs to buy purple flowers at the store by repeating to herself that the top of the letter "P" in purple is round, just like a flower, and also like the container that she wants to plant them in. Therefore, she is using the shape of a circle to help her remember what she needs to buy at the store. Items and information can be grouped by color, size, shape, function, origins, etc.

- *Mental retracing*: This is when a person retraces steps in his/her mind. For example, "I can't find my keys. I thought they were on the table. Let me think. When I came home, I took the mail out of the mailbox and then opened the door. I walked inside and put the mail down on the hutch. Oh, I maybe I put the keys down with the mail on the hutch."

- *Visual imagery*: The client closes his/her eyes and pictures in the mind's eye the information, the task, or the action. For example, the client pictures herself in the locker room at the YWCA and walks through the process of re-dressing to help her to remember all of the items she needs to take with her — hairdryer, towel, change of clothes, lock for the locker, soap, etc.

- *Story method*: The client forms a story about the words or phrases s/he is to remember. For example, if a client has to remember to call his friend Dave, buy dog food, and call the water department, he might remember it by making up a story, such as "Dave ate the dog food and then needed a drink of water."

- *Association*: This is when two new pieces of information are associated or when new information is associated with old information. For example, when being introduced to "Brenda," the client might associate the name "Brenda" with "Brown" since Brenda has brown hair. Associating two pieces of new information will help her remember Brenda's name. The client might also associate "Brenda" with the name of a current friend, "Brendan," to help her remember Brenda's name, using association to connect new information with old information. Associations can be made from all sensory modalities (e.g., relating information to a particular smell or sound). An emotional association can also assist in recall.

- *Pegging*: This is when a word is developed from the first letters of things that need to be recalled (e.g., DEEP: D: deep breathing, E: eat right, E: exercise, P: play).

External Strategies

External strategies are tangible things that a client can use to compensate for cognitive impairments. External strategies, in addition to serving as compensatory strategies, can be used as a transitional aid to move to an internal strategy. For example, a client may start out using a written list that outlines the sequential steps for transferring a seedling into the garden. When repetitively practicing the task, the client can be prompted to say the steps aloud and create a visual image of each step as it is spoken, with the goal of eventually getting rid of the list and using the self-talk and imagery techniques to recall the steps involved. In addition to the common external strategies that are reviewed below, there are a variety of commercially available memory aids. The therapist should always remember to fit the aid to the client and not the other way around.

Non-Electronic Aids

When using non-electronic aids, consideration must be given to the placement of the aids to maximize their effectiveness. For example, if a client has to remember to put bills in the mailbox the next morning, a reminder note could be taped at eye level on the door to serve as a reminder when leaving the house. Likewise, if a client needs to remember the sequential steps to perform a task, then the steps should be easily visible in the location in which the task is routinely performed, such as placing written steps to play a game inside the game box.

Memory book: The use of a memory book is a common compensatory strategy to help clients with memory. A memory book is developed by the therapist to meet the needs of the client. The size and form of the book, the number of sections, the labeling of the book, the location where the book is kept, and the information in the book vary depending on the client's needs and abilities. In an inpatient rehabilitation setting, a binder is typically used to make a memory book that contains four tabbed sections

labeled "calendar," "people," "therapy schedule," and "things to do." The calendar section has a copy of the current month. The client crosses off each day to help track the current day, month, and year. The people section is typically made up of two subsections, one titled "therapists" and the other titled "family and friends." A picture of each person the client needs to remember is placed in the appropriate section. Under each picture the person's name and relationship to the client is written to help the client identify and remember people in his/her life. The therapy schedule section contains a printout of the client's therapy schedule for the day. Every morning the client puts in the new schedule and throws away the previous schedule to promote awareness of time and related appointments. The things-to-do section contains sheets of blank or lined paper. It is a place for the client to write down things that s/he needs to remember to do, such as calling his sister after lunch or ask the nursing aid for an extra blanket. After each task is accomplished the client is prompted to strike a line through the item. Training begins by teaching the client what the notebook is, what it's used for, and the sections of the notebook. Training can be done using errorless learning (see the separate chapter on "Errorless Learning") or simple question and answer rehearsal (e.g., "This is your memory notebook. What is this?", "The memory notebook is used to help you remember things. What is the memory notebook used for?", "In the things-to-do section, write down things you want to remember to do. Where do you write down the things you want to remember to do?"). Once the client demonstrates a basic understanding of the notebook, the therapist can then facilitate the use of the notebook during clinical sessions. For example, at the beginning of the therapy session, the therapist reviews the client's schedule with him and provides needed assistance. For example, "Hi John! It's good to see you. Before we get started, can you tell me what therapy you had before me today?" The therapist then assists the client in locating the daily schedule in the notebook and finding the answer. The therapist might additionally ask, "Do you remember what therapy this is? Do you remember my name?" and subsequently prompt the client as needed to use the memory book to find information the client is unable to recall. Following the session, the therapist prompts and assists the client to identify his/her next appointment by looking at the calendar section and reviews the things-to-do section to draw lines through items that have been completed and add new items to the list. Some memory notebooks might also containing a "daily log" section where the therapist and client write down what they did during the therapy session to help the client recall the activities from the day. The amount of assistance or guidance from the therapist will vary depending on the client, but the goal is to facilitate optimal independence. Once the client is able to demonstrate basic use of the notebook, the client is challenged further to utilize the notebook in settings and situations outside of the clinic environment. A client might be asked to write down the name of the place he is going to for community integration training with the therapist, make notes about upcoming appointments, or make notes about what he did over the weekend outside of therapy sessions. Memory books are typically carried by the client in the hand or in a backpack or placed next to client on the wheelchair. Although memory books can be helpful, they can also be potentially bothersome, confusing, and disorienting to the client if they are not properly maintained and designed to fit the lifestyle of the client. For example, if a memory book is not cleaned out, too many pages can accumulate, confusing and disorienting the client further. Also, a large white binder that contains mostly therapy information can become cumbersome to transport and not correlate with the client's post-therapy lifestyle. The client might even perceive the large, white memory book as embarrassing or it may be difficult to carry when trying to carry a bag of groceries and use a cane at the same time. Consequently, memory books are often changed when planning for discharge from a large white binder to a small organizer. The therapist also helps the client identify adaptations for managing the book, such as carrying it in a thin backpack. Changing the style and layout of a memory book can be problematic for some clients who may have difficulty generalizing information from one type of memory book to another. Therefore, the therapist who designs the memory book should be keenly aware of this issue and design a book that can transition from one setting to another with minimal changes.

Signs and Post-It notes: Signs or Post-It Notes can be posted in key locations to help the client remember specific things that occur in common locations. For example, on the inside of the front door

a sign could be posted saying, "Remember your keys!" Too many signs however, can cause the environment to be cluttered and can become disorienting and confusing to the client.

Picture cards: A sequential set of picture cards can guide the client through a particular task. For example, if a client has difficulty remembering how to fill the birdfeeder, a laminated sheet of paper with pictures depicting the steps involved can be placed near the bird feeder. The sheet might have a picture of the birdseed in the client's outdoor shed (as a cue to remember where the birdseed is kept), followed by another picture that shows a hand unscrewing the lid on the bird feeder (as a cue to remember how to open the bird feeder). The picture of the client walking with the birdseed in his hand back towards the shed might be the last picture (as a cue to remember to put the birdseed back in the shed). Whenever possible, the pictures should reflect the actual people, equipment, and environment of the client to avoid the added challenge of association.

Lists: Lists can be a helpful memory aid if they are placed in easily accessible and visible locations. Lists can be posted on the refrigerator (e.g., keep a running list on the refrigerator of food items that need to be purchased), in a computer (e.g., keep a list of items that need to be packed when going to the shore house, camping, or a simple day trip), in a smart phone, or any other key locations where they will serve as a trigger, such as on the dining room table.

Calendars: Paper calendars, such as wall calendars or small pocketbook calendars, can be helpful for those who have difficulty using electronic calendars.

Electronic Aids

Electronic aids are used for a set of external strategies. Devices to consider include the following:

Recorders: A small recorder can be a helpful memory aid. The client can record bits of information that need to be recalled and have pre-establish set times to review the recordings, for example, lunchtime and dinnertime. The client can write down recorded information and then attend to the information as appropriate (e.g., transfer notations onto the wall calendar in the kitchen or cross off items that are completed). Recorders can also be used to capture verbal instructions and can be played back to remember the instructions.

Alarms and calendars: Watches with alarms (or alarms on smart phones) can be preset for multiple times during the day and serve as a helpful reminder for daily activities and appointments as varied as taking medicine, performing weight shifts, trying to use the bathroom, calling a sister, and engaging in 20 minutes of leisure time physical activity. In addition to setting separate alarms, alarms can set for tasks that are placed on the calendar, such as setting an alarm to go off one hour before a scheduled appointment as a reminder to get ready.

iPads: The use of iPads and other, similar devices as a tool to address cognitive impairments, as well as serve as a compensatory strategy for cognitive deficits, is gaining in popularity. See the Appendix for specific information about the use of iPads in therapy.

Specific Approaches

Errorless learning: Trial-and-error learning can be counterproductive to learning, as clients may perseverate on misinformation. The goal of errorless learning is to teach the client only the correct information to minimize the chances of error and subsequently decrease the chances of learning and perseverating on wrong information. In errorless learning, the therapist provides the client with a true statement and then asks the client a simple question about the statement. For example, the therapist might state, "Today is Monday" and then immediately ask the client, "What day is today?" The therapist might also show the client a specific task and then ask the client to repeat it. For example, the therapist might demonstrate how to use a gardening shovel and then provide the client with the gardening shovel and ask him to repeat the movement. The therapist might also chose to use a more complex method by verbalizing a statement or demonstrating a task with a condition and then asking the client what he would do under that specific condition. For example, "When you meet someone new, introduce yourself. What should you do when you meet someone new?" or "When walking over uneven surfaces, make sure the cane is planted firmly on the ground. What should you do with the cane when you are walking on uneven surfaces?"

Spaced retrieval: Spaced retrieval is the same as errorless learning except the client is challenged to remember the information or task for a longer period of time, for example after a one-minute delay. Prior to implementing spaced retrieval, the therapist needs to make sure that the client is successful with the errorless learning by being able to recall the information with no delay.

Chaining: Clients learn how to complete a sequential task by breaking down the complex task into single specific steps. Each step is learned in a sequenced manner using procedural memory. The client may not have the ability to recognize that all of the sequence steps when put together result in a meaningful task, but are rather learning how individual tasks chain together with each step serving as a cue to begin the next step. There are two types of chaining:

- *Forward chaining*: The therapist introduces the first step (e.g., turn on the hose). Once the client is able to perform the first step, the second step is introduced and paired with the first step, creating a "chain" (e.g., turn on the hose, walk the hose to the garden). Once the client is able to perform to first and second step, the third step is added to the chain (e.g., turn on the hose, walk the hose to the garden, water the tomato plant), then a forth step (e.g., turn on the hose, walk the hose to the garden, water the tomato plant, walk the hose back to the hose bib), a fifth step (e.g., turn on the hose, walk the hose to the garden, water the tomato plant, walk the hose back to hose bib, turn off the hose), and so on until all of the steps have been successfully learned in the chained sequential order. When teaching each step and chaining each step together, the therapist uses a variety of teaching methods including cueing, modeling, picture cards, etc., depending on the needs of the client.
- *Backward chaining*: The therapist demonstrates all of the sequenced steps in the task (e.g., turn on the hose, walk the hose to the garden, water the tomato plant, walk the hose back to hose bib, turn off the hose). After demonstrating the entire task, the therapist omits the last step and guides the client in performing the last step. This continues until the client completes all of the steps. For example, in a five-step task, the therapist will demonstrate steps one through four and then guide the client in completing step five. After the client is successful in completing step five with the therapist demonstrating steps one through

four, the therapist completes steps one through three and guides the client in completing the last two steps. Once the client is able to complete steps four and five after the therapist completes steps one through three, the therapist completes steps one and two and guides the client in completing the last three steps. This process continues until the client is successfully able to complete (chain) all five steps. When guiding the client through each step, the therapist uses a variety of teaching methods, including cueing, modeling, picture cards, etc., to facilitate learning.

Other Problem-Specific Interventions

Group interactive structured treatment (GIST) for social competence: GIST consists of the use of a structured small group format to work on social skills. There are six sequential steps in each group session: review of homework, a brief introduction of the topic and target skill to be addressed, a guided discussion, small group practice with therapist modeling and/or role-play, group problem solving and feedback, and a homework assignment. Topics might include basic communication skills, initiation of conversation, maintaining conversation, coping with conflicts, maintaining personal space, etc. The use of video recording can be helpful to review performance and provide feedback. Community outings also provide opportunities for real-life practice. Group work helps to facilitate support because it shows the client s/he is not the only one who has difficulties with social competence due to cognitive impairments. Positive social reinforcement helps build confidence and motivation for continued practice. Each client sets individual goals with specific steps to achieve each goal. This is done with the therapist in a collaborative fashion to emphasize self-awareness, self-monitoring, and self-assessment.

Emotional perception training: Secondary to cognitive deficits, clients may have difficulty reading the emotions of others in facial expressions, nonverbal language, or tone of voice. This impairs the formation and maintenance of social relationships. Training often begins with discussion and knowledge about emotions associated with particular situations as varied as giving a speech, breaking a favorite item, talking with someone after a loved one dies. The client is then asked to judge a person's emotions based on simple line drawings. This then progresses

to identifying a person's emotions in a photograph and then video recordings. The video recordings begin with visual stimuli only (no sound), then with visual stimuli and sound, and then with visual stimuli, sound, and context of the situation. This challenges the client to attune to other contextual stimuli that help in figuring out the person's emotions. The use of errorless learning can be helpful if the client doesn't know the emotion or states that s/he doesn't know. The therapist would then tell the client the person's emotion, avoiding problems with getting confused by incorrect guesses.

Limb activation strategies: Strategies include:

- *Spatio-motor strategies*: These promote awareness and subsequently promote return of motor abilities. The client is encouraged to look at and move the involved upper extremity before and during visual training tasks. For example, prior to scanning the left side of the environment and during the scanning activity, as appropriate, the client is encouraged to move the left hand (e.g., make a fist and then stretch out fingers, tap table), left arm (e.g., elbow flexion and extension), and left shoulder (e.g., shoulder shrugs).

- *Visuo-spatial-motor strategies*: This strategy combines visual scanning and motor strategies into a single task, which promotes awareness of the limb and subsequently promotes return of motor abilities. For example, when completing a tabletop task, the client places his left hand on the table at the far left end of the task (e.g., at the far left margin of the book). When scanning to the left the client verbalizes, "Scan to the hand." When said repeatedly, the verbalization can trigger the incorporation of the left hand into the task, as well as the scanning behavior. The best activities to use are those that inherently require scanning, such as reading, using a computer keyboard, coloring, copying, writing, drawing, puzzles, scanning the hallway for signs, etc.

- *Imagined limb activation*: If the client has no movement in the limb, the client is prompted to imagine movement of the limb. The client is first directed to perform a number of movements with the unaffected limb (e.g., wiggle fingers, make a fist, open hand, rotate wrist, flex wrist, bend elbow, raise arms, shrug shoulders) and then directed to repeat the movements again. Following this, the client is asked to imagine these movements in the unaffected limb and then to imagine these movements in the affected limb. Visualization of limb movement helps to stimulate attention to the limb, which can aid in regaining motor function. Recreational therapists might consider using movements that relate to the specific activity instead of standard movements. For example, if the task is drawing a picture, the client could be instructed to perform task-related movements, such as picking up the pencil, moving the wrist to draw a circle, and putting the pencil back in a box on the far right, repeating this two times. Then ask the client to imagine these movement again, first with the unaffected upper extremity and then with the affected upper extremity.

Predict-perform procedure: This is used to help clients identify issues or impairments that are impacting performance. The client is presented with a task, such as open and read email. Prior to engaging in the task, the client is asked to predict his/her performance on the task and identify possible problems and solutions. The client then engages in the task and is subsequently asked to self-evaluate the performance. Following the client's self-evaluation, the therapist's observations are shared with the client, and a discussion ensues with the goal of identifying strengths and weaknesses, as well as strategies to improve performance.

Neglect protocols: Clients with right cerebral hemisphere lesions often have left neglect, also referred to as hemispatial neglect or unilateral neglect. This is when the brain does not recognize stimuli on the left side of the body despite have intact visual ability. Therapists can utilize

- *Anchoring*: This is a verbal or visual cue that begins at the extreme left side of the page or table to indicate the starting position — e.g., placing a strip of red construction paper at the far left side of the table, providing a verbal cue to the client to find the extreme left edge of the book. Improvement is noted when the anchor is used by the client.
- *Pacing*: Despite the use of an anchor, clients still have a tendency to drift their attention to the right side of the environment. To minimize this, the client is taught to slow down the pace of the activity to increase attention to the total environ-

ment (e.g., decreasing activity speed, reciting the steps of the activity out loud).

- *Density*: Awareness of stimuli decreases when items are closer together, therefore spacing items further apart and increasing the size of the stimuli can aid in decreasing errors.
- *Information load*: The more items that need to be located in the environment, the more challenging the task. Therefore minimizing the number of items will help improve performance.
- *Performance prediction and feedback*: The therapist asks the client to predict his/her performance on the task, as well as provide feedback on performance after the task. This helps increase the client's awareness and attention to the task.
- *The lighthouse technique*: The client is taught to visualize himself/herself as a lighthouse that illuminates the environment by scanning side to side. The client turns his/her head to the far right and then slowly turns the head to the far left to scan the entire environment. The visual imagery of the lighthouse can serve as a cue to trigger the scanning behavior.

Time pressure management training: Time pressure management is used when a client has difficulty processing information and consequently feels overwhelmed with resulting difficulty in performing tasks. To use this method, the client must recognize that his/her mental processing is impaired. Consequently, helping the client to recognize the impairment and realize its effect on functional task performance may need to be addressed before teaching this method. It begins by identifying a specific problem (e.g., difficulty communicating needs when under pressure). The client is then taught how to avoid or minimize such situations using strategic and tactical planning. Strategic planning consists of developing a plan prior to engaging in the challenging task to minimize the problems (e.g., bringing paper and pen to write down thoughts when verbalizations fail; considering alternative ways to convey needs, such as gesturing and demonstrating, if verbalizations fail). Tactical planning consists of moment-to-moment decisions based on the situation (e.g., allowing the next person in line to go ahead of the client while he gains his thoughts, taking slow deep breaths to decrease feelings of anxiety). Once strategies are identified and practiced in a safe clinical environment, the client is challenged to apply the strategies to more difficult real-life settings and situations.

Caregiver Education and Training

Regardless of the strategies utilized, it is imperative that caregivers are educated and trained on how to provide the client with the assistance needed to continue to facilitate continued improvement post discharge through cognitive rehabilitation. Changes in the brain can occur over an extended period of time. The potential for further recovery is still there. This is why it is important to educate caregivers about the function of the brain and their role in assisting the client with further recovery. Failure to educate caregivers on this process can limit the client's recovery. Additionally, education helps the caregiver understand the importance of activity beyond the psychosocial benefits, thus promoting greater carryover of activities after discharge and greater assistance from the caregivers in helping the client to participate in activities.

Outcomes and Documentation

Haskins (2012) recommends that treatment objectives related to cognitive rehabilitation include the (1) type of task (impairment-oriented tasks such as divided attention tasks or memory tasks or function-oriented tasks such as specific leisure or community tasks), (2) complexity of task (simple, moderate, complex), (3) level of cueing or assistance needed (none, mild, moderate, maximum), (4) type of strategy employed (the specific internal or external strategy utilized), and (5) measure of success (e.g., percent right, speed, accuracy). For example, "Pt to perform simple (2) gardening task (1) utilizing self-instructional strategy (3) with minimal verbal cues and a sequential step list (4) with 100% accuracy (5)."

Outcomes can also be documented by noting the changes in ICF codes between initial assessment and the current point in treatment.

Resources

For more cognitive rehabilitation techniques, refer to Haskins (2012) in the reference list, as well as the following text: Gillen, G. (2009). *Cognitive and perceptual rehabilitation: Optimizing function.* St. Louis, MO: Mosby Elsevier.

Appendix: iPad Issues, Resources, and Apps

This appendix provides some basic information regarding the use of the iPad in therapy, along with resources and apps that could be helpful with cognitive rehabilitation. A web search will give you the latest information about the item. iPad-specific information can be found at support.apple.com

This is not meant to be an exhaustive list. Other electronic devices may also be used, especially if the client is more familiar with their functioning.

Medical Concerns

The iPad has a magnet in it, so it can't be used near someone who has a shunt or pacemaker because it can change the settings.

HIPAA Concerns

Skype is not HIPAA compliant, as it is easily hacked. Facetime is HIPAA compliant. If talking about client info, use Facetime.

Keeping the iPad safe and clean

- Big Grips
- Seal Shield
- Eva iPad cases
- Large Ziploc freezer bag, make slit for speaker, protects from drool and goop.
- Mobile Cloth: Cloth to clean iPhones, iPads, computer screens, etc. Removes 98% of bacteria and germs. Great product when sharing devices among clients. Cloth is washable.

iPad Accessibility Features

- Zoom
- Large text
- Invert colors
- Speak selection
- Assistive touch

iPad Adaptations

- PVC transformer for the iPad
- How to make an iPad stand (video) (www.iod.unh.edu/PriorityAreas/assistivetechnology/default.aspx)

- Bubcap: Prevents hitting home button by accident
- Pererro: Using a button to scan through iPad
- iPad holder: Get a piece of plastic the width of the iPad. Stick the piece of plastic onto the back of the iPad using "u-glue dashes" (strong glue dots, comes on a roll). Cut two pieces of industrial Velcro about 2" by 2" (self-stick, hook side). Stick each piece to the outer edges of the piece of plastic. Cut a piece of Velstretch (stretchy Velcro) the length of the iPad, stick a piece of 2" by 2" industrial Velcro on the end of the Velstretch (loop side). Press the loop pieces to the hook pieces. Slide palm of hand through the strap to hold iPad.

Mounting iPad

- Mountn Mover
- Ram Mounts
- Modular Hose (Loc Line)
- GripGo: Very inexpensive (about $15). Think about how to use this creatively, such as clamp it onto a table or suction it to a computer monitor or onto a wheelchair laptop tray, etc.

Keyboard

- Big Keys
- iKeyboard: A tactile overlay for the iPad keyboard. Provides tactile sensation for preciseness of touching keyboard keys.

Reminder and Scheduling

- ReQall
- Nudge: Can pair it with a sound, in case someone has difficulty reading but can remember associations.
- VoCal: Can make a voice reminder with your own voice; good for those who have vision or reading problems.
- First Then Visual Scheduler: Add your own pictures to create a "schedule" for the day, along with voice reminder and text.
- Cozi
- iPrompts Pro
- "Forgetful" app: Times videos to play on your iPhone or iPad at chosen times (e.g., "Time to feed the cat" with a video showing where the cat food is stored).

- Epil: Vibrating watch reminder (but could also just set an alarm on the iPad or iPhone).
- Pebble: For people who put down the iPad or iPhone and forget where it is, consider having them wear a Pebble watch instead to perform some of the same tasks as an iPad.

Vital signs

- Blood Pressure app: BP cuffs that plug into the iPad/iPhone.
- Instant Heart Rate app: Measures heart rate.

Adaptations for functional limitations

- Taking pictures of hard to see areas. Attach the iPhone to a Swiffer with a rubber band, place it on video mode, and video record the hard to see areas (e.g., backside, underside of residual limb). Can also take a screen shot from the video and then send the picture to a healthcare provider for guidance or help.

Finding items (Search for "Bluetooth finders" for more)

- Pocket Finder
- Stick and Find
- Chipolo

Behavior Tracking

- Behavior Tracker Pro
- ABC Data Pro

Task transitioning

- Time Timer app: Helps with transitioning, circle gets smaller and smaller to show time left.

Communication/speech

- Take pictures of common items and tasks. Place them in an associated picture album in the iPad.
- Pictello: Create visual stories and talking books, e.g., share your vacation. Can also be used to create social stories.
- Sonic Pics: Turns pictures into a narrated slide show.
- PhotoTell: Narrative with each picture.
- Blurb Mobile
- Scene Speak
- Abilipad
- iMean: Letter board.
- Touch Chat
- Prologuo2go

- Sonoflex
- Speak It: Can store phrases.
- Assistive Chat
- Phrase Board
- Sounding Board
- My Talk Tools

Writing

- iWordq: Word prediction.

Spelling

- Chicktionary: Game.
- Spellboard: Practice.

Reading (Audio books/text to speech)

- Learning Ally
- Voice Dream: Converts to different languages.

Hearing

- UHear: Screening.
- EARs: Turns iPad into a hearing aid.

Sensory Processing and Self-Regulation Apps

- Pinterest site (www.pinterest.com/csleynse/apps-for-sensory-processing-self-regulation/)
- Teaching new skills
- Educreations
- Show Me Interactive Whiteboard
- Teaching skills from the person's point of view: Put a helmet on your head. Attach the iPad or iPhone to the helmet with Velcro and/or u-glue. Open the video app and begin recording. Provide verbal directions as you complete the task. When you're done, stop recording. You now have a video from the "do-er's" point of view which can be very helpful when teaching someone a new skill, especially if the person is in another location, setting up a "how-to" video on the web, etc.

Memory games

- Monster Hunt: Game.
- Personal Photo Match: Game. Traditional memory card match game, but you can insert your own pictures.

Social Skills/Behavior

- Sosh
- Inside Voices app

Feelings/Relaxation

- Mood Touch
- At Ease: Deep breathing, breath awareness.
- BrainWave
- UZU
- Coy Pond

Physical Abilities

- Dexteria: fine motor skills development
- UP band and Fitbit band: A band that you wear on your wrist that records data to help you live an optimal healthy lifestyle (activity, mood, sleep, diet, etc.). If working with a client who has the UP band or Fitbit band (or you purchase it and have client wear it during rehab), they can download the free app onto their iPhone and start tracking. Once you have baselines, try interventions to positively impact the baselines (e.g., meditation, decreasing caffeine, etc.). To learn more, go to www.fitbit.com and https://jawbone.com/up.

Daily Living

Using video

- Create video memory books (e.g., how to make cookies, how to attach a piece of adaptive equipment, how to perform a specific wheelchair skill).
- Create your own social skills training videos (e.g., video tape an interaction and discuss).

Cooking

- Photo Cookbook: Could create your own photo cookbooks for clients with pictures and voice-over in picture albums.

Finding a bathroom

- Restroom, bathroom, toilet finder app

Environmental Control

- Switchamajig
- Belkin WeMo

References

Koehler, R., Wilhelm, E., & Shoulson, I. (2011). *Cognitive rehabilitation therapy for traumatic brain injury: Evaluating the evidence*. Washington, DC: The National Academies Press.

Riccio, C. (2007). *Cognitive retraining.* In *Encyclopedia of special education: A reference for the education of children, adolescents, and adults with disabilities and other exceptional individuals.* Retrieved from http://search.credoreference.com.libproxy.temple.edu/content /entry/wileyse/cognitive_retraining/0.

Haskins, E. C. (2012). *Cognitive rehabilitation manual: Translating evidence based recommendations into practice.* American Congress of Rehabilitation Medicine: Reston, VA.

23. Community Participation: Integration, Transitioning, and Inclusion

Heather R. Porter

To begin the discussion of the very complex topic of community participation, we must first define it. The word "community" is often thought of in terms of a place. We think of living in the community as opposed to living in a long-term care facility. This view of community, however, is limiting and does not reflect the broader context of the term. Community is more appropriately defined as a group of people that share a common locality and/or characteristic. There are, in fact, many different types of communities. Some examples of communities include a neighborhood community, a school community, a Native American community, a residential senior living community, a religious community, an online community, a homeless community, a profession-specific community, or a gang community. As individuals, we are commonly a part of many communities. Some we are aware of and others that we participate in without realizing the extent of the community we are in. We also might be viewed by outsiders as being a part of a specific community depending on outward appearance or other variables, such as career or place of residence. We may or may not identify, or even want to identify, with the community others put us in.

As recreational therapists, we are keenly aware of the benefits of being an active member of healthy communities and the importance of building strong communities to support the needs of people. Among the benefits are social interaction, social support, and resources. For example, data from 16,849 adults from the Third National Health and Nutrition Examination Survey and the National Death Index were used to examine the relationship between social isolation and mortality compared to traditional clinical risk factors (Pantell et al., 2013). Findings indicated that socially isolated men and women had worse unadjusted survival curves than less socially isolated individuals. Social isolation predicted mortality for both genders, as did smoking and high blood pressure. Among men, individual social predictors included being unmarried, participating infrequently in religious activities, and lacking club or organization affiliations. Among women, significant predictors were being unmarried, infrequent social contact, and participating infrequently in religious activity. The authors summarized by stating, "The strength of social isolation as a predictor of mortality is similar to that of well-documented clinical risk factors" (p. 2056).

Despite the evidence of the benefits of social interaction with others, it's also important to note that problematic and non-supportive interactions with others can have an adverse effect (Seeman, 1996). Not all communities support the positive growth of their members. Some communities can have very serious negative effects that can result in, among other things, incarceration, death, destruction of property, and damaged emotional health. The degree to which a community supports the healthy growth of its members can vary greatly, and therapists must be careful not to evaluate the health of a community's members based on what the community is perceived as being. For example, a community group that provides activities for children with disabilities might appear to be an excellent community for involvement given the nature of the group. However, it does not guarantee that the community is safe or able to meet the needs of a particular child.

Additionally, being a self-identified member of a community does not always equate with participation. Levels of participation can vary greatly from being a spectator to being actively involved (see

Table 13, later in this chapter), thus influencing the outcomes experienced. For example, a person might belong to a university community. If the person doesn't talk to anyone during class time, goes directly home after class, and doesn't participate in any school activities, the person is getting very few benefits from the community. Another person, however, might actively engage in conversation with others at school and be actively involved in school activities with the corresponding benefits.

Terminology

In the field of recreational therapy, as well as healthcare in general, there are a variety of terms related to community participation:

Community Presence

A person with a disability is physically present in an integrated community setting and occupies the same social space as individuals without disabilities (Thorn et al., 2009).

Community Integration

Although not clearly defined in the literature, community integration is the process of integrating (assimilating, participating, fitting, joining, taking part) into all aspects of community life including employment or productive activity, independent living, and social activity (Sander, Clark, & Pappadis, 2010). It has been described by Thorn and colleagues (2009) as the "full amalgamation of a person's life into the community" (p. 894), and further described by Yasui and Berven (2009) as "a function of various factors (e.g., individual and contextual) [that] involves multiple dimensions (e.g., physical, social, and psychological), [and that] advancement in research in this area should, in turn, contribute to planning and implementation of interventions directed at individual and societal levels, including relevant policymaking" (p. 761).

Community integration is referred to as both an intervention, such as an order for community integration training, and an outcome, such as successful community integration. In clinical practice, it most often refers to helping a client assimilate into his or her real-life environment or community, as well as helping the community assimilate to the individual through the provision of education and training. Since people desire to integrate into a variety of communities, community integration commonly focuses on helping individuals integrate into their everyday environments and communities. This may include their neighborhood community (e.g., shopping centers); recreation, leisure, and play communities (e.g., recreation centers, activity-specific groups); residence communities (e.g., long-term care community); and work or school communities. How to measure successful community integration is often debated, as participation alone doesn't necessarily equal a feeling of connection and belonging within the community. For example, an adolescent with a disability might go to school every day and participate in after-school activities, but emotionally might not feel a sense of connection with others in the school community. Community integration interventions will vary depending on the framework of the community integration model being used. See the Protocols and Processes section of this chapter for specific community integration models and intervention programs for recreational therapy.

Community Reintegration

In clinical practice, the terms community integration and community reintegration are often used synonymously, however there is a slight distinction. The prefix "re" means "back" or "again." Consequently, the term community reintegration implies integration back into a community where the individual was previously integrated. For example, an adult client who was previously integrated into his neighborhood community requires community *reintegration* into the neighborhood community after having a traumatic brain injury. Community reintegration, like community integration, refers to the intervention of integrating into one's community, as well as an outcome of successfully reintegrating.

Transitioning

Transitioning is a process (e.g., moving from one life situation to another life situation), an intervention (e.g., an order for transitional services), and an outcome (e.g., the client successfully transitioned from school life to adult life). In the U.S. educational system, transitioning refers to the process of moving an individual from student life to adult life. The educational system helps students with disabilities develop a transition plan and work toward accomplishing a successful transition.

Transition services are provided by many professionals in the education system, including therapists. The Individuals with Disabilities Education Act (IDEA) defines transition services as "a coordinated set of activities for a child with a disability that is designed to be a results-oriented process, that is focused on improving the academic and functional achievement of a child with a disability to facilitate the child's movement from school to post-school activities, including post-secondary education, vocational education, integrated employment (including supported employment), continuing and adult education, adult services, independent living, or community participation that is based on the individual child's needs, taking into account the child's strengths, preferences, and interests, and includes instruction, related services, community experiences, the development of employment and other post-school adult living objectives, and, if appropriate, acquisition of daily living skills and functional vocational evaluation" (U.S. Department of Education, 2007). Transition services must be included in all Individualized Education Plans (IEPs) once the student reaches age 16 and may be included for young students if deemed appropriate by the IEP team (Bateman, 2015). Transition services must include instruction, related services, community experiences, and development of employment and other post-school adult living objectives, as well as daily living skills and functional vocation evaluation if appropriate (Bateman, 2015). Below are examples of each of the five components (Center on Community Living and Careers, 2011):

Instruction: Learn and practice social skills, self-determination, self-advocacy, employability skills, budgeting and money management, anger management, time management, study skills, transportation skills, computer and technology skills, self-management, problem-solving, communication, coping, recreation and leisure skills, decision-making skills, etc. It also entails enrolling in and taking courses that offer instruction, such as SAT prep, parenting, finance, driver's education, CPR or first aid, and babysitting courses, as well as researching instruction-based opportunities related to colleges, career choices, or requirements.

Related services: These are supports that a student might need for accessing more integrated work, education, and living environments. Tasks in this area include exploration of supports beyond high school, identifying potential providers of such services, how to access identified services. Such services might include therapies, assistive technology, orientation and mobility services, audiology services, interpreter services, vehicle modification, service animals, and substance abuse or mental health programs.

Community experiences: These are experiences outside of the school building that contribute to the transition to adult life. Skill training involves activities like practicing shopping skills, using transportation, accessing local community resources, exploring new ways to use leisure time, and learning about dangers of accepting goods or services from strangers. Active participation experiences may include planning and participating in community activities, participating in work or volunteer experiences, touring colleges and apartments, obtaining a driver's license, participating in community recreation centers or extracurricular activities, and taking a community education course.

Development of employment and adult living objectives: These activities focus on the development of work-related behaviors, job seeking and keeping skills, career exploration, skills training, and actual employment in an integrated work setting that pays a competitive wage or at least minimum wage. This area also includes engagement in volunteer work, as it provides important skills and experiences that could lead to integrated employment or supported employment. Some of the activities may include participating in a work-study program, an apprenticeship, or an internship program; applying to vocational rehabilitation services; going on work interviews; participating in community work experiences; practicing completing job applications and interviewing skills; attending career fairs; learning about social security work incentives; researching careers; learning and practicing skills needed to access job search services; and developing a resume, cover letter, and thank you letter. Beyond job-related skills there is a focus on adult living skills, such as banking or renting an apartment. Activities in this component might include exploring college grants, loans, or scholarships; applying for housing assistance; opening a bank account; learning how to personally manage health and fitness; and exploring residential options.

Acquisition of daily living skills, including a functional vocational evaluation: This area focuses on the development of skills related to activities of daily living and the person's ability to complete these tasks in a real-life setting. This might include cooking, operating a washer or dryer, using an ATM machine, meal preparation, grocery shopping, purchasing and caring for clothes, practicing basic self-care, communicating personal information appropriately, managing a daily schedule, banking, learning emergency procedures and phone numbers, taking a class on family planning, learning medication self-management, planning for outings, choosing appropriate clothing, listening to weather forecast and planning accordingly, and demonstrating safety skills in various settings.

It's clear from these definitions that recreational therapy is well suited to provide transition service. However, recreational therapy is often underutilized in the education system, not only in transitional service provision, but also in the school system in general. Recreational therapy is included as a related service in Individuals with Disabilities Education Act of 2004, as can be seen from this definition:

> Related services means transportation and such developmental, corrective, and other supportive services as are required to assist a child with a disability to benefit from special education, and includes speech-language pathology and audiology services, interpreting services, psychological services, physical and occupational therapy, recreation, including therapeutic recreation, early identification and assessment of disabilities in children, counseling services, including rehabilitation counseling, orientation and mobility services, and medical services for diagnostic or evaluation purposes. Related services also include school health and school nurse services, social work services in schools, and parent counseling and training (U.S. Department of Education, ND).

Furthermore, section 11 of IDEA specifically states, "Recreation includes assessment of leisure function, therapeutic recreation services, recreation programs in schools and community agencies, and leisure education" (U.S. Department of Education, ND). Bullock and Johnson (1998), as cited in Hawkins et al. (2012), further note that recreational therapists assist in achieving educational outcomes by performing the following job tasks in education settings:

> (a) assessing functional skills, impairments, and recreation/leisure skills, knowledge, and attitudes; (b) planning appropriate interventions and programs based on assessment findings; (c) conducting leisure education programs to promote successful transition from school to work and life situations; (d) providing resource and consultative assistance to teachers in regular and special education to include leisure education in their curricula; (e) promoting and providing recreation participation in inclusive school and community settings; (f) providing supportive/resource services to special education classroom teachers and resource room teachers who incorporate recreation and play into their curriculum to increase functional skills; and (g) collaborating with multiple disciplines, professionals, and family members invested in students' education and supportive services. (p. 135)

A review of the literature by Hawkins and colleagues (2012) yielded potential explanations for under-representation of recreational therapy in the school system including poor support of recreation and leisure services by the public school systems; lack of awareness of recreational therapy as a related services in IDEA by recreational therapists, school teachers, administrators, and parents; low advocacy for the inclusion of recreational therapy in the school system by recreational therapists; lack of communication about the benefits and outcomes of recreational therapy in the school system and how such outcomes differ from other services; lack of clear communication about requirements to provide recreational therapy services, such as the need for a CTRS credential; and difficulty in getting related services approved because schools are forced to weigh the necessity of the service with logistics of providing the service. Even if they are aware of the benefits of recreational therapy services, parents who advocate for the services are often required to put significant effort into their struggle to overcome ignorance on the part of the school systems, power differences between school officials and parents, and denial of services by school officials. Recommendations to remediate these challenges include (Hawkins et al., 2012):

- Professional-based recommendations, such as educating school systems, parents, and teachers about recreational therapy; advocating for the inclusion of recreational therapy in the school system by the American Therapeutic Recreation Association; strongly communicating and demonstrating the value of recreational therapy services currently being provided in the school system; and increasing opportunities for recreational therapy students to specialize in child development and education rather than a general education program.

- Education system and policy recommendations, such as ensuring that only properly licensed or certified recreational therapists are employed; including the specific requirement of the CTRS credential for recreational therapists in IDEA so schools are held accountable for hiring appropriately qualified recreational therapists; including recreational therapists in teacher training programs to increase knowledge of services and collaboration; seeking out recreational therapy educators and/or recreational therapists practicing in other schools to educate the school system on the benefits and outcomes of recreational therapy services; and advocating for the term "therapeutic recreation" to be changed to "recreational therapy" within IDEA to more accurately reflect services provided.

Although transition services are strongly associated with the education system, transitions occur frequently throughout life. We may transition from one life stage to another, as when we move through childhood, adolescence, adulthood, and old age. We may transition from one environment to another, as a child transitioning from being at home with a parent all day to being at full-day pre-school or from being a free member of society to being incarcerated. We also transition from one situation to another, such as from being single to being married, from being unpopular to being popular, from not having a disability to having a disability, from being in a relationship to not being in a relationship, or from having no children to having children. Some of these transitions are a normal and expected part of life that brings a sense of joy and excitement, whereas other transitions, even if

normal and expected, can be overwhelming and difficult to negotiate. Consequently, as therapists, we should be continually aware of transitions that clients are experiencing and incorporate transitional needs into the treatment plan. Recreational therapists should also recognize that part of community integration and reintegration requires transitioning.

Inclusion

Inclusion is defined by the National Council for Therapeutic Recreation Certification (NCTRC) as "a planning process in which individuals have the opportunity to participate fully in all community activities offered to people without disabilities. Inclusion requires providing the necessary framework for adaptations, accommodations, and supports so that individuals can benefit equally from an experience" (National Council for Therapeutic Recreation Certification, 2015).

Inclusion could be considered an intervention, as in provision of inclusion training for a facility or program. It is most often referred to as an ideal, a goal, or optimal state, such as providing an inclusive recreation program, working towards inclusion of individuals with disabilities, or marketing a service as being inclusive. Recreational therapists provide education and training to community programs to facilitate inclusion, teach clients about their rights related to inclusion (see the Disability Rights chapter), form partnerships with community programs to foster inclusive practices (see the Protocols and Processes section of this chapter for examples), and assist clients in integrating and transitioning into inclusive settings. Community inclusion "encompasses a greater emphasis on community connectedness" (Thorn et al., 2009, p. 894). Therefore, the provision of inclusive programming alone does not get to the heart of the true meaning of inclusion. At the most basic level, individuals should feel accepted by others, play a meaningful role, have something to contribute, and feel a sense of belonging. Consequently, in addition to developing a strong framework with adaptations and accommodations that support inclusion, attention also needs to be given to the interpersonal nature and facilitation of the program.

It is also important to note that, although inclusion is viewed in a very positive light, always participating in an inclusive setting might not be desired by the client or family. For example, a mother who has a child with autism might prefer participating in a swimming class that is only for children with autism, as it provides the mother with a support group and lessens anxiety about having to explain her child's behavior. Not to say that everyone thinks this way, but it is important for therapists to understand the needs and desires of the client and family. Therapists should not impose their ideals on their clients.

General guidelines for developing an inclusive program can be found in the *Guidelines for Disability Inclusion in Physical Activity, Nutrition, and Obesity Programs and Policies: Implementation Manual* (Kraus & Jans, 2014) developed for the National Center on Health, Physical Activity, and Disability (NCHPAD) through a Centers for Disease Control and Prevention (CDC) grant. See the Resources section in this chapter for information on obtaining a free copy of the manual.

The principal investigator in the development of this manual was James Rimmer, a leading voice on physical activity and disability and highly recognized researcher. The manual provides nine guidelines to assist in the updating of community health programs and policies to allow them to be inclusive of the needs of people with disabilities. These guidelines were generated based on previously recommended guidelines and structure input and review from a panel of national experts (p. 2).

1. Objectives include people with disabilities: Program objectives should explicitly and unambiguously state that the target population includes people with a range of different disabilities (cognitive, intellectual or other developmental disabilities, mobility, visual, hearing, and mental health disabilities).

2. Involvement of people with disabilities in development, implementation, and evaluation: Program development, implementation, and evaluation should include input from people with a range of different disabilities and their representatives (e.g., community members or other experts with disabilities, potential participants with disabilities and their family members, personal assistants, and caregivers).

3. Program accessibility: Programs should be accessible to people with disabilities and other users socially, behaviorally, programmatically, in communication, and in the physical environment.

4. Accommodations for participants: Programs should address individual needs of participants with disabilities through accommodations that are specifically tailored to those needs.

5. Outreach and communication to people with disabilities: Programs should use a variety of accessible methods to outreach and promote the program(s) to people with disabilities.

6. Cost considerations and feasibility: Programs should address potential resource implications of inclusion (including staffing, training, equipment, and other resources needed to promote inclusion).

7. Affordability: Programs should be affordable to people with disabilities and their families, personal assistants, and caregivers.

8. Process evaluation: Programs should implement process evaluation (with transparent monitoring, accountability, and quality assurance) that includes feedback from people with disabilities and family members, personal assistants, caregivers, or other representatives, and a process for making changes based on feedback.

9. Outcomes evaluation: Programs should collect outcomes data, using multiple disability-appropriate measures.

Recreational therapists can utilize the above guidelines in several ways: (1) as a guide to evaluate current inclusive practices of an agency or program as it relates to client needs; (2) as a guide to educate community facilities that offer play, recreation, and leisure opportunities about the process of evaluating the provision of inclusive services; and (3) to determine areas where intervention is needed within a particular program and then further assess the specific needs or issues related to the identified area, with the provision of subsequent education, training, and counseling services to agency staff to remediate identified inclusion deficits.

Indications

Community integration has been incorporated into disability-related public policy and legislation and is at the core of deinstitutionalization efforts (Yasui & Berven, 2009). It is also "frequently referred to as the ultimate goal of rehabilitation for individuals with a variety of disabling conditions" (Yasui & Berven, 2009, p. 761). Rehabilitation, however, goes beyond the typical inpatient and outpatient services that many people associate the term. Kreutzer and Wehman (1990) note, "The rehabilitation process must be concerned with capacities to engage in education, vocation, recreation, social interaction, and community activities. For this reason, the rehabilitation process … extends beyond the intensive care unit and the inpatient rehabilitation unit into facilities and programs whose focus is on teaching the necessary skills to both the … survivor and his or her family in order to achieve optimal community integration" (p. xi).

Community integration is also not a process, intervention, and/or outcome only for individuals with diagnosed disabilities. Other people without a formal diagnosis can benefit as well when difficulties are experienced integrating, reintegrating, or transitioning into a community. For example, approximately 44% of military service members and veterans report a range of difficulties readjusting to civilian life (Committee on the Assessment and Readjustment Needs of Military Personnel, Veterans, and Their Families, 2013).

If community integration is not successful, it could exacerbate other problems. For example, a review of the literature by Crocker and colleagues (2014) found that difficulty with community integration is associated with worse overall mental health (PTSD, anxiety, depression, alcohol and substance abuse, increased rate of suicide, homelessness) impacting self-care, employment, education, relationships, finances, marriages, and home, civic, and community life. Consequently, community integration should be considered and promoted in non-disabled populations, as well, to prevent health conditions and related complications. Some possible clients include community dwelling older adults who are lonely, a shy student in the classroom who is having trouble making friends, or a parent who has become socially isolated because she is taking care of a child with a disability. Community participation has been frequently studied in the literature as it relates to other variables, such as impairment and quality of life. It has also been incorporated into health and wellness models, including the ICF. To only consider community integration, inclusion, and transitioning for those with diagnosed health conditions is an injustice that should be featured more in the literature.

Contraindications

Contraindications to community integration, transitioning, and inclusion are not clearly outlined in the literature. However, there are a variety of factors to consider that could potentially contraindicate integration, transitioning, or inclusion interventions for certain environments where harm could come to the client. These include cases where the client is a flight risk, the environment triggers extreme panic attacks, or the hot temperature of the location is contraindicated for the client due to a heat-sensitive diagnosis. Consequently, therapists must have a full understanding of the client's medical history, precautions, and parameters, as well as obtaining the appropriate clearances and orders.

Negative effects could also be experienced if a client is not ready for integration, transitioning, or inclusion, or if the client prefers to participate in more segregated environments. For example, a client who sustained a recent spinal cord injury might not be emotionally ready to integrate back into the sports community, or a mother of a young child with autism might not want to participate in an inclusive martial arts program, but prefers to participate in a special martial arts program for children with autism. Consequently, therapists need to have a full understanding of the client's needs and preferences.

Loss of opportunity also presents a risk of harm to clients. Therapists need to ensure that the client possesses the skills and resources (or that resources are available) to support continued integration, transitioning, and/or inclusion when treatment ends. Consequently, therapists must possess a full understanding of client-specific intrapersonal, interpersonal, and structural facilitators and barriers, as obtained through a detailed and comprehensive activity and task analysis, to ensure the safety of the client, as well as maximize the likelihood of continued participation and positive outcomes. For example:

- Are supports in place to foster continued and successful participation? For example: Is there support from caregivers to make sure the client gets to the bus on time? Do the activity program leaders have the skills and knowledge to provide for and adapt to the needs of the client?
- Does the client's skill level at discharge from integration or transitioning services match that which is required for continued and successful

participation? For example, if a client needs physical assistance for a task or cueing for a behavior, are these challenges highly likely to yield negative outcomes once treatment ends? Has the client developed a feeling of connection and belonging in the community, so emotional and psychological support from the therapist is no longer needed?

- Does the client possess the resources necessary to sustain participation, including a strong social support network, money, and reliable transportation?

Protocols and Processes

As reviewed earlier in the chapter, the terms community integration, transitioning, and inclusion, do not have standard and universal definitions. In the literature the terms are sometimes used synonymously. Trying to separate interventions by these categories also poses a challenge, because one could argue that interventions could be a blend of approaches. For example, interventions aimed at improving a youth's "transition" from school life to community life also involves strengthening the youth's community integration skills in new situations and/or community reintegration skills into prior life situations that may have been discarded due to challenges. Consequently, when reading the material that follows, please pay more attention to the processes, techniques, and outcomes than to the specific words used to describe the treatment used to improve community participation.

Models

Community integration, inclusion, and transitioning are complex and multi-dimensional constructs. Consequently, successful community integration, transitioning, and inclusion can be viewed from various perspectives. This informs the type of model chosen to serve as a framework for services provided.

A review of the literature by Yasui and Berven (2009) found three overarching community integration models:

Functional independence model: Community integration is achieved if the client is able to demonstrate functional independence in environments that are outside of the treatment setting. Measures related to this model include the *Reintegration to Normal*

Living Index (RNL Index) and the *Community Integration Questionnaire* (CIQ).

Acculturation model: Community integration is achieved if the client's unique characteristics are recognized and supported by the larger community and the client is actively involved in the larger community. A measure related to this model is the *Assimilation, Integration, Marginalization, Segregation Interview* (AIMS). Buell (2003) provides a framework for the acculturation perspective related to individuals with developmental disabilities. The framework asks two questions: (1) Is it considered to be of value to recognize and support the unique characteristics of persons with developmental disability? and (2) Is it considered valuable for persons with developmental disability to maintain relationships with others groups? If the answer is yes to both questions, then integration results. As Buell (2003) says, "The smaller group wishes to maintain cultural identity and characteristics while maintaining positive relations with the dominant culture" (p. 224). If the answer to both questions is no, then marginalization is present. "The smaller group's distinctiveness (cultural identity) is not valued or retained, and therefore becomes confused, and maintaining relations with the dominant culture is not valued or sought and is therefore ambiguous" (p. 224). If it is considered valuable to recognize and support the person's unique characteristics, but the individual doesn't value relationships with other groups, then segregation occurs. "The smaller group wishes to maintain their cultural identity and distinctive characteristics independent of relations with the larger group" (p. 224). If the opposite occurs (it is not considered valuable to recognize and support the person's individual characteristics, but the person values relationships with other groups), then assimilation occurs. "The smaller group minimizes distinctiveness and shares positive relationships with the dominant group" (p. 224).

Normalization model: Community integration is successful if individuals with disabilities have access to everyday living conditions that are as close as possible to the regular circumstances and way of life of the society. Measures related to this model include the *Program Analysis of Service Systems' Implementation of Normalization Goals* (PASSING), the *Subjective Index of Physical and Social Outcomes* (SIPSO), the *Community Integration Measure*, and the *Participation Objective, Participation Subjective* (POPS).

Only the acculturation model takes into consideration the client's perspective of successful community integration. A person can function independently in the community (functional independence model), value her own unique disability characteristics and that of the larger community (acculturation model), and have access to normative community living conditions (normalization model), but that doesn't mean the person actually *feels* integrated into the community. In an attempt to understand community integration from the person's perspective, McColl and colleagues (1998) conducted a qualitative study, consisting of 116 interviews with people with moderate to severe brain injuries, resulting in the identification of common themes related to successful community integration, commonly referred to as *McColl's Nine Themes of Community Integration*:

1. *Conformity*: Knowledge of how to, and ability to, conform with individuals in a community.
2. *Acceptance*: Perception of being accepted by a community in which the person seeks to be integrated.
3. *Orientation*: Knowing one's way around and feeling oriented to the community.
4. *Close relationships*: Ability to develop and maintain relationships with whom the person cares about, such as a spouse or parents.
5. *Diffuse relationships*: Ability to develop and maintain relationships with individuals seen on a daily basis (such as store employees or bus drivers) that are not characterized by closeness, reciprocity, mutuality, or intimacy.
6. *Productivity*: Being able to make a contribution, have a sense of purpose, have daily structure, and receive economic rewards and respect from others through education, employment, and/or volunteer work.
7. *Leisure*: Participation in leisure opportunities within the community.
8. *Independence*: Being able to have autonomy in decision-making and being independent in the ability to complete tasks.
9. *Living situation*: Living at a place that allows for autonomy, living independently (not in a facility or institution), and having control over one's living situation.

Based on these themes, Passmore (2012) suggested six potential recreational therapy treatment areas: (1) community barriers, such as perceived competency and ability to overcome personal and environmental barriers; (2) perception of opportunities for participation in the community, (3) functional skills that directly relate to community participation, such as mobility, self-esteem, and social skills; (4) perception of engagement and participation with people in the community who have and do not have a disability; (5) perception of quality of life, and (6) perception of success in leisure and other functional areas.

Additional literature highlights the need to view community integration from a blended approach. Wong and Solomon (2002) conducted a review of the literature to identify factors that influence community integration for individuals with psychiatric conditions. From the review, they identified three key dimensions of community integration, which they termed the *Community Integration Model for Individuals with Psychiatric Conditions*:

Physical integration: "The extent to which an individual spends time, participates in activities, and uses goods and services in the community outside his/her home or facility in a self-initiated manner" (p. 18).

Social integration: An interactional dimension: "The extent to which an individual engages in social interactions with community members that are culturally normative both in quantity and quality, and that take place within normative contexts" (p. 18) and social network dimension: "The extent to which an individual's social network reflects adequate size and multiplicity of social roles and the degree to which social relationships reflect positive support and reciprocity, as opposed to stress and dependency" (p. 19).

Psychological integration: "The extent to which an individual perceives membership in his/her community, expresses an emotional connection with neighbors, and believes in his/her ability to fulfill needs through neighbors, while exercising influence in the community" (p. 19).

The authors state that the model is based on an ecosystems perspective, where interdependence and interrelatedness of the three components influence community integration.

There are also discipline specific models for community integration, such as the *Ecological Model of Community-Focused Therapeutic Recreation and Life Skills*. King, Curran, and McPherson (2012) note that "community-based therapeutic recreation initiatives are on the increase because of a shift from institutional to community-based care, growing awareness of the importance of promoting health and wellness, a broadened view of health, and recognition of the importance of involving community members in community development efforts" (p. 235). In response to this shift, the Holland Bloorview Kids Rehabilitation Hospital, Canada's largest pediatric rehabilitation teaching hospital developed the Ecological Model of Community-Focused Therapeutic Recreation and Life Skills to guide adaptive recreation program planning and development and to articulate principles and strategies to support community-focused *therapeutic recreation* and *life skills* services. The framework of this model "supports [the] change from [an] individually focused deficit approach to a strength-and resources-based approach aimed at community development and sustainable community services ... [with the goal of] developing *community capacity* to provide inclusive recreation and leisure participation opportunities, thereby encouraging positive community attitudes and social inclusion" (p. 329, italics added, see Table 8 for definitions).

Table 8: Definitions of Services

Therapeutic recreation: Services that aim to encourage leisure awareness and support clients' participation in community-based recreation and leisure programs and activities, including sports, recreation, leisure, and arts activities (King et al., 2012, p. 326).

Life skills: Services that aim to teach children and youth the skills they need to manage life demands and reach their full potential in adulthood, such as problem solving and social skills (King et al., 2012, p. 326).

Community capacity building: Increasing the knowledge and skills of individuals and the community (e.g., their awareness of community resources and problem-solving abilities) through strategies such as direct training, resource sharing, nurturing their strengths and resources, and facilitating

experiential learning through participation in change initiatives (King et al., 2012, p. 326).

The model is based on four principles:

1. *Community-based therapeutic recreation*: Defined as "a resource-based approach to creating more receptive communities, in which service providers [recreational therapists] provide advice, guidance, and material support to members of community organizations, assisting them to provide direct services at a variety of community venues to families" (p. 326). The authors note that communities often lack the resources to provide recreation and leisure experiences for children with disabilities, hence community-based recreational therapy services play a critical role.

2. *Community development*: Defined as "the process of supporting groups in identifying their health issues, planning and acting upon their strategies for social action or social change, and helping them to gain increased self-reliance and decision-making power as a result of their activities" (p. 326). A review of the literature by the authors indicates that community development projects empower clients, families, and local communities to work together to identify sustainable solutions to self-identified issues; increase connections between community members; raise awareness of community assets; encourage collective identification of priorities for action; improve target health outcomes; allow for better reach of the target population and more efficient use of resources; increase local competence and commitment for health action and change; and improve community attitudes towards people with disabilities. This approach focuses on identifying existing community capacities (rather than deficits) and often uses a scaffolding approach where the supportive structure is gradually withdrawn as community capacity builds to foster greater independence.

3. *Community health promotion*: Defined as "an approach that emphasizes the central importance of empowerment and wellness and encourages a broadened view of health encompassing physical well-being, activity participation, and involvement in community life. This approach addresses determinants of health through larger entities,

such as service organization and communities, which affect how people interact and their opportunities for employment and recreation" (p. 326). The authors note that shifting the focus from individual change and curing disease to community-level change and adopting the broader concept of health results in longer-lasting widespread behavior change, as it additionally builds community capacity and knowledge. Additionally, the greater the amount of community involvement, the greater the impact on individual health behavior change. In healthy communities, individuals also have opportunities for meaningful participation and roles in various settings, allowing for enhancement of self-efficacy and resilience to cope with stress, more years of good health, and other rippling effects including functional improvements and quality of life. Community-based participatory strategies assume that the "community members have the best knowledge for improving the health of their community, changes are more likely to occur when the people affected are involved in the change process, and a culturally appropriate holistic approach based on community assets contributes to sustainable and transferable outcomes" (p. 330).

4. *Client/family-centered care*: Defined as "a philosophy and method of service delivery that recognizes people's expertise concerning their own needs, promotes partnerships in achieving change, and supports community members in making ultimate decisions about services in their communities" (p. 326). The authors additionally recognize that all individuals and families are unique and that optimal functioning occurs within a supportive family and community context.

The model consists of four *integrated* pillars that provide a well-rounded community focused therapeutic recreation and life skills strategy for an organization, with the goals of building community capacity, skills transference, and promotion of public health and well-being (King et al., 2012). The pillars are

1. *Community outreach services*: Defined as "the delivery of direct services in the community in partnership with local service providers, drawing

on the specialized resources of rehabilitation centers" (p. 326). This includes the provision of services in a client's home and community that address targeted skills related to meaningful activities, such as playing at the park with friends, using transportation, and engaging in hobbies.

2. *Community development services*: Defined as "services that support community groups to identify their health issues and plan and act upon their strategies for change, thereby helping them to gain increased self-reliance and decision-making power" (p. 326). This involves heightening community service providers' and community members' awareness of disability and integration, assisting communities to identify areas of need, and developing structured recreation programs through consultation and training processes.

3. *Resource sharing*: Defined as "sharing of physical materials, such as adapted recreational equipment, and educational materials, such as videotapes, information pamphlets, and training workshops provided for members of other community organizations" (p. 326). This includes the loan of adapted recreation equipment to empower youth and families to access recreation opportunities, along with the provision of information about recreation and leisure, community consultation and development, and sharing of research.

4. *Center as a community facility*: Defined as "providing an adapted physical space for community programs to occur, along with specialized instruction" (p. 326). This involves providing physical space for community programs to provide recreation opportunities for youth with disabilities at the health center, along with specialized instruction from recreational therapists. This acts as a stepping-stone program to help clients and families gain skills and confidence to experience success, foster self-efficacy, and transition into community programs. This also heightens the public's awareness of the health center, highlights the center's community-focused philosophy, and allows the public to gain a better understanding of people with disabilities if the recreation program integrates individuals with and without disabilities.

Specific Programs and Studies

The rest of this section will look at the protocols and processes for specific programs and studies related to community participation.

Promoting Access, Transition, and Health (PATH)

Northeast Passage is a non-profit organization founded in 1990 whose mission is "to create an environment where individuals with disabilities can enjoy recreation with the same freedom of choice, quality of life, and independence as their non-disabled peers" (Northeast Passage, 2015). Northeast Passage provides a variety of recreational therapy services, including PATH. PATH is delivered by state-licensed recreational therapists and guided by Healthy People 2020 concepts, the World Health Organization's ICF health framework, and Bandura's self-efficacy theory (Wilder et al., 2011). Recreational therapists are reimbursed for services rendered at the competitive regional rate for community-based therapeutic interventions.

The intent of PATH is for participants to engage more fully in the life of their community, to experience greater life quality, and to become aware of and make choices that lead to a healthy lifestyle, thereby decreasing their healthcare utilization due to a decrease in occurrence and/or severity of secondary conditions (Sable & Gravink, 2005).

The PATH program consists of six interventions (Sable & Gravink, 2005):

1. *Individualized fitness program*: Based on client interests and the individual situation, this includes all components leading to active participation, such as identification of resources, development of skills, and community integration training.

2. *Wellness education*: Education varies depending on the needs of the client, but may include nutrition, stress management, weight management, dealing with fatigue, smoking cessation, pain management, and preventing skin breakdowns.

3. *Advanced functional skill development*: Skills such as higher-level transfer skills and mobility are developed through recreation activities and community involvement.

4. *Community reintegration and engagement*: This takes place in the client's home and surrounding communities through exploration of home communities; identification of accessible restaurants, stores, attractions, and places of business; and how to advocate (with and without support) for accessibility when necessary. It translates skills learned in rehab to the clients' home communities.

5. *Network and resource development*: The client learns the processes for finding resources and develops a resource file that includes support agencies, accessibility guidelines, adapted recreation programs, adapted equipment resources, low interest loans, transportation, and state agencies. Clients also explore personal networks for ongoing support in fitness and social and community involvement. To aid in transition, clients have unlimited access to Northeast Passage's call-in resource and referral service, which includes an extensive database of programs, adaptive equipment, and practitioner expertise to assist with problem solving. In certain cases Northeast Passage may recommend the client employ an aide to follow through on long-term fitness and community goals. Northeast Passage provides training for aides, and clients have access to a referral bank of trained peer mentors to discuss issues and experiences pertinent to living with a disability.

6. *Individual and family recreation skill development*: The recreational therapist learns from the assessment about the recreation enjoyed by clients prior to the acquisition of their disabilities, including the identification of specific recreation activities and the value the activities had. The recreational therapist then works with the family to identify adapted or alternative activities, equipment, and resources that return recreation to its role in the family.

The program has been used with adults who have recently sustained a spinal cord injury and are transitioning from rehab to their home community and natural supports (Sable & Bocarro, 2004), individuals living in the community with a variety of physical mobility disabilities, such as spinal cord injury, amputation, multiple sclerosis, muscular dystrophy, cerebral palsy, post-polio syndrome, spina bifida, and stroke (Sable & Gravink, 2005), and veterans (Wilder et al., 2011). Martin's Point Health Care (MPHC), a not-for-profit physician-led organization and third party payer that manages the Uniform Service Family Health Plan for retired military and military families in New Hampshire and Southern Maine, also contracted with Northeast Passage to deliver a pilot test of PATH to approximately 75-100 MPHC clients (Sable & Gravink, 2005).

In the transitioning program for individuals with spinal cord injury (Sable & Bocarro, 2004), the recreational therapist met with the participant three weeks prior to his/her discharge date from rehabilitation to introduce PATH, obtain leisure lifestyle information, and discuss any issues or concerns. One week prior to discharge, the recreational therapist returned to the rehabilitation facility, met with the participant and family, and conducted a chart review and/or met with the inpatient treatment team for clarification of issues or concerns. One-to-one interventions began in the participant's home one to two months post-discharge and lasted for 12 months. During that time, six treatment intervention areas were employed, based on the client assessment and goals. Shortened PATH protocols have also been utilized (Sable & Gravink, 2005) for individuals living in the community with a variety of physical mobility issues. These protocols consist of three to ten home and community visits with a recreational therapist with each session lasting approximately four hours, including drive time.

Qualitative findings from the spinal cord injury study found improved physical health, improved quality of life, improved independence, feelings of less isolation and more confidence, more motivation to sustain healthy behaviors that supported their community participation, re-engagement in recreation and social activities, discovery of new outlets for physical and social engagement, alleviation of boredom and depression, increased physical activity, increased confidence in the client's ability to control the environment, altered attitudes and beliefs about recreation as a health promoting behavior, altered normative beliefs about physically and socially active behavior, and greater sense of control.

To learn more about PATH, visit Northeast Passage at www.nepassage.org.

Therapeutic Recreation Empowering Kids (TREK)

TREK is a school- and community-based recreational therapy program designed to support the educational, developmental, and transitional needs of students with intellectual and developmental disabilities in the K-12 public school system in New Hampshire (Wilder, Craig, & Frye, 2014). The program

currently provides services to 30+ elementary, middle, and high schools in the state. The purpose of TREK's transition-based program is to "prepare students with disabilities in the ... public school system for successful post-school outcomes by facilitating inclusion in the school curriculum, sports and recreation opportunities, after school or summer programs, family and community life, and by providing supports for positive career development and early work experiences" (p. 36). The program aligns with best practices in transition, including "(a) meaningful interagency service collaboration; (b) an individualized, strengths-based, and ecological approach to learning and task performance in a variety of environments; (c) parental/family involvement; (d) participation in community experiences that foster recreational and social skill instruction, self-determination, and independence; and (e) supports for postsecondary education and/or vocation" (p. 37). Each of these is explained in detail in Wilder, Craig, and Frye (2014). Services are delivered by a state-licensed recreational therapist who facilitates valued transition outcomes. The recreational therapist "uses purposefully and systematically designed recreation and leisure-based interventions to facilitate the development of knowledge, skills, and abilities to use leisure time constructively, to improve quality of life, and to address or otherwise ameliorate the effects of illness or disability" (p. 34). Services are tailored to support the specific educational goals identified in the Individualized Education Plan (IEP) where recreational therapy has been classified as a related service under U.S. public education law since 1975.

TREK is a multifaceted program that includes school-based services, school trip facilitation, and similarity awareness.

School-based services: These include recreational therapy and transition interventions. There are individual or group-based recreational therapy services for students who receive special education or IEP services from elementary school to post graduate studies and/or transition-based services for ages 14-21. Services include recreation assessment, recreational therapy treatment planning, intervention, and evaluation delivered in natural settings with a focus on community integration and meaningful inclusion in school and community settings

School trip facilitation: These services address barriers to full inclusion in school-based field trips or other off-site recreational events such as hiking, canoeing, ropes courses, cycling, skating, and skiing. Planning strategies and adaptive equipment instruction are provided to mitigate barriers to inclusion.

Similarity awareness: This intervention includes lecture, discussion, video, and experiential activities to promote an awareness and appreciation for the positive aspects of diversity among students, teachers, staff, and administration. Participants are encouraged to explore and embrace a sense of community that is inclusive of all abilities.

TREK's concept of transition is grounded in Halpern's definition of transition (Halpern, 2012):

Transition refers to a change in status from behaving primarily as a student to assuming emergent adult roles in the community. These roles include employment, participating in postsecondary education, maintaining a home, becoming appropriately involved in the community, and experiencing satisfactory personal and social relationships. The process of enhancing transition involves the participation and coordination of school programs, adult service agencies, and natural supports within the community. (p. 116)

Although transitioning services in the public school system typically beings at age 14, TREK's transition services begin in elementary and middle school and advance to higher-level independent living skills in high school. The transition program consists of three interrelated recreational therapy intervention strategies that build on each other to facilitate positive postsecondary outcomes for students with disabilities (p. 36):

IEP-related recreational therapy intervention: During elementary and middle school this emphasizes basic and intermediate recreational and social skill development, which are two important pre-requisite skill sets for progress in transition.

Pre-transition recreational therapy intervention: This is an introduction to the concepts of self-sufficiency and independence for students in the early high school years, a bridge between the basic and intermediate skill development emphasized during the elementary and middle school years.

Transition services: These provide a more intensive independent-living focus during the later high school transition years. They are delivered to students whose IEP includes specific transition goals emphasizing independent living skills, advanced social and recreational skill development, and/or exploration of vocational or postsecondary education opportunities.

To learn more about TREK, visit Northeast Passage at www.nepassage.org.

Home Leisure Educational Program (HLEP)

A review of the literature by Nour et al. (2002) found that older adults who sustain a stroke often have difficulties adjusting to home life, particularly in the areas of leisure and social activities. These difficulties appear to be closely linked to poor psychosocial outcomes such as depression and poor quality of life. Consequently, the authors conducted an experimental study with a control group to measure outcomes related to participation in a home leisure education program. The home-based program was provided to individuals 55 and older who had a stroke, had been discharged from a healthcare center, were retired, and did not present with major communication or cognitive impairments that would make it difficult to answer questionnaires or follow the program. Individuals were assigned to a control group (a friendly visit one time a week for one hour for 10 weeks; n = 7) or an experimental group (HLEP; n = 6). In the HLEP program, participants progressed along 12 steps and were given homework to complete outside of sessions.

Step 1: Self-Awareness. Is leisure important to you? If yes, move to Step 2. If not, Step 1A: Leisure Awareness (How can leisure be beneficial).

Step 2: Self-Awareness. At the present time, is your leisure practice satisfactory? If yes, move to Step 3. If not 2B: Self-Awareness. What place could leisure activities take in your life?

Step 3: Self-Awareness. Which leisure activities would you like to do?

Step 4: Self-Awareness. What do these activities give you?

Step 5: Self-Awareness. How did you do it?

Step 6: Self-Awareness. Can you still do it this way? If yes, move to step 9A. If no, go to Step 7.

Step 7: Competency-Development. Can you do it another way? If yes, move to step 9A. If no, go to Step 8.

Step 8: Leisure Awareness. What can you do instead?

Step 9A through Step 11: Competency Development

- Step 9A: Self-Awareness. What are the barriers limiting your participation?
- Step 9B: Self-Awareness. What are the ways to get around the perceived barriers?
- Step 10: Self-Awareness. What abilities are required?
- Step 11: Self-Awareness. What resources are available?

Step 12: Competency Development. Autonomous practice and leisure satisfaction.

The participants receiving the HLEP performed significantly better on physical and total quality of life measures than individuals in the control group.

Family Centered Community Stroke (FCCS) Program

This was an eight-week multidisciplinary group therapy program for couples. One partner had one or more strokes and had been living at home for at least six months after discharge from a healthcare facility. A maximum of six couples participated during each eight-week session for a total of 17 couples. The program worked on strengthening family relationships post stroke (Ryan et al., 2008).

The program was held twice a week for four hours (eight hours a week in total) for eight weeks. It included couple therapy, recreational therapy, leisure education, physiotherapy, exercise therapy, speech therapy, recreation participation, and informal peer contact. The authors reported on the outcomes of the recreational therapy component of the program related to perceived leisure competence, perceived leisure barriers, and participation in active, community-based leisure activities. All participants completed the *Leisure Diagnostic Battery*, a recreation life history, received five group leisure education sessions that focused on the "development of a cognitive understanding of leisure, a positive attitude towards leisure experience, various participatory and decision making skills, and knowledge of and the ability to utilize resources" (Ryan et al., 2008, p. 125). Topics in the sessions included attitudes and values awareness, interests, barriers, resources, and

planning. Following the leisure education sessions, the participants and activity programmer provided opportunities for the couples to engage in leisure activities including bocce ball, word puzzles, cards, painting, horticulture, and walks outside.

At the end of the program, each participant collaborated with the recreational therapist to design an individualized recreational therapy intervention plan that focused on the community reintegration process and recommendations for future recreation. The individualized treatment plan included a participant profile; a list of past recreation and activity interests; participant strengths and areas of concern; goals and outcome and performance measures for the three recreational therapy treatment sessions and the end of the FCCS Program eight-month follow-up; and future recreation and leisure program and activity options. At the eight-month follow up, participants had increased their perception of opportunities for leisure and increased involvement in community programs. Additionally, the spouses' perception of leisure competence increased.

Independence through Community Access and Navigation (I-CAN)

A review of schizophrenia spectrum disorders (SSD) literature by Snethen, McCormick, and Van-Puymbroeck (2012) found that social integration correlated with leisure activities (Sorgaard et al., 2001), improved overall functioning (Graham, Arthur, & Howard, 2002), and earlier treatment of symptoms (Yilmaz et al., 2008). It was also found that individuals with SSD who participate in fewer social leisure activities experience greater social isolation (Graham, Arthur, & Howard, 2002). To increase social integration of individuals with SSD, the Independence through Community Access and Navigation (I-CAN) intervention program was developed and pilot tested with seven individuals with SSD receiving services from a local community mental health center. This was a nine-week recreational therapy intervention modeled after the individualized placement and treatment (IPT) model to support community-based recreation participation, matching clients with interest-based activities to promote autonomy, and providing onsite training through co-participation. Perceived outcomes from the intervention included increased community involvement, development of planning skills, and the development of coping skills. All of these were facilitated by the therapeutic relationship between the client and recreational therapist. In 2013, Snethen received a three-year $600,000 National Institute on Disability and Rehabilitation Research (NIDRR) grant to further explore the outcomes of the I-CAN intervention. The I-CAN program for increasing community participation in adults with schizophrenia is currently funded by NIDRR as Project Number H133G130137 (National Rehabilitation Information Center, 2013).

Inpatient Rehabilitation Recreational Therapy Community Integration Training for Spinal Cord Injury (SCIRehab)

The SCIRehab Project, which gathered information from 1032 individuals with spinal cord injury (SCI) across six rehabilitation centers found that increased time spent on community outings led by a recreational therapist resulted in higher social integration and mobility scores on the *Craig Handicap Assessment and Reporting Technique* (CHART), less re-hospitalization at the one-year mark post injury, decreased pressure ulcers, increased prediction of sports involvement and outdoor activities one year post discharge, and higher *Functional Independence Measure* (FIM) motor scores at discharge (Backus et al., 2013).

Further analysis of this data found that increased recreational therapy during inpatient rehabilitation was positively associated with higher social integration scores. More time in inpatient recreational therapy and receipt of post-discharge peer support and vocational services were associated with a greater likelihood of school enrollment or employment at one year post injury. More recreational therapy post discharge was associated with higher satisfaction with life. It is also noteworthy that only one-third of the study participants received post-discharge recreational therapy, compared to 87.3% who received physical therapy (PT) and 68.5% who received occupational therapy (OT), "yet neither inpatient or post discharge PT or OT were associated with positive outcomes in social integration or satisfaction with life. The potential benefits of both inpatient and post discharge [recreational therapy] services should be studied further to determine which aspect of [recreational therapy] services provides positive benefits, how receipt of services may be expanded, and what the cost benefit is associated with these services. Dissemination of these findings

must also include payer groups, and therefore if there are positive benefits to be gained from [recreational therapy] services, there might also be reimbursement for these services. Few centers provide post discharge [recreational therapy] services, and more centers might be inclined to do so if the provision of these services will not only lead to improved outcomes for people with SCI, but are also reimbursable services that profit their programs" (p. S172).

Integration of International Refugees and Immigrants

Refugees are individuals who are forced to flee their country for survival, have limited choice as to where they will relocate, and often are unable to return to their country due to imminent danger. Immigrants, on the other hand, choose to leave their country, have choices regarding where they relocate, and are able to return to their homeland without fear. During the 2004-2005 academic year, a non-governmental organization (NGO) assisting Vietnamese and Cuban refugees in a mid-western community in the U.S. approached an interdisciplinary group of healthcare students, professionals, and educators from three universities to assist a group of refugees integrate into the community (Kensinger et al., 2007). They used Anderson and McFarlane's (2000) systems theory, which states that the subsystems of the physical environment, education, safety, transportation, politics and government, communication, economics, and recreation all interact and must be controllable by the individual in order to successfully navigate life. If any of the subsystems are excluded, the individual's life will be lacking and necessary services will be ignored (Anderson & McFarlane, 2000, as cited in Kensinger et al., 2007).

The recreational therapy students were asked to address communication, transportation, and community resources. To identify the specific needs of the group, a recreational therapy student conducted one-to-one visits with the refugees for 90 days and shared findings with fellow recreational therapy students. The students then conducted an ecological assessment of the community in which the refugees settled. This included the identification of two major bus routes near the refugee housing and identifying community resources along the bus routes including banks, pharmacies, shopping centers, grocery stores, churches, parks and recreation facilities, health centers, gas stations, post offices, libraries, schools, city and state buildings, and resource centers (e.g., pregnancy/women centers, English as a second language (ESL) classes, daycare, employment agencies, etc.). The students created a resource manual that provided a list of the resources with information on the hours open, location, and services.

Standardized assessment tools, including the *Bus Utilization Skills* test and the *Rapid Travel Training Program*, and informal questionnaires were utilized to measure outcomes.

Twenty recreational therapy students and two recreational therapy professors facilitated a two-hour training session for eleven participants twice a week for seven weeks. The students conducted an assessment of the assigned individual to determine the person's specific needs, designed and implemented interventions, and measured outcomes.

In the area of transportation, students taught participants how to obtain a valid driver's license and how to use public transportation, including basic bus skills, sign recognition, money management for ticket purchase, finding bus routes and schedules, proper bus etiquette, social skills, and safety techniques. Students accompanied participants on the bus to participant-selected destinations, such as a shopping mall.

In the area of communication, students helped participants find, access, and register for ESL classes, interpret signs and symbols, read classified ads and apply for jobs, including finding employee assistance programs in their native language. The students took participants on trips to retail locations to demonstrate and explain services. A variety of resources were utilized including translators, flashcards, demonstrations, and role-playing.

In regards to community resources and money management, participants were taught about low-cost services, such as childcare, libraries, parks and recreation centers, and shopping malls, and practiced accessing such services through community integration training sessions. Students also addressed writing checks, reading and paying bills, and identifying and exchanging currency. Money exchange games were used in addition to individual instruction and community integration sessions to practice generalizing skills into real-life environments. Although detailed outcomes from formative and summative evaluation procedures were not shared in the article, it was noted that the program was a valuable asset to the refugee settlement process.

Community Participation and Disaster Relief

Life can be drastically changed when a community disaster, such as a flood, hurricane, terrorism, mudslide, fire, volcano, or tornado, strikes. People not only lose homes, but they also lose their communities leading to a loss of stability, security, and health. The community can be changed in an instant and transitioning from pre-disaster to post-disaster brings a host of challenges. In October 1999, immediately following Hurricane Floyd, which destroyed much of eastern North Carolina, recreational therapy professionals and pre-professionals assisted in the disaster relief mission (Russoniello et al., 2002). A total of 450 fourth and fifth graders were displaced from the Pattillo Elementary School. Teachers noted behavioral problems, resulting in a social worker seeking help from recreational therapy professionals and students from East Carolina University.

The recreational therapy students and professors provided services to the school three times a week. A graduate assistant was appointed to help coordinate the project and various groups were contacted to donate items including recreation equipment, sportswear, school supplies, tickets to see a play, and prizes for students excelling in school. The recreational therapy group delivered a stress management seminar for the teachers and stress management training sessions for the students. The project consisted of four tiers: (1) acquisition of recreation supplies and materials to facilitate growth and development, (2) planning and construction of a new playground for the children at the school to foster community participation and developmental growth, (3) provision of hands-on training of recreational therapy students to utilize the concept of learn and serve through supervised service delivery, and (4) provision of systematic interventions to address the effects of natural disasters on the lives and functional performance of school aged children. Tier 4 involved the use of the I'm in Charge of Me (I-C Me) program, a biopsychosocial program strategy that utilizes cognitive behavioral stress control to aid in managing stress and increase self-concept.

In addition to this program, the recreational therapy students integrated biopsychosocial recreational activities into the strategy to promote normalization. All of the interventions were delivered to classroom groups. Students identified to be high-risk by a teacher-rating scale received one-on-one and small group treatment and recreation activities. The I-C Me is a five-week program that helps children identify stress symptoms and teaches coping skills to ameliorate such symptoms (Week 1: What is Kid Stress, Week 2: The Power of Positive Thinking, Week 3: Breathing for Health, Week 4: Dealing with Stress: Coping Activities, Week 5: Expressing Emotions).

The interventions resulted in positive behavioral changes, including increased attentiveness, positive assertiveness, improved attention span, and decreased hyperactive behavior. Grade testing demonstrated greater growth than for all other county elementary schools. This project demonstrated a shift of paradigm for the recreational therapy profession in the area of disaster relief. As disaster relief "becomes more defined, it is becoming increasingly evident that recreation and leisure services can and should play an integral role in disaster recovery [and] be included as an integral component of extended disaster relief" (Russoniello, 2002, p. 81).

Partnership F.I.V.E. (Fostering Inclusive Volunteer Efforts)

Community inclusion is about being a *part* of the community, not just functioning *within* the community. Volunteering is one way for an individual to foster and build a sense of belonging in the community. Volunteering is a form of leisure activity, as it is freely chosen, intrinsically motivating, and performed during one's free time (Cnaan, Handy, & Wadsworth, 1996, as cited in Miller et al., 2005). A review of the literature by Miller and colleagues (2005) found that volunteering yields extensive benefits including increased self-esteem, life satisfaction, self-knowledge, personal growth and efficacy, self-acceptance, empathy, likelihood of taking responsible action, happiness, positive educational trajectories, understanding of others, appreciation for diversity, and sense of control over one's life. It also leads to decreased alienation, depression, antisocial behavior, engagement in risky behaviors, and negative stereotypes. Specifics included reductions in teen pregnancy, course failure, school suspensions, dropping out, drinking, and taking drugs. Volunteering was also found to decrease mortality rates, result in improved functional ability, and lead to greater perceived health.

Most of this research has been done with adolescents, adults, and older adults who do not have disabilities. In regards to individuals with disabilities,

the research is more limited. However, a review of the literature by Miller et al. (2005) found that volunteer work can lead to positive behavior change with increased appropriate behavior and decreased disruptive behavior, improved academic performance, improved functional skills, increased verbalizations and facial expressions, more positive attitudes about service recipients, improved self-confidence, increased sense of the ability to act on and influence the world, improved social skills, increased social networks, development of practical and work skills, increased enjoyment, increased involvement and eagerness to participate, decreased self-stimulatory behaviors, increased sense of purpose, increased verbal communication and social interaction, social relationship development with nondisabled peers, increased sense of empowerment, increased belief in self, and increased sense of responsibility. "Given the potential breadth and veracity of these benefits, volunteerism by people with disabilities could significantly impact their levels of independence, functioning, physical and mental health, employability, positive use of free time, and overall quality of life" (Miller et al., 2005). To foster inclusive volunteering it is recommended that recreational therapists utilize the Partnership F.I.V.E's six-component Process to Inclusive Volunteering that was developed by the U.S. Department of Education, Rehabilitative Services Administration:

Recruitment and preparation: Individuals with disabilities, family members, care providers, volunteer coordinators, nondisabled partners, and nonprofit agency staff are recruited and prepared for inclusive volunteering. Knowledge is imparted, such as what is volunteering, why people volunteer, what people do as a volunteer, the benefits of volunteering, and the responsibilities of being a volunteer. Parents and care providers are additionally educated on how to best support the individual in this endeavor, and agency staff are trained on how to successfully engage volunteers at various functional abilities. Individuals without disabilities are also recruited to serve alongside the person who has a disability and work together as partners. After recruitment and preparation are completed, the individual is asked if s/he is interested in volunteering. If yes, move on to the next step.

Assessment: Assess the person's abilities, preferences, and needed supports. Forms of volunteer work should match the client's interests and skill ability. Leisure and recreation interests should also be explored to determine if interests can be converted into a volunteer opportunity.

Matching: Following the assessment, the individual is matched to a volunteer task in the community. Volunteer opportunities are identified through the "recruitment" phase and/or through outreach to community volunteer centers.

Building supports: This includes implementing individualized supports that were identified as needs during the assessment process. "Supports should be as natural and nonintrusive as possible so as not to interfere with opportunities for social inclusion or call attention to their limitations" (p. 24). Supports might include task or equipment adaptations, alternative training formats, transportation strategies, identification of a mentor or peer partner, etc. See Miller et al. (2005) for case study examples regarding use of supports.

Communication: This consists of identifying and maintaining open communication channels for problem solving among the volunteer, peer partner (if applicable), volunteer coordinator, and family members. Although Miller et al. (2005) identifies that communication is predominantly used for problem solving, it is also thought that communication about strengths, opportunities for advancement to new roles, and achievement should additionally be conveyed to foster psychological and emotional benefits, as well as reinforce and thank the family and caregiver for their continued support.

Evaluation: Feedback is gathered and discussed to evaluate the success of the volunteer match regarding all involved parties. Questions that may be discussed include: Is the individual enjoying the volunteer experience? Does the individual feel valued? Do the agency staff and/or peer partner feel comfortable working with the volunteer? Do any changes need to be made?

Other Approaches

Strengths-Based Approach

Engagement in a productive lifestyle is a key component of community integration. Petrella and colleagues (2005) conducted semi-structured interviews with six individuals who have been living with a brain injury for an average of 14 years. Results revealed that engagement in productive activities were directly linked to opportunities to try, support from others, and feedback from others (extrinsic factors), along with experimenting, fighting for identity, and reconciling abilities and disabilities (intrinsic factors). All of these were facilitated through activity engagement that allowed for exploration, vulnerability, and self-awareness (learning about capacity). The authors note, "Perceived capacity is influenced over the course of people's lives [and therefore] support services need to be available on an on-going basis. This literature supports this view for long-term, possibly life-long, services" (p. 654).

Sports

A study of 90 individuals with SCI (C5 or below, majority 10 years post injury) was divided into two groups based on self-reported sports participation (45 sports, 45 non-sports) (McVeigh et al., 2009). Sports participants had to participate in recreational, organized competitive, elite, or professional sport at least one time a month. Non-sport participants were individuals who reported no regular sports participation since onset of SCI. Findings indicated that the *Community Integration Questionnaire* (CIQ) and *Reintegration to Normal Living Index* (RNL) total mean scores were higher among sport participants vs. non-sport participants.

Training Support Staff

Thorn and colleagues (2009) conducted a nine-month study of 556 individuals with intellectual disability (ID) living in a residential facility. (Nine had mild ID, 32 had moderate ID, 69 had severe ID, and 418 had profound ID; 315 males, 241 females, mean age of 54; mean length of residence 28 years.) The study consisted of three parts:

Therapeutic milieu: Every interaction between an individual and staff has learning opportunities. Staff were educated about skills learned in the traditional academic classroom and those in the client's support plan. Staff were taught how to generalize the skills to the evenings and were given quick reference cards. The staff were mentored to competency to implement skills reinforcement and generalization in contextually appropriate activities in the residence.

Community presence: The researchers identified and worked through barriers to going out into the community, taught staff the value of community presence and presence in community integrated activities, taught staff basic concepts of functional learning context and the difference in teaching skills based on living in a residential setting vs. teaching transportable skills from the person's support plan in community integrated activities.

Community participation: Focused on promoting more individual involvement and participation while in the community, which was identified in the literature as a highly desired outcome for individuals with intellectual disabilities. Staff were trained on how to facilitate activities that improved from simply going to a place in the community to socially interacting with people in the community; were educated about the value of partaking in routine activities in the community and functionally interacting in integrated settings, leading to increased community-based abilities; were taught how to identify potential community integrated learning opportunities and link these to the individual's likes and preferences; were taught how to identify a functional skill from the individual's support plan to be generalized and implemented based on the context of the community integrated activity preferred; and were taught how to utilize the quick reference cards (which were continually updated) to identify skills to reinforce during the community integrated activity.

"True participation in community integrated activities creates an endless continuum of functional learning opportunities in which an individual can learn and practice new skills, and staff can capitalize on skill reinforcement, generalization and incidental learning opportunities" (p. 896). Relative to baseline evaluation data, this process resulted in a significant increase in the number of people experiencing community integrated activities, the degree to which participants actively joined and shared in community activities, opportunities for choice, access to community resources, meaningful interactions with people in the community not associated with the service provider, and more types of interactions and social involvement, social roles, and discharges from the large residential facility to smaller facilities. "Literature has indicated that the higher an individual's ability level the more access they have to community activities. This work highlights the advantages of creating a therapeutic milieu for fostering learning and practicing functional skills in real-life activities and how this translates to increased community integration success for individuals with significant ID" (p. 899).

The authors recommend that this framework could be enhanced with more focus on chaining skill acquisition opportunities together and organizing community integrated activities as a sequence of opportunities in which individuals can chain learning events together in a rhythm of life activity. One possibility is working on money management, then going to a restaurant that carries over money management learning but now introduces dining skills, to then shopping at a store to add in the component of social skills.

Diagnosis-Specific Recommendations

Stumbo and colleagues (2015) reviewed recent community integration research for multiple diagnoses related to scope of recreational therapy practice. They highlighted client needs, treatment strategies, and implications for recreational therapy practice by diagnosis. Based on the literature, the authors recommended the following:

Stroke or traumatic brain injury: For individuals who had a stroke or traumatic brain injury, community integration services should be planned and structured. The therapist should be mindful of stage of injury, have well formulated goals that are shared with the client's social network, and focus on psychological and social needs.

Intellectual or developmental disability: For individuals who have an intellectual or developmental disability, community integration services should be geared towards facilitation of being a valued and integral member of the community, be delivered in the communities where the client lives, collaborate relationships with key services, address active community participation to combat risk of obesity, and involve the client's social support network.

Mental illness: For individuals with mental illness, community integration services should focus on the development of positive social interaction and active involvement with friends, family, and social supports, identification and integration of assets that support and aid recovery instead of only focusing on deficits, and empowering clients to take greater control in making choices related to desired health outcomes.

Spinal cord injury: For individuals with spinal cord injury, community integration services should incorporate peer mentors, develop independence, incorporate resources that maximize independence, and promote physical activity and self-efficacy.

Aging: For aging individuals with chronic conditions, community integration services should focus on creating open environments for engagement with others, providing transitional services to lesser levels of care, improving community involvement, increasing knowledge of resources, and providing opportunities for engagement in community settings for those residing in long-term residential care.

General leisure participation

Salzberg and Langford (1981) point to the importance of leisure activities as a vehicle for increasing involvement in the community, developing skills, and making friends. Thus the focus need not be entirely on productive activities, so long as the activities chosen are meaningful to the individual. Both Crapps and Stoneman (1989) and Kruzich (1985) also stressed the importance of getting involved in activities outside the home, activities that require becoming more familiar with the community and more comfortable interacting in the community.

Outcomes and Documentation

One of the challenges in measuring community participation is the lack of a consensual definition of what constitutes successful community participation (Resnik et al., 2012), as successful community participation can mean different things to different people. For example, one person might view the attainment of employment as successful community participation, whereas another person might view having a sense of belonging in one's community as successful community participation. Consequently, community participation includes both objective and subjective measurements, and there is currently no gold standard of measurement (Resnik et al., 2012).

It has been proposed that the *International Classification of Functioning, Disability, and Health* (ICF) is the best available classification system for the *objective* measurement of community integration through the use of participation scores in the Activity and Participation codes. This would involve using the degree of difficulty a person has with a particular life task, such as employment. To assist clinicians in identifying relevant Activity and Participation codes, research has been conducted to identify specific codes that are most relevant to particular disability populations. For example, Resnik and colleagues (2012) recommended specific Activity and Participation codes for clinicians to consider when addressing

community integration with veterans. The downside to the ICF, however, is that it does not allow for the *subjective* measurement of community integration. In other words, it doesn't acknowledge the person's perspective. To be sensitive to the person's perspective, the assessment needs to also ask: How important is this task to the person? What characteristics are present in the participation, such as the extent that a person feels a sense of belonging within the activity? (Brown, 2010).

Brown (2010) reviewed three common assessment instruments utilized in community participation research and discussed the extent to which they include the *subjective* component of participation assessment. All are available at www.tbims.org.

Community Integration Questionnaire (CIQ) and *Craig Handicap Assessment and Reporting Technique (CHART)*: Both measure the frequency of engagement in activity indicating that the more frequently one participates in activity and approaches normative levels the better. Increased frequency equals better integration.

Participation Objective, Participation Subjective (POPS): The POPS measures the frequency of participation, as well as how important the activity is to the person and whether or not the person wishes to increase the frequency, decrease the frequency, or not change the frequency at all. Desire for change is called saliency. A change in either direction indicates dissatisfaction. The POPS generates two scores: (1) the degree to which the person's frequency of participation varies from normative data and (2) the degree to which the person is satisfied with the level of engagement in activities that are important to the person. The POPs is a step in the right direction in regards to subjective measurement, but it only allows the person to comment on a set list of activities. There is no individualized process in identifying the activities that are important to the person. It also contains limited qualifiers: the extent to which the activity is important and whether or not the person wishes to change the frequency of participation in the activity.

Brown et al. (2010) recommends that clinicians consider the use of *Goal Attainment Scaling* (GAS) in the assessment and goal planning process. GAS is an individualized measurement approach where the clinician, client, and family jointly identify treatment goals that are important and meaningful to the client.

Outcomes related to each goal are then identified along a five-level scale shown in Table 9 (McDougall & Wright, 2009). In order for the goal to be clinically meaningful, only one variable should change along the five levels (see Table 10). It is additionally believed that the GAS can be easily paired with related ICF codes and clinicians are encouraged to consider adopting this approach (McDougall & Wright, 2009). See Table 11 and Table 12.

Table 9: Goal Attainment Scaling Levels

-2: the client's baseline

-1: improvement that is less than the expected level of attainment after intervention

0:   the expected level of attainment after intervention

+1: attainment that is somewhat more than expected after intervention

+2: attainment that is much more than expected after intervention

Table 10: Sample Goal Attainment Scaling with One Variable of Change.

-2 (client's baseline): When at the neighborhood playground, client initiates conversation with peers with **maximum multi-modal prompting.**

-1 (less than expected): When at the neighborhood playground, client initiates conversation with peers with **moderate multi-modal prompting.**

0 (expected): When at the neighborhood playground, client initiates conversation with peers with **minimal multi-modal prompting.**

+1 (somewhat more than expected): When at the neighborhood playground, client initiates conversation with peers with **increased time.**

+2 (much more than expected): When at the neighborhood playground, client initiates conversation with peers **independently.**

Table 11: Sample ICF Codes Paired with GAS with One Variable of Change

Targeted ICF goal area: d3500 Starting a Conversation with support from e355 Health Professionals

ICF component: Participation restriction and environmental factor

Time frame: 2 months

-2 (client's baseline): When at the neighborhood playground, client initiates conversation with peers with **maximum multi-modal prompting.**

-1 (less than expected): When at the neighborhood playground, client initiates conversation with peers with **moderate multi-modal prompting.**

0 (expected): When at the neighborhood playground, client initiates conversation with peers with **minimal multi-modal prompting.**

+1 (somewhat more than expected): When at the neighborhood playground, client initiates conversation with peers with **increased time.**

+2 (much more than expected): When at the neighborhood playground, client initiates conversation with peers **independently.**

Table 12: Sample ICF Codes Paired with GAS with Two Variables of Change

Targeted ICF goal area: Engagement in d9200 Play with e1401 Assistive Products and Technology for Culture, Recreation, and Sport

ICF component: Participation restriction and environmental factor

Time frame: 3 months

-2 (client's baseline): During play group, client engages in shared cooperative play for **10 minutes** with **moderate verbal cues.**

-1 (less than expected): During play group, client engages in shared cooperate play for **15 minutes** with **moderate verbal cues.**

0 (expected): During play group, client engages in **20 minutes** of shared cooperative play with **moderate verbal cues.**

+1 (somewhat more than expected): During play group, client engages in 20 minutes of shared cooperative play with **minimal verbal cues.**

+2 (much more than expected): During play group, client engages in 20 minutes of shared cooperative play with **increased time.**

As an alternative or to augment the GAS, Brown et al. (2010) recommend expanding the range of qualifiers applied to a standard list of activities when assessing participation. Some examples include:

- The extent the person feels welcomed in the activity and the level of satisfaction with social contact in home and community activities. For this recommendation, recreational therapists should consider utilizing the *Leisure Meanings Gained and Outcomes Scale* that measures the extent that a person experiences personal meaning in activities. If you are interested in utilizing this scale, contact Dr. Heather Porter at hporter@temple.edu.

- The extent the person is engaged in the activity — attending vs. participating. For this recommendation, recreational therapists might consider use of Dehn's Levels. See Table 13.

Table 13: Dehn's Levels of Participation

Cathartic Level: The person's participation reaches a point of catharsis, makes a measurable change in the person's life.

Level 4: The person's participation involves creativity, invention, imagination, taking nothing and making something, not following a plan or instruction.

Level 3: The person's participation involves physical, social, and/or cognitive activity that follows instruction, a plan, or rules, and participation is on an emotional level.

Level 2: The person is a spectator who is emotionally involved.

Level 1: The person is a spectator with no emotional involvement.

Level 0: The person is preoccupied in thought or feeling and just going through the motions of the activity. Participation could be forced, obligated, duty, with no internalization of participation.

Level -1: The person is harmed physically, mentally, or emotionally (e.g., substance abuse, dangerous high-risk activities, self-abuse, excessive exercising).

Level -2: The person affects others (family, friends, community) in a harmful or hurting manner (physical, emotional, mental).

Lost Freedom: The person harms himself/herself or others and behavior causes a lack of freedom to choose one's own leisure. Often negatively affects the leisure of others (e.g., family, victims).

Dehn, 1998, p. 564

- The perceived fit between the skills the person thinks are demanded for participation in an activity and the skills the person brings to the activity to identify and address skill development needs. For this recommendation, recreational therapists should consider the extent to which the client experiences flow during the activity. The *Flow Short Scale* consisting of 11 items is clinically easy to administer. See Jackson, Martin, and Eklund (2008) for a copy of the scale.

Increased inclusion of the person's perspective during the assessment, goal setting, and planning process holds much value, including:

- With the inclusion of what is important and salient to the person, better information can be obtained about the person's values and goals.

- Encouraging the person to share his or her perspective in the assessment process reflects an equalization of power and allows the clinician to solicit and identity participation goals.

- Participation goals established by drawing on the person's perspective can help shape and sharpen the treatment plan so that it addresses goals that are important and meaningful to the person. If the person's perspective is not included in the clinical model, functional changes (despite being positive) may or may not add value to the person's life, as perceived by the person.

- Participation data reflecting the person's perspective would substitute for or augment the one-size-fits-all approach, such as seen in the *Functional Independence Measure* (FIM). For example, the FIM tells clinicians very little about the degree to which the treatment plan was helpful in preparing the person to function at home or in the community in successful and meaningful ways as defined by the person.

- Gathering perspective on participation from many individuals with the same characteristics could contribute to the identification of external barriers and internal challenges that commonly need attention in a particular population.

Therapists who are seeking additional community participation assessment instruments that align with ICF components should consider the 17 instruments identified in the systematic review conducted by Chang, Coster, and Helfrich (2013). The CIQ, CHART, and POPS are reviewed above, and were identified in the systematic review as aligning with some of the ICF components. Additional instruments include the *Activity Card Sort*; *Client's Assessment of Strengths, Interests and Goals*; *Community Participation Indicators*; *Frenchay Activities Index*; *Guernsey Community Participation and Leisure Assessment*; *Independent Living Skills Survey*; *Index of Community Involvement*; *Katz Adjustment Scale*, *Keele Assessment of Participation*; *Late-Life Function and Disability Instrument*; *Maastricht Social Participation Profile*; *Participation Assessment with Recombined Tools — Objective*; *Instrument of Home and Community Participation*; and *Social Functioning Scale*. The authors determined that none of the instruments covered the full breadth of community participation domains as reflected in the ICF, but that each tool addressed community participation to some extent. The authors concluded that new instruments that evaluate community participation more comprehensively are needed. Another measure not identified in the study is the *Community Reintegration of Service-Members* (CRIS).

For billing purposes, the American Medical Association (AMA) Current Procedural Terminology (CPT) code 97537 "Community/work Reintegration (e.g., shopping, transportation, money management, avocational activities and/or work environment modification analysis, work task analysis, use of assistive technology device/adaptive equipment)" (American Medical Association, 2011) can be utilized as one of several possible CPT codes related to community integration, transitioning, and inclusion interventions.

Resources

Resources related to community integration are often diagnosis, age, location, and/or setting specific. Conduct a search using such key terms to identify relevant resources.

A Community for All Children: A Guide to Inclusion for Out-of-School Time
By Kimberly Miller, Ph.D., CTRS
www.ces.ncsu.edu/depts/fourh/old/afterschool/comm
unityforall1.pdf

Center for Parent Information and Resources
www.parentcenterhub.org/
Under "Resources," "K-12 Issues," you will find a link to "Transition from School to Adult Life." Contains resources and links.

Guidelines for Disability Inclusion in Physical Activity, Nutrition, and Obesity Programs and Policies: Implementation Manual
www.nchpad.org/fppics/Guidelines%20Implementati
ons%20Manual.pdf
National Center on Health, Physical Activity, and Disability (NCHPAD)

Institute for Human Centered Design
www.adachecklist.org/checklist.html
Community integration, inclusion, and transitioning require therapists to be knowledge of disability rights and laws (see the Disability Rights chapter) and demonstrate competency in assessing the physical accessibility of buildings and recreational areas. The New England ADA Center, a project of the Institute for Human Centered Design, developed a website that provides printable checklists based on 2010 ADA accessibility standards.
More information can also be found at www.ada.gov.

Pacer's National Parent Center on Transition and Employment
www.pacer.org/transition/
Resources related to transition and employment.

Transition Coalition
http://transitioncoalition.org/transition/file.php?path=
files/docs/47365_FINAL_WEB1213214133.pdf
The Community Transition Program: Experiences Starting a Community-Based Program for Students. Ages 18-21 is an 85-page manual to assist individuals in developing a transition program.

U.S. Department of Education, Office of Special Education Programs
http://idea.ed.gov/explore/view/p/,root,dynamic,Topi
calBrief,17.
Reviews IDEA regulations related to secondary transition.

Wrights Law
www.wrightslaw.com/info/trans.index.htm
Transition, Transition Services, and Transition Planning contains information on definitions, articles, cases, publications, etc.

References

American Medical Association. (2011). *CPT professional 2012.* Chicago, IL: American Medical Association.
Anderson, E. T. & McFarlane, J. (2000). *Community as partner: Theory and practice in nursing.* Philadelphia: Lippincott, Williams, and Wilkins.

Backus, D., Gassaway, J., Smout, R. J., Hsieh, C., Heinemann, A. W., DeJong, G. & Horn, S. D. (2013). Relation between inpatient and postdischarge services and outcomes 1 year postinjury in people with traumatic spinal cord injury. *Archives of Physical Medicine and Rehabilitation, 94*(4 Suppl 2), S165-74.

Bateman, B. (2015). *Legal requirements for transition components of the IEP.* Retrieved from www.wrightslaw.com/info/trans.legal.bateman.htm.

Brown, M. (2010) Participation. The insider's perspective. *Archives of Physical Medicine and Rehabilitation, 91*(9, Suppl 1), S34-7.

Buell, M. K. (2003). Integration as acculturation: Developmental disability, deinstitutionalization, and service delivery implications. *International Review of Research in Mental Retardation, 26,* 221-260.

Bullock, D. E. & Johnson, C. C. (1998). Recreational therapy in special education. In F. Brasile, T. Skalko, & J. Burlingame (Eds.), *Perspectives in recreational therapy: Issues of a dynamic profession* (pp. 107-124). Ravensdale, WA: Idyll Arbor.

Center for Community Living and Careers. (2011). *Transition services: Definitions and examples.* Retrieved from www.iidc.indiana.edu/styles/iidc/defiles/INSTRC/Transition%20Services_and_Activities_Definition_and_Examples.pdf.

Chang, F., Coster, W. J., & Helfrich, C. A. (2013). Community participation measures for people with disabilities: A systematic review of content from an international classification of functioning, disability, and health perspective. *Archives of Physical Medicine and Rehabilitation, 94,* 771-81.

Cnaan, R. A., Handy, R., & Wadsworth, M. (1996). Defining who is a volunteer: Conceptual and empirical considerations. *Nonprofit and Voluntary Sector Quarterly, 25,* 364-383.

Committee on the Assessment and Readjustment Needs of Military Personnel, Veterans, and Their Families; Board on the Health of Select Populations. (2013). *Returning home from Iraq and Afghanistan: Assessment of readjustment needs of veterans, service members, and their families.* Washington, DC: Institute of Medicine of the National Academies, the National Academies Press.

Crapps, J. M. & Stoneman, J. (1989). Friendship patterns and community integration of family care residents. *Research in Developmental Disabilities, 10*(2), 153-169.

Crocker, T., Powell-Cope, G., Brown, L. M., & Besterman-Dahan, K. (2014). Toward a veteran-centric view on community (re)integration. *Journal of Rehabilitation Research and Development, 51*(3), xi-xvii.

Dehn, D. (1998). *Leisure step up.* Enumclaw, WA: Idyll Arbor.

Graham, C., Arthur, A., & Howard, R. (2002). The social functioning of older adults with schizophrenia. *Aging and Mental Health, 6,* 149-152.

Halpern, A. S. (2012). The transition of youth with disabilities to adult life: A position statement of the division on career development and transition, the council for exceptional children. *Career Development for Exceptional Individuals, 17*(2), 115-124.

Hawkins, B. L., Cory, L. A., McGuire, F. A., & Allen, L. R. (2012). Therapeutic recreation in education: Considerations for therapeutic recreation practitioners, school systems, and policy makers. *Journal of Disability Policy Studies, 23*(3), 131-139.

Jackson, S., Martin, A., & Eklund, R. (2008). Long and short measures of flow: The construct validity of the FSS-2, DFS-2, and new brief counterparts. *Journal of Sport and Exercise Psychology, 30,* 561-587.

Kensinger, K., Gearig, J., Boor, J., Olson, N., & Gras, T. (2007). A therapeutic recreation program for international refugees in a Midwest community. *Therapeutic Recreation Journal, 41*(2), 148-157.

King, G., Curran, C. J., & McPherson, A. (2012). A four-part ecological model of community-focused therapeutic recreation and life skills services for children and youth with disabilities. *Child: Care, Health, and Development, 39*(3), 325-336.

Kraus, L. E. & Jans, L. (2014). *Implementation manual for guidelines for disability inclusion in physical activity, nutrition, and obesity programs and policies.* Center on Disability at the Public Health Institute: Oakland, CA.

Kreutzer, J. S. & Wehman, P. (1990). *Community integration following traumatic brain injury.* Baltimore, MD: Paul H Brookes.

Kruzich, J. M. (1985). Community integration of the mentally ill in residential facilities. *American Journal of Community Psychology, 13*(5), 553-564.

McColl, M. A., Carlson, P., Johnston, J., Minnes, P., Shue, K., Davies, D., & Karlovits, T. (1998). The definition of community integration: Perspectives of people with brain injuries. *Brain Injury, 12*(1), 15-30.

McDougall, J. & Wright, V. (2009). The ICF-CY and goal attainment scaling: Benefits of their combined use for pediatric practice. *Disability and Rehabilitation, 31*(16), 1362-1372.

McVeigh, S. A., Hitzig, S. L., & Craven, B. C. (2009). Influence of sport participation on community integration and quality of life. A comparison between sport participants and non-sport participants with spinal cord injury. *Journal of Spinal Cord Medicine, 32*(2), 115-124.

Miller, K. D., Schleien, S. J., Brooke, P., Frisoli, A. M., & Brooks, W. T. (2005). Community for all: The therapeutic recreation practitioner's role in inclusive volunteering. *Therapeutic Recreation Journal, 39*(1), 18-31.

National Council for Therapeutic Recreation Certification. (2015). Certification standards part V: NCTRC national job analysis. Accessed via website https://www.nctrc.org/documents/5JobAnalysis.pdf.

National Rehabilitation Information Center. (2013). *Increasing community participation in adults with schizophrenia.* Retrieved from http://search.naric.com/research/redesign_record.cfm?search=1&type=all&criteria=recreational%20therapy&phrase=no&rec=3264.

Northeast Passage. (2015). *About Northeast Passage.* Retrieved from http://nepassage.org/about/.

Nour, K., Desrosiers, J., Gauthier, P., & Carbonneau, H. (2002). Impact of a home leisure educational program for older adults who have had a stroke (Home Leisure Educational Program). *Therapeutic Recreation Journal, 36*(1), 48-64.

Pantell, M., Rehkopf, D., Jutte, D., Syme, S. L., Balmes, J., & Adler, N. (2013). Social isolation: A predictor of mortality comparable to traditional clinical risk factors. *American Journal of Public Health, 103*(11), 2056-62.

Passmore, T. (2012). Community integration/reintegration: A recreational therapy intervention. *American Journal of Recreation Therapy, 11*(4), 7-13.

Petrella, L., McColl, M. A., Krupa, T., & Johnston, J. (2005). Returning to productive activities: Perspectives of individuals with long-standing acquired brain injuries. *Brain Injury, 19*(9), 643-655.

Resnik, L., Bradford, D., Glynn, S., Jette, A., Hernandez, C., & Wills, S. (2012). Issues in defining and measuring veteran community reintegration: Proceedings of the working group on community reintegration, VA rehabilitation outcomes conference. Miami, Florida. *JRRD, 49*(1), 87-100.

Russoniello, C. V., Skalko, T. K., Beatly, J., & Alexander, D. B. (2002). New paradigms for therapeutic recreation and recreation and leisure service delivery: The Pattillo A+ Elementary School disaster relief project. *Parks and Recreation, 37*(2), 74-81.

Ryan, C. A., Stiell, K. M., Gailey, G. F., & Makinen, J. A. (2008). Evaluating a family centered approach to leisure education and community integration following a stroke. *Therapeutic Recreation Journal, 42*(2), 119-131.

Sable, J. & Bocarro, J. (2004). Transitioning back to health: Participants' perspective of Project PATH. *Therapeutic Recreation Journal, 38*(2), 206-224.

Sable, J. & Gravink, J. (2005). The PATH to community health care for people with disabilities: A community-based therapeutic recreation service. *Therapeutic Recreation Journal, 39*(1), 78-87.

Salzberg, C. L. & Langford, C. A. (1981). Community integration of mentally retarded adults though leisure activity. *Mental Retardation, 19*(3), 127-131.

Sander, A., Clark, A., & Pappadis, M. (2010). What is community integration anyway? Defining meaning following traumatic brain injury. *Journal of Head Trauma Rehabilitation, 25*(2), 121-127.

Seeman, T. E. (1996). Social ties and health. The benefits of social integration. *Annals of Epidemiology, 6*(5), 442-451.

Snethen, G., McCormick, B. P., & VanPuymbroeck, M. (2012). Community involvement, planning and coping skills: Pilot outcomes of a recreational therapy intervention for adults with schizophrenia. *Disability and Rehabilitation, 34*(18), 1575-1584.

Sorgaard, K. W., Hansson, L, Heikkila, J. Vinding, H. R., Bjarnason, O., Bengtsson-Tops, A., Merinder, L., et al. (2001). Predictors of social relations in person with schizophrenia living in the community: A Nordic multicenter study. *Social Psychiatry and Psychiatric Epidemiology, 36,* 13-19.

Stumbo, N. J., Wilder, A., Zahl, M., DeVries, D., Pegg, S., Greenwood, J., & Ross, J. (2015). Community integration: Showcase the evidence for therapeutic recreation services. *Therapeutic Recreation Journal, 49*(1), 35-60.

Thorn, S. H., Pittman, A., Myers, R., & Slaughter, C. (2009). Increasing community integration and inclusion for people with intellectual disabilities. *Research in Developmental Disabilities, 30,* 891-901.

U.S. Department of Education. (2007). *IDEA regulations: Secondary transition.* Accessed via website http://idea.ed.gov/explore/view/p/,root,dynamic,TopicalBrief, 17.

U.S. Department of Education. (ND). *Sec. 300.34 related services.* Retrieved from http://idea.ed.gov/explore/view/p/,root,regs,300,A,300%252E 34.

Wilder, A., Craig, P., & Frye, M. (2014). Therapeutic recreation empowering kids: Exploring best practices in transition. *American Journal of Recreation Therapy, 13*(2), 33-48.

Wilder, A., Craig, P., Sable, J., Gravink, J., Carr, C., & Frye, J. (2011). The PATH-way home: Promoting access, transition, and health for veterans with disabilities. *Therapeutic Recreation Journal, XLV*(4), 268-285.

Wong, Y. & Solomon, P. (2002). Community integration of persons with psychiatric disabilities in supportive independent housing: A conceptual model and methodological considerations. *Mental Health Services Research, 4*(1), 13-28.

Yasui, N. & Berven, N. (2009). Community integration: Conceptualisation and measurement. *Disability and Rehabilitation, 31*(9), 761-771.

Yilmaz, M., Josephsson, S., Danermark, B., & Ivarsson, A. B. (2008). Participation by doing: Social interaction in everyday activities among persons with schizophrenia. *Scandinavian Journal of Occupational Therapy, 15,* 162-172.

24. Community Problem Solving

Heather R. Porter

Community problem solving is the knowledge of, and ability to problem solve for, physical and non-physical barriers in a real-life setting (work, home, school, community). The client learns about barriers that may be experienced in a real-life setting and how to problem solve for these barriers. The specific material reviewed depends on the identified barriers for the task. This could include a combination of community accessibility training, Americans with Disabilities Act education, or a tailored focus on a specific problem (e.g., self-catheterizing in a public restroom). This protocol, although it incorporates the use of other forms of education and training, was included because it addresses the client's ability to integrate a variety of protocols for the task of community problem solving.

Therapists who address these issues proactively will maximize a client's problem-solving skills, resource awareness, and functional application skills. Should a client encounter barriers that s/he is unable to solve, unhealthy consequences may occur. This could include the development of secondary disability, such as deconditioning due to decreased activity level, emotional adjustment issues, and decreased quality of life, such as not pursuing personal life goals because of perceived insurmountable barriers.

Indications

Community problem solving should be considered for a client who verbalizes concerns about his/her ability to function in a real-life environment, exhibits difficulty identifying anticipated barriers, or does not adequately solve for barriers resulting in undesirable outcomes including safety concerns. The client may have a deficit in problem solving indicated by ICF code d175 Solving Problems. If the client is going into the community, community problem solving would be indicated as one of the interven-

tions to help deal with the deficit. Often the problem is with specific aspects of community involvement. Deficits in ICF codes as they relate to the community, such as d230 Carrying Out Daily Routine, d4 Mobility, and d5 Self-Care, suggest a need for community problem-solving interventions.

Contraindications

Community problem solving is not appropriate for a client who has significant cognitive impairments that impact his/her ability to recall, retain, or apply verbal, pictorial, or demonstrative education. If significant cognitive impairments are evident, the therapist will need to educate the client's caregivers since they will be the ones to facilitate community activities.

Protocols and Processes

The length and frequency of community problem-solving sessions will vary depending on the identified needs and abilities of the client. Barriers are identified through activity and systematic analysis of each task that will be a part of the client's activity pattern.

Education should take place in a quiet, non-distracting environment to promote concentration. The therapist should have relevant materials including specific handouts for review and reference during the session along with paper and pen to write down barriers and identified solutions. Additional sessions should be scheduled to allow for evaluation of activity performance in a real-life environment. This is typically done in the form of community integration training.

The process for presenting information will vary depending upon the information reviewed. Typically, education is provided verbally along with a written handout that is given to the client for future reference. (See the Appendices in this chapter for examples.) The handouts in the Appendices are not meant to be complete. They are a sample of common problems, which should give you a good idea of what to look for and address when your clients are faced with other kinds of barriers. We encourage you to write specific community problems and possible solutions in a manner that is tailored to the needs of the individual client. Therapists are welcome to use the worksheets provided and alter them to meet the needs of their clients.

Therapists may also need to educate and train clients on other issues that could cause problems for the client in the community. Other issues may include, but are not limited to, wheelchair mobility, walking techniques, energy conservation training, anger management, relaxation and stress reduction, leisure resource awareness, the Americans with Disabilities Act, activities of daily living, assertiveness training, dietary precautions management, pain management, anxiety management, and social skills training.

After education, the client is asked to verbally apply information and skills learned to solve a proposed situations ("what would you do if…"). Following this intervention, clients are scheduled for community integration training to more fully evaluate the client's ability to apply the information and skills in a real-life environment.

Material should be presented carefully and gently to the client, especially the what-if questions. The therapist does not want to scare the client about possibilities, yet wants to educate and inform so that these barriers do not pose a threat to the client's continuing activity and community involvement and working towards his/her life goals.

Outcomes and Documentation

The therapist documents the specific education provided and the client's ability to verbally apply information to proposed situations as well as the client's ability to perform learned techniques in a real-life environment. *Example*: Post education on problem solving for weather conditions, the client was able to verbally apply information at modified independence secondary to increased time (capacity). However, in a community environment (performance), the client required minimal verbal cues to

make adjustments for weather conditions because "I'm just not used to doing it."

If a client has an assessed deficit in solving problems (d175 Solving Problems), the therapist documents changes in the client's ability to problem solve for community barriers using this specific ICF code. The client will also have documented deficits in activities required to go into the community that are impacted by problem solving deficits such as d230 Carrying Out Daily Routine, d420 Transferring Oneself, d530 Toileting. Treatment and outcomes for these deficits should be documented using the ICF code of the deficit.

Appendix A: Community Problem-Solving Techniques

Carrying and Transporting Items

There are several ways to carry things if you are using a wheelchair, walker, or cane:

Backpack: If you are using a wheelchair, hook each arm strap of the backpack over the back of the wheelchair. If you are using a walker or cane, wear the backpack. Here are several characteristics of a good backpack: waterproof, a dark color that won't show a lot of dirt, and several roomy compartments that are easy to open. A thin arm strap may be more comfortable to lean against if you are putting it on the back of a wheelchair. A thick arm strap may be more comfortable if you are wearing it.

Clothing: Use clothing pockets, a waist pack, or a small pocketbook with a large strap that you can wear across your shoulders.

Custom bags and baskets: You can make one or purchase one from a medical catalog. A small cloth bag or basket can be hung on the front bar or the side of a walker. A small nylon bag can attach to a cane or crutch with Velcro. Small cloth bags can attach to a wheelchair armrest. Be careful not to put items in the bags that are too heavy, as they could cause the walker to tip over. In addition, the more weight you add to the walker or cane the more difficult it will be to move so you will tire more quickly.

Shopping baskets: If you are using a wheelchair, you can put a store basket on your lap. However there are several things that must be considered: (1) *Sensation*: If sensation in your legs is impaired, you will not be able to feel the basket on your lap nor will you realize that it may be digging into your skin if it is overloaded with heavy items. This could cause skin breakdown. If you have poor sensation in your legs and want to use a basket, take a towel along with you (keep it in your backpack), lay it down on your lap, and then put the basket on top of the towel. Also, do not load it with heavy items. (2) *Type of mobility device*: If you are sitting in a wheelchair at a 90° angle, the basket may have a tendency to slide off your lap. If you are sitting on an angle that is less than 90°, your knees will be slightly higher than your hips. This position will keep the basket on your lap much more easily. If you are using a walker, you should not use a handheld basket at the same time. It is not safe. You need both hands on the walker handles. If you are using a cane, you can use a handheld basket provided you have enough strength in the other hand and arm to hold it, as well as the balance to compensate for the weight.

Store carts: A standard store cart can be pushed with one hand while propelling the wheelchair with the other hand. It takes a bit of practice but it can be done provided you have enough upper body strength and endurance. If you are using a walker or a cane, do not put your device into a cart and push the cart. The cart handle is higher than your walker or cane, so the cart is only supporting your upper body, not your lower body. As a result you may find yourself leaning on the cart. This is not good. If you cannot walk upright while using the cart, you are not ready to use it.

Electric scooters: Many stores have electric scooters for their customers to use. They are hand-operated. Ask at the customer service counter for a key and instructions. They are usually free and you do not have to prove that you have a disability to use them. After you transfer to the scooter, ask the customer service representative to take your assistive device back to the customer service counter and hold it for you. When you go through the checkout lane, ask the cashier to get a customer service representative to bring out your device and help you get your packages into the car.

Ask for help: Under the Americans with Disabilities Act (ADA) you are entitled to have "reasonable accommodations." Asking for assistance to carry items it considered reasonable.

Rain

If it is raining outside and you are using a wheelchair:

Choose your clothing carefully. If you are wearing good clothes and shoes (e.g., going to a wedding) and you don't want to get them wet, consider taking your good clothes with you and changing when you get there.

When you are in the house (before you transfer into the wheelchair), waterproof the wheelchair cushion. This is very important. You do not want to wind up having to sit on a wet cushion and it will get wet from the rain when loading the wheelchair into the car. Wet cushions are dangerous. If the water seeps out of the cushion, through your pants, and moistens your skin, you are at a higher risk for developing skin breakdown. Skin is fragile when it is wet and is much more likely to break down, especially if you are putting pressure on the skin by sitting on it. To keep the cushion dry, slip the cushion into a clean kitchen trash bag. Slip the cushion that is now inside the kitchen trash bag into a snug fitting cloth pillowcase. The plastic will become a water barrier and the cloth pillowcase will keep you from slipping off the cushion when you sit on it. Transfer into the car. Pull the cushion into the car immediately. If the pillowcase is wet, take it off and put on a dry one. When transferring out of the car, quickly put the cushion on the wheelchair and transfer onto it. If you are with someone, ask the person to hold an umbrella over the wheelchair to keep it as dry as possible. Once you enter the building, you can continue to sit on the pillowcase if it is not wet. If it is wet, have yet another pillowcase with you or simply take both the trash bag and the pillowcase off. Remember to repeat this process before you leave if it is still raining. Also, wear a poncho. A poncho will provide the most protection from the rain. Do not sit on the poncho. Put the back part over the back of the wheelchair. It will keep the wheelchair and backpack drier. An umbrella is not feasible. Even clip-on umbrellas have had limited success. Raincoats do not work well either, as they will not cover the back of your chair and they may be slippery to sit on.

If it is raining outside and you are walking:

Choose your clothing carefully, as stated in the previous scenario.

Wear a raincoat with a hood. The raincoat will not get in your way and will provide maximum protection from the rain. An umbrella is not feasible because you want both of your hands available to hold an assistive device or to assist with keeping your balance. A poncho is not feasible either; it will get in your way when you are walking. Ponchos have too much material.

Clothing

Carefully consider the clothes that you wear when you go out. Here are some things to think about:

- Can you easily manipulate clothing for using the bathroom?
- Are they weather appropriate? If your sensation is impaired, it is important to be aware of the weather. For example, you may not notice that your cotton pants aren't protecting your skin well on a very cold day.
- If you are using a wheelchair, you may want to purchase pants that are an inch or two longer than you normally would have purchased. The extra length will allow your pants to cover your ankles when you are in a seated position. Purchasing pants that are one size larger in the waist might also be more comfortable when sitting for prolonged periods of time.
- If you are using a wheelchair, you may want to purchase shirts with a longer shirttail if you plan on tucking them in, so that they do not work their way out of the back of your pants.

Parking

Do you have a handicap parking placard or tag? Do you need one? Talk with your therapist for more information on how to apply for one. Handicap parking spaces are close to the front door or accessible entrance and they are also wider to allow adequate room to get in and out of the car. If there are no handicap parking spaces available, you have several options:

Park in the middle of two regular parking lot spaces and display your handicap parking placard or tag. Some people fear that other customers may become angry if you take up two parking spaces, so get a piece of poster board and write on it "I'm allowed to park here. There were no handicap parking spaces available. Thank you for understanding." This will usually avoid any confrontations.

If someone else is driving, you have two options. (1) Have the driver pull halfway into a regular parking spot and put on the hazard lights. Transfer out of the car and then have the driver pull the rest of the way into the spot. Vice versa for when you leave. (2) Have the driver let you off up front if it is safe and appropriate.

A word of caution: Do not enter or exit a car from a curb if at all possible. Getting in and out of the car by a curb can be very difficult because your wheelchair will be higher up making the transfer more difficult. If you are not using a wheelchair, your knees will be higher than your hips because you feet will have to be on the sidewalk making that transfer more difficult as well. Even if there is enough room between the car and the curb to place your feet on the street, there is limited space for mobility, which may increase your risk of falling.

Social Posture

If you have poor sensation in your legs, you must be aware of your posture because skin breakdown is a concern. It is very common for skin breakdown to occur in places besides your bottom. For example, resting your ankle or foot on the opposite knee can cause skin breakdown on the top of your knee. Crossing your ankles can cause skin breakdown on your ankle.

If your sensation is impaired, you will not be able to feel the discomfort that others feel from increased pressure. If you do rest your foot on your knee or cross your ankles, be aware of the length of time that you are in this position and vary your posture regularly. Remember to do a weight shift at least every 30 minutes. Some people have found it helpful to wear a watch and set it to beep every 30 minutes as a reminder.

Flat Tire

Most wheelchair tires have a solid insert so flats will not happen. However, if you do choose a tire that inflates with air, be sure to ask for instruction on how to change a tire. Be sure that you carry the repair supplies with you in your backpack. If you are unable to change the tire by yourself and you plan on being out by yourself a lot, you may want to choose a different type of tire.

Dead Battery

If you have a power wheelchair, make sure the battery is fully charged before you go out. You may wind up being out later than you anticipated and use up more battery power than expected. If you do find yourself in a position where the battery is dead, change the wheelchair to manual mode. You will require assistance to push the chair. If you are by yourself, ask a passerby to push you to a safe area and call someone for help. This is a prime example of the importance of having a cell phone.

Emergency (Cell Phone, Road Assistance)

It is a very good idea to carry a cell phone with you at all times in case of an emergency (e.g., flat tire, a fall, car breaks down). It is also advisable to carry a 24-hour roadside assistance program just in case the car breaks down.

Medication

If you are taking medication on a regular basis, it would be a good idea to take it with you when you go out. This way, if you want to say out later, you can. If it is a narcotic, it must stay in its original prescription bottle to be verified as being legal.

Bowel and Bladder

Using a public bathroom is not always an easy feat. It may not be accessible to your needs. Here are several things to consider.

If you are self-catheterizing

Make self-catheterization packs. Put everything that you need for one self-catheterization session into a plastic grocery bag, fold it over, and put it into your backpack. It is good to take a few extra packs just in case you stay out later or you drink more fluid. Remember, the more you drink, the more often you will need to self-catheterize.

If it is feasible for you to learn how to self-catheterize from a seated position, you should do it. There are not many places to lie down and self-catheterize in a public environment. Inform your nurse and therapists of your desire to learn and practice this skill.

If you are self-catheterizing in a public bathroom, pull up to the urinal or toilet, take out a self-catheterizing pack from your backpack, hook one of the plastic bag handles onto your wheelchair, and let the other end of the bag hang open. Get yourself into the correct position to self-catheterize and then reach into the bag to get your supplies. A bungee cord works well to hold your pants open. Unzip your pants and hook one end of the bungee cord to the pant flap and then hook the other end to someplace on your wheelchair. Now you have both hands available for self-catheterizing. You could also use a bungee cord to keep the bathroom door shut. Sometimes there is not enough room to turn around to lock the door, so on your way in, hook the door somewhere (bottom, side) and then hook the other end somewhere else in the bathroom (toilet paper holder, wheelchair, side of stall).

If You Can Void on Your Own

If you are male, keep a plastic bottle with a good leak-proof lid in your backpack. If you are unable to stand, you may still be able to sit to use the bottle, and then dump it in the urinal or toilet. It also comes in handy when bathrooms are on the second floor (e.g., private home). Find a private area to use the bottle and then ask someone to take it upstairs to dump it or you could put it back into your backpack and empty it at home. If you prefer to do this, you may want to pull a dark sock over the bottle. This way, anyone who goes into your backpack is none the wiser that the bottle contains urine.

If you are female, you will want to call ahead to make sure the public bathroom meets your specific needs. If it does not, or there is no way to determine ahead of time if the bathroom is accessible, wear a protective pad especially made for holding urine just in case you can't get into the bathroom.

Bowel

Know your bowel routine and try to be at home at that time.

If you anticipate having to use the bathroom when you are out, call ahead to make sure it is accessible and be sure to have help with you so you can use the bathroom if necessary.

Pack an extra change of clothes, as well as clean-up supplies and a Ziploc bag, in your backpack just in case of a bowel or bladder accident.

When you are in the hospital, your nurse will set you up on a bowel program at a certain time of the day. This will help train your bowels to move at a particular time. Be sure to discuss your lifestyle with your nurse and set up a time that will work best with your lifestyle after discharge rather than your inpatient therapy routine.

Appendix B: Lower Extremity Amputation Community Problem Solving

Something Doesn't Feel Quite Right While You Are Walking

Stop what you're doing, sit down, take off the prosthetic, and inspect your skin and prosthetic.

Did the prosthetic shift position? Readjust the prosthetic.

Is there any skin reddening? Some reddening is normal. It should resolve within 30 minutes. If it does not resolve, call your physician immediately as it may be a beginning sign of ulceration.

You Find a Skin Opening

If there is a skin opening, you need to keep the prosthetic off. If you continue to wear it, it will make the opening worse. However, you also need to make it back to the car and into your house safely. Here are some ideas:

Find out if a wheelchair is available

Is there a wheelchair for customers to use (e.g., at a store)? Ask your friend to get it for you. If you are by yourself, ask an employee to get it for you. If you are able, push the wheelchair yourself or request assistance to push the wheelchair back to the car.

Once you arrive home you will need to exit the car and get into the house. Do you need to wear the prosthetic to get into the house? If you still have your walker or crutches in the home, can someone go inside the home and bring it out to you so that you can "hop" into the house? If you are by yourself or "hopping" is not safe for entering your home, put the prosthetic back on and enter your home as you did before. As soon as you get in the door, take the prosthetic off.

If no wheelchair is available

If you are using a walker or crutches, is it possible to "hop" back to the car?

If you are not using a walker or crutches but you did in the past, is it possible to keep it in the trunk of your car in case of an emergency? Ask someone to go out to the car and get it for you.

Is there some sort of transportation available to get you back to the car? For example, if you are at an arboretum, an employee may be able to drive you back to your car in one of their carts.

If the previous options do not work, put the prosthetic back on and walk directly back to your car. Take the prosthetic off, drive home, and then follow the previous suggestions for entering your home.

Walking on Uneven Surfaces

If you do a lot of walking on uneven surfaces (e.g., hiking), it is important to check your skin regularly for any irritation, since walking on uneven surfaces challenges the fit of the prosthetic. The prosthesis may also shift when you are walking, so it might need to be readjusted or repositioned periodically.

Sunburn

It is particularly important to avoid sunburn on your residual limb.

Sunburn can cause blisters. Friction from the prosthetic may cause the blisters to open. Once the skin has an opening, you may be restricted from using the prosthetic until the skin heals. If you are diabetic, it could take quite some time for the opening to heal due to circulation problems.

Sunburn makes your skin more sensitive. This can cause pain when wearing the prosthetic.

Beware of using sunburn-soothing agents (e.g., aloe vera). Putting a wet substance on your residual limb will cause your skin to become more fragile and more prone to breakdown. Also, you do not want to use a sunburn-soothing agent on an open wound since it can cause an infection.

If your residual limb becomes sunburned, evaluate the severity of the burn. If it is just slightly pink and there are no blisters, you can try wearing your prosthetic. Check your skin frequently for irritation. If it causes any pain or discomfort, remove the prosthetic until the sunburn heals. If it is moderate to severe and there is a blister, it is recommended that you do not wear your prosthetic until the sunburn heals. You will have to problem solve for alternative ways to get around (e.g., crutches, wheelchair).

Water

It is important that the skin on your residual limb is totally dry before putting on the socks and prosthetic. Wet skin is fragile and can increase your risk of skin breakdown from the friction of wearing the prosthetic. Remember to fully dry your skin after showering, swimming, sitting in the sun (if the residual limb is sweaty), being out in the rain, etc. The correct procedure is to dry the limb with a towel and to let it air dry for at least 20 minutes. High periods of activity may cause your socks to become soaked with perspiration. Take extra socks with you at all times and change them regularly to prevent skin breakdown.

Socks

The volume (circumference) of your residual limb changes throughout the day so you will need to change your socks frequently to ensure a proper prosthetic fit. Because the number of plies you need will change, it is important to have a variety of sizes with you.

Traveling via Airplane

Some people report that their residual limb swells after flying due to air pressure changes and seems to take one full day to resolve. This may cause the prosthetic to not fit properly. Be prepared by taking thinner socks to wear with the prosthetic. Also, it might be helpful to consider light activities for your first day after flying (e.g., sedentary activities such as watching a show) which may provide you with easier alternatives for getting around if you are unable to use your prosthetic.

Kneeling

If you have a one-limb amputation (e.g., leg or arm), you may be able to kneel without much discomfort. However, it is important to make sure that you can do this in a safe manner and that it does not irritate the skin or the prosthetic. Work on this skill with your therapist. Do not attempt this for the first time on your own. Kneeling is not recommended for someone who has two or more limb amputations.

Appendix C: Spinal Cord Injury Problem Solving Worksheet

One useful type of handout is a question and answer sheet. Here is one listing problems associated with a spinal cord injury.

Questions

1. What would you do if you were out with two friends and you wanted to get into a building that had five steps? What if you were with one friend?
2. What would you do if you were up on the second floor and the elevator died?
3. What would you do if you couldn't open a heavy manual door at a store?
4. What would you do if you fell out of your wheelchair in the middle of the mall?
5. What would you do if there were no handicap parking spaces? What would you do if someone who didn't have a handicap tag or placard was parked in a handicap parking space?
6. What would you do if you were a passenger in a car and the passenger side of the car was parked along a curb? How would you get out of the car?
7. What would you do if there was no curb cut and you were with another person? What if you were by yourself?
8. How would you get over a thick gravel driveway? If you still couldn't get over it, what could you do?
9. What would you do if your friends asked you to go on a deep-sea fishing trip and you were unsure as to how you would get on and off the boat? Let's say you really want to go along.
10. What would you do if you were out in the community and you got a flat tire?
11. How would you go out somewhere and not get wet if it was raining outside?
12. What would you do if you had to use the bathroom and the bathroom was not accessible? What would you do if you were at someone's house and the bathroom was on the second floor?
13. What would you do if your wheelchair would not fit between the clothing racks at the store and you wanted to look at a particular sweatshirt?
14. What would you do if something broke on your wheelchair (e.g., a hand rim)?

15. What should you put in your backpack?

16. What would you do if you experienced a dysreflexic episode in the community?

17. What would you do if you had to empty your Foley bag and there was no bathroom around?

18. What would you do if you realized that your Texas catheter has fallen off and you were in the middle of a store? What if you didn't realize that it fell off and you had a bladder accident?

19. What should you carry with you at all times in your backpack in regards to your bowel and bladder needs?

20. Come up with three other questions about things that could happen when you are out in the community. List possible solutions.

Answers

1. Prior to attempting the steps, find out if there is a portable ramp that can be placed over the steps. If a portable ramp is not available, instruct your two friends on how to assist you in bumping up and down the steps, if that is safe and appropriate. If you are with only one friend, ask for assistance from security personnel, if they are available and able. Provide verbal training on how to provide assistance. If no one is available to help or it is not safe for your friends or employees at the location to help, do not attempt the steps.

2. Ask how long it is going to be out of service. If you can wait, wait. If not, ask if there is another elevator available for you to use (public, freight). If there is no other elevator, you will need to use the stairwell. Do not allow untrained people to assist you in bumping up and down the steps. If needed, call local emergency service and they will take you down the steps in a blanket carry.

3. Ask for assistance.

4. If you can, get back in the wheelchair by yourself or with the help of other people who know how to assist you. If you are unable to get back into the wheelchair, instruct someone to call the local emergency service for help. Do not allow untrained people to help you. If something seems "wrong" (e.g., broken leg, shooting pain), do not attempt to get into the wheelchair. Call the local emergency service.

5. Park in the middle of two standard parking spaces. Inform security or the store or office manager. The violators should be fined. Some people find satisfaction by making their own "tickets" and putting them on the windows of vehicles that are not legally parked in handicap spaces. For example, "This is a warning. You are parked illegally in a handicap parking spot. Consider yourself lucky. Next time I will call the police and you will be ticketed."

6. Look around for a parking garage or parking lot. If there isn't a parking garage, consider having the driver pull into a parking spot at an angle, put on the hazard lights, transfer out of the car into the street between the car and the curb, bump up the curb, and then have the driver park the vehicle correctly. Avoid this situation by calling ahead to locate safe parking.

7. If you are unable to bump up and down the curb yourself, look for an alternative route. If there isn't an alternative route, ask your friend to bump you up and down the curb, provided the person knows how to do this. It is not safe to have an untrained person assist you. If there is no alternative route and you are unable to get up the curb, you will not be able to access the building. This could possibly be avoided by calling ahead.

8. Pull the wheelchair over it backwards or look for an alternative route (e.g., grass on the side of the gravel driveway).

9. Call the charter boat company and ask them if they offer assistance getting on and off the boat. Ask detailed questions. Possible questions include: Is it a floating dock so the ramp is somewhat even with the boat deck? How wide is the ramp? Are there safety rails on the ramp? The main point: if you want to do something and you are not sure how to do it, explore it. Don't make assumptions. You could wind up denying yourself opportunities or you could put yourself in a dangerous situation.

10. Fix it. If you are unable to fix it and you are close to a place of safety, such as your home or car, ride on it for the short distance and then fix it. You could also seek assistance from local establishments (e.g., bike shop, garage) or call someone to help you.

11. Poncho.

12. Find a private area and use a bottle (male). Plan ahead and wear a protective pad (female).

13. Ask a store employee to move the racks if possible — many are on wheels. If this is not possible, the store employee should get the sweatshirt and bring it to you. This is a reasonable accommodation under the Americans with Disabilities Act.

14. Call the wheelchair vendor. Get this information from your physical therapist. Do not attempt to fix the wheelchair yourself. It may void the warranty.

15. Bowel and bladder supplies; cell phone; medication; water bottle; and a medical card with your physician name, phone number, your health history, and any allergies.

16. Call for emergency medical help. While you are waiting for help to arrive, you should try to resolve the problem yourself by checking for irritants such as a full bladder, full rectum, unrecognized injury, or tight clothing.

17. Use a bottle in a private area.

18. Immediately find a private area (e.g., bathroom) and put it back on. Change your clothes. Keep extra clothes in your backpack. If you don't have extra clothes, lay something over your lap, such as a jacket or package, and head back home to change. You could also purchase clothes when you are out and change into them.

19. As it pertains to your situation: self-catheterizing supplies in packs, wipes, Ziploc plastic bag, and change of clothes.

20. Additional possible questions: What would you do if a child asked why you are using a wheelchair? What if a server makes assumptions about your intelligence because you are using a wheelchair and asks your companion what you want to order? What would you do if it was time to take your medication and you didn't have water or, even worse, forgot to bring your medication?

25. Constraint-Induced Movement Therapy

David M. Morris, Edward Taub, and Mary Bowman

Constraint-Induced Movement Therapy or CI therapy is a multi-component rehabilitation approach that has been shown to promote large improvements in functional skills in adults with a variety of physical disabilities. Though applied to a variety of functional limitations, the approach has been employed most often to improve upper extremity (UE) use with adults recovering from stroke and with children with cerebral palsy. CI therapy involves a variety of intervention components used to promote increased use of a more-impaired extremity in the research laboratory or clinic and, most importantly, in the home setting (Taub et al., 1993; Taub, Uswatte, & Pidikiti, 1999; Taub, Uswatte, & Elbert, 2002; Taub, 2004; Morris & Taub, 2001; Morris, Crago, DeLuca, Pidikiti, & Taub, 1997; Morris, Taub, & Mark, 2007; Taub & Uswatte, 2006; Mark & Taub, 2004).

The CI therapy protocol has its origins in basic animal research, conducted by Taub. He used surgery to cut the sensory nerves where they come out of the spinal cord (dorsal rhizotomy) to a single forelimb in monkeys. This series of studies where Taub cut the sensory (afferent) nerves led him to propose a behavioral mechanism that can interfere with recovery from a neurologic insult — learned nonuse (Taub, 1977; Taub, 1980).

When CI therapy is implemented by a therapist, it directly addresses the mechanism of learned nonuse of the specified limb to promote improved functional use of the more affected limb in everyday life as a way to overcome learned nonuse. In more recent years, a linked but separate mechanism, use-dependent brain plasticity, has also been proposed as partially responsible for producing positive outcomes from CI therapy (Liepert et al., 1998; Liepert et al., 2000; Kopp et al., 1999; Bauder et al., 1999; Wittenberg et al., 2003; Levy et al., 2001; Mark, Taub, & Morris, 2006; Gauthier et al., 2008).

For more than 25 years, a substantial body of evidence has accumulated to support the efficacy of CI therapy for hemiparesis following chronic stroke and for children born with cerebral palsy. These findings have led several authorities to endorse CI therapy as one of the few rehabilitation approaches whose efficacy is evidence-based. One of the most important components of the CI therapy is termed the "transfer package," a set of behavioral techniques designed to induce transfer of the therapeutic gains achieved in the clinic to activities of daily living in the community setting (Taub et al., 2013a, 2013b).

While typically applied by physical and occupational therapists to improve UE use with basic activities of daily living (e.g., eating, bathing, grooming), the recreational therapist (RT) could be an important member of the healthcare team applying CI therapy, especially in the implementation of the transfer package. The skills of an RT could be particularly helpful in encouraging clients to use their weaker extremities during leisure and community-based activities. Also, the RT could be helpful in helping to assure continued use, via hobbies and meaningful activities, after the CI therapy intervention period.

The purposes of this chapter are to: (1) describe the key components and strategies most often employed in the CI therapy treatment protocol; (2) discuss the characteristics that make it unique as a rehabilitation approach; (3) describe considerations for selecting appropriate clients for CI therapy; and (4) discuss implications for RT practice. In this chapter the purposes will be achieved by discussing the CI therapy protocol used in an outpatient rehabilitation setting for adults recovering from stroke and applied to improving UE use. The principles can also be applied to individuals with other disabling conditions, including cerebral palsy, traumatic brain injury, and multiple sclerosis, and to improving other functions, such as walking and speech.

Indications

CI therapy was originally developed for upper extremity (UE) recovery with individuals having mild to moderate body structure limitations following stroke (b730 Muscle Power Functions, b735 Muscle Tone Functions, b740 Muscle Endurance Functions, b760 Control of Voluntary Movement Functions, d440 Fine Hand Use, d445 Hand and Arm Use). More recent research has shown successful application to individuals with more profound hemiparesis following stroke, with other disabling conditions, including cerebral palsy, traumatic brain injury, multiple sclerosis, and with other functional problems, such as walking and speech (d450 Walking, b3 Voice and Speech Functions). Specific inclusion criteria have been used to select individuals for participation in the research studies and are described in more detail later in this chapter under the sections titled Protocols and Processes and Identifying Clients Best Suited for CI therapy. As noted above, the expanding research has shown effective application of CI therapy with individuals with greater movement deficits, different medical conditions, and greater co-morbidities. Therefore, the inclusion criteria provided primarily describe the range of conditions where research has been conducted. It is possible, and probably likely, that CI therapy could be successfully applied with individuals with even more significant disability. To assure a positive outcome, however, we recommend using the most current research inclusion criteria when selecting individuals appropriate for CI therapy.

Contraindications

To date, absolute contraindications to CI therapy have not been clearly identified. However, conditions that present challenges to applying the intervention, including safety issues, have been identified. These factors are described later in this chapter under the sections titled Identifying Clients Best Suited for CI Therapy and Safety Issues with Using the Mitt Restraint. Some of these factors, especially when mild in nature, can be addressed through modifications in the CI therapy protocol without sacrificing positive outcomes. Future research should provide more insight into these issues.

Protocols and Processes

CI therapy is a "therapeutic package" consisting of a number of different components. Some of these intervention elements have been employed in neu-rorehabilitation before, although it was usually as individual procedures and at a reduced intensity compared to CI therapy. The main novel features of CI therapy are the introduction of a number of techniques designed to promote transfer of the therapeutic gains achieved in the clinic or laboratory to the home environment and the combination of these treatment components and their application in a prescribed, integrated, and systematic manner for many hours a day for a period of two or three consecutive weeks (depending on the severity of the initial deficit) to induce a client to use a more-impaired extremity.

The CI Therapy Protocol

In the University of Alabama at Birmingham (UAB) CI Therapy Research Laboratory and Taub Training Clinic, clients are categorized according to their ability to achieve minimal movement criteria with the UE prior to treatment. To date, six categories, referred to as "grades," have been described (See Appendix A). During initial evaluation, additional aspects for a client's inclusion in CI therapy protocol (other than range of motion) are assessed by therapists including use deficit of the more affected limb or function, cognition, mobility, balance, presence and status of pain, presence of comorbities, and medical stability.

CI therapy has undergone modification over the two plus decades. However, most of the original treatment elements remain part of the standard procedure. The present CI therapy protocol, as applied in our research and clinical settings, consists of three main elements with multiple components and subcomponents under each (See Appendix B) (Taub et al., 1993; Morris, Taub, & Mark, 2007; Mark & Taub, 2004). These include: (1) intense repetitive, task-oriented training of the more-impaired UE for several hours a day for 10 or 15 consecutive weekdays (depending on the severity of the initial deficit); (2) motor training by means of systematic strategies (i.e., shaping or task practice) and (3) applying a transfer package of adherence-enhancing behavioral methods designed to transfer gains made in the research laboratory or clinical setting to the client's real-world environment. Each of the elements, component, and subcomponent strategies are described in the following sections.

Repetitive, Task-Oriented Training

On each of the weekdays during the intervention period, clients receive training under the supervision of a therapist for several hours each day. The original protocol called for six hours per day for this training. More recent studies indicate that a shorter daily training period (three hours per day) is as effective for certain clients scored as Grade 2 or 3 (Kunkel et al., 1999; Sterr et al., 2002). Two distinct training procedures are employed as clients practice functional task activities: shaping and task practice.

Shaping is a training method based on the principles of behavioral training (Skinner, 1968; Panyan, 1980). In this approach a motor or behavioral objective is approached in small steps by "successive approximations." For example, the task can be made more difficult in accordance with a client's motor capabilities, or the requirement for speed of performance can be progressively increased. Each functional activity is performed for a set of ten timed (often 30- to 45-second) trials while explicit, immediate feedback is provided regarding the client's performance after each trial (Taub et al., 1994). When increasing the level of difficulty of a shaping task, the progression parameter selected for change should relate to the client's movement problems. For example, if the client's most significant movement deficits are with thumb and finger flexion and adduction (i.e., making a pincer grasp) and an object-flipping task is used, the difficulty of the task would be increased by making the object progressively smaller. If the movement problem involved thumb and finger extension and abduction (i.e., releasing a pincer grasp), the difficulty of the task would be increased by making the object progressively larger. As another example, if there is a significant deficit in elbow extension and a pointing or reaching task is used, the shaping progression might involve placing the target object at increasing distances from the client to promote increased elbow extension.

The shaping task is typically made progressively more difficult as the client improves in performance. Generally, only one shaping progression parameter at a time should be varied. The increase in difficulty should be such that it is likely that the client will be able to accomplish the task, though with slight effort.

This often makes it possible to achieve a given objective that might not be attainable if several large increments in progression of motor performance were required. Another advantage of this approach is that excessive client frustration is avoided, assuring continued motivation to engage in the training.

Task practice is the other repetitive, task-oriented training procedure. It is less structured than shaping. It involves functionally based activities performed continuously for a period of 15-20 minutes (e.g., wrapping a present, writing) and the tasks are not set up to be carried out as individual trials of discrete movements. In successive periods of task practice, the spatial requirements of activities, or other parameters, such as duration, can be changed to require more demanding control of limb segments for task completion. Global feedback about overall performance is provided at the end of the 15-20 minute period.

Therapists are encouraged to provide four forms of interaction during the shaping and task practice activities: modeling, feedback, encouragement, and coaching. Each type of interaction is briefly described in Appendix C. Training tasks are selected for each client considering (1) specific joint movements that exhibit the most pronounced deficits, (2) the joint movements that therapists believe have the greatest potential for improvement, and (3) client preference among tasks that have similar potential for producing specific improvement. Frequent rest intervals are provided throughout the training day and intensity of training — the number of trials per hour or the amount of time spent on each training procedure — is recorded. If needed, upper extremity stretches are performed by the therapist to enable to client to move optimally, but is not typically done for prolonged periods of time with Grade 2 or Grade 3 clients.

Adherence-Enhancing Behavioral Methods (Transfer Package)

One of the overriding goals of CI therapy is to transfer gains made in the research or clinical setting to the client's real-world environment in home and community settings. To achieve this goal, we employ a set of techniques that we term a "transfer package," which has the effect of making the client accountable for adherence to the requirements of the therapy. This is the aspect of CI therapy that the RT could be particularly helpful in carrying out. Through the transfer package, clients become responsible for their own improvement. The client must be actively engaged in (and adherent to) the CI therapy protocol without constant supervision from a therapist, especially in a life situation where the therapist is not present. Adherence has several aspects. One aspect is using the more-impaired UE during functional tasks and obtaining appropriate assistance from caregivers, if present. The assistance is to prevent clients from struggling excessively, while allowing them to try as many tasks by themselves as is feasible. The other aspect of adherence includes wearing the restraint (the mitt) as much as possible when it is safe to do so. Evidence indicates that the transfer package of techniques is largely responsible for the large increase in spontaneous use of a more-affected UE in the life situation (Taub et al., 2013a).

Potential solutions to these adherence challenges have been used to increase compliance to exercise programs in older adults, the population most commonly experiencing stroke and therefore most likely to receive CI therapy (Dominick & Morey, 2006). Two psychological factors, self-efficacy and perceived barriers, have been identified as the strongest and most consistent predictors of adherence to physical activity in older adults. Self-efficacy is defined as an individual's confidence in his/her ability to engage in the activity on a regular basis and is related to both the adoption and maintenance of a target behavior (Trost et al., 1996; Dishman, 1994; Sallis & Owen, 1999). Studies have demonstrated that self-efficacy can be enhanced through training and feedback (King, Blair, & Bild, 1992; McAuley, 1992; Rejeski, Brawley, & Ambrosius, 2003, McAuley et al., 2003). Perceived barriers may incorporate both objective and subjective components (Trost et al., 1996; Dishman, 1994). Objective obstacles can be reduced through environmental and task adaptation. Subjective barriers may be reduced by such interventions as confidence building, problem solving, and refuting the beliefs that hinder activity.

A number of individual intervention principles have been successfully applied to enhance adherence to exercise and physical function-oriented behaviors. The four most relevant ones used in the adherence-enhancing behavioral components of CI therapy are monitoring, problem solving, behavioral contracting, and social support.

Monitoring is one of the most commonly used strategies and involves asking clients to observe and document performance of target behaviors (Dominick & Morey, 2006). Clients can be asked to record a variety of aspects of these behaviors including mode of activity, duration, frequency, perceived exertion, and psychological response to the activity. Clients should be asked to submit their monitoring records to therapists to facilitate consistency and completeness of records, but most importantly to promote adherence to the self-monitoring strategy.

Problem-solving interventions involve partnerships between the therapist and client that ultimately teach individuals to identify obstacles that hinder them, generate potential solutions, select a solution for implementation, evaluate the outcome, and choose another solution if needed (Dishman, 1994).

Behavioral contracting involves asking clients to write out specific behaviors they normally carry out during the course of a day and then entering into an agreement with the therapist as to which will be carried out by the client and in what way they will be carried out. Verification of the execution of the contract occurs as part of the monitoring aspects of the procedure.

Social support by way of educating and enlisting the caregiver to provide the optimal amount of support is important to successfully using the mitt restraint and more-involved UE when in the home and community setting (DiMatteo, 2004). The caregiver is instructed to encourage the client's independence with tasks as much as possible but also assist the client when absolutely necessary to prevent frustration on the part of the client. This social support is optimized by reviewing the terms of the behavioral contract and requesting a caregiver contract with anyone who spends a significant amount of time with client.

Monitoring, problem solving, contracting, and social support interventions have been used successfully, alone or in combination, to enhance adherence to physical activity in a variety of client groups with a variety of physical conditions. These are essential aspects of the CI therapy approach.

The full range of adherence-enhancing behavioral subcomponents currently employed in the CI therapy protocol include behavioral contracts with the client and the caregiver independently; daily administration of the *Motor Activity Log* (MAL), a structured, scripted interview that elicits information on how well and how often the more affected UE was used in 30 important activities of daily life; a client-kept home diary keyed to what the client has agreed to carry out in the behavioral contract; problem solving between the therapist, client, and possibly a caregiver; a daily schedule constructed by the therapist; home skill assignment; home practice; and post-treatment contact (Taub et al., 1993, Uswatte, Taub, Morris, Barman, & Crago, 2006; Uswatte, Taub, Morris, Vignolo, & McCulloch, 2006; Uswatte, Taub, Morris, Light, & Thompson, 2006; Van der Lee et al., 2004). Each transfer package subcomponent is listed and aligned with its main behavior management approach or approaches as shown in Appendix D. A full description of each component is beyond the scope of this chapter. Each subcomponent is described in more detail in several key resources written by members of this team (Morris, Taub, & Mark, 2007; Taub et al., 2013a).

Constrained Use of the More-Impaired UE

The most commonly applied CI therapy treatment protocol has incorporated use of a restraint (most often a heavily padded protective safety mitt) on the less-impaired UE to prevent clients from succumbing to the strong urge to use that UE during most or all of the functional activities, even when the therapist is present. The protective safety mitt has been preferred for restraint as it prevents functional use of the less-impaired UE for most purposes while still allowing protective extension of that UE in case of falling. It also permits swinging the limb during ambulation to help maintain balance.

Clients are taught to put on and take off the mitt independently, and decisions are made with the therapist as to when its use is feasible and safe. The goal for mitt use for clients with mild to moderate motor deficits is 90% of waking hours. This so-called "forced use" is arguably the most visible element of the intervention in the rehabilitation community and is frequently and mistakenly described as synonymous with "CI therapy." However, Taub (1999) has stated "there is … nothing talismanic about use of a sling, protective safety mitt, or other restraining device on the less-affected UE" as long as the more-impaired UE is exclusively engaged in repeated practice. "Constraint," as used in the name of the therapy, was not intended to refer only to the application of a physical restraint, such as a mitt, but also

to indicate a constraint of opportunity to use the less-impaired UE for functional activities (Taub, Uswatte, & Pidikiti, 1999). As such, any strategy that encourages exclusive use of the more-impaired UE is viewed as a "constraining" component of the treatment package. For example, shaping was meant to constitute a very important constraint on behavior; either the client succeeds at the task or s/he is not rewarded (e.g., by praise or knowledge of improvement).

Preliminary findings by Sterr et al. (2002) indicate a significant treatment effect using CI therapy without the physical restraint component. Likewise, our laboratory has obtained similar findings with a small group of clients (n = 9) when a CI therapy protocol without physical restraint was employed (Taub, Uswatte, & Pidikiti, 1999; Morris et al., 1997; Uswatte et al., 2006). However, our study suggested that this group experienced a larger decrement at the two-year follow-up testing than groups where physical restraint was employed. If other treatment package elements, developed in our laboratory, are not used, our clinical experience suggests that routine reminders to not use the less-affected UE alone, without physical restraint, would not be as effective as using the mitt. Consequently, we use the mitt to minimize the need for the therapist or caregiver to keep reminding the client to remember to limit use of the less-impaired UE during the intervention period.

Unique Aspects of CI Therapy as a Rehabilitation Approach

In rehabilitation today, three general approaches are commonly employed to improve motor function after stroke (Shumway-Cook & Woollacott, 2001). The first, compensation, refers to modification of activities of daily living (ADL) such that they can be performed primarily with the less-affected side of the body. In this way, the more-affected extremities would, at most, be used as a prop or assist. This approach is believed to be particularly useful when spontaneous recovery of function has plateaued and further recovery seems doubtful. In more recent years, however, a more optimistic view has been adopted. As a result, emphasis on regaining movement on the more-affected side of the body has been advocated. With one such approach, true recovery, a specific function is considered "recovered" if it is performed in the same manner and with the same efficiency and effectiveness as before the stroke. With a substitution approach, the more-affected extremities may be used to perform a functional task in a new way, compared to before the neurologic insult. The question regarding which approach to rehabilitation is most effective has been an ongoing debate in the neurorehabilitation field for many years.

In a sense, the CI therapy approach cuts through the long-standing discussion. Trends apparent in the content of popular physical rehabilitation textbooks, evaluative criteria for professional educational programs, and topics commonly addressed in continuing education courses suggest that conventional physical rehabilitation still includes a predominance of true recovery, substitution, or compensation approaches to intervention. The CI therapy approach to stroke rehabilitation bypasses compensation entirely and does not emphasize the requirement for the exact replacement of normal or pre-stroke coordination to produce improved motor function and functional independence. Quality of movement is addressed in feedback to clients and it does improve, but it is not the emphasis of the treatment. Further, due mainly to reimbursement policies, most intervention is delivered in short treatment periods, relative to CI therapy, and in a distributed manner. If applied clinically, the CI therapy approach, as used in the UAB research laboratory, represents a substantial paradigm shift for conventional physical rehabilitation. The CI therapy approach is inconsistent in a variety of ways with the more conventional compensation and functional recovery approaches, as discussed below.

Use of More-Affected Extremity

Use of the protective safety mitt prevents clients from performing ADL and training activities with the less-affected extremity, unless use of the less-affected UE is necessary for safety or to avoid having the restraining device wet with water, even if the less-affected UE would normally be used for that function. For example, if the less-affected UE was the dominant UE before the stroke and the task was typically performed by the dominant UE (e.g., picking up small objects), the CI therapy protocol still requires the client to perform the task with the more-affected, non-dominant UE. This remains true for tasks that are bilateral in nature, such as folding clothing. Instead of removing the mitt and performing the task with both UEs, the clients perform the

task, in a modified fashion, with the more-affected UE exclusively, or enlist the assistance of a caregiver to serve as a "second UE." Many of the CI therapy clients' ADLs are modified during the training period. In this way, the CI therapy protocol does not allow compensation and deviates from a functional recovery approach where all ADLs would be attempted in the "typical" manner they were performed before the stroke.

The purpose of the strict adherence to use of the protective safety mitt is not to encourage a permanent change in the way the client performs ADLs. Rather, use of the protective safety mitt requires the concentrated and repetitive use of the more-affected UE. This concentrated use leads both to overcoming the strongly learned habit of nonuse and to use-dependent cortical plasticity. Once the treatment period of two to three weeks has ended, clients return the protective safety mitt to the laboratory staff and perform ADLs in the most effective manner possible with enhanced use of the more-affected UE. Interestingly, anecdotal observations suggest that after treatment many clients with more-affected, non-dominant UEs begin using the more-affected, non-dominant UE for tasks previously performed with the dominant, less-affected UE. Such observations warrant further investigation.

Importance of Concentrated Practice

While the most-often used CI therapy protocol includes some sort of restraint on the less-affected UE, variations in this approach (e.g., shaping only, intensive physical rehabilitation) do not (Taub, Uswatte & Pidikiti, 1999; Uswatte et al., 2006). There is nothing magical about the use of a restraining device on the less-affected UE. The common factor in all of the techniques, producing an equivalently large treatment effect, appears to be repeatedly using the more-affected UE in meaningful activities. This factor is likely to produce the use-dependent cortical plasticity found to result from CI Therapy and is presumed to be the basis for the long-term increase in the amount of use of the more-affected limb.

Researchers have also shown that repetitive practice is an important factor in stroke rehabilitation interventions (Butefisch et al., 1995; Hesse et al., 1994). Conventional physical rehabilitation, regardless of setting (inpatient or outpatient) or stage of rehabilitation (acute, sub-acute, or chronic), does not provide a sufficient concentration of practice. The conventional schedule falls short not only in absolute time where using the more-affected UE is required, but also in the consecutive nature of the practice periods. Clinical application of CI therapy will likely require a change in the typical scheduling pattern for rehabilitation. Episodes of care will likely need to be modified from short treatment sessions held several times a week for several months to up to six-hour sessions carried out daily for consecutive days over a two to three week period. Financial feasibility of this type of approach requires changes in payment structures and policies in reimbursement agencies.

Shaping as a Training Technique

CI therapy studies in the laboratory have predominately used either task practice or shaping for training activities. Preliminary data suggests that a predominance of shaping in the training procedures is more effective for lower functioning clients than a predominance of task practice. Use of either technique for higher functioning clients appears to be beneficial, though even here use of shaping appears to confer a therapeutic advantage (Taub et al., 1994). Thus, shaping would seem to be an effective training procedure for enhancing use of the more-affected UE in the life situation.

While there are many similarities between shaping and the conventional training techniques used by therapists, important differences also exist. Shaping procedures use a highly standardized and systematic approach to increase the difficulty level of motor tasks attempted. Also, feedback provided in shaping is immediate, specific, quantitative, and emphasizes only positive aspects of the clients' performance. In this way, the therapist's input and continuous encouragement motivates the client to put forth continued and maximal effort. Tasks are used that emphasize movements in need of improvement yet with a slight demand or challenge for the client, such that the task is slightly beyond what can be accomplished easily. Excessive effort is avoided as it may bring about a de-motivating effect for the client. The focus of shaping is to keep clients motivated and increase the amount of use of their UE during training. The main objective is to get the client to use the more-affected UE repeatedly in a concentrated, massed-practice fashion to overcome learned nonuse and to induce use-dependent cortical plasticity.

Use of a Transfer Package

It is our belief that most clients (and therapy professionals) view rehabilitation as occurring primarily as a hands-on intervention under the direct supervision of the rehabilitation professional. However, we believe that continued use and practice, for many hours daily, away from the rehabilitation facility is critical to achieving permanent changes in CNS plasticity and motor function. A unique aspect of the CI therapy approach involves an emphasis on the use of adherence-enhancing behavioral techniques (the transfer package) to facilitate more-affected UE use. While the use of similar behavioral techniques has been described in the physical rehabilitation literature, they are not as intense or concentrated as CI therapy. The use of the transfer package provides multiple opportunities for systematically increasing attention to more-affected UE use, enhancing confidence in using the more-affected limb, promoting clients' accountability for adhering to the CI therapy protocol, and providing structured problem solving between clients and clinical personnel. Intensive contact with the therapist establishes an important rapport between therapist and client which helps in getting the client to take home-practice and mitt-wearing requirements of the therapy very seriously.

Taken together, the behavioral techniques result in improved adherence to the required CI therapy procedures. Evidence from our research laboratory suggests that this transfer package may be the most important component of the CI therapy protocol (Gauthier et al., 2008; Taub et al., 2013a). A possible explanation for this could be successful carry-over of the behavioral techniques used during the treatment period to promote adherence, even when at home and not in contact with research personnel. These findings highlight the importance of the "out of laboratory" activities and subsequently the behavioral techniques needed to assure clients' adherence to them.

Main Effect of CI Therapy: Increased Use

Since a true recovery approach promotes performance of specific functional tasks in a manner similar to before the stroke, quality of movement would seem to be an important, if not primary, indicator of successful rehabilitation. Results from CI therapy research, as evidenced by the *Wolf Motor Function Test*, suggest that clients significantly improve their quality and skill of movement. A more powerful change, however, has been demonstrated with increased amount of use of the more-affected UE in the life situation, as evidenced by the *Motor Activity Log* and the *Actual Amount of Use Test*. Clients may well be developing new movement strategies to accomplish functional tasks. If so, this would further distinguish CI therapy from recovery-oriented therapies.

Relevance to Recreational Therapy

The RT specializes in adapting leisure and community-based activities so that they can be performed by individuals with physical disabilities. These skills, when applied along with a CI therapy protocol, could enhance treatment gains and promote retention of these gains long after the CI therapy intervention period. It should be noted, however, that during the CI therapy intervention period, the protocol is applied throughout the client's waking hours and to all functional skills. As such, the approach was designed to be delivered in a team approach including healthcare professionals with a wide array of skills who bring to bear several different scopes of practice that encompass procedures addressing the many needs of the client engaged in this comprehensive therapeutic approach.

Many safety issues and co-morbid medical conditions must also be considered when applying the CI therapy protocol. The RT, working as part of the CI therapy team, should be thoroughly educated on the CI therapy protocol and should consider the following points when executing professional duties.

Identifying Clients Best Suited for CI Therapy

While research concerning CI therapy has demonstrated benefits for a wide range of individuals, client inclusion criteria have been carefully considered in these studies. Applying the approach to individuals not meeting these criteria could be ineffective and possibly harmful. The following client characteristics should be considered when determining appropriateness for engaging in the protocol.

Active movement of the more-affected UE prior to treatment. The CI therapy research at UAB has been conducted with individuals with a minimum amount of active movement (see Appendix A). As such, individuals with less movement may not respond optimally to the treatment protocol or may need a modified treatment approach (Bowman et al., 2006; Taub et al., 2013b).

Passive range-of-motion of the more-affected UE: Individuals with severe joint limitations are not included in the research studies at UAB. The following minimum inclusion criteria are used for UE joint passive range of motion: Shoulder Flexion: > 90°; Shoulder Abduction: > 90°; Shoulder External Rotation: > 45°; Elbow Extension: -30° contracture or less; Forearm Supination: 45° or more from neutral; Forearm Pronation: 45° or more from neutral; Wrist Extension: To neutral or more; and MCP Extension: -30° contracture or less.

Balance and mobility skills: In order to participate in CI therapy research at UAB, clients must demonstrate the ability to stand up independently and stand for two minutes. In doing so, they can use their stronger arm to push up and steady themselves in standing. The therapist determines if a client has a history of falls or other safety concerns which would require problem solving especially with regard to use of the restraint. However, it is possible to successfully treat a client who is wheelchair dependent while optimizing safety.

Cognitive skills: The research laboratory uses a cut off score of 24 on *Mini-Mental State Examination*. This cut off is in the moderately impaired range. If a client has a supportive caregiver, then it may be possible to treat someone with more cognitive deficits but with more input and support from a caregiver especially with regard to the transfer package.

Unstable medical conditions: Because the intervention is relatively intense and requires participation during all waking hours, individuals with unstable medical conditions are excluded from participation.

Pain (acute or chronic): Since the more affected UE is used extensively during the intervention period, individuals with acute or chronic pain in any joints of the more-affected UE and/or the spine (i.e., cervical, thoracic, or lumbar spine pain) are excluded from participation.

Safety Issues with Using the Mitt Restraint

While other strategies (e.g., reminders, rewards) can encourage use of the more-affected UE, use of a mitt restraint on the less-affected UE is frequently used as part of the CI therapy protocol. When incorporating restraint into the program, safety issues should be identified and discussed with the client.

One of the primary goals of the behavioral contract procedure is to assure safe participation in the therapy. Using the behavioral contract procedure, the therapist asks the client about the functional activities that make up the client's daily routine. Using their understanding of specific movement requirements of the functional skills reported and their analysis of the client's pre-treatment movement skills, the therapist counsels the client about how they can safely engage in the CI therapy protocol. This is accomplished by suggesting: (1) modifications to the functional task itself (e.g., eating breakfast first then reading the newspaper instead of doing both at the same time; having sliced fruit that can be managed with the fingers instead of cereal and milk, which requires manipulation of a spoon in the impaired hand); (2) use of adaptive equipment, such as spill-proof cups, plate guards, build-ups for eating utensils; and (3) having a caregiver assist with the task. If none of the above is a reasonable or safe alternative, the client is advised to remove the mitt and carry out the task using the less affected extremity. It is important to note that the mitt is removed only when absolutely necessary and for only the period of time needed to complete the task.

Applying Shaping and Task Practice Principles to Leisure and Community-Based Activities

The principles of the shaping and task practice training procedures can be applied to leisure and community-based activities and then integrated into the CI therapy protocol. The motivation and enjoyment experienced in such activities could significantly enhance clients' engagement in the intervention. Incorporating these activities into the home practice program used after the conclusion of the in-clinic phase of CI therapy could also lead to better retention of gains achieved during the intervention period. A few suggestions about applying these motor training principles to leisure and community-based activities are listed below.

Shaping: Since shaping is very systematically delivered, utilizes short bouts of activities over 10 timed trial sessions, and focuses primarily on using parts of functional tasks, these motor training principles are less likely to be directly applicable to leisure and community-based activities. Instead, the RT and PT or OT should consult about the client's preferred leisure and community-based activities to identify the specific movement skills needed to effectively execute the skill. For example, if a client needs better forearm supination to play card games, a shaping task that promotes that movement should be utilized. If

the difficulty is in flipping cards over or dealing the cards, the RT and PT or OT may confer and decide to incorporate forearm supination shaping tasks into the motor training part of the intervention. Communication between professionals is important for selecting the shaping tasks that will lead to optimal outcomes.

Task Practice: The professional skills of the RT can be of particular benefit to the clients' program when considering task practice activities. Since these activities are more continuous, delivered over longer periods of time (15 to 30 minutes), and are more functionally based, leisure and community-based activities are appropriately used with this type of motor training. Again, the RT and PT or OT should collaboratively assess the client's movement needs and activity preferences and then incorporate the leisure and community-based activities into a task-practice training format that will most likely assure client motivation and engagement. The RT will also be helpful for identifying adaptive equipment and strategies that will assure client success with the activity. It should be noted, however, that the typical progression through the intervention involves a reduction in such assistance as the client gains skill with the activity.

Outcomes and Documentation

Two main outcome measures are used in the CI therapy research projects at UAB: the *Motor Activity Log* (MAL) and the *Wolf Motor Function Test* (WMFT).

The MAL is a semi-structured interview during which respondents are asked to rate how much and how well they use their more affected arm for 30 ADL items in the home over a specified period. As such, the MAL focuses on activity limitations and participation issues. The MAL is administered independently to the client and an informant (often the caregiver). The tasks include such activities as brushing teeth, buttoning a shirt or blouse, and eating with a fork or spoon. For each item the client must report how often and how well (on six-point scales) each activity was performed during a specified period. Information is gathered about motor activity in the week and year prior to the person's participation in the project, the days before and after the intervention, and at the one and two-year follow-up time points. Informants complete the MAL just prior to the beginning of treatment, on one of the testing days just after the completion of treatment, and two times in follow-up. ICF codes that record similar information are found primarily in d4 Mobility, d5 Self-Care, and d6 Domestic Life.

The WMFT primarily addresses body structure limitations and was developed by Dr. Steven Wolf and was modified by Taub and co-workers to quantify motor function in persons with stroke and TBI. Performance time (up to 120 seconds), strength (for lifting and handgrip), and quality of motor function (six-point scale of functional ability) are assessed. The WMFT consists of 17 items, two of which involve strength measures and 15 of which involve timed performances on various tasks. The first half of the test involves simple limb movements, primarily of the proximal musculature. The second half of the test involves tasks performed in the life situation using the distal musculature. The WMFT has been deemed reliable when used with individuals with hemiplegia due to stroke (Morris et al., 2001; Wolf et al., 2001; Wolf et al., 2005).

The WMFT is administered in entirety to the less-affected UE first and then to the more-affected UE. It is conducted pre-treatment, immediately post-treatment, and during the two-year follow-up. The WMFT is filmed and rated later by a panel of therapists who are blinded to the treatment condition and testing session.

Both outcome measures typically demonstrate substantial and statistically significant improvements with research clients. The largest improvements, however, are realized with the MAL, suggesting that the most significant effect of CI therapy is on real-world use of function following the intervention. For this reason, the primary outcome measure used in the UAB Taub Training Clinic is the MAL. The WMFT is not used clinically as the required administration time and equipment needed makes it clinically infeasible.

Conclusion

Over the last 20 years, a large body of evidence has accumulated in support of using CI therapy for hemiparesis following chronic stroke (> one year). CI therapy is believed to produce positive effects through two separate but linked mechanisms: overcoming learned nonuse and use-dependent cortical plasticity. As a result, the CI therapy approach represents a significant paradigm shift in physical rehabilitation. With continued investigation, elaboration, and application to clinical settings, CI therapy would appear to hold great promise for the field of physical rehabilitation. The RT, as part of a collaborative healthcare team, can participate in using CI therapy principles in their therapeutic interventions. The RT is likely to enhance outcomes, as they are experts in assisting their clients to fully engage in leisure and community-based activities. Such activities are more likely to motivate the CI therapy client and, therefore, enhance client engagement in activities that involve spontaneous use of the more affected extremity.

Resources

Constraint-Induced Movement Therapy Research Group, University of Alabama at Birmingham
www.uab.edu/citherapy/
Description of CI therapy, bibliography, training resources, current research projects, and clinical services.

The Brain Fitness Program (Video) PBS Home Video
www.shoppbs.org/product/index.jsp?productId=2966842
The Brain Fitness Program is based on the brain's ability to change and adapt, even rewire itself. In the past two years, a team of scientists has developed computer-based stimulus sets that drive beneficial chemical, physical, and functional changes in the brain. Dr. Michael Merzenich of the University of California and his colleagues share their scientifically based set of brain exercises in this life-altering program.

The Brain that Changes Itself. By Dr. Norman Doidge
www.normandoidge.com/normandoidge.com/MAIN.html
Dr. Norman Doidge introduces principles we can all use to overcome a number of brain limitations and explores the profound brain implications of the changing brain in an immensely moving book that will permanently alter the way we look at human possibility and human nature.

Appendix A: Grade Criteria – Minimum Active ROM and Motor Activity Log (MAL) Scores

Grade 2 Impairment (MAL < 2.5 for AS and HW scale)

Shoulder: Flexion $\geq 45°$ and abduction $\geq 45°$
Elbow: Extension $\geq 20°$ from a 90° flexed starting position
Wrist: Extension $\geq 20°$ from a fully flexed starting position
Fingers: Extension of all MCP and IP (either PIP or DIP) joints $\geq 10°$*
Thumb: Extension or abduction of thumb $\geq 10°$

Grade 3 Impairment (MAL < 2.5 for AS and HW scale)

Shoulder: Flexion $\geq 45°$ and abduction $\geq 45°$
Elbow: Extension $\geq 20°$ from a 90° flexed starting position
Wrist: Extension $\geq 10°$ from a fully flexed starting position
Fingers: Extension $\geq 10°$ MCP and IP (either PIP or DIP) joints of at least 2 fingers[†]
Thumb: Extension or abduction of thumb $\geq 10°$

Grade 4 Impairment (MAL < 2.5 for AS and HW scale)

Shoulder: Flexion $\geq 45°$ and abduction $\geq 45°$
Elbow: Extension $\geq 20°$ from a 90° flexed starting position
Wrist: Extension $\geq 10°$ from a fully flexed starting position
Fingers: Extension of at least 2 fingers $> 0°$ and $< 10°$[†]
Thumb: Extension or abduction of thumb $\geq 10°$

Grade 5 Impairment (Low MAL < 2.5 for AS and HW scale)

Shoulder: At least one of the following: flexion $\geq 30°$ abduction $\geq 30°$ scaption $\geq 30°$
Elbow: Initiation[‡] of both flexion and extension
Wrist, Fingers, and Thumb: Must be able to either initiate[‡] extension of the wrist or initiate extension of one digit

Notes: Each movement must be repeated three times in one minute. Grade 6 clients would fall below the minimum Grade 5 criteria. Grade 1 participants are individuals who are too high functioning for meeting research inclusion criteria. This is primarily determined by scoring higher than a mean of 2.5 on the MAL. These individuals are not included in the research, as we would expect a ceiling effect on their outcome measures. Grade 1 participants may be accepted in the UAB Taub Training Clinic if they wish to achieve a higher level of function.

* Informally assessed when picking up and dropping a tennis ball.
[†] Informally assessed when picking up and dropping a washcloth.
[‡] Initiation is defined for the purposes of criteria as minimal movement (i.e., below the level that can be measured reliably by goniometer).

Appendix B: Components and Subcomponent of the CI therapy Protocol

1. Repetitive, task-oriented training
   a. Shaping
   b. Task practice
2. Adherence-enhancing behavioral strategies (i.e., transfer package)
   a. Daily administration of the *Motor Activity Log* (MAL)
   b. Home diary
   c. Problem solving to overcome apparent barriers to use of the more affected UE in the real-world situation
   d. Behavioral contract
   e. Caregiver contract
   f. Home skill assignment
   g. Home practice
   h. Daily schedule
   i. Weekly phone calls for the first month after treatment to administer the MAL and problem solve
3. Constrained use of the more-affected UE
   a. Mitt restraint
   b. Any method to continually remind the client to use the more-affected UE

Appendix C: Forms of Therapist/Client Interaction Used During Shaping and Task Practice

Feedback

Definition: Providing specific knowledge of results about a client's performance on a shaping trial or task practice session (e.g., the number of repetitions in a set period of time or time required to perform a task or specific number of repetitions).

Use in Shaping: Provided immediately after each trial.

Use in Task Practice: Provided as global knowledge of results at the end of the entire task practice activity.

Coaching

Definition: Providing specific suggestions to improve movements. Aspects of this procedure are described in the behavioral literature as cueing and prompting.

Use in Shaping: Provided liberally throughout all shaping trials.

Use in Task Practice: Provided throughout entire task practice session, though not as often as in shaping.

Modeling

Definition: When a trainer physically demonstrates a task.

Use in Shaping: Provided at the beginning of shaping activity. Repeated between trials as needed.

Use in Task Practice: Provided at the beginning of a task practice activity.

Encouragement

Definition: Providing enthusiastic verbal reward to participants to increase motivation and promote maximal effort (e.g., "that's excellent, that's good, keep trying").

Use in Shaping: Provided liberally throughout all shaping trials.

Use in Task Practice: Provided throughout entire task practice session though not as often as in shaping.

Appendix D: Adherence-Enhancing Intervention Principles Emphasized in Each CI Therapy Transfer Package Component

Motor activity log: monitoring

Behavioral contract: problem solving, behavioral contracting, social support

Caregiver contract: behavioral contracting

Home diary: monitoring, problem solving

Home skill assignment: problem solving, behavioral contracting

Daily schedule: *monitoring*, social support

Home practice: monitoring, behavioral contracting

References

Bauder, H., Sommer, M., Taub, E., & Miltner, W. H. R. (1999). Effect of CI Therapy on movement-related brain potentials. *Psychophysiol, 36*(S), 31.

Bowman, M. H., Taub, E., Uswatte, G., Delgado, A., Bryson, C., Morris, D., McKay, S., & Mark, V. W. A treatment for a chronic stroke patient with a plegic hand combining CI therapy with conventional rehabilitation procedures: Case report. *Neurorehabil, 21*, 167.

Butefisch, C., Hummelsheim, H., Kensler, P., & Mauritz, K-H. (1995). Repetitive training of isolated movements improves the outcome of motor rehabilitation of the centrally paretic hand. *J Neurol Sci, 130*, 59-68.

DiMatteo, M. R. (2004). Social support and patient adherence to medical treatment: A meta-analysis. *Health Psychology, 23*(2), 207.

Dishman, R. K. (1994). Determinants of participation in physical activity. In: Bourchard, C., Shephard, R. J., Stephens, T., Sutton, J. R., & McPherson, B. D., (Eds.) *Physical activity, fitness and health: International proceedings and consensus statement*. Champaign, IL: Human Kinetics.

Dominick, K. L. & Morey, M. (2006). Adherence to physical activity. In: Bosworth, H. B., Oddone, E. Z., Weinberger, M. (Eds.) (2006). *Patient treatment adherence: Concepts, interventions, and measurement*. Mahwah, NJ: Lawrence Erlbaum Assoc.

Gauthier, L. V., Taub, E., Perkins, C., Ortmann, M., Mark, V. W., & Uswatte, G. (2008). Remodeling the brain: Plastic structural changes produced by different motor therapies after stroke. *Stroke, 39*, 1520.

Hesse S., Bertelt C., Schaffrin A., Malezic M. S., & Mauritz K-H. (1994). Restoration of gait in nonambulatory hemiparetic patients by treadmill training with partial body-weight support. *Arch Phys Med Rehabil, 75*, 1087-1093.

King, A. C., Blair, S. N., & Bild, D. E. (1992). Determination of physical activity and interventions in adults. *Med Sci Sports Exerc, 24*, S221.

Kopp, B., Kunkel, A., Muhlnickel, W., Villringer, K., & Taub, E., & Flor, H. (1999). Plasticity in the motor system related to therapy-induced improvement of movement after stroke. *Neuroreport, 10*, 807.

Kunkel, A., Kopp, B., Muller, G., Villringer, K., Villringer, A., Taub, E., & Flor, H. (1999). Constraint-Induced Movement therapy for motor recovery in chronic stroke patients. *Arch Phys Med Rehabil, 80*, 624.

Levy, C. E., Nichols, D. S., Schmalbrock, P. M., Keller, P., & Chakeres, D. W. (2001). Functional MRI evidence of cortical reorganization in upper-limb stroke hemiplegia treated with Constraint-Induced Movement therapy. *Am J Phys Med Rehabil, 80*, 4.

Liepert, J., Bauder, H., Wolfgang, H. R., Miltner, W. H., Taub, E., & Weiller, C. (2000). Treatment-induced cortical reorganization after stroke in humans. *Stroke, 31*, 1210.

Liepert, J., Miltner, W. H., Bauder, H., Sommer, M., Dettmers, C., Taub, E., & Weiller, C. (1998). Motor cortex plasticity during Constraint-Induced Movement therapy in stroke patients. *Neurosci Lett, 250*, 5.

Mark, V. M. & Taub, E. (2004). Constraint-Induced Movement therapy for chronic stroke hemiparesis and other disabilities. *Res Neurol and Neurosci, 22*, 317.

Mark, V. W., Taub, E., & Morris, D. M. (2006). Neural plasticity and Constraint-Induced Movement therapy. *Europa Medicophysica, 42*, 269.

McAuley, E. (1992). The role of efficacy cognitions in the prediction of exercise behavior in middle-aged adults. *J Behav Med. 15*, 65.

McAuley, E., Jerome, G. J., Marquez, D. X., Elavsky, S., & Blissmer, B. (2003). Exercise self-efficacy in older adults: Social, affective, and behavioral influences. *Ann Behav Med, 25*, 1.

Miltner, W. H., Bauder, H., Sommer, M., Dettmers, C., & Taub, E. (1999). Effects of Constraint-Induced Movement Therapy on patients with chronic motor deficits after stroke: A replication. *Stroke, 30*, 586.

Morris, D. M., Crago, J. E., DeLuca, S. C., Pidikiti, R. D., & Taub, E. (1997). Constraint-Induced (CI) Movement Therapy for motor recovery after stroke. *Neurorehabil, 9*, 29.

Morris, D. M., Shaw, S. E., Mark, V. W., Uswatte, G., Barman, J., & Taub, E. (2006). The influence of neuropsychological characteristics on the use of CI therapy with persons with traumatic brain injury. *NeuroRehabilitation, 21*, 131.

Morris, D. M. & Taub, E. (2001). Constraint-induced therapy approach to restoring function after neurological injury. *Top Stroke Rehabil, 8*, 16.

Morris, D. M., Taub, E., & Mark, V. W. (2007). Constraint-induced movement therapy: Characterizing the intervention protocol. *Europa Medicophysica, 42*, 257.

Morris, D. M., Uswatte, G., Crago, J. E., Cook, E. W., & Taub, E. (2001). The reliability of the Wolf Motor Function Test for assessing upper extremity function after stroke. *Arch Phys Med and Rehab, 82*, 750.

Panyan, M. V. (1980). *How to use shaping.* Lawrence, KS: HH Enterprises.

Rejeski, W. J., Brawley, L. R., & Ambrosius, W. T. (2003). Older adults with chronic disease: Benefits of group-mediated counseling in promotion of physical active lifestyles. *Health Psychol, 22*, 414.

Sallis, J. F. & Owen, N. (1999). *Physical Activity and Behavioral Medicine.* Thousand Oaks, CA: Sage Publications.

Shumway-Cook, A. & Woollacott, M. (2001). *Motor control: theory and practical applications.* Philadelphia, PA: Lippincott.

Skinner, B. F. (1968). *The technology of teaching.* New York: Appleton-Century.

Sterr, A. Elbert, T., Berthold, I., Kolbel, S., Rockstroh, B., and Taub, E. (2002). CI therapy in chronic hemiparesis: The more the better? *Arch Phys Med Rehabil, 83*, 1374.

Taub, E. (1977). Movement in nonhuman primates deprived of somatosensory feedback. *Exercise and Sports Sciences Reviews, 4*, 335.

Taub E. (1980). Somatosensory deafferentation research with monkeys: Implications for rehabilitation medicine. In: Ince, L. P. (Ed.): *Behavioral psychology in rehabilitation medicine: Clinical applications.* New York: Williams & Wilkins.

Taub, E. (2004). Harnessing brain plasticity through behavioral techniques to produce new treatments in neurorehabilitation. *Am Psychologist, 59*, 692.

Taub, E., Crago, J. E., Burgio, L. D., Groomes, T. E., Cook, E. W., DeLuca, S. C., & Miller, N. E. (1994). An operant approach to rehabilitation medicine: Overcoming learned nonuse by shaping. *J Exp Anal Behav, 61*, 281.

Taub, E., Miller, N. E., Novack, T. A., Cook, E. W., Fleming, W. C., Nepomuceno, C. S., Connell, J. S., & Crago, J. E. (1993). Technique to improve chronic motor deficit after stroke. *Arch Phys Med Rehabil, 74*, 347.

Taub, E. & Uswatte, G. (2006). Constraint-induced movement therapy: Answers and questions after two decades of research. *NeuroRehabilitation, 21*(2), 93.

Taub, E., Uswatte, G., Bowman, M. H., Mark, V. W., Delgado, A., Bryson, C., Morris, D., & Bishop-McKay, S. (2013b). Constraint-Induced Movement Therapy combined with conventional neurorehabilitation techniques in chronic stroke patients with plegic hands: A case series. *Arch Phys Med Rehabil, 94*, 86.

Taub, E., Uswatte, G. & Elbert, T. (2002). New treatments in neurorehabilitation founded on basic research. *Nat Rev Neurosci, 3*, 228.

Taub, E., Uswatte, G., Mark, V. W., Morris, D. M., Barman, J., Bowman, M. H., Bryson, C., Delgado, A., & Bishop-McKay, S. (2013a). Method for enhancing real-world use of a more affected arm in chronic stroke: Transfer package of Constraint-Induced Movement Therapy. *Stroke, 44*, 1383.

Taub, E., Uswatte, G., & Pidikitti, R. (1999). Constraint-induced movement therapy: A new family of techniques with broad application to physical rehabilitation – a clinical review. *J Rehabil Res Dev, 36*, 237-251.

Trost, S. G., Owen, N., Bauman, A. E., Sallis, J. F., & Brown, W. (2002). Correlates of adults' participation in physical activity: Review and update. *Med Sci Sports Exer. 34*, 1996.

Uswatte, G. & Taub, E. (2005). Implications of the learned nonuse formulation for measuring rehabilitation outcomes: Lessons from Constraint-Induced Movement Therapy. *Rehabil Psychol, 50*, 34.

Uswatte, G., Taub, E., Morris, D., Barman, J., & Crago, J. (2006). Contribution of the shaping and restraint components of Constraint-Induced Movement Therapy to treatment outcome. *NeuroRehabil., 21*(2), 147.

Uswatte, G., Taub, E., Morris, D., Light, K., & Thompson, P. (2006). The Motor Activity Log-28: Assessing daily use of the hemiparetic arm after stroke. *Neurology, 67*, 1189.

Uswatte, G., Taub, E., Morris, D. M., Vignolo, M., & McCulloch, K. (2006). Reliability and validity of the upper-extremity motor activity log-14 for measuring real-world arm use. *Stroke, 36*, 2493.

Van der Lee, J. H., Beckerman, H., Knol, D. L., deVet, H. C., & Bouter, L. M. (2004). Clinimetric properties of the motor activity log for the assessment of arm use in hemiparetic patients. *Stroke, 35*, 1410.

Wittenberg, G. F., Chen, R., Ishii, K., Bushara, K. O., Eckloff, S., Croarkin, K. O., Taub, E., Gerber, L. H., Hallett, M., & Cohen, L. G. (2003). Constraint-induced therapy in stroke: Magnetic stimulation motor maps and cerebral activation. *Neurorehabilitation & Neural Repair, 17*, 48-57.

Wolf, S. L., Catlin, P. A., Ellis, M., Link, A., Morgan, B., & Piacento, A. (2001). Assessing the Wolf Motor Function Test as an outcome measure for research with patients after stroke. *Stroke, 32*, 1635.

Wolf, S. L., Thompson, P. A., Morris, D. M., Rose, D. K., Winstein, C. J., Taub, E., Giuliani, C., & Pearson, S. (2005). The EXCITE Trial: Attributes of the Wolf Motor Function Test in patients with subacute stroke. *Neurorehabil Neural Repair, 19*, 194.

26. Disability Rights: Education and Advocacy

Terry Dean Long, Jr.

One of the many roles of a recreational therapist is to educate and advocate in the realm of disability rights (d940 Human Rights, d950 Political Life and Citizenship). Through recreational therapy services, clients can be equipped with knowledge and skills that enable them to fully exercise their rights as citizens and as human beings. Successful transition and integration into the community is often contingent upon an individual's ability to recognize and exercise his/her rights. In cases where a client cannot self-advocate, recreational therapists may act on the client's behalf. Whether on behalf of an individual or the disability community in general, advocacy should be an inherent part of the recreational therapists daily activities, particularly in regard to the right to recreation programs and services, community involvement, and the active engagement with and contribution to society. At the same time, recreational therapy services can focus on educating clients to self-advocate in their daily lives.

Client deficits in connections with the community can be documented with ICF codes in d6 Domestic Life, d8 Major Life Areas, and d9 Community, Social, and Civic Life. Self-advocacy often involves d7 Interpersonal Interactions and Relationships. Problems in the environment that may need to be addressed are found in many of the Environmental Factors codes, especially e1 Products and Technology for assistive devices and accessibility issues; e3 Support and Relationships for assistance and healthcare; e4 Attitudes for making the community aware and accepting of disability rights; and e5 Services, Systems, and Policies for policies about accessibility.

As educators and advocates, recreational therapists can consider disability rights from both a civil rights perspective and a human rights perspective. Civil rights pertain to a person's right to equality as a citizen, and often are established on behalf of specific segments of society such as women, people of color, or persons with disabilities. Civil rights laws are typically enacted at the federal level, but can also be enacted through state or local government. Human rights, on the other hand, refer to the rights that a person has simply based on the fact that they are human beings. Citizenship is not required. Human rights, by their nature, reflect a global perspective and are legally established at the international level through organizations such as the United Nations. The applicability of both civil and human rights to recreational therapy practice is important to consider.

The Persistence of Inequity

Despite significant positive change over the past 50 years, persons with disabilities are often overlooked, forgotten, and even intentionally ostracized, neglected, or abused. In the United States, there are daily violations of the Americans with Disabilities Act, the Individuals with Disabilities Education Act, and many other disability-related laws. Beyond the law, society struggles to rid itself of misunderstanding, stereotypes, fear, and cruelty.

The consequences of such inequities have been documented in the findings of the National Organization on Disability's (NOD) 2010 survey of Americans with disabilities (NOD & Kessler Foundation, 2010). Overall, respondents were found to score somewhat behind or far behind people without disabilities on 12 of 13 quality of life indicators considered in the survey. In addition, the survey indicated that, since the first NOD survey in 1986, gaps between persons with and without disabilities have widened on five of ten social and economic indicators. In the 2010 survey, persons with disabilities reported lower employment rates (21% vs. 59%), higher poverty rates (34% vs. 15%), and lower high school completion rates (83% vs. 89%).

The 2007 American Community Survey (ACS) also found that non-institutionalized working aged (21-65) persons with a disability were less likely to be employed compared to persons with no reported disability (37% vs. 80% employment rate; Erickson & Lee, 2008). Only 22% of ACS respondents with disabilities indicated being employed full time for at least one full year, compared to 57% of respondents reporting no disability (Erickson & Lee, 2008). This finding is consistent with the 2010 NOD finding. Employment is a complex issue that can be directly impacted by disability-related impairments; however, there is no doubt that inequities exist for people with disabilities.

There is also a significant disadvantage for persons with disabilities regarding access to healthcare. NOD survey results indicated that 19% of respondents who had disabilities reported that they did not get needed medical care in the past year, compared to 10% of individuals without disabilities. Research suggests that the disability community is less likely than the general population to participate in routine health screenings and routine checkups (Altman & Bernstein, 2008). The unfortunate irony of this disparity is that persons with disability are more likely to experience health-related difficulties than the general population. When they do seek out healthcare services, individuals commonly find themselves experiencing barriers including inaccessible facilities and medical equipment, lack of transportation, inadequate accommodations regarding communication, inappropriate attitudes among medical staff, and a lack of knowledge among healthcare providers regarding the unique health-related needs of persons with disabilities (Centers for Disease Control and Prevention, 2006; Drainoni et al., 2006; Kroll et al., 2006; Lezonni et al., 2004; McIlfatrick, Taggart, & Truesdale-Kennedy, 2011; National Council on Disability, 2009; Pereira & Fortes, 2010).

In the social realm, the 2010 NOD survey findings indicated that persons with disabilities were less likely to socialize with close friends or family at least twice a month (79% vs. 90%). They were also less likely to regularly attend a worship service (50% vs. 57%) or eat at a restaurant at least twice a month (48% vs. 74%).

Federal Law and Civil Rights

Throughout the latter half of the 20th century, American society was transformed by the Civil Rights movement. One of the ostracized groups in America to be empowered through this movement was the disability community. In addition to advocacy efforts from inside and outside of the disability community, a series of federal acts led to the recognition of rights for persons with disabilities. The Americans with Disabilities Act (ADA) of 1990 is the most contemporary and comprehensive disability rights law in existence today. The Individuals with Disabilities Education Act, with its most recent reauthorization in 2004, has been equally impactful in the realm of education. Both laws have direct implications for recreational therapy practice and will be the focus of discussion for the remainder of this section.

Americans with Disabilities Act of 1990

The Americans with Disabilities Act (ADA) made it illegal to discriminate on the basis of disability in the areas of employment, public services, public accommodations, transportation, and telecommunications. Prior laws had included mandates pertaining to some of these areas, as well, though not in such a comprehensive and enforceable manner. The ADA applies to people who have a physical or mental impairment that substantially limits one or more major life activities, such as dressing, bathing, working, and shopping.

Therapists need to be very familiar with the ADA to facilitate successful community integration and empower and educate clients about their civil rights. Clients are usually very interested in the ADA because it addresses their ability to participate in life tasks such as work and recreation. Question that the ADA answers include: Is my employer supposed to let me work a flexible workweek? Is the YMCA supposed to have a ramp out front? Is it reasonable to ask the grocery store to provide me with assistance in getting my groceries into the car? Is the city bus supposed to have a wheelchair lift? Therapists should know the answers to these questions or know how to find out the answers to help facilitate positive changes and compliance with the ADA. The therapist might call the grocery store about available assistance or the YMCA to inquire about putting a ramp out front, or teach the client how to ask those questions.

Therapists should have copies of the ADA technical manuals (I, II, III) and information on specific modes of transportation and telecommunications related to ADA compliance. Therapists must have a copy of the "Americans with Disabilities Act Accessibility Guidelines" and the "Uniform Federal Accessibility Standards." Both of these come in a checklist format and make assessment of facilities quite easy. Additionally, therapists should have copies of "ADA Accessibility Guidelines for Play Areas" and "ADA Accessibility Guidelines for Recreation Facilities." Both are very helpful in clinical practice. Contact information for acquiring these resources is provided in the Resources section.

Educating clients, caregivers, and the community about the ADA increases their insight into changes that have been made in our society. People who have a new disability are often not aware of this federal law that protects their civil rights and prohibits discrimination against them in regard to employment, transportation, telecommunication, and accessibility to buildings and programs. Knowledge of the ADA is a tool that can leverage change. It can expand a client's perception about what s/he can do in the community (work, recreation, travel), dispel disability myths (there are more opportunities and access than people usually expect), and empower the client to seek needed changes in his/her own life tasks (e.g., contact employer to discuss accommodations). This knowledge may also aid in decreasing anxiety (e.g., knowing that an employer needs to make reasonable accommodations lessens anxiety over what the client is going to do about a job), lifting feelings of depression (e.g., knowing that many places in the community are now wheelchair accessible and provide services to help someone who has a disability), and fostering an internal locus of control (e.g., knowing what s/he is entitled to under the ADA gives the client a knowledge base to assert change in his/her community). ADA education is one of many interventions that can increase the activity level of the client. Maintaining a healthy activity level decreases the client's risk for developing secondary complications.

ADA Titles

The following brief description of the elements of the ADA, referred to as "Titles," can be used to educate clients about their rights under the law. It is not a full account of all compliance requirements.

Therapists and clients should consult the ADA technical assistance manuals and contact the appropriate organizations when more information is needed. Information on how to obtain these manuals and the organizations that can assist you in understanding the ADA is provided in the Resource section. One resource found to be particularly helpful is *The Americans with Disabilities Act: Your Personal Guide to the Law*, which is a free booklet put out by the Paralyzed Veterans of America. Therapists can ask clients to call and request their own free copy, or the therapist (in anticipation of reviewing this information with the client) can call on behalf of the client and have it mailed to the facility in time to review it with the client. See the Resource section for contact information.

Title I: Employment: If a person with a disability is qualified for the position and can perform the job requirements with or without reasonable accommodations, the employer cannot deny the person employment solely based on the fact that s/he has a disability. Employers who have 15 or more employees must abide by this law and make reasonable accommodations unless it is a proven hardship for the company. An undue hardship means that the accommodations would be unduly costly, disruptive, or extensive or would fundamentally alter the nature or operation of the business. In this situation, the person with the disability should be allowed to provide the accommodation (e.g., will supply the desk) and/or pay for the portion of the accommodation that is above the employer's ability. Tax incentives are available for employers who make accommodations for a person with a disability (tax credits and deductions). Reasonable accommodations could include job restructuring, modified work schedules, acquisition or modification of equipment, provision of readers or interpreters, and any other accommodation that is deemed as being reasonable. Employees with disabilities are held to employment standards and termination could occur if they are not met (e.g., use of illegal drugs, inability to perform job even with accommodations). Employers who have less than 15 employees are not required to comply with this law. They are not required to comply because they will often lack the resources to make reasonable accommodations. State and local government employers with less than 15 employees do not have this exemption and must comply with the ADA

Title II: Public Services: Any state or local government service, program, activity, or building must comply with the ADA. This includes the courts, town meeting halls, police and fire departments, voting locations and machines, emergency assistance (including 911), and motor vehicle licensing. The person who has a disability cannot be denied access to a service, program, or activity because of disability. Integrated services must be implemented unless separate services are needed to ensure equal opportunity. Programs must be held in accessible locations in the building, such as the first floor rather than the second floor when there is no elevator. Public entities may choose between two technical standards for accessible design: the Uniform Federal Accessibility Standards (UFAS) or the Americans with Disabilities Act Accessibility Guidelines (ADAAG). Free copies of both of these guides can be obtained from the U.S. Architectural and Transportation Barriers Compliance Board. Public entities are required to provide alternative forms of communication (e.g., interpreter, large print materials) when needed.

Title III: Public Accommodation: A public accommodation is defined as a facility operated by a private entity that affects interstate commerce and falls within at least one of these categories:

- Places of lodging, such as inns, hotels, and motels, except establishments in which the proprietor resides and rents out no more than five rooms.
- Establishments serving food or drink, such as restaurants and bars.
- Places of exhibition or entertainment, such as theaters, auditoriums, and stadiums.
- Places of public gatherings, such as auditoriums, convention centers, and lecture halls.
- Sales or rental establishments, such as grocery stores, bakeries, clothing stores, and shopping centers.
- Service establishments, such as dry cleaners, banks, beauty shops, hospitals, and offices of health-care professionals, lawyers, and accountants.
- Stations used for specified public transportation, such as terminals and depots.
- Places of public display, such as museums, libraries, and galleries.
- Places of recreation, such as parks, zoos, and amusement parks.

- Places of education, such as nursery, elementary, secondary, undergraduate, and postgraduate private schools.
- Social service centers, such as day-care or senior citizen centers, adoption programs, food banks, and homeless shelters.
- Places of exercise or recreation, such as gymnasiums, health spas, bowling alleys, and golf courses.

Such accommodations include making any new construction accessible (including remodeling), providing accessible parking spaces, a ramp at the entrance, accessible seating, access to elevators, Braille markings, note takers, and interpreters. Private clubs and religious organizations are exempt from public accommodation requirements.

Transportation regulations: Transportation regulations fall under both Title II and Title III of the ADA, although the technical manual for transportation is kept separate. The ADA provides specific requirements for city buses, taxis, paratransit services, trains, airplanes, over-the-road (intercity or interstate) buses, university bus systems, vanpools, and subways. There are different regulations for each mode of travel depending on whether or not they are private or public, the number of people who are able to be seated in the mode of transportation, and the type of system (e.g., fixed route, demand responsive). Therapists can consult the various technical assistance manuals from the U.S. Architectural and Transportation Barriers Compliance Board. There is a manual for each mode of transportation.

Title IV: Telecommunications: A nationwide telephone relay service has been established through the use of text-based telephones called Telecommunication Devices for the Deaf (TDDs). A TDD is a device with a keyboard and a message display that connects to a specially equipped telephone. Some TDDs have printers that print out the message as it is received rather than a screen. Sometimes they are referred to a Text Typewriters (TTs) or Teletypewriters (TTYs). Before the ADA, a person with a hearing or speech impairment typed a message into the TDD and the message appeared on the TDD screen of the person s/he was calling. This meant that the other person also had to have a TDD. Now, because of the ADA, there is a nationwide telephone relay service so the other person does not have to have a TDD. The person who has a hearing or speech impairment types a message into the TDD and it is sent to a relay operator. The relay operator reads the message to the other party. The person responds to the message verbally by speaking to the relay operator. The relay operator sends the response to the person with the hearing or speech impairment through the TDD. This exchange continues for as long as the two parties wish to communicate and there are no restrictions on the content of the messages. Relay operators are not allowed to intentionally alter any part of the communication and they are prohibited from disclosing the content or nature of the calls. TDD calls cannot be limited or refused by the phone carrier. Service is available 24 hours a day. Therapists who are interested in acquiring a TDD for a client should contact their local phone company for further information. As technologies have advanced, more sophisticated means of communication have developed. In fact, proposed revisions to ADA could soon change wording in the law to include other voice, text, and video-based telecommunications products and systems, including TTYs, videophones, and captioned telephones or other equally effective telecommunications systems. As an example, video technology allows for individuals using sign language to make "calls" via a live interpreter. The sign language interpreter communicates through a video relay with the caller from a remote location, and then relays the message to the call recipient. Video systems also allow two individuals using sign language to have direct, and more effective, conversation than a text-based system would permit. Another important area of communications related accommodation is closed-captioning. All public service announcements that are federally funded or produced must have closed-captioning on the television screen. Closed-captioning is text on the bottom of the television screen similar to movie subtitles that allows a person to read what is being said on the television. All television sets that have screens larger than 13" have a built-in decoder chip to enable the set to display the captioning. Televisions that have this chip can be programmed to show closed-captioning on the screen when it is provided. Most programs now provide closed captioning.

ADA Legal Issues

The right to accessible programs and services: The ADA is recognized by most as a law that requires buildings and facilities to be constructed in a manner that provides physical accessibility. What is less known is that the ADA guarantees equal access to not only facilities, but also to any service provided by government-funded agencies. Essentially, this aspect of the ADA mandates the right to inclusive participation, as the opportunity to participate in programs and services must be provided in the most integrated setting possible. For example, Title II of the ADA ensures access to government-funded parks and recreation programs and services. Educating clients about the services aspect of the ADA is critical, as is informing them of the limitations of these rights. For example, accommodations can be denied when the accommodation creates an unreasonable economic or administrative burden, presents a safety risk, or would otherwise change the inherent nature of the program. In addition, all participants, regardless of disability, can be required to meet "essential eligibility requirements" pertaining to age restrictions, pre-registration requirements, or providing their own transportation. Having a disability does not exempt a person from being required to meet these requirements. However, selectively applying these requirements to only certain individuals is a violation of the ADA. For example, requiring a person who uses a wheelchair to arrange for his own transportation when others are provided transportation would not be allowed.

The Olmstead decision: When relevant to client circumstances, education and training regarding the ADA should include a discussion of 1999 Olmstead ruling (Olmstead v. L.C., 527 U.S. 581), otherwise known as the Olmstead Act. In this case, the Supreme Court interpreted Title II of the ADA as requiring states to place persons with disabilities in community settings rather than in institutions whenever appropriate. The Court ruled that offering institutionalization as the only option for care violated the right to access services in the most integrated setting possible. This law is relevant to individuals in institutions who would prefer not to be there, as well as those who are at risk of institutionalization. States are required to meet their obligations regarding the Olmstead decision by developing a comprehensive work plan for placing qualified persons in "less restrictive settings." The end result is a variety of different community-based service opportunities. Therapists can educate clients in this realm, as well as personally advocate for the appropriate fulfillment of this obligation by the state.

ADA complaints and enforcement: Procedures for filing a complaint regarding an ADA violation depend on the Title under which the violation occurs. For example, Title I complaints are filed with the Equal Employment Opportunity Commission. Other types of complaints are filed with the Department of Justice. In addition, private lawsuits can be filed. Except for circumstances involving employment, private lawsuits seek to force compliance rather than obtain monetary awards for the plaintiff. The exact method for pursuing a complaint, like many legal actions, can be fairly complex. Seeking guidance from the Department of Justice and legal counsel is typically the best route, as they can assist with solving the problem and/or filing a complaint.

Individuals with Disabilities Education Act

The Individuals with Disabilities Education Act (IDEA) provides the right to a free and appropriate public education. Originally referred to as the Education for All Handicapped Children Act (1975), the law had four initial purposes (U.S. Department of Education, 2007):

to assure that all children with disabilities have available to them…a free appropriate public education which emphasizes special education and related services designed to meet their unique needs

to assure that the rights of children with disabilities and their parents … are protected

to assist States and localities to provide for the education of all children with disabilities

to assess and assure the effectiveness of efforts to educate all children with disabilities

The reauthorization of the law in 1990 changed the title to IDEA, with subsequent reauthorizations in 1997 and 2004 resulting in the current IDEA requirements. IDEA is a federal law, but is monitored and implemented at the state level. Thus, programs and associated regulations may vary from state to state. Key elements of IDEA that each state must ensure include the zero reject principle, the right to a non-discriminatory evaluation, provision of the least restrictive environment, the right to due process, and the parent/student participation principle. These elements are mentioned here because they are critical to successfully advocate among parents and service providers. Zero reject ensures no eligible child will be denied special education services, regardless of cost or other circumstances. Non-discriminatory evaluation ensures fairness and parental consent when determining if the child has a disability and identifying any necessary special education services. Least restrictive environment means that schools must provide academic services in the setting that best allows for student achievement. In other words, segregation from other students should not occur beyond what is absolutely necessary for successful learning. The parent/student participation principle ensures that the family is directly involved and an equal party in educational decisions. This principle is sometimes referred to as the "50% rule," meaning the parents hold 50% of decision-making power, and that no decision regarding special education eligibility, placement, or services goes unchecked. Due process allows for third party arbitration when it comes to academic placement and planning decisions. Due process provides a mechanism for fair resolution to be exercised when disagreements occur between school and parent.

As an example, the state of Missouri has published the *Parents Guide to Special Education in Missouri*. This resource outlines federal and state-specific rights, rules, and regulations regarding special education. It also includes a listing of the following parental rights under IDEA (Missouri Department of Elementary and Secondary Education, 2008, p. 16):

1. All children with disabilities must be provided a free and appropriate public education.
2. The special education services for each identified, eligible child with a disability should be designed to meet the child's unique needs, and the parents cannot be required to pay for those special education services.
3. The school program for a child with a disability must be based on a complete and nondiscriminatory evaluation of the child.
4. Parents must give their permission for their child to be evaluated if the assessment or tests are not administered to all students in the same class, grade, or school.

5. Parents must give their permission for their child to receive special education services for the first time.

6. Parents have the right to participate in decisions about the identification, eligibility, provision of a free appropriate public education, and placement of their child with a disability.

7. Parents must be notified in writing of any proposed change in their child's IEP before it occurs.

8. Parents must be informed, by receiving a copy of the Procedural Safeguards, how they may challenge and appeal any decisions or proposed actions concerning identification, evaluation, free appropriate public education, or placement of their child.

These rights are core elements of IDEA, but other Missouri-specific elements are included in the handbook as well, such as eligibility guidelines, deadlines for completing evaluations, and procedures for developing individualized education programs. States often vary on specifics such as these. It is critical that recreational therapists familiarize themselves with the guidelines of the state where clients receive their education.

Three aspects of education that might be especially relevant to recreational therapists as they work with children and their families to understand and utilize related resources are early childhood programs, after-school programs, and transition planning. IDEA requires the development of an Individualized Family Service Plan (IFSP) for infants and toddlers who are eligible for services before they reach school age. This plan is intended to address developmental delays as early as possible, so that critical developmental milestones and associated goal areas can be addressed at the appropriate and most beneficial time. The IFSP often involves programs that are outside of the school system and recreational therapy could potentially be built into this system of intervention. Likewise, after school programs may be considered an extension of the school day, and educational goals and objectives may be relevant to this setting as well, even though outside entities may be involved in the planning and implementation of such programs. Finally, preparing for the transition to adulthood and post-education life requires the development of a Transition Plan. School officials sometimes work with outside agencies and professionals to prepare the student in all areas of functioning for life as an adult. Recreational therapists are potential partners as transition plans are put into place, typically around the age of 16. Finally it should be noted that, in some cases, recreational therapists are employed in the school system to provide recreational therapy services to children receiving special education services; however, most schools do not provide such services in their school-day curriculum.

The extent to which recreational therapy is a part of the student's actual educational program will vary from state to state, and even district to district. Generally speaking, recreational therapy is sometimes provided as part of special education, but IDEA does not require recreational therapy for all special education students. Still, recreational therapists will work with school-aged clients and their parents, and educating them about their educational rights is an area that can be addressed through disability rights education. As with ADA, there are many misperceptions and inaccurate assumptions regarding IDEA, and families are often hesitant to question school officials. They may not even realize that IDEA applies to their child. Unfortunately, IDEA is grossly underfunded, which creates scenarios that make compliance difficult and typically obtained at only a minimal level. Parents, and eventually their children, must be able to advocate for their right to a free and appropriate public education.

International Law and Human Rights

The concept of human rights, in theory, goes beyond civil rights in that human rights pertain to every human being, regardless of location or circumstance. It is often said that a human right only exists when it applies to all humans. This would include individuals with a disability of any type. By their very nature, human rights are identified and enacted on an international scale (either regionally or globally). This fact creates some challenges in regard to ensuring human rights, as historical and cultural views within individual societies often conflict with one another or with the philosophy that all humans have such rights.

To illustrate this challenge, consider the *Convention on the Rights of the Child*. This international treaty (or law) is intended to protect the human rights of children throughout the world, requiring governments to enact laws that protect the best interest of the child (United Nations, 1997). The United States helped developed this treaty and signed it in 1995, but has yet to ratify the treaty more than 15 years later. Essentially, this means that the U.S. supports the development of this treaty, but will not allow for the associated laws to be enforced, by outside parties, within its own borders. At first glance, the position of the U.S. Government on this treaty seems inhumane, but the reason for declining to ratify the treaty is complex. Concerns related to ratification of this treaty include the potential for international courts to determine American policies regarding child custody disputes, abortion, stem cell research, and the right to home-school children. As of 2010, the United States and Somalia were the only two countries that had not ratified this treaty (Amnesty International, 2011).

The above case illustrates that human rights are a theoretically ideal, but the diverse array of world-views regarding virtually every human rights issue creates significant challenges regarding widespread adoption and monitoring of international law. Despite these challenges, the establishment of human rights is an important element of the disability rights movement and an important educational topic to explore with recreational therapy clients. The following section discusses existing international law pertaining to individuals with disabilities, its potential application, and related limitations.

Convention on the Rights of Persons with Disabilities

A series of international declarations that address the human rights of individuals with disabilities has been developed during the past 50 years. For the most part, these declarations are position statements and lack mechanisms for enforcement. The first and only globally established international law regarding disability is the United Nations Convention on the Rights of Persons with Disabilities. This treaty was signed by the United Nations General Assembly in 2006 and by the United States in 2009 (United Nations, 2010). As with other treaties, the United States has been hesitant to ratify this convention, with much of the debate focusing on potential incompatibility with the ADA, the feasibility of enforcement, and the potential for external entities to impact or override domestic law.

Because the convention has not been ratified through a two-thirds majority vote of the U.S. Senate, any legal benefits or resources for persons living in

the United States have yet to manifest. However, the level of international commitment to this treaty has significant implications. In essence, the treaty is a reflection of worldwide societal and cultural changes regarding attitudes and actions toward persons with disabilities. By signing this Convention, the U.S. has endorsed its principles and should honor them as a society. Recreational therapists can empower clients to recognize this commitment and advocate for their rights as citizens and as human beings. Furthermore, it may be that the near future will bring U.S. ratification of the treaty and the development of associated protocols for enforcement. At the very least, awareness of the convention's existence and what it entails communicates to individuals with disabilities an ideal of equality that can be empowering even when not fully realized.

Principles of the Convention

The CRPD is the first legally binding international treaty that specifically provides comprehensive protection of the rights of persons with disabilities. General principles of the convention, as described in Article 3, include the following:

- Respect for inherent dignity, individual autonomy, including the freedom to make one's own choices and independence of persons
- Non-discrimination
- Full and effective participation and inclusion in society
- Respect for difference and acceptance of persons with disabilities as part of human diversity and humanity
- Equality of opportunity
- Accessibility
- Equality between men and women
- Respect for the evolving capacities of children with disabilities and respect for the right of children with disabilities to preserve their identities

Specific rights falling under these principles include:

- Equality before the law without discrimination
- Right to life, liberty, and security of the person
- Equal recognition before the law and legal capacity
- Freedom from torture
- Freedom from exploitation, violence, and abuse
- Right to respect of physical and mental integrity
- Freedom of movement and nationality

- Right to live in the community
- Freedom of expression and opinion
- Respect for privacy
- Respect for home and the family
- Right to education
- Right to health
- Right to work
- Right to an adequate standard of living
- Right to participate in political and public life
- Right to participate in cultural life (United Nations, 2010)

In regard to recreational therapy, many of these principles and rights should be a common focus of discussion and intervention in practice. The CRPD framework can be utilized as a context for explaining the importance of understanding and acting upon one's rights and advocating for those rights whenever necessary. Once again, gaining knowledge of one's rights can be tremendously empowering, as clients are encouraged to see themselves as justified in their desire to experience a fulfilling life.

Indications

Any individual with a newly acquired disability can benefit from the opportunity to learn about their rights as a member of society, as a human being, and as a person with a disability. Furthermore, significant changes in life circumstances may warrant additional education, training, and advocacy. Education is also necessary for those who may have lived with a disability for years, but were never given the opportunity to learn about their disability-related rights. Finally, additional education may be necessary as laws and treaties continue to evolve, particularly in regard to the continued development of ADA codes and the potential ratification of CRPD.

Contraindications

A client who has significant cognitive impairment may experience difficulty with retention, recollection, and application of material presented to them regarding human rights and advocacy opportunities. Other clients may struggle to advocate in a productive, rather than destructive, manner. If significant cognitive impairments are evident, the therapist can work to educate the client's caregivers, as they may be in a position to advocate for or with the care recipient. Careful consideration and adequate

justification should occur before dismissing the potential of any individual to advocate for himself/herself. Underestimating a person's potential to develop and apply such skills can be extremely harmful. Always maximize client opportunities, no matter how small, to learn about their rights and to engage in both self and social advocacy

Protocols and Processes

The length and frequency of disability rights training sessions will vary depending on the identified needs and abilities of the client. On average, training takes about one hour (one half hour to review information pertaining to civil and human rights and another half hour to practice applying the information through role-playing and phone calls). The exact nature of the presented material may vary based on the client circumstances, but common concepts would include reviewing IDEA principles with school-aged clients and their parents, the titles of the ADA, and even the basic principles of international law. Also to be included in this session and subsequent sessions is the topic of advocacy skills and dealing with circumstances where rights are being violated. This is not to say that a client will be fully proficient in knowledge and application of these laws and concepts in one hour, but the client who does not have cognitive impairments should be able to obtain a basic understanding of the law and its application.

Education should take place in a quiet, non-distracting environment to promote concentration, consideration of the implications of the act, and retention of information. The therapist should have relevant materials (e.g., ADA booklet from the Paralyzed Veterans Association, paper and pen to write down barriers and identified solutions). Additional sessions should be scheduled to allow for evaluation of the client's ability to apply learned information in a real-life environment. This is typically done in the form of community integration training on scheduled outings into the community.

The general process of disability rights education is reflected in the outline below. Therapists should alter this process as needed to best meet the needs of the client.

What is it? Tell the client that disability rights pertain to their rights as a citizen and as a human being and prohibit discrimination on the basis of disability.

How does it affect the client? Discuss with the client their particular circumstances and how relevant laws guarantee the right to aspects of life such as equal employment opportunities, communication, transportation, public services, and recreation participation. Being aware of what is supposed to be available is very important so that clients can make plans to do things without running into problems. Unfortunately, despite the many changes that have already been made, barriers still exist and clients will undoubtedly encounter them. When these occur, they will need to problem solve and talk with people to come up with a solution. The more the clients know, the better they will be able to problem solve for these situations.

Review specific rights: Educate the client about his/her rights under federal law and international treaty. Use the document descriptions provided in this chapter when applicable.

Problems: Ask the client what problems s/he foresees and help the client problem solve (e.g., worksite is not accessible, can't get into the bathroom at the gym, no accessible parking spots at the local store). When appropriate, advocate for the client.

Questions and manuals: If the therapist does not know the answer to a particular problem or question, call the corresponding government office, as listed in the Resources section. In addition to queries directed to the appropriate office representative, various manuals and other resources are available at minimal or no cost to assist in training and troubleshooting. Once the information is received it can be put into a binder for later reference.

Application: Recreational therapists help clients apply the information that they have learned about the ADA. This is usually done through phone calls and outings, as well as through spontaneous and planned opportunities to self-advocate. The therapist may ask the client to identify a place in the community where s/he wishes to go and needs to know its level of accessibility and the services it offers to someone who has a disability. Draw up a list of questions to ask before the phone call is placed. The amount of assistance a client needs with this task will vary. Set a realistic goal for applying disability rights law and re-explain the purpose of setting this goal, if needed. A possible goal might be. "Client to require minimal verbal cues to apply ADA information through telephone inquiries." Next, plan an outing

with the plan of working on the application of the ADA in a community environment. This might include finding out where the accessible bathroom is located, evaluating the bathroom to determine if it truly meets accessibility guidelines, identifying the bathroom challenges for the client, and then problem solving for a solution. Clients should be encouraged to identify problem areas, seek out assistance to overcome a specific barrier, and identify architectural or service changes that could increase his/her function. Challenge the client further with "what if" questions, such as: What would you do if you were told there was an accessible bathroom and when you got there you found out that it was a low toilet instead of a high toilet and now you require assistance? What would you do if the elevator was broken and you were on the second floor? Challenging practical problem-solving skills is important for successful community transitioning.

The therapist documents the specific education provided and the client's ability to recall the information, verbally apply information to proposed situations, and demonstrate application of learned material in a real-life environment (activity performance).

Example: Client educated on the ADA. Client able to recall 75% of ADA material at modified independence (increased time and use of written reference — PVA booklet). Client able to contact a community facility via telephone and explore its level of accessibility and available disability services with minimal assistance. During community integration session to Home Depot, client independently requested assistance from an employee to retrieve and carry large items.

In addition to the ICF codes discussed earlier, the therapist may also score the specific problems that make it difficult for the client to enjoy human rights (e.g., b1266 Confidence, d166 Reading). Client and therapist work to resolve the environmental factors that were noted earlier should also be documented.

Conclusion

Addressing disability rights should be an ongoing element of recreational therapy services. Empowering clients to master and utilize their civic and human rights may be the most powerful tool we can offer them in regard to life-long, active participation in society and healthy living in general. Disability rights education is presented here as a specific technique for practice, but ideally should be an inherent part of all comprehensive programs and the systems through which they are delivered. Sylvester (2011) emphasizes this point when stating,

> The ICF is designed to assess functioning at three levels: individual, institutional, and social (WHO, 2002). At the social level, it pointedly asks, "Will guaranteeing rights improve functioning at the societal level?" (p. 6). While the ADA has resulted in some improvements, significantly more progress is necessary for citizens with disabilities to substantially achieve rights comparable to citizens who, at least at the time, do not have disabilities. Consequently, professions must do more than offer counsel on laws and rights. They must assess, plan, and intervene to effect change at the social level. (p. 26)

Disability rights (d940 Human Rights) are at the heart at the ICF philosophy, which goes beyond "clinical diagnosis, treatment, and medical outcomes to how people with health conditions are actually able to live in their communities" (Sylvester, 2011, p. 1). The ability to utilize rights, disability-related or otherwise, must be recognized as a key element of our comprehensive understanding of health. Furthermore, disability rights education and advocacy should be a primary element of any effort to positively influence health status, including recreational therapy services.

Resources

Equal Employment Opportunity Commission (EEOC)
www.eeoc.gov
1801 L Street NW
Washington, DC 20507
800-669-EEOC (Voice/TDD)
Provides free copies of the technical manual for Title I of the ADA (employment) and provides assistance understanding and interpreting this title.

U.S. Department of Justice, Civil Rights Division
www.ada.gov
950 Pennsylvania Ave, NW
Disability Rights Section NYAV
Washington, DC 20530
800-514-0301 (Voice)

800-514-0383 (TDD)
Provides free copies of the technical manuals for Title II (public services) and Title III (public accommodations) of the ADA and provides assistance with understanding and interpreting these titles.

United States Access Board
www.access-board.gov
1331 F Street, NW, Suite 1000
Washington, DC 20004-1111
Phone (voice): 800-872-2253
Phone (TTY): 800-993-2822
Fax: 202-272-0081
E-mail: info@access-board.gov
Provides free copies of the "Americans with Disabilities Act Accessibility Guidelines," the "Uniform Federal Accessibility Standards," technical assistance manuals for each mode of transportation, "ADA Accessibility Guidelines for Play Areas," "ADA Accessibility Guidelines for Recreational Facilities," and "Recommendations for Outdoor Developed Areas."

Federal Communications Commission
Common Carrier Bureau
TRS Complaints
1919 M Street, NW
Washington, DC 20554
202-418-0500 (Voice)
202-632-6999 (TDD)
Provides information on telecommunication regulations and is responsible for the enforcement of Title IV of the ADA (telecommunications).

Paralyzed Veterans of America
www.pva.org
801 18th St., NW
Washington, DC 20006
800-424-8200 (Voice)
800-795-4327 (TDD)
Provides "The Americans with Disabilities Act: Your Personal Guide to the Law."

UN Enable
www.un.org/disabilities/index.asp
Secretariat for the Convention on the Rights of Persons with Disabilities
Two United Nations Plaza, DC2-1382
New York, NY 10017
United States of America
Email: Enable@un.org

UN Enable provides detailed information on the Convention on the Rights of Persons with Disabilities, as well as many other resources related to disability rights and the disability issues.

References

Altman, B. & Bernstein, A. (2008). *Disability and health in the United States, 2001-2005*. Hyattsville, MD: National Center for Health Statistics.

Amnesty International. (2011). *Convention on the rights of the child.* Retrieved from www.amnestyusa.org/children/convention-on-the-rights-of-the-child/page.do?id=1101777.

Centers for Disease Control and Prevention. (2006, December 8). Environmental barriers to health care among persons with disabilities — Los Angeles County, California, 2002-2003. *Morbidity and Mortality Weekly Report, 55*(48), 1300-1303. Retrieved from www.cdc.gov/mmwr/preview/mmwrhtml/mm5548a4.htm.

Drainoni, M., Lee-Hood, E., Tobias, C., Bachman, S. S., Andrew, J., & Maisels, L. (2006). Cross-disability experiences of barriers to health-care access: Consumer perspectives. *Journal of Disability Policy Studies, 17,* 101-115. DOI:10.1177/10442073060170020101.

Erickson, W. & Lee, C. (2008). *2007 Disability status report: United States*. Ithaca, NY: Cornell University Rehabilitation Research and Training Center on Disability Demographics and Statistics. Retrieved from http://digitalcommons.ilr.cornell.edu/edicollect/1256/.

Kroll, T., Jones, G. C., Kehn, M., & Neri, M. T. (2006). Barriers and strategies affecting the utilisation of primary preventive services for people with physical disabilities: a qualitative inquiry. *Health and Social Care in the Community 14*(4), 284-293. DOI: 10.1111/j.1365-2524.2006.00613.x.

Lezonni, L. I., O'Day, B. L., Killeen, M., & Harker, H. (2004). Communicating about health care: Observations from persons who are deaf or hard of hearing. *Annals of International Medicine, 140*(5), 356-362.

McIlfatrick, S., Taggart, L., & Truesdale-Kennedy, M (2011). Supporting women with intellectual disabilities to access breast cancer screening: A healthcare professional perspective. *European Journal of Cancer Care 20*(3), 412-420. DOI.1111/j.1365-2354.2010.01221.x.

Missouri Department of Elementary and Secondary Education. (2008). *Parent's guide to special education in Missouri.* Retrieved from www.dese.mo.gov/divspeced/Compliance.

National Council on Disability, (2009). *The current state of healthcare for persons with disabilities.* Washington, DC: Author. Retrieved from www.eric.ed.gov/PDFS/ED507726.pdf.

National Organization on Disability & Kessler Foundation, (2010). *ADA: 20 years later*. Retrieved from www.2010disabilitysurveys.org/pdfs/surveyresults.pdf.

Pereira, P. C. A. & Fortes, P. A. C. (2011). Communication and information barriers to health assistance for Deaf patients. *American Annals of the Deaf, 155*(1), 31-37.

Sylvester, C. (2011). Therapeutic recreation, the International Classification of Functioning, Disability, and Health, and the capability approach. *Therapeutic Recreation Journal, 45*(2), 85-104.

United Nations. (1997). A summary of United Nations agreements on human rights. Retrieved from wwww.hrweb.org/legal/undocs.html.

United Nations. (2010). *Monitoring the convention on the rights of persons with disabilities: Guidance for human rights monitors* — professional training series No. 17. New York: Author.

U.S. Department of Education. (2007). *Twenty-five years of progress in educating children with disabilities through IDEA*. Washington, DC: Author. Retrieved from www2.ed.gov/policy/speced/leg/idea/history.html.

27. Energy Conservation Techniques

Heather R. Porter

Individuals with a disability, illness, or injury may fatigue easily during physical activity due to deconditioning, physical limitations, such as lower extremity amputation or knee replacement, and impaired body functions, including poor cardiac or respiratory functions. Some clients may additionally have specific parameters set by the physician that limit their energy expenditure, such as needing to stop physical activity if blood pressure, pulse, or oxygen saturation reaches a particular level. (See the chapter on Parameters and Precautions for more information about limitations.) Keeping energy requirements within appropriate limits is needed to prevent harm and injury, minimize fatigue to maximize participation in meaningful activity, promote self-efficacy, and contribute to quality of life. Consequently, teaching and employing energy conservation techniques can be a helpful intervention.

Indications

Energy conservation techniques are taught and implemented with clients who have medical conditions or symptoms that exacerbate with physical exertion. These include chronic obstructive pulmonary disease, multiple sclerosis, cardiac conditions, asthma, lung cancer, obesity, and Guillain-Barré syndrome. Techniques are also taught to clients who are severely deconditioned and require the use of energy conservation techniques to safely perform activities, or demonstrate compromised endurance due to the normal aging process. For example, approximately 78% of individuals with chronic obstructive pulmonary disease (COPD) experience dyspnea (shortness of breath) that interferes with "professional, family, and social activities, as well as activities of daily living, leading to depression and anxiety, as well as to a significant reduction in quality of life" (Velloso & Jardim, 2006, p. 581). Energy conservation techniques, including adaptation of the environment and appropriate posture in activities have been shown to be efficient in reducing the sensation of dyspnea, oxygen consumption, and production of carbon dioxide and heart rate, thus improving activity performance (Velloso & Jardim, 2006). Blikman and colleagues (2013) conducted a systematic review and meta-analysis of the literature on the effectiveness of energy conservation techniques in reducing fatigue in individuals with multiple sclerosis. They found that energy conservation technique training was more effective than no treatment in reducing the impact of fatigue and improving health-related quality of life in physical, social, and mental health domains. And, as a final example, Schrack (2011) notes that "as individuals age, a greater proportion of daily energy is needed purely for survival and the availability of energy for instrumental daily activities and recreational pursuits progressively shrinks" (p. 145). Although the author did not explore the utilization or effectiveness of energy conservation techniques, it can be deducted that the use of such techniques might be helpful.

Looking at ICF codes provides another set of indications for teaching energy conservation techniques. Education and training are suggested when deficits in b410 Heart Functions, b440 Respiration Functions, b455 Exercise Tolerance Functions, b730 Muscle Power Functions, b740 Muscle Endurance Functions, or b770 Gait Pattern Functions are documented. The techniques might be used to address deficits in d230 Carrying Out Daily Routine and d570 Looking After One's Health. Techniques can also be used to address any activity-specific code, such as those found in d4 Mobility, d5 Self-Care, and d9 Community, Social, and Civic Life.

Contraindications

Energy conservation techniques should only be taught and implemented when indicated. Individuals who can safely perform activities without utilization of energy conservation techniques should be encouraged to do so, as conserving energy that otherwise should be spent to maintain and improve health can yield negative outcomes, such as weight gain, muscle atrophy, and cardiopulmonary deconditioning.

Protocols and Processes

Energy conservation techniques are taught by various disciplines that focus on their area of clinical expertise. For example, physical therapists instruct clients how to conserve energy related to mobility, whereas occupational therapists instruct clients how to conserve energy in self-care activities, such as dressing. In recreational therapy, therapists address energy conservation and fatigue management in leisure, play, and community activities. Recreational therapists who work in hospitals and rehabilitation predominately focus on instruction. Recreational therapists who provide therapeutic activities in community settings incorporate energy conservation techniques into the activities they provide, as appropriate.

Prior to teaching energy conservation techniques, the recreational therapist obtains information regarding the client's limitations, abilities, precautions, and parameters related to physical activity, as well as the client's desired activity pattern (e.g., activity preferences, level of engagement, frequency, locations) and baselines related to such participation. This information is judged against an activity analysis for each specific activity to determine opportunities for the utilization of energy conservation techniques.

Once the therapist has preliminary energy conservation technique ideas, the therapist engages in a conversation with the client to explain the purpose of energy conservation techniques as they relate to the client's health situation and the activities that s/he desires to participate in. Energy conservation ideas are explored to gauge their feasibility. Clients may not be open to some of the recommended energy conservation techniques due to individual preferences and tolerances. For example, although parking in a handicap parking space could reduce the car-to-door distance, a teenager might rebel against it for fear of looking "un-cool." Consequently, in the conversation

the therapist must be open to understanding the particular preferences and needs of the client and take a joint problem-solving approach.

In some cases, the therapist might also encounter resistance to activity participation, despite the helpfulness of energy conservation techniques, due to feared consequences of fatigue, such as fear of falling or fear of using energy that is needed for a self-care routine. Consequently, education about the consequences of inactivity and the benefits of activity engagement related to health, functioning, independence, and quality of life may need to be added.

When teaching energy conservation techniques, review the five P's as described below (Porter & burlingame, 2006; Falvo, 2013) and tailor the suggestions to the particular recreation, leisure, play, or community activities. The therapist might also opt to create an individualized handout for the client that explains the specific energy conservation techniques at each step in the activity to maximize recall and application.

Prioritize

Clients may put too many activities requiring a high amount of physical energy into one day or one part of the day. There is not only a risk of injury or harm, but it can also lead to frustration, depression, or anxiety when the client is unable to complete the desired tasks. This, in turn, could cause the individual to give up participation in healthy activities, thus giving rise to secondary complications from a less active lifestyle. For example, "It is too much work to go shopping, so I'll just let my husband do it." Encourage clients to make a list of all of the things that they want to accomplish in a day or week and prioritize the activities based on their deadlines, needs, and desires.

It is important to note however, that when energy levels are compromised, clients have a tendency to prioritize activities that have to be done (e.g., housecleaning, doctors' appointments, grocery shopping), rather than personally meaningful recreation, leisure, and community activities. Consequently, clients may require education about the importance of such activities for recovery, health promotion, and quality of life. For example, the therapist might say, "It is very important that you continue to go to the senior center because that is where you get to be with all of your friends. You might not realize this now, but having people to talk to will help you get through tough times. It is actually very good for you to laugh and have fun because when you laugh and have fun your body releases endorphins that actually help to reduce pain."

Plan

Once a client is able to prioritize a healthy activity list for the day or week, the therapist talks to the client about planning techniques for each activity that reduce the amount of energy expended to a level that is appropriate for the client. Some suggestions for planning include:

Time: Figure out what time of day the client has the most energy. This is the best time to schedule activities that require a lot of energy. Although this is not always possible (e.g., client relies on her daughter to take her to the knitting shop and she is only available on Saturday afternoons), it is encouraged whenever possible.

Activity analysis: Do an activity analysis of each activity and identify techniques that can be used. For example:

- The client can apply for and use a parking placard so that the client can park in a handicap parking space. This will reduce the amount of walking or wheelchair propulsion to the front door. Handicapped parking spaces are also wider (at least they are supposed to be), allowing the client extra room to open the car door and easily enter and exit the car.
- The client should plan a travel route. Some appropriate questions include: Where do you need to go in the building and what do you need to do when you are there? How far will you need to walk or propel the wheelchair? Are there places along the travel route to sit and rest? Planning out a travel route will reduce the chances of backtracking or spending unnecessary energy (e.g., walking down an aisle at the store that does not have an item the client needs). Clients are encouraged to use mall directories, aisle signs, and assistance from customer service whenever possible.
- Encourage clients to assert needs and ask for assistance with tasks that are above their energy limits, such as carrying heavy bags or retrieving an item at the end of the aisle.

- The client should use adaptive equipment, if needed, such as an electric scooter in the store. They are available at many grocery stores, large store chains, malls, and even some amusement parks and other recreational spots. Explain the process of using a scooter. Explore other personal adaptive equipment that could aid in energy conservation including a reacher, walker bag, or backpack.

Pace

Rushing can put the client in a dangerous situation that could lead to injury or harm. Common situations include trying to keep up with another person, trying to walk quickly across a parking lot so as not to hold up a car that is waiting, moving quickly in the home when trying to get ready for an outing, or not sitting and taking a rest because time is short or needing to rest is embarrassing. Some common pacing techniques include:

Build in extra time: Clients are encouraged to build in extra time when getting ready to go out. Extra time is often needed to get ready due to limitations and impairments. It is also important to build in additional time to allow rest periods when getting ready. So, if a client currently requires one hour for getting ready, then it would be best for the client to give herself an hour and a half to get ready.

Don't rush: Clients are educated about the dangers of allowing their energy expenditure to be influenced by others (e.g., having to rush in line because someone behind the client is waiting, not wanting to sit and take a rest because he knows that his shopping partner is in a rush to get home). It is often helpful to validate that these feelings are normal, but that the client needs to take care of himself/herself. Otherwise the resulting injury or harm may affect important and meaningful life activities even more negatively.

Sit before becoming tired: Clients are encouraged to sit *before* feeling tired. Once tired, it can be difficult to recover and go on with the activity. For many clients, however, taking a rest break before feeling tired is difficult because it feels unnatural. To help with this, clients are encouraged to look for places to sit while walking and when a place is spotted, perform a time check ("How long have I been walking?") and judge whether or not it would be beneficial to take advantage of the opportunity. Some places don't have many places to sit. Outside of the traditional chairs and benches, some creative places to sit and rest in the community include the bathroom, stairwell, dressing room, shoe department, furniture department, sport department (e.g., open up a folding sport chair), or ledge. Tell the client if s/he has been looking for a place to sit and has not been successful in finding one, to be assertive and ask someone to bring a chair or anything else that may be suitable to rest on. Encourage clients to explain the urgency of the situation so that action is taken immediately. The request could be something like, "Excuse me. I am not feeling so great and I really need to sit down because I am afraid I am going to fall. Could you please get me something to sit down on?"

Position

Body mechanics, posture, items being carried, and positions relative to the current task all have an impact on energy expenditure. Common techniques include:

Body mechanics: Reasons for using good body mechanics include muscles work best when used correctly; pulling, pushing, and lifting are easier; unnecessary fatigue and strain are reduced; it saves energy and prevents injury (Simmers, 2008). There are eight basic rules of good body mechanics: (1) maintain a broad base of support by keeping feet shoulder-width apart (about eight to ten inches), place one foot slightly forward with weight placed evenly on both feet, and point toes in the direction of movement, (2) bend from the hips and knees to get close to the object and keep the back straight (don't bend at the waist), (3) use the strongest muscles to do the job, such as the shoulders, upper arms, hips, and thighs (back muscles are weak), (4) use the weight of your body to help push or pull an object (whenever possible push or slide, rather than pull or lift), (5) carry heavy items close to the body, (6) avoid twisting (turn the feet and then the entire body to change direction), (7) avoid bending for long periods of time, and (8) if an object is too heavy, use equipment to reduce the amount of weight that needs to be lifted and/or seek assistance (Simmers, 2008).

Posture: Sitting or standing with good posture uses the least energy. It also opens up the lungs and allows for better oxygen intake for energy expenditure.

Sitting: Perform activities in a seated position when possible instead of a standing position (e.g., sit at the table when chopping or preparing food).

Objects: Place objects in places where they are easy to reach (e.g., put coupons in a waist pack so they can be easily accessed instead of in a backpack, store commonly used items in easy-to-reach areas). Consider using alternative methods for transporting objects to eliminate energy expenditure, such as a backpack, cart, rolling bag, or fanny pack.

Environment: Design environments that reduce energy expenditure. For example, organization reduces the amount of energy needed to find things and limited furnishings reduce the amount of energy needed to negotiate around things. When in environments that can't be manipulated, look for the best line of approach for the task to minimize energy expended. For example, in an art class that requires the client to get up and down multiple times to retrieve supplies, it would be best to choose a table that is close to the supplies to minimize the amount of walking.

Pounds

Carrying extra weight requires the client to expend more physical energy. Body weight and items being carried both add to energy expenditure. Common recommendations include:

Lose extra body weight: Encourage clients who are overweight or obese to strive for a healthy body weight.

Analyze extra weight carried: Clients can place carried items on a scale to find out how much weight they are actually carrying.

Prioritize items: Prioritize what is needed, such as limiting the number of things that are carried in a pocketbook or tote bag.

Exchange: Exchange heavy items for lighter ones, such as carrying a nylon jacket in a backpack instead of a heavy sweatshirt, using a lightweight plastic gardening trowel instead of a heavy metal one. Another common problem is using a heavy and cumbersome pocketbook. Not only is it in the way, making it more challenging to maintain balance, it also has a tendency to slide off the shoulder. Clients should opt for a smaller and lighter pocketbook that has a long strap so that it can be worn across the chest.

Carry or transport heavy items by different methods: For example, carrying a five-pound item in a backpack puts less stress on the cardiovascular system than carrying it in the arms because the load is being carried through larger muscle groups and more efficient skeletal structures. Other examples include using a suitcase with wheels instead of one with a handle or going to the grocery store, picking out and paying for the groceries, and then requesting the items be delivered to the home.

Outcomes and Documentation

Knowledge of energy conservation techniques can be assessed via verbal recall of the energy conservation techniques for a particular activity and/or application shown by implementing the energy conservation techniques in the activity. Note the level of cueing required for recall or implementation. When using the ICF, score changes in the codes that triggered the need for teaching energy and conservation techniques, as discussed in the Indications section.

References

Blikman, L. J., Huissted, B. M., Kooijmans, H., Stam, H. J., Bussmann, J. B., & van Meeteren, J. (2013). Effectiveness of energy conservation treatment in reducing fatigue in multiple sclerosis: A systematic review and meta-analysis. *Archives of Physical Medicine and Rehabilitation, 94*, 1360-76.

Falvo, D. (2013). *Medical and psychosocial aspects of chronic illness and disability*. Burlington, MA: Jones & Bartlett Publishers.

Porter, H. & burlingame, j. (2006). *Recreational therapy handbook of practice: ICF based diagnosis and treatment*. Ravensdale, WA: Idyll Arbor, Inc.

Schrack, J. A. (2011). Aging and the conservation of energy. *Environmental Abstracts, 72*, 145.

Simmers, L. M. (2008). *Diversified health occupations*. Clifton Park, NY: Delmar Cengage Learning.

Velloso, M. & Jardim, J. R. (2006). Functionality of patients with chronic obstructive pulmonary disease: Energy conservation techniques. *J Bras Pneumol, 32*(6), 580-586.

28. Errorless Learning

Donna L. Long

Individuals with severe memory deficits often have difficulty learning. Errorless learning is a technique which relies on implicit or procedural memory where information is unconsciously recalled. Some examples include riding a bike, putting on a shirt, and throwing a ball. This is different from explicit or declarative memory where information is consciously recalled, such as recalling a phone number or appointment time or recalling the answer to a test question (Haskins et al., 2012). Errorless learning has been used effectively to teach individuals with severe memory impairments new information, specific skills, or procedures (Cohen et al., 2010).

Indications

Individuals with severe memory impairments often do not benefit from trial and error learning because they are unable to recall their errors and what the correct responses were. Therefore, the errors are strengthened through repetition and the individual learns the error instead of the correct response (Pitel et al., 2006). Errorless learning (EL) ensures that the individual avoids repeating the errors, thus learns only the correct response.

ICF codes that might indicate a need for EL include b144 Memory Functions, b164 Higher-Level Cognitive Functions, d155 Acquiring Skills, and d210 Undertaking a Single Task.

EL is a practical strategy that can be implemented in a variety of settings. Recreational therapists who understand the EL technique are able to consider its application when determining which learning strategy will be most effective for a particular task and a given individual.

Protocols

The principle of EL is that individuals should be prevented from making mistakes during learning (Pitel et al., 2006). When using the EL technique, teaching should occur in a highly structured manner following clearly delineated routines. Learning trials should occur frequently (Haskins et al., 2012) and the information or skills are taught the same way each time.

Processes

EL may be achieved by implementing a variety of strategies:

- Break down the information, skill, or procedure into small, discrete steps or units using task analysis (Clare & Jones, 2008; Pitel et al., 2006).
- Teach only one step or piece of information at a time.
- Provide a model before asking the individual to perform step or skill (Clare & Jones, 2008; Haskins et al., 2012).
- Use a forward or backward chaining technique. A chaining technique can be used to teach an individual the sequence of steps or components that make up a task. Chaining is most successful when each step of the task is strongly linked to the next one (Haskins et al., 2012). Each step of the task is learned as an isolated unit then linked to the step before and after (Haskins et al., 2012). When using forward chaining, the therapist guides the individual in performing the first step of the task (Haskins et al., 2012); the therapist then completes the rest the task. Once the individual is able to perform the first step, the second step is added and the individual is then guided through the performance of both steps together.

This continues until all the steps of the task are linked together. When using backward chaining, the steps are taught from the last step in the sequence to the first. The therapist completes all but the last step or component of the task. The individual then performs the last step with guidance from the therapist. As each step is mastered, another step or component of the task is added to the individual's performance until s/he is able to perform the whole sequence (Haskins, 2012).

- Avoid guessing and trial and error learning (Clare & Jones, 2008; Haskins et al., 2012).
- Provide the amount of cueing and/or physical assistance needed to prevent an error from occurring.
- If an individual begins to make an error, immediately stop him/her. Intervene to prevent errors (Clare & Jones, 2008).
- Guide learning using a cueing hierarchy and fade cues and prompts as performance improves (Haskins et al., 2010; Sohlberg, Ehlhardt, & Kennedy, 2005). When using a cueing hierarchy, provide the least intrusive level of cueing needed for the person to perform the task (Clare & Jones, 2008). Fade the level of cueing from most to the least intrusive as the person's performance improves. For example, move from hand-over-hand assistance to partial physical assistance or tactile cueing to gestural cues then verbal cues with the goal of the client performing the task independently.
- Present the information, skill, or procedure to be learned in the actual setting or context in which it will be used (Haskins et al., 2012).

Although research on EL has yielded mixed results, evidence suggests that individuals with severe memory deficits following an acquired brain injury can benefit from EL (Clare & Jones, 2008). Several studies have shown positive results with the use of EL. Pitel et al. (2006) found EL to be effective in teaching individuals with severe memory deficits complex semantic information and procedures needed to program an electronic organizer. Kelly and Nikopoulos (2010) demonstrated the effectiveness of EL and strategy training in reducing the amount of assistance needed by participants with severe brain injuries to complete targeted personal activities of daily living.

Other individuals with severe memory deficits may also benefit from EL. Although Clare and Jones (2008) found that individuals with early-stage Alzheimer's disease appear to do equally well with EL and trial-and-error methods, Kessels and Olde Hensken (2009) found EL of a procedural task resulted in a better performance than learning from errors for individuals with dementia.

A literature review by Clare and Jones (2008) found that tasks with the following characteristics are likely to benefit from EL: Tasks involving a single cognitive domain and a single component of behavior, or those amenable to being broken down into a series of discrete learning steps. Tasks should not require flexibility of response. Completion of the task should require attention only to the correct response. The behavior or response to be trained should already exist in the participant's behavioral repertoire, although if it does not, pre-training could be undertaken.

Outcomes and Documentation

EL can be an effective learning strategy for individuals with severe memory impairments (Whyte et al., 2010). Initially, cues and/or physical assistance may be required for each step of the task to prevent errors. Cues and/or physical assistance are gradually faded as the individual begins to initiate more of the actions correctly (Whyte et al., 2010).

The weakness of EL is that these skills typically do not generalize. For example, if an individual has learned how to use one type of cell phone, this does not mean that s/he will be able to use another type. The strength of the EL technique is that an individual with severe memory impairments can be taught new information, skills, or procedures when all other methods fail. These individuals can learn the task even if they are unable to consciously recall it.

Document changes noted in the ICF codes discussed in the Indications section, in the specific skills taught, and in the ability of the client to generalize what was learned to other situations.

References

Clare, L. & Jones, S. P. (2008). Errorless learning in the rehabilitation of memory impairment: A critical review. *Neuropsychological Review 18*, 1-23.

Cohen, M., Ylvisaker, C., Hamilton, J., Kemp, L., & Claiman, B. (2010). Errorless learning of functional life skills in an individual with three aetiologies of severe memory and executive function impairment. *Neuropsychological Rehabilitation, 20*(3), 355-376.

Haskins, E. C., Cicerone, K., Dams-O'Connor, K, Eberle, R., Langenbahn, D, & Shapiro-Rosenbaum, A. (2012). *Cognitive rehabilitation manual: Translating evidence-based recommendations into practice,* (pp. 42-55). Reston, VA: ACRM Publishing.

Kelly, F. & Nikopoulos, C. K. (2010). Facilitating independence in personal activities of daily living after a severe traumatic brain injury. *International Journal of Therapy and Rehabilitation, 17*(9).

Kessels, R. P. C. & Olde Hensken, L. M. G. (2009). Effects of errorless skill learning in people with mild-to-moderate or severe dementia: A randomized controlled pilot study. *NeuroRehabilitation, 25,* 307-312.

Pitel, A., Beaunieux, H., LeBaron, N., Joyeux, F., Desgranges, B., & Eustache, F. (2006). Two case studies in the application of errorless learning techniques in memory impaired patients with additional executive deficits. *Brain Injury, 20*(10), 1099-1110.

Sohlberg, M. M., Ehlhardt, L., & Kennedy, M. (2005). Instructional techniques in cognitive rehabilitation: A preliminary report. *Seminars in Speech Language Pathology, 26,* 268-279.

Whyte, J., Ponsford, J., Watanabe, T., & Hart, T. (2010). Traumatic brain injury. In DeLisa et al. (Eds.), *Rehabilitation medicine: Principles and practices* (5th ed.) (pp. 575-623). Philadelphia: Lippincott Williams & Wilkins.

29. Group Psychotherapy Techniques

Glenn A. Kastrinos

The delivery of activities in group structures oriented to client treatment issues has been one of the foundations of recreational therapy. It has also been accepted in the healthcare arena as a cost-effective and viable way to work with client problems and issues. In order to run effective groups, the recreational therapist should be competent in both activity and thematic dialogue and processing of client interaction. This is a challenge considering all the factors that play into group leadership. In addition, many recreational therapists work in short-term units that may have a length of stay of seven days or less. Consequently, the purpose of this chapter is to address group therapy on short-term units, such as inpatient psychiatric units.

Therapy groups are commonly described as being closed-ended or open-ended. Closed-ended groups refer to having the same group composition over several sessions. Group members stay the same and the group develops over time. Open-ended groups, on the other hand, have a changing population and the group members will usually be different each group. For example, an open-ended group may consist of new members, members who have attended a couple of groups in the program already, and members who are attending their last group session. This changing group atmosphere requires the leader to use a different set of techniques than the closed-ended group. These techniques will be discussed later in this chapter. The open-ended group can feel chaotic and anxiety provoking for both the therapist and the clients. Without an active leader the group can quickly become ineffective (Yalom, 1983; Kastrinos, 1994; Brabender & Fallon, 2009).

Inpatient stays have become shorter and shorter over the last thirty years. This is driven by high healthcare costs and studies that demonstrate the success of brief therapy techniques. Such short-term techniques include the use of fast-paced treatment such as cognitive therapies, as well as cognitive-behavioral therapies, often delivered in groups. Many inpatient psychiatric hospitals have become more centered on crisis intervention than acute care (Kastrinos, 1994). This has many impacts on delivery of recreational therapy groups including (Emer, 2004):

All groups are open ended. This means that each group will have different clientele and the group experience becomes an entity unto itself in the therapy framework.

Most clients will exhibit high anxiety levels. Iatrogenic anxiety, or anxiety related to a situation, is common. If this is the case in a group setting, groups will usually need to be highly structured with a therapist actively leading the group.

Short-term goals and self-regulation is required. Short-term goals regarding groups must be user friendly. However, clients must still be responsible for their self-regulation.

Being client-centered is challenging. If the therapist waits for the client to trust him/her, the client may be gone before anything is done. The therapist has to be challenging, take a few more risks, and not wait until the client is ready to work. Engaging the client in the group to be present, focused, and work with the group is of highest importance.

The group structure has to be highly structured with few interruptions. The system has to be supportive of groups, and it is imperative that a client does not become overwhelmed by chaos that can occur in the short-term unit. If clients are consistently taken from groups for outside appointments, they will invariably not be able to focus on what is going on in the group.

Recidivism can be high. Clients will commonly be leaving and returning to the unit. The therapists have to be careful not to get frustrated by this and pick up where they left off last time with the returning client. Often clients will return to the short-term unit because of lack of support outside the unit (Emer, 2004).

Due to the nature of short-term stays, Yalom (1983) and Kastrinos (1994) make the case for short-term inpatient groups having a different set of demands. Yalom (1983) cites four points on the unique nature of inpatient therapy groups:

- Inpatient groups exist as a part of a larger treatment system.
- Clients in inpatient units live together, so discussions concerning their in-group therapy will typically arise. In outpatient groups, clients are asked to keep information confidential, but Yalom suggests that in inpatient groups, clients can learn through carrying what they are working on into other inpatient groups. For instance, if they develop a treatment goal for the day in group therapy, they can gain benefit by carrying that goal into the rest of their groups that day.
- The inpatient group therapist has access to considerably more information than what is supplied by the client.
- Hospitalized clients are more deeply troubled and tend to have high anxiety about being in the hospital setting. This means that they will need high structure by the therapist in order to feel safe in this new setting.

Brabender and Fallon (2009) agree with Yalom's view that the inpatient and short-term group structure has to be viewed very differently. In their book, *Group Development in Practice* (Brabender & Fallon, 2009) they contrast the structure of open-ended groups with the five stages that closed-ended groups go through. The stages of closed-ended groups are

Stage 1. Formation and Engagement: This is the opening stage of group development, where clients begin to get to know each other and are trying to figure out what they can accomplish in the group and what others may be trying to accomplish.

Stage 2. Conflict and Rebellion: At this stage, clients question the leader's abilities and/or get into conflicts with other group members. This is often an uncomfortable stage but is needed for the group to progress to deeper meaning.

Stage 3. Unity and Intimacy: At this stage, clients begin to find they are not alone with their problems

and want to find common themes with other group members.

Stage 4. Integration and Work: At this stage, clients work through their issues using the group dynamic and the group takes on a work-like structure.

Stage 5. Termination: This is the last stage, and clients try to make the transition from what they learned in the group settings to future situations.

Brabender and Fallon (2009) note that an open-ended group, with members changing all the time, clients rarely go past the second stage of development and most likely will stay in the first stage of development, Formation and Engagement. This contrasts markedly with a closed-ended group, where clients go through the five developmental stages. They state that the major task necessary for stage one in open-ended groups is for members to engage with one another and the therapist. With this in mind, the therapist should be active in fostering engagement through diminishing resistance wherever possible and strengthening attraction to being involved. Yalom's points about inpatient groups working together outside the group itself can make the task easier.

This active approach, focusing on engagement, helps frame therapist behaviors in the acute setting. Suggested therapist behaviors include:

Foster identification among members. It is imperative to have clients want to work together and the therapist needs to take the lead in this area. Helping clients find out more from each other through questioning and caring for one another is critical. It is also important for the therapist to model these behaviors. If the therapist doesn't appear interested, it will definitely affect the group negatively.

Encourage positive changes among members. The therapist is supportive of clients in making initial changes in the group and trying to substitute positive behaviors for negative ones.

Avoid high level of focus on individual members. The therapist must help clients reach out to each other and not focus on purely individual problems. Yalom and Leszcz (2005) recommend therapists help clients move from a personal problem to an interpersonal problem and then to a here-and-now problem that the group can focus on. Long explanations of individual problems can make the group feel helpless and stagnant.

Focus on the present. In a short-term unit, focusing on the present helps clients work on each other's issues in the present. If a client states he has trouble communicating with his boss, it will take a long process to figure out the problem itself let alone addressing issues. However, if the client is redirected to look at his/her communication issues in the group, the problem becomes observable and can be worked on more easily. This can be modeled once again by the therapist keeping a present-oriented focus.

Support members' hopefulness about group. It is critical that clients hold the view that a group can be helpful to their problems and show them ways to get out of their feelings of helplessness (Brabender & Fallon, 2009). This is critical, because clients who come in with the feeling that the group will help them typically do try and use the group in a productive way. Secondly, if they gain something from the group, they have a better chance of seeking out a group on an outpatient basis (Brabender & Fallon, 2009).

Yalom (1983), Kastrinos (1994), and Brabender and Fallon (2009) advocate for an active approach by the therapist to insure clients' feelings of safety and help. The therapists are also responsible for urging clients to engage in interactions with other group members. This active approach has implications for the recreational therapist. If they are searching for the stages of development that are taught during most group training sessions, they will usually be missing the mark. There can be situations where a group of individuals in short-term inpatient care go further in development, but it is not a common theme that occurs in the inpatient unit. Since recreational therapists use an active approach followed by processing, it can create a structure that is suitable for the inpatient group. Yalom's call for focusing on the present should be something recreational therapists feel very comfortable with. Recreational therapists value spontaneity and bringing the person out in an activity, so this fits with the first group stage and the acute inpatient setting. The concept of focusing on strengths and fostering identification between members is also a competency recreational therapists are well versed in and continue to learn about. It is imperative for the recreational therapist to make sure the group continues to participate, and also to take control of group matters, such as stopping a person who is monopolizing the conversation.

Indications

Short-term inpatient recreational therapy groups can help clients feel less iatrogenic anxiety about being in rehabilitation (anxiety about a novel situation such as being in a new rehabilitation facility) and be used to help clients recover from a crisis (d240 Handling Stress and Other Psychological Demands). Inpatient therapy groups can engage people in "problem spotting" (d175 Solving Problems) (Yalom, 1983), or frame a difficulty they are having so that they are provided with a more positive outlook (b126 Temperament and Personality Functions) that helps them believe they can overcome the problem over time. The inpatient group can provide opportunities for clients to see that they are not alone in having problems and have the opportunity to share with other people going through similar feelings and situations.

Therapy groups run by recreational therapists are usually through modalities such as stress management (d240 Handling Stress and Other Psychological Demands), exercise (b455 Exercise Tolerance Functions), adventure-type initiatives (b130 Energy and Drive Functions), games (d710 Basic Interpersonal Interactions, d910 Community Life), and relaxation (d920 Recreation and Leisure). A lot of clients who come into short-term units will have unique problems that fall under one of these modalities. The recreational therapist will develop goals for the client that can be worked on in groups. Clients then can get helped through talking through their issues in relation to the topic of the group. For instance, a client who is struggling with high anxiety on a regular basis could benefit from talking with other clients about anxiety and getting ideas on how to cope better with anxiety issues. Since other clients may have similar issues, a group led by an experienced therapist can give them the opportunity to learn new coping skills from one another.

Contraindications

Inpatient groups can be counterproductive for manic clients or other clients who cannot follow rules or respond to limit setting (e.g., d720 Complex Interpersonal Interactions). According to the DSM-5 (APA, 2013), clients in a manic episode "may talk continuously and without regard for others' wishes to communicate, often in an intrusive manner or without concern for the relevance of what is said." This would not be productive for the group, and the client would not be able to limit responses so the group could be run efficiently.

Inpatient groups also would not be a place to work on long standing issues that will take a lot of time to turn around. Clients who cannot express themselves (b167 Mental Functions of Language) because of their condition's severity may also not gain much from the inpatient group because participants in inpatient group approaches need to communicate issues and treatment goals with other clients in the group.

Lastly, some clients with borderline disorders who have great difficulty with emotional regulation (d720 Complex Interpersonal Interactions) may not be appropriate for this group level. According to the DSM-5 (APA, 2013), clients with borderline disorders may have affective instability due to marked reactivity of mood and exhibit frantic efforts to avoid real or imagined abandonment. It is extremely difficult to run an effective inpatient group with a client who can change drastically in the course of one session, such as idealizing the therapist or other clients in the group one minute and then totally devaluing them the next. Since personality disorders are rigid and difficult to change, usually clients with borderline disorders need a supportive group over an extended period of time (Freeman & Stewart, 2006).

Processes

Each group should be in a one-session format. People who may be coming to a second thematic group, such as stress management, can be engaged in a different topic or allowed to take stress management to another level. Considerations for the one-session format are

Start and finish on time. It is imperative to have high structure in this setting.

Start every group with introductions. For the benefit of new clients, in particular, as well as those with memory impairments.

Have a few simple rules. Don't over limit people, but explain the group rules to every group. If one of the group's rules is to start and finish on time, state that at the beginning of each group. Another simple rule would be to maintain respect for other clients in the group through having one person speak at a time and not to interrupt others when they are speaking.

Another rule may be that if a client leaves, s/he cannot return to the group because it is disruptive.

Groups have to work on individual issues that can be worked on in group format. Individual goals for groups need to be addressed every session. For example, what is each person meant to be working on in stress management today?

Keep distractions to a minimum. If groups are an inherent part of the program, interruptions should be minimized at all costs.

Think inside the group. If clients get caught up in outside problems, the group will not have the time to address major issues. Yalom (1983) states that clients will bring their problems with them, so engaging with other group members about those problems will be more productive than problem solving outside material. This should fall into line with recreational therapy delivery.

Lead with other therapists. Co-leading can be a great way to share information and learn from other therapists. Having at least two leaders can also give clients more security and allow one leader to take the lead while the other watches for client interactions. Although this may be less cost efficient, it can be very effective in giving clients a more thorough and therapeutic group experience and improve leader competency.

Use daily/hourly experiences to address issues. If a client wants to make a lifestyle change, start with that in the group meeting and have each person discuss how it is going. You are trying to get the person to experiment with change and process it in the group.

Pay attention to three group processes. Yalom and Leszcz (2005) state that there are three group processes which go on at all times. They are (a) therapist interventions, (b) facilitation of group interactions, and (c) what the group is doing as a whole. As stated earlier, the therapist needs to be active in the process, and often clients look to the therapist for structure and guidance. The therapist seeks to actively encourage group members to talk with one another and share their thoughts and feelings with the group for help. The group as a whole may not develop, but establishing an environment where the group feels safe and work-like is equally important. If people are doing any maladaptive behaviors, it will quickly break down the group process.

Outcomes and Documentation

Charting should be done daily or after each session. With a shortened stay, what is happening during in-group sessions should be documented frequently. If a client is in the unit for five days, you need to document status/progress at least once a day. It can also be helpful to have the clients document on their perceived progress or regression. For example, a unit may have a section in the clients' chart where clients can write and reflect on their group experiences. This, in turn, can be very helpful information for the team.

Thematic groups should be in line with common therapeutic issues. When a client comes to stress management, they should be working on a stress management or coping issue that was discussed in assessment or prior to group. Themes should be general but directly relate to what the clients are being treated for. Some inpatient psychiatric centers will change their group schedule every week to accommodate a changing population.

Outcomes for inpatient units should reflect getting a person out of crisis and problem formulation. The system is not designed to cure, relieve the person of major symptomology, or make a life-altering change, simply because of the short-term nature of the therapy. However, clients can benefit from identifying with others and seeing they are not alone in their problems. Clients can also be enticed to continue therapy after leaving the facility to allow them to continue to work on their issues.

Groups should reflect the current struggles of the clients on the unit. Themes of groups can change quickly based on the client population.

Miscellaneous

Aside from working on an acute unit for seven years, the author has seen many acute psychiatric units and some of the struggles recreational therapists and their colleagues have in this challenging situation. Some of the issues to watch for can include:

Therapist becomes purely educationally or pre-scriptively focused. The therapist begins to do the same thing over and over again. Stress management may have an initiative that works and because of the fast change in population, they continue to do that same initiative over and over, not thinking about clients' needs in the group. The other situation is when in-group meetings change into a more lecture-based session, where clients are told what they need to do for stress. Both of these issues can lead to the therapist viewing groups as looking the same and an increased chance of burnout. It is imperative that the recreational therapist focuses on issues of individual clients related to the theme of the group.

There is no connection between group therapy and other groups run on the unit. If clients don't see the connection among groups, clients may think that only certain groups are "important" and that the rest are time wasters. If the RT is not a part of the other group therapy sessions, the RT will need to find out what happened in the other sessions so they can assist the clients in seeing the full picture of treatment. According to Yalom (1983) and Kastrinos (1994) communication between staff is vital on the short-term unit.

Everyone starts looking the same. The short-term inpatient units can be so fast paced that sometimes therapists forget how each group and each client is different, and they start seeing things diagnostically rather than descriptively. They may start looking for "borderlines" and major depressive episodes rather than a client with a unique set of problems on the unit. This can very quickly lead to burnout. It is very important to have a fresh outlook on every group.

Documentation becomes prohibitive. With a large caseload and high client turnover, documentation can become time consuming and overwhelming, resulting in late and/or low-quality documentation. Documentation needs to be an expedient and time-efficient process, just like the therapy that is delivered on the unit. For example, it is not uncommon for a recreational therapist to have four to seven new clients admitted each day to a unit. If the recreational therapist conducted a one-hour assessment on each client, therapy sessions would be severely limited.

Groups are optional. Although this provides clients a chance to be intrinsically motivated, with this setup clients will often choose not to come to groups. Clients are often uncomfortable as is, and to ask them if they would choose to come to a group or stay in their room or a more comfortable space, usually the client will try to stay with the more comfortable situation.

Individual therapy is done in group. This defeats the purpose of having groups and clients will want the therapist to help them but no one else. Therapists work on individual issues but encourage the group to help each other with their issues.

Groups spend a lot of time processing arrival and discharge. This certainly is important, but if the group takes this on, virtually every group will be on people coming and going, and other issues will not have any time in the discussion.

Resources

Most universities and some medical centers offer training in group therapy, but often they are focused on the closed-ended group. Brief therapy models including cognitive therapy, cognitive behavioral therapy, and brief therapy, can also be useful background for leading groups in the inpatient unit. Some websites related to training include:

Psychotherapy.net

www.psychotherapy.net

A great resource for books and articles on psychotherapy and leading psychotherapy groups.

International Association for Group Psychotherapy

www.iagp.com

A valuable resource for group psychotherapy literature. Both articles and books are included.

Mindfulness Based Cognitive Therapy

www.mbct.com

A mindfulness cognitive therapy based resource which can be useful in leading groups with a short-term focus.

Positive Psychology Center

www.ppc.sas.upenn.edu

A great resource for positive psychology, which can be integrated effectively in RT groups. Includes web pages, books, and articles.

Solution Focused Brief Psychotherapy Association

www.sfbta.org

Includes training possibilities and resources for brief therapy.

Beck Institute for Cognitive Behavior Therapy

www.beckinstitute.org

An excellent resource for cognitive behavioral therapy including finding out information on how to deliver cognitive therapy in group formats and where to get training in cognitive therapy.

References

APA (2013) *Diagnostic and statistical manual of mental disorders* (5th ed.). Washington DC: American Psychiatric Association.

Beck, A. P. & Lewis, C. M. (2000). *The process of group psychotherapy: Systems of analyzing change.* Washington, DC: American Psychological Association.

Brabender, F. (2009*). Group development in practice: Guidance for clinicians and researchers on stages and dynamics of change.* Washington, DC: American Psychological Association.

Emer, D. (2004). The use of groups in inpatient facilities: Needs, focus, successes, and remaining dilemmas. In J. L. Delucia-Waak, D. A. Gerrity, C. R. Kalodner, & M. T. Riva (Eds.) *Handbook of group counseling and psychotherapy* (pp. 351-351) Thousand Oaks CA: Sage.

Freeman, A. & Steward, J. L. (2006) Personality disorders. In P. J. Bieling, R. E. McCabe, & M. M. Antony (Eds.) *Cognitive-behavioral therapy in groups* (pp. 324-338). New York: Guilford.

Kastrinos, G. (1994). Implications for inpatient group psychotherapy models and therapeutic recreation in acute psychiatric settings. In D. Compton and S. Iso-Ahola (Eds.), *Leisure and Mental Health.* Park City, UT: Family Development Resources.

Woody, R. (2004). *Group therapy: An integrative cognitive social-learning approach.* Sarasota, FL: Professional Resource Press.

Yalom, I. (1983). *Inpatient group psychotherapy.* New York: Basic.

Yalom, I. & Leszcz, M. (2005). *The theory and practice of group psychotherapy* (5th ed.). New York: Basic Books.

30. Leisure-Based Stress Coping

Susan L. Hutchinson

Coping is what people do to try to manage or eliminate stressful situations. In the context of living with a chronic health condition, for example, coping is what people do to manage the emotional consequences and effects of illness or impairment on their abilities to carry out normal roles and activities (Coulter & Ellins, 2007). How well people adapt to changes in their life situation or health condition depends in large part on how well they cope with or manage a myriad of stressors they may encounter in their everyday lives, whether these are illness symptoms or relationship conflicts.

Although there are hundreds of thousands of articles and books on coping in both the scientific and self-help literature, most contemporary definitions, models, and studies of coping can be traced to the seminal work of Lazarus (1966). Lazarus argued for a contextual or transactional approach to the study of coping, in which there is recognition of a reciprocal influence between persons and their environments. Context refers not just to a specific situation someone finds himself/herself in but also to the personal (e.g., personality, socioeconomic status, age), social (e.g., social network), and sociocultural (e.g., unsafe neighborhood) environments in which people view themselves and their immediate situation. Most contemporary models of coping appear to have adopted this cognitive and contextualized approach.

From this transactional perspective, coping is viewed a "constantly changing cognitive and behavioral effort to manage [that is, to master, tolerate, reduce, minimize] specific external and/or internal demands [and conflicts among them] that are appraised as taxing or exceeding the resources of the person" (Lazarus & Folkman, 1984, p. 141, cited in Aldwin, 2011, p. 22). In Lazarus and Folkman's model, coping involves a primary appraisal of the situation as threatening, benign, or manageable and then secondary appraisal, which involves the decision about how to respond to the situation depending on an appraisal of resources or capacities to manage the situation. This secondary appraisal leads to the selection of different coping strategies.

Hood and Carruthers (2002) highlighted implications for recreational therapy in this definition. For example, the idea of constantly changing efforts implies that people will need to: (1) develop a repertoire of coping strategies to draw on in response to a stressor, and (2) know how to assess a situation in order to decide which coping strategy will be most effective. As Hood and Carruthers (2002) noted, "A fundamental component of the coping process is appraisal.... For therapeutic recreation specialists who are trying to impact coping skills, it is important to recognize the importance of the appraisal process throughout the coping experience" (p. 139).

Different research groups have identified various ways to categorize coping strategies. For example, Lazarus and Folkman (1984) categorized coping strategies as *problem-focused* (efforts to change the situation) or *emotional-focused* (efforts to manage one's emotional state). Folkman and Lazarus (1980) suggested that most people use emotional- and problem-focused strategies together in the majority of situations. Skinner and colleagues identified five basic types of coping strategies: *problem solving*, *support seeking* (reaching out to others to receive instrumental or emotional support), *avoidance*, *distraction* (positive behaviors and cognitions to minimize stress), and *positive cognitive restructuring* (reinterpreting situations and benefit finding) (Skinner, Edge, Altman, & Sherwood, 2003). A final overarching way to categorize coping strategies is dividing them in *approach-focused* strategies (efforts to control the situation) and *avoidance-focused* strategies (distancing oneself from the stressor). The latter do include some maladaptive responses to stress, such as procrastination, excessive eating, or alcohol use. Table 14 provides examples of coping strategies organized in terms of whether they are behaviorally or cognitively focused, and adaptive or maladaptive.

Table 14: Coping Strategies

Behavioral Strategies

Positive (Adaptive) Strategies

- Exercise
- Relaxation techniques
- Use of aids (e.g., walker, brace, assistive devices): For example, to manage declining memory, aids such as calendars, lists, notes, written instructions, and asking others for reminders may be used.
- Modifying activities: For example, reducing time, space, or effort needed for different activities; creating and following routines.
- Receiving education from professionals and peers.
- Seeking and establishing social connections, being with similar people getting help.
- Expressing emotions and thoughts, including self-disclosure. For example, deciding who, when, and how to talk about the situation.
- Humor, laughing, and joking.
- Maintaining important activities that affirm identity and give life meaning. For example, family roles, leisure, work, and volunteering.
- Alternative therapeutic treatments related to the disease condition or situation. For example, massage therapy.
- Establishing connection with God by praying, seeking spiritual guidance, or asking God for help in restoring health.
- Refraining from or avoiding former activities or habits, such as smoking and alcohol.

Negative (Maladaptive) Strategies

- Inappropriate self-medication.
- Use of alcohol and illicit drugs.
- Negative self-statements.
- Negative emotions or avoiding showing emotions.
- Isolating self; withdrawing from or avoiding social contacts.
- Refusing help.
- Refraining from seeking information and help.

Cognitive Strategies

Positive (Adaptive) Strategies

- Taking personal responsibility for the situation and health.
- Maintaining hope and a positive outlook.
- Focusing on or reminding self of positive aspects of life despite the illness or situation.
- Anticipating. Preparing self for the situation, including anticipating potential problems or barriers.
- Positive self-statements.
- Living one day at a time.
- "Fighting spirit." For example, determination and perseverance.
- Not thinking about the illness to maintain as normal a life as possible.
- Coming to terms with the disease or situation. For example, thinking that there is no point worrying because "you can't do anything about it." Accepting the reality of the situation while maintaining sufficient optimism to carry on from day to day.
- Positive reinterpretation. Seeing value in situations and being grateful for the things one can do.
- Revising goals to match abilities and interests.

Negative (Maladaptive) Strategies

- Negative thoughts about self or situation.
- Ruminating.
- Overgeneralization about situation.
- Avoidance strategies, such as denying, minimizing, and distancing or avoiding thinking and planning ahead.

Over the last two decades there has been a significant shift in attention away from managing distress (or the negative consequences of stress) to focusing on the role of positive emotions in the stress appraisal and coping process (Folkman, 1997; Folkman & Moskowitz, 2000) and on the positive emotions and outcomes, such as resilience, that can result from coping responses to stress (Fredrickson & Joiner, 2002). As well, an important focus of coping interventions has been on self-regulatory beliefs and behaviors. Self-regulation is the process through which people control and direct their own actions in order to meet their goals. In self-regulation theory, goal-setting, problem solving (e.g., anticipating and planning ways to overcome barriers to goal accomplishment), and action planning (e.g., making specific plans to meet goals) are viewed as important determinants of actual performance (Carver & Scheier, 1998). Proactive coping theory offers a useful framework for such planning (Aspinwall, 1997, 2004; Aspinwall & Taylor, 1997). Proactive coping implies that people can go beyond reaction to threats. They can anticipate situations and prevent them from interfering with their goals in the future.

Leisure and Coping

An extensive review of the literature related to leisure and coping and implications for recreational therapy practice can be found in Hood and Carruthers (2002) and Hutchinson, Bland, and Kleiber (2008); consequently only a brief overview will be provided. Coleman and Iso-Ahola (1993) were the first to conceptualize the relationships between leisure and stress. They suggested that leisure-generated social supports and "self-determination dispositions," such as beliefs in personal abilities to take action on issues that matter, would buffer the relationships between life stress and physical and mental health. Perceived freedom, competence, and control associated with leisure are viewed as contributing to beliefs in one's abilities to be self-determined. In turn, these beliefs will help people more effectively turn to their leisure to help them cope with stress. Since then numerous researchers have tested and expanded on these propositions.

Iwasaki and Mannell (2000) developed and tested a leisure-coping model that distinguishes leisure coping beliefs from leisure coping strategies. Similar to self-determination dispositions, *leisure coping beliefs* reflect the extent to which people believe they can use their leisure to cope in times of stress. Beliefs about the availability of leisure-based social supports as well as feelings of self-determination, empowerment, and competence developed through leisure pursuits can enhance leisure coping beliefs. *Leisure coping strategies* are the situational leisure-based responses to stressful or challenging situations. They can be either cognitive or behavioral.

Juniper (2005) recommended the following three leisure-based stress coping techniques to preemptively counteract stress. The first two are cognitive strategies and the last is behavioral.

1. Distraction: Creating distance between the problematic situation and the person. This can be done intuitively by individuals or can be facilitated by developing use of:

- Visualization, such as visualizing a happy moment or positive experience to facilitate attention shifting.
- Thought handling or positive reappraisal: Interrupting self-denigrating, situation-negative thoughts and concentrating instead on positive ideas and images associated with past or current leisure experiences.

2. Anticipation: Having something positive to look forward to. Similar to distraction, anticipation involves the ability to visualize positive upcoming events or actions and the potential positive consequences of these events or actions. Techniques to facilitate anticipation include:

- Planning future recreation activities, focusing on anticipated thoughts and feelings.
- Keeping an activity log, in which the client records "the pleasure potential" of selected activities before and after the experience.

3. Confrontation: This is problem-oriented coping, wherein people take action to address the problem directly, such as swimming to counteract negative effects of overeating. Juniper (2005) suggested that engaging in activities that require physical or cognitive investment of effort and energy can disrupt previous behavioral patterns and can be a means for stimulus control. For example, the cues for drinking might be removed by being in a different social or physical environment.

In the context of coping with chronic stressors such as those associated with acquired disability or chronic illness, Kleiber and colleagues (Hutchinson, Loy, Kleiber, & Dattilo, 2003; Hutchinson & Kleiber, 2005; Kleiber, Hutchinson, & Williams, 2002) identified similar ways that leisure could be a resource for coping (self-protection) and adaptation (self-restoration):

Self-protection: This has two aspects:

- Leisure that is a *positive distraction* can help people take their minds off their problems, experience positive emotions, and feel renewed and better able to return to the problem. Included in this is mental distraction, such as reading a book, and distancing oneself from the physical or social environment or situation, such as going for a walk.

- Leisure that is a source of motivation can sustain coping efforts. Included in this is *anticipating* benefits from leisure which can provide people with something to look forward to and remember, and experiencing *immediate successes* in leisure which can generate optimism about the future.

Self-restoration: Opportunities to experience a sense of mastery, achievement, or normalcy — and connect people with previous sources of meaning and identity — can promote adaptation in the face of losses and change by *affirming life goals, values and self-attributes*.

Hutchinson et al. (2008) concluded that almost any leisure or recreation activity, whether done alone or with others, has the potential to be a coping resource if it addresses coping goals — a notable exception is extended amounts of television watching. Activities that contribute to self-restoration tend to provide immediate benefits while being less physically, emotionally, or cognitively demanding. A myriad of leisure pursuits can be positive distractions when they enable people to take their minds off their problems, even momentarily, and to experience positive emotions.

Leisure activities that occur in social contexts can generally help people feel a sense of belonging, solidarity, or support, even when not directly addressing problems (Hutchinson et al., 2003). More active forms of leisure or recreation (those that require some investment of physical, social, emotional, or cognitive resources) seem to be most beneficial for restoring a sense of self, especially when, as noted above, they enable people to optimize talents and abilities and to affirm life goals or values. Examples include more demanding forms of physical activities; hobbies; playing an instrument; self-development or self-care activities, such as journaling or reading a self-help book; or learning new leisure skills. As Iwasaki et al. (2006) noted, "one key essence of active leisure coping involved meaning

creation … provid[ing] an opportunity for gaining one's highly valued meanings, such as: social, spiritual, cultural, altruistic, and/or empowerment" (p. 174). However, casual forms of leisure can also be restorative when they affirm individual, family, and cultural beliefs and values (Hutchinson & Kleiber, 2005).

Indications

These interventions should be considered when deficits in ICF code d240 Handling Stress and Other Psychological Demands are seen. The interventions may also be indicated when portions of ICF code b126 Temperament and Personality Functions are cited as concerns.

Most of the evidence indicates immediate and enduring benefits of recreation or leisure participation, including participation in facilitated group recreation programs, for coping with daily hassles, or acute or chronic stressors, for a wide variety of populations including:

- Younger adolescents (Hutchinson, Baldwin, & Oh, 2006) and older adolescents (Cassidy, 2005; Passmore & French, 2000), including children and adolescents of families in transition (Doyle, Wolchik, Dawson, & Sandler, 2003).

- University students (Iwasaki, 2001; Iwasaki & Mannell, 2000; Pantry, Blanchard, & Mask, 2007).

- Adults (Iso-Ahola & Park, 1996; Iwasaki, 2006), including adults in high-stress work roles (Iwasaki, Mannell, Smale, & Butcher, 2005; Trenberth & Dewe, 2002).

- Marginalized and nondominant groups including persons who identify as gay or lesbian and Aboriginal populations living with diabetes (Iwasaki, Bartlett, & O'Neil, 2005; Iwasaki & Bartlett, 2006; Iwasaki & Ristock, 2004).

- Women (Hutchinson, Yarnal, Sanford-Son, & Kerstetter, 2008; Werner & Shannon, 2013), including women who are homeless (Klitzing, 2003).

- Persons living with acquired disabilities or chronic health conditions (Hutchinson & Kleiber, 2005; Hutchinson, Loy, Kleiber, & Dattilo, 2003; Lee & McCormick, 2002) including persons living with cancer (Shannon & Bourque, 2005).

- Caregivers of persons living in residential settings (Dupuis & Pedlar, 1995).

- Families experiencing divorce and/or remarriage (Hutchinson, Afifi, & Krause, 2007).

Notably in the above research, individuals have identified and experienced coping benefits from participation *without* intervention from a recreational therapist.

Coping Interventions

There are numerous coping skills interventions that may or may not involve recreational therapists or may or may not or include a focus on leisure-based stress coping. For example, Creed, Machin, and Hicks (1999) recommended recreation participation as a coping strategy for youth living with long-term unemployment; and Lochman, Boxmeyer, and Powell (2009) utilized play and recreation activities in a cognitive-behavioral intervention for aggressive children. Although neither of these studies utilized a recreational therapist, they employed the use of recreation and play for stress coping. Most interventions have been developed for people with similar diagnoses, such as chronic pain (e.g., Kratz et al., Schreurs et al., 2003) or experiencing similar life situations, such as caregiving (McMillan et al., 2013). Coping skills interventions for children have targeted children presenting challenging behaviors or those who are seen as at risk (e.g., Puskar, Sereika, & Tusaie-Mumford, 2003). Consequently, recreational therapists are advised to review literature for condition-specific stress-coping interventions across various fields of study.

Although there is the suggestion that many people could benefit from strengthening their internal and external resources and abilities to better cope with acute or chronic stressors in their lives (e.g., Hood & Carruthers, 2002; Hutchinson et al., 2008), evidence of specific populations for whom recreational therapy coping interventions are indicated is limited.

Leisure counseling is recommended for individuals with a "range of existing but inadequate coping skills" (Juniper, 2005, p. 27) and for building these key skills when they are absent. Juniper recommended that leisure-based distraction, anticipation, or confrontation techniques (described previously) can be developed through leisure counseling to address:

- Phobias.
- Panics.

- Stress and tension states.
- Traumatic episodes. ("The technique of choice is the determined retrieval of a pre-traumatic hobby, activity, or interest, and, once retrieved, its intense development.... Its objective is the recreation of a familiar mood-state with intent to soothe and stabilise trauma's emotional disruption." p. 33.)
- Mood maintenance. ("systematic planning of a continuous series of future pleasurable events...." p. 33.)
- Habits, impulses, obsessions.

Recreational therapy coping skills interventions have been developed and/or recommended for:

- Persons living with HIV/AIDS (Caroleo, 1999).
- Persons in recovery from substance abuse (Carruthers & Hood, 2002).
- Caregivers who are experiencing high rates of caregiver stress and burden (Hughes & Keller, 1992; Hutchinson, Doble, Warner, & MacPhee, 2011).
- Persons who have experienced trauma (Aria, Griffin, Miatello, & Greig, 2008; Griffin, 2005).
- Individuals who have difficulties managing anger (Gongora, McKenney, & Godinez, 2005). Also see the chapter in this book on Anger Management.

Contraindications

Evidence of specific populations for whom coping interventions are contraindicated is limited. Hutchinson et al. (2008) cautioned that leisure-based coping interventions may not be beneficial for the following populations:

- Individuals who are experiencing acute levels of distress or grief for whom a focus on leisure may be viewed as trivializing their situation.
- Individuals whose cognitive abilities are not sufficient to undertake the tasks of problem solving, organizing thoughts, and remembering because the protocols included in this chapter are cognitively based and rely on the individual's appraisals to guide problem solving, decision making, and taking action.
- Individuals who do not believe leisure could be beneficial for coping with stress.

Protocols and Processes

It may be that people engage in behavioral or cognitive coping strategies — like information seeking or positive reappraisal — in order to engage in valued leisure pursuits. If this is the case, then leisure participation may not be the coping strategy, but rather the *outcome* of successful coping. Recreational therapy practitioners are advised to develop a large knowledge and skill base related to general behavioral and cognitive coping strategies, as shown earlier in Table 14, and to utilize goal setting, planning, and problem-solving processes to ensure clients are self-directed in developing knowledge, skills, and confidence to address stressors, including stressors which serve as barriers to leisure participation.

The recreational therapy coping protocols recommended by Hood and Carruthers (2002) and Hutchinson et al. (2008) have been summarized in combination in Figure 1. Both are generic protocols, designed to be applied with any population in individual or group recreational therapy interventions to address stress coping. However, neither specifies the frequency or duration of interventions that will result in positive change. Recreational therapists are en-

couraged to review each article for more detailed practice guidelines. It is also strongly recommended that therapists are informed about potential stressors associated with the presenting problems and diagnoses of their client population prior to planning individual or group coping interventions.

Assessment

Hutchinson et al. (2008) provided examples of standardized tools that can be used for individual assessment and care planning (e.g., the *Brief COPE*, Carver, 1997) but none have specifically incorporated a focus on leisure-based coping. The *Leisure Coping Beliefs* and *Leisure Coping Strategies* scales developed by Iwasaki and Mannell (2000) do assess leisure coping but they have not been validated for use in recreational therapy settings.

In order to guide decisions about individual treatment planning related to stress coping, it is recommended that recreational therapists assess the following:

Situational stress appraisal: How stressful people perceive their current situation to be, including how stressful they perceive leisure to be in the

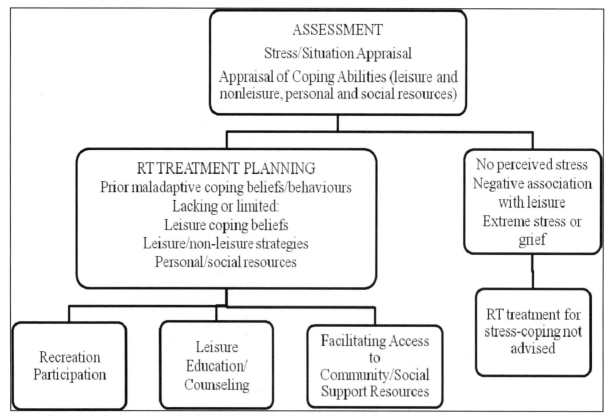

Figure 1: Overview of the APIE Process for Stress-Coping Interventions in Recreation Therapy

context of their current situation.

Appraisal of coping abilities (based on appraisal of prior experiences and resources): To what extent people perceive leisure has helped them in the past or could currently help them cope with stress in their lives; how people have coped with stressful situations in the past (and currently), including using leisure to cope with stress; and to what extent people perceive they have the personal or social resources to cope with stress, including the ability to use their leisure to cope with stress.

If clients do not perceive their situation to be unduly stressful, then recreational therapy treatment related to stress coping is not warranted. If clients perceive they possess adequate personal or social resources to manage stress on their own, then individual treatment is also not needed. Instead, it may be sufficient to ensure they have access to equipment, supplies, or opportunities to be self-directed in coping with stress in their lives. Individual treatment planning related to leisure-based stress-coping is warranted if clients perceive their situation to be stressful *and* they: believe leisure has been or could be a coping resource for them; do not possess adequate knowledge, skills, or resources to use their leisure to cope with stress; and have engaged in unhealthy leisure behaviors to cope in the past.

Juniper (2005) recommended that to amplify the benefits of leisure-based coping with stress there is a need to address the following, in order of priority: reduce phobias, panics, stress, tension states, and aftermath of trauma; enhance positive mood states; and contain or limit destructive habits or impulses.

If clients perceive their situation to be extremely stressful or believe leisure may exacerbate their perceived stress, then recreational therapy treatment goals focused on leisure-based coping may not be appropriate. Instead, it may be advisable to refer clients for grief counseling or psychotherapy, or to assist them in developing other non-leisure coping strategies, such as thought-stopping strategies to manage anxiety in social situations, in collaboration with other healthcare professionals with expertise in cognitive-behavioral therapies.

Planning

In general, the scope of services related to stress coping will be determined by the overall departmental or agency goals and overarching client needs.

Regardless of the setting, in most cases a leisure-based stress-coping intervention will focus on helping clients learn about the benefits of leisure for coping with stress, develop and use their leisure-coping repertoire, and build their personal and/or social leisure-coping resources. One goal is to increase the range of leisure pursuits perceived to be personally beneficial in times of stress.

In some settings, such as residential care, this may mean providing opportunities for people to engage in a variety of leisure activities, alone or in group settings, that they perceive to be beneficial for coping with stress.

Hood and Carruthers' (2002) coping skills intervention focuses on planning for skills and knowledge development and resource enhancement in order to reduce negative demands of stressful situations and to increase positive resources that can prevent or reduce the impact of stress on physical or mental health. Notably, many of the skills and resources they recommend are not specific to leisure. Hood and Carruthers recommend helping clients develop the following coping strategies that can directly address problematic or stressful situations or help in managing the negative emotional consequences of stressful situations:

- Problem solving skills including decision making, time management, assertiveness, and relationship skills.
- Cognitive restructuring including positive reappraisal.
- Stress management skills.
- Relaxation techniques.
- Distraction strategies — both mental and behavioral.

In addition to addressing the stressful situation, Hood and Carruthers (2002) recommended that clients be assisted in developing their internal and external (e.g., social) resources that can prevent or reduce the impact of stress on physical or mental health, including:

Physical: including overall fitness and energy.

Psychological: including hope, optimism, self-esteem, self-efficacy, and perceptions of control.

Social: including increasing social support, extending social network, and strengthening quality of relationships.

Lifestyle: including the ability to experience pleasure and enjoyment in leisure and other life areas, community involvement, and civic participation.

Implementation

Overall, experiential activities; cognitive-behavioral, leisure education, and leisure counseling interventions; and supporting clients in accessing community or social resources are the most frequently recommended techniques for improving people's stress-coping skills and resources. Specifically, when creating individual recreational therapy coping-related care plans, the following therapeutic modalities or techniques are recommended (summarized from Hood & Carruthers, 2002, and Hutchinson et al., 2008):

Recreation Participation

Facilitating experiential opportunities in conjunction with debriefing (e.g., leisure sampling or recreation participation) is recommended for clients who lack knowledge or awareness of the coping-related benefits of leisure. This is especially useful for helping clients to develop distraction strategies.

Helping clients to identify and participate in activities that provide a sense of competence and control, and enable them to experience positive emotions and success more generally, will enhance leisure coping beliefs that leisure can be a useful coping strategy and also enhance psychological resources, such as self-efficacy, hope, and optimism. When clients experience for themselves how much better they feel as a result of participating in an enjoyable and personally meaningful leisure activity, they may be more likely to identify its stress-coping benefits.

Leisure Education and/or Counseling

Recommended for clients who do not possess adequate knowledge, skills, or resources for leisure-based coping, or for those who previously engaged in unhealthy leisure coping behaviors. Depending on assessed client needs, education and/or counseling techniques will focus on helping clients identify perceived benefits of leisure for coping, beliefs about leisure for coping, problem solving and decision making to address perceived stressors and/or barriers to leisure, and/or personal and social resources for coping.

To enhance leisure coping beliefs, it may be necessary to help people identify self-limiting beliefs, potential benefits of leisure for stress coping, and/or develop an ethic of leisure-based self-care.

As noted earlier, a self-regulatory process is recommended, with an emphasis on planning (identifying stress triggers, goal setting, decision making) and problem solving (including anticipating and planning strategies to address potential stressors or stress triggers).

Practicing coping skills with debriefing or other opportunities for reflection is essential to enhance coping self-efficacy.

Cognitive behavioral therapy techniques are recommended for teaching clients other general coping skills, such as thought stopping, positive reappraisal, visualization, stress management, etc. Cognitive-behavioral techniques are important to help clients see the connections between their thoughts and actions, specifically the connections between stress appraisals, leisure coping beliefs, and leisure coping strategies.

For those who have relied on unhealthy or maladaptive coping strategies in the past, the focus is on teaching substitute skills and activities that fulfill similar needs.

Leisure-related skills development (including physical activity and relaxation skills) is recommended for clients who do not possess a leisure repertoire that they perceive could be beneficial in coping with stress. It is also recommended to strengthen clients' physical, social, and lifestyle resources.

Also see the chapter on Leisure Education and Counseling in this book.

Facilitating Access to Community and Social Resources

Recommended for clients who believe their leisure can help them cope, and/or possess adequate knowledge and skills for leisure participation, but who may not have strong social or leisure networks for social support or leisure companionship.

Connecting individual clients with peers, as either supports or participation partners (e.g., Peers for Progress, 2013) for mutual support, shared participation, and/or information sharing is recommended.

Information provision (e.g., about available leisure, community, support resources) or teaching specific adaptive strategies (e.g., to overcome barriers to leisure participation) may be needed to support self-directed participation in leisure for stress coping.

Outcomes and Documentation

From the review of the leisure coping research there is evidence that leisure contributes to immediate outcomes such as reduced distress (d240 Handling Stress and Other Psychological Demands), improved mood (e.g., b126 Temperament and Personality Functions), and longer term outcomes related to improved physical and mental health and psychological well-being (Iwasaki, 2001, 2006). In the context of living with an acquired disability or chronic health condition, leisure participation contributes to psychological resilience and enables people to feel more capable of managing ongoing stressors in their lives (Hutchinson et al., 2003; Kleiber et al., 2002).

To measure outcomes of leisure-based stress-coping interventions the following measures or processes are recommended. Their use will depend on the goals of the intervention.

Standardized tools: Standardized measures can be used to assess various aspects of coping. Some examples include: The *Positive and Negative Affect Schedule* [PANAS] assesses self-reported changes in perceived stress and positive and negative affect (Watson, Clark, & Tellegen, 1988). Perceived leisure coping beliefs can be measured by the *Leisure Coping Beliefs* scale. General or leisure-based coping strategies are covered with the *Brief COPE* or *Leisure Coping Strategies* scale identified previously. Other standardized measures used by the department or agency may also be used to assess changes in mental health or psychological well-being.

Observable behavior: Recreational therapists may also assess and track data related to changes in behaviors and/or perceptions in relation to client stress-coping goals. Examples of data include frequency and type of participation, the extent to which the client was able to anticipate stressful situation and use a leisure-based coping strategy to cope, and perceived benefits of leisure-based stress coping. These data will be gathered primarily during individual or group sessions, for example: achievement of assigned tasks; qualitative statements during sessions or post-session debriefing; and client journals, worksheets, or participation records.

References

Aldwin, C. (2011). Stress and coping across the lifespan. In S. Folkman (Ed.), *Oxford handbook of stress, health, and coping*. New York: Oxford University Press.

Aria, S., M., Griffin, J., Miatello, A., & Greig, C. L. (2008). Leisure and recreation involvement in the context of healing from trauma. *Therapeutic Recreation Journal, 42*(1), 37-55.

Aspinwall, L. G. (1997). Where planning meets coping: Proactive coping and the detection and management of potential stressors. In S. L. Friedman & E. Kofsky Scholnick (Eds.). *The developmental psychology of planning: Why, how and when do we plan?* (pp. 285-320). New York: Erlbaum.

Aspinwall, L. G. (2004). Dealing with adversity: Self-regulation, coping, adaptation, and health. In M. B. Brewer & M. Hewstone (Eds.), *Applied social psychology* (pp. 3-27). Malden, MA: Blackwell.

Aspinwall, L. G. & Taylor, S. E. (1997). A stitch in time: Self-regulation and proactive coping. *Psychological Bulletin, 121*, 417-36.

Caroleo, O. (1999). The impact of a therapeutic recreation program on the use of coping strategies among people with AIDS. *Annual in Therapeutic Recreation, 8*, 22-32, 82-83, 87.

Carruthers, C. P. & Hood, C. D. (2002). Coping skills program for individuals with alcoholism. *Therapeutic Recreation Journal, 36*(2) 154-171.

Carver, C. S. (1997). You want to measure coping but your protocol's too long. Consider the Brief COPE. *International Journal of Behavioral Medicine, 4*, 92-100.

Carver, C. S. & Scheier, M. F. (1998). *On the self-regulation of behavior.* Cambridge, MA: Cambridge University Press.

Cassidy, T. (2005). Leisure, coping and health: The role of social, family, school and peer relationship factors. *British Journal of Guidance & Counselling, 33*(1), 51-66.

Coleman, D. & Iso-Ahola, S. E. (1993). Leisure and health: The role of social support and self-determination. *Journal of Leisure Research, 25,* 111-128.

Coulter, A. & Ellins, J. (2007). Effectiveness of strategies for informing, educating, and involving patients. *British Medical Journal, 335*, 24-27.

Creed, P. A., Machin, M. A., & Hicks, R. E. (1999). Improving mental health status and coping abilities for long-term unemployed youth using cognitive-behaviour therapy based training interventions. *Journal of Organizational Behavior, 20,* 963-978.

Doyle, K. W., Wolchik, S. A., Dawson, M. S. R., & Sandler, I. N. (2003). Positive events as a stress buffer for children and adolescents in families in transition. *Journal of Clinical Child and Adolescent Psychology, 32,* 536-545.

Dupuis, S. L. & Pedlar, A. (1995). Family leisure programs in institutional care settings: Buffering the stress of caregivers. *Therapeutic Recreation Journal, 29*(3), 184-205.

Folkman, S. (1997). Positive psychological states and coping with severe stress. *Social Science and Medicine, 45*(8), 1207-1221.

Folkman, S. & Lazarus, R. S. (1980). An analysis of coping in a middle-aged community sample. *Journal of Health and Social Behavior, 21,* 219-239.

Folkman, S. & Moskowitz, J. T. (2000). Stress, positive emotions, and coping. *Current Directions in Psychological Science, 9*(4), 115-118.

Fredrickson, B. L. & Joiner, T. (2002). Positive emotions trigger upward spirals toward emotional well-being. *Psychological Sciences, 13,* 172-175.

Gongora, E. L., McKenney, A., & Godinez, C. (2005). A multidisciplinary approach to teaching anger coping after sustaining a traumatic brain injury: A case report. *Therapeutic Recreation Journal, 39*(3), 229-240.

Griffin, J. (2005). Recreation therapy for adult survivors of childhood abuse: Challenges to professional perspectives and the evolution of a leisure education group. *Therapeutic Recreation Journal, 39*(3), 207-228.

Hood, C. & Carruthers, C. (2002). Coping skills theory as an underlying framework for therapeutic recreation services. *Therapeutic Recreation Journal, 36*, 137-153.

Hughes, S. & Keller, J. M. (1992). Leisure education: A coping strategy for family caregivers. *Journal of Gerontological Social Work, 19*, 115-128.

Hutchinson, S. L., Afifi, T., & Krause, S. (2007). The family that plays together fares better: Examining the contribution of shared family time to family resilience following divorce. *Journal of Divorce and Remarriage, 46*(3/4), 21-48.

Hutchinson, S. L., Baldwin, C. A., & Oh, S. S. (2006). Adolescent coping: Exploring adolescents' leisure-based responses to stress. *Leisure Sciences, 28*(2), 115-131.

Hutchinson, S. L., Bland, A., & Kleiber, D. A. (2008). Leisure and stress-coping: Implications for therapeutic recreation practice. *Therapeutic Recreation Journal, 42*(1), 9-23.

Hutchinson, S. L., Doble, S., Warner, G., & MacPhee, C. (2011). Lessons learned from Take Care: A brief leisure education intervention for caregivers. *Therapeutic Recreation Journal, 45*(2), 121-134.

Hutchinson, S. L., Loy, D. P., Kleiber, D. A., & Dattilo, J. (2003). Leisure as a coping resource: Variations in coping with traumatic injury and illness. *Leisure Sciences, 25*, 143-162.

Hutchinson, S. L. & Kleiber, D. A. (2005). Gifts of the "ordinary": Considering the contribution of casual leisure to health and well-being. *World Leisure Journal, 47*(3), 2-16.

Hutchinson, S. L., Yarnal, C. M., Sanford-Son, J., & Kerstetter, D. (2008). Beyond fun and friendship: The Red Hat Society® as a coping resource for older women. *Ageing & Society, 28*(7), 979-999.

Iso-Ahola, S. E. & Park, C. (1996). Leisure-related social support and self-determination as buffers of the stress-illness relationship. *Journal of Leisure Research, 28*(3), 169-187.

Iwasaki, Y. (2001). Contributions of leisure to coping with daily hassles in university students' lives. *Canadian Journal of Behavioural Science, 33*(2), 128-141.

Iwasaki, Y. (2006). Counteracting stress through leisure coping: A prospective health study. *Psychology, Health & Medicine, 11*(2), 209-220.

Iwasaki, Y. & Bartlett, J. G. (2006). Culturally meaningful leisure as a way of coping with stress among Aboriginal individuals with diabetes. *Journal of Leisure Research, 38*(3), 321-338.

Iwasaki, Y., Bartlett, J., & O'Neil, J. (2005). Coping with stress among Aboriginal women and men with diabetes in Winnipeg, Manitoba. *Social Science and Medicine, 60*(5), 977-988.

Iwasaki, Y. & Mannell, R. C. (2000). Hierarchical dimensions of leisure stress coping. *Leisure Sciences, 22*, 163-181.

Iwasaki, Y., Mannell, R. C., Smale, B. J. A., & Butcher, J. (2005). Contributions of leisure participation in predicting stress coping and health among police and emergency response services workers. *Journal of Health Psychology, 10*(1), 81-101.

Iwasaki, Y. & Ristock, J. (2004). Coping with stress among gays and lesbians: Implications for human development over the lifespan. *World Leisure Journal, 46*(2), 26-37.

Iwasaki, Y., Mackay, K. J., & Mactavish, J. B. (2006). Leisure from the margins: Stress, active living, and leisure as a contributor to coping with stress. *Leisure Sciences, 28*, 163-180.

Juniper, D. (2005). Leisure counselling, coping skills and therapeutic applications. *British Journal of Guidance & Counselling, 33*(1), 27-36.

Kleiber, D. A., Hutchinson, S. L., & Williams, R. (2002). Leisure as a resource in transcending negative life events: Self-protection, self-restoration, and personal transformation. *Leisure Sciences, 24*, 219-235.

Klitzing, S. W. (2003). Coping with chronic stress: Leisure and women who are homeless. *Leisure Sciences, 25*, 163-181.

Kratz, A. L., Molton, I. R., Jensen, M. P., Ehde, D. W., & Nielson, W. R. (2011). Further evaluation of the Motivational Model of Pain Self-Management: Coping with pain in multiple sclerosis. *Annals of Behavioral Medicine, 41*, 391-400.

Lazarus, R. S. (1966). *Psychological stress and the coping process.* New York: McGraw-Hill.

Lazarus, R. S. & Folkman, S. (1984). *Stress, appraisal, and coping.* New York: Springer.

Lee, Y. & McCormick, B. P. (2002). Sense making process in defining health for people with chronic illness and disabilities. *Therapeutic Recreation Journal, 36*(3), 235-246.

Lochman, J. E., Boxmeyer, C., & Powell, N. (2009). The role of play within cognitive behavioral therapy for aggressive children: The Coping Power program. In A. A. Drewes (Ed.), *Blending play therapy with cognitive behavioral therapy: Evidence-based and other effective treatments and techniques* (pp. 179-197). Hoboken, NJ: John Wiley & Sons.

McMillan, S. C., Small, B. J., Haley, W. E., Zambroskio, C., & Buck, H. G. (2013). The COPE intervention for caregivers of patients with heart failure. *Journal of Hospice & Palliative Nursing, 15*(4), 196-206.

Pantry, D. A., Blanchard, C. M., & Mask, L. (2007). Measuring university students' regulatory leisure coping styles: Planned breathers or avoidance? *Leisure Sciences, 29*, 247-265.

Passmore, A. & French, D. (2000). A model of leisure and mental health in Australian adolescents. *Behavior Change, 17*(3), 208-221.

Peers for Progress. (2013). Peers for Progress: A program of the American Academy of Family Physicians Foundations. Retrieved from: http://peersforprogress.org/

Puskar, K., Sereika, S., & Tusaie-Mumford, K. (2003). Effect of the Teaching Kids to Cope (TKC) program on outcomes of depression and coping among rural adolescents. *Journal of Child & Adolescent Psychiatric Nursing, 16*(2), 71-80.

Schreurs, K., Colland, V. T., Kuijer, R. G., de Ridder, D., & van Elderen, T. (2003). Development, content, and process evaluation of a short self-management intervention in patients with chronic diseases requiring self-care behaviours. *Patient Education and Counseling, 51*, 133-141.

Shannon, C. & Bourque, D. (2005). Overlooked and underutilized: The critical role of leisure interventions in facilitating social support through breast cancer treatment and recovery. *Social Work in Health Care, 42*(1), 73-92.

Skinner, E. A., Edge, K. A., Altman, J., & Sherwood, H. (2003). Searching for the structure of coping: A review and critique of category systems for classifying ways of coping. *Psychological Bulletin, 129*(2), 216-269.

Trenberth, L. & Dewe, P. (2002). The importance of leisure as a means of coping with work-related stress: An exploratory study. *Counselling Psychology Quarterly, 15*(1), 59-72.

Watson, D., Clark, L. A., & Tellegen, A. (1988). Development and validation of brief measures of positive and negative affect: The PANAS scales. *Journal of Personality and Social Psychology, 54*(6), 1063-1070.

Werner, T. L. & Shannon, C. S. (2013). Doing more with less: Women's leisure during their partners' military deployment. *Leisure Sciences, 35*, 63-80.

31. Leisure Education and Counseling

Colleen Deyell Hood and Cynthia Carruthers

Leisure education is a central focus of recreational therapy professional practice. The field is grounded in the notion that leisure involvement contributes to the optimal functioning, health, and well-being of individuals (Stumbo & Peterson, 2008). However, the accrual of the benefits of leisure may be impacted by illness and disability. People with illnesses or disabilities may not have access to the full range of opportunities and supports necessary to engage in satisfying leisure. Additionally, like many other people in society, those with disabilities or illnesses may not fully appreciate the contribution of leisure engagement to well-being and quality of life. Through leisure education, individuals recognize the potential value of leisure and the knowledge and skills necessary to reap its full benefits. It is important to note that leisure education is not limited to RT services and settings. While other professionals may provide leisure education programs in schools, general recreation agencies, health promotion settings, and many other places, this section will focus on leisure education as it fits in RT practice.

A focus on leisure education is consistent with many recent shifts in the fields of healthcare, youth development, social work, and psychology, where there is an increasing recognition of the importance of helping individuals build their capacities and strengths, as well as resolve their difficulties. Positive psychology, in particular, emphasizes the importance of frequent experiences of positive emotion combined with the recognition and use of personal strengths and capacities as essential practices in creating a life of meaning and fulfillment (Seligman, 2002). Leisure experience can support both of these thrusts in that leisure can be an important source of positive emotion, as well as a context and experience through which to discover, develop, and express personal strengths (Carruthers & Hood, 2007; Hood

& Carruthers, 2007). In a spiral of positive evolution, these strengths, in turn, allow individuals to more effectively address future challenges in their lives.

Indications

Leisure education is appropriate for any individual who does not recognize the value of leisure for recovery, coping (d240 Handling Stress and Other Psychological Demands), health (d570 Looking After One's Health), meaning making (b126 Temperament and Personality Functions), happiness (b152 Emotional Functions), well-being, or other valued outcomes of recreational therapy practice (Caldwell et al., 2004; Hood & Carruthers, 2013). Disability and illness often result in a reduction in leisure involvement (d920 Recreation and Leisure) increased boredom (b126 Temperament and Personality Functions, b152 Emotional Functions), and lessened social interaction (d7 Interpersonal Interactions and Relationships, d9205 Socializing) (Rogers, Lee, & Yang, 2007; Vuillerot et al., 2010). Thus it is also appropriate for individuals who, as a result of illness or injury, may need to rediscover an interest in leisure and/or adapt or modify leisure engagement in order to accommodate disability or limitation (Coyle, Shank, & Vliet, 2010). Finally, leisure education is also congruent with the notion of "positive interventions" — those interventions that are designed to move people beyond normal functioning to optimal functioning, as leisure is an important source of positivity in one's life (Biswas-Diener, 2008).

The needs addressed in leisure education vary based on the characteristics and experiences of the particular clients being served.

For older adults, issues such as isolation (d7 Interpersonal Interactions and Relationships), reduced activity levels (d230 Carrying Out Daily Routine), pain (b280 Sensation of Pain) (Finch, 2006), and boredom (b126 Temperament and Personality Functions, b152 Emotional Functions) are all challenges that necessitate leisure education interventions (Dattilo, 2008; Janssen, 2004; Lovell, Dattilo, & Jekubovich, 1996).

For individuals with cognitive or intellectual impairments, some issues that suggest the need for leisure education include lack of leisure skills and awareness (d920 Recreation and Leisure), low levels of involvement in physically active leisure (d920 Recreation and Leisure), boredom (b126 Temperament and Personality Functions, b152 Emotional Functions), lack of opportunities to pursue valued goals (b130 Energy and Drive Functions), lack of social skills (d7 Interpersonal Interactions and Relationships), and lack of independence (e.g., d940 Human Rights) (Dattilo, 2002; Dattilo, 2008; Dattilo, Williams, & Cory, 2003; Hoge & Dattilo, 1999; Hoge, Dattilo, & Williams, 1999; Hoge & Wilhite, 1997).

For individuals with mental health problems, the issues that give rise to the need for leisure education services include such things as isolation (d7 Interpersonal Interactions and Relationships) and stigma (e4 Attitudes), lack of engagement in community activities (d910 Community Life), poor health habits, such as smoking or lack of exercise (d570 Looking After One's Health), social discomfort (e.g., d710 Basic Interpersonal Interactions), anhedonia (b126 Temperament and Personality Functions, b152 Emotional Functions), and lack of autonomy (e.g., d940 Human Rights) (Dattilo, 2008; Davidson et al., 2006; McKenney et al., 2004; Mitchell, 1998; Mueller & Volker, 2005).

For individuals with physical disabilities, leisure education interventions could address such things as coping with a change in functioning (d240 Handling Stress and Other Psychological Demands), fatigue (b4552 Fatigability), the necessity to adapt or replace previously valued activities (d920 Recreation and Leisure), pain (b280 Sensation of Pain), and lack of knowledge of adapted community leisure resources (d9 Community, Social, and Civic Life) (Broach, Dattilo, & McKenney, 2007; Desrosiers et al., 2007; Hutchinson et al., 2003; Ryan et al., 2008; Santiago & Coyle, 2004).

Other client groups that could benefit from leisure education interventions include: individuals with substance abuse problems (Aquadro et al., 2010;

Hood, 2003); incarcerated or at-risk youth (Caldwell et al., 2010; Robertson, 2001); and caregivers of older adults with physical or cognitive limitations (Bedini & Guinan, 1996; Carbonneau, Caron, & Desrosiers, 2011; Carter et al., 2001; Charters & Murray, 2006; Hughes & Keller, 1992; McMahon & Wardlaw, 2011).

As with any RT intervention, the issues addressed should be determined based on the results of an assessment process (Stumbo & Peterson, 2008). Assessments can be used to determine leisure-related needs and barriers as well as strengths and capacities related to leisure involvement. It is important to assess both deficits and capacities in order to plan for the most effective leisure education intervention. This twofold focus in assessment and planning will allow clients and therapists to identify client aspirations, the barriers that create challenges in achieving those aspirations, and the capacities the client already has that can be mobilized towards reaching his/her aspirations (Anderson & Heyne, 2012).

Contraindications

There are no documented contraindications for leisure education. However, a level of cognitive capacity is needed to learn skills, concepts, and practices related to leisure (d1 Learning and Applying Knowledge, d155 Acquiring Skills). As such, individuals with severe intellectual limitations may require significant educational supports and adaptations. These educational supports may include computer-assisted instruction and experiential learning activities (Cory, Dattilo, & Williams, 2006), memory aids, communication aids, and technological supports (Ramella, Tennis, & Yoshioka, 2009).

Protocols

There are a number of ways to approach leisure education. Mundy (1998) suggested that leisure education can be incorporated into existing recreation programs through the infusion method. In this approach, information about leisure is incorporated informally into existing recreation activities. For example, during a skiing instructional program, the RT professional might discuss the resources and facilities necessary for continued engagement in skiing.

The more common form of leisure education is a more direct approach, where systematic programs related to leisure are developed and delivered to a specific targeted group. There are a number of models in the fields of RT that identify common content areas for leisure education, such as the Leisure Ability Model (Stumbo & Peterson, 2008), Healthy Living through Leisure (Shank & Coyle, 2002), the Scope and Sequence Model (Mundy, 1998), and Leisure Wellness (McDowell, 1983). Most of these models identify knowledge, attitudes, and skills related to leisure that are needed for meaningful independent involvement in leisure. These models include information related to the value and benefits of leisure for all individuals, the vast variety of possible leisure activities, examination of personal values as they relate to one's own leisure, personal interests and experiences related to leisure, information related to accessing and engaging in leisure at home and in the community, leisure activity skills, social interactional skills, and planning and participation skills. These models assume that if people know how to participate in leisure and recognize its benefits, they will participate.

In more recent years, there has been increased recognition that RT professionals should focus their leisure education efforts on not only helping clients engage in leisure, but also on the quality of the leisure experience and potential outcomes of engagement. Dattilo, Kleiber, and Williams (1998) proposed a service delivery model of RT that shifted the leisure education emphasis toward self-determination and enjoyment. They suggested that RT services should support the development of intrinsic motivation towards leisure by helping clients manage challenge, invest their attention in the experience, and make choices. Engaging in intrinsically motivated experiences results in an increased feeling of self-determination and enjoyment. Hood and Carruthers (2007), in their Leisure and Well-Being Model (LWM), suggest that there are a set of capacities related to leisure involvement that enhance the value of leisure in creating a life of well-being. They suggest that people can participate in leisure and not receive the benefits if they are not attending to the experience or are not making choices that generate optimal experience. Thus, in the LWM, the emphasis of leisure education is on both developing basic capacities related to leisure involvement and supporting people to reap the greatest reward from leisure involvement. The LWM proposes five areas to

address in leisure education (Hood & Carruthers, 2007).

The first component, Savouring Leisure, refers to focusing on the positive aspects of the leisure experience. In Savouring Leisure, participants learn a set of strategies designed to help them to attend to and reap the benefits of the positive aspects of leisure experience. Savouring Leisure strategies include such things as looking for and concentrating on the positive emotion producing aspects of the experience (senses, memories, etc.), sharing the experience with others through story-telling, building memories (photos and keepsakes), counting blessings and gratitude, and reflection on the successes and satisfactions associated with involvement (Bryant & Veroff, 2007; Hood & Carruthers, 2007).

The second component, Mindful Leisure, refers to being fully present in the current moment (Hood & Carruthers, 2007). In Mindful Leisure, participants learn strategies to slow their minds and to become more fully present in the current moment. They may learn about traditional mindfulness practices, such as meditation and yoga, to assist them to slow their minds, or they may learn that certain leisure choices draw them into full engagement and total absorption, thus creating mindfulness in the moment.

The third component, Authentic Leisure, refers to making leisure choices that are personally meaningful. Authentic Leisure is based on the notion that developing and expressing a congruent identity is central to well-being and that activity engagements that "fit" are likely to create more benefits than those that do not "fit." Thus in Authentic Leisure, the focus is on participants' exploration and engagement in leisure experiences that encourage the discovery, development, and expression of their true selves.

The fourth component, Leisure Gratifications (Hood & Carruthers, 2007), refers to engagement in leisure experiences that optimally challenge the individual and facilitate the development of personal strengths and capacities. Leisure Gratifications are those activities that allow a person to become completely absorbed in the experience and that draw that person back to the activity time after time. These types of experiences often foster flow and, as such, lead to the enjoyment and evolving complexity of the individual. In Leisure Gratifications, participants learn how to select activities that are personally relevant and that afford degrees of skilled performance — creating the possibility of flow experiences.

Finally, the fifth component, Virtuous Leisure, refers to using one's personal strengths and abilities in the services of something greater than oneself. To promote Virtuous Leisure involves helping individuals to identify opportunities to be of service in their communities that are a match for their talents and which they would find meaningful.

Processes

The processes of planning for leisure education interventions has been well documented (Dattilo, 2008; Mundy, 1998; Stumbo & Peterson, 2008) and are specific to the client group being served and the unique characteristics of that group (age, ethnicity, gender, etc.). Specific program planning, a term used by Stumbo and Peterson (2008), describes a systematic process of planning that includes identifying the purpose, goals, objectives, and performance measures of the leisure education program, as well as the content and processes necessary to achieve them. In planning, it is important to start with the desired outcome in mind and then identify the content that must be taught and the manner in which the information will be taught (process). Table 15 provides an example of a typical program plan.

Table 15: Sample Leisure Education Program

Purpose of Program

To enhance positive emotion on a daily basis through engagement in meaningful leisure experiences.

Goals of Session

To facilitate the development of skills necessary for savoring leisure.

Performance Measures

After a leisure experience, the client will demonstrate the ability to consciously focus on the positive emotion-generating aspects of the experience by identifying three aspects of the experience that resulted in positive emotion.

Content

There are several strategies suggested that support savoring. One strategy is sensory perceptual

sharpening (Bryant & Veroff, 2007). This involves looking for aspects of the experience that generate positive emotion (e.g., sights, smells, sounds, movement, memories, etc.) and then focusing purposeful attention on those aspects to gain the greatest appreciation for those experiences. Oftentimes, just going into an experience with this focus is enough to create greater awareness of the positive emotion-producing elements of an experience. Asking yourself questions is also a technique for sensory perceptual sharpening. The questions include: What do I notice (see, hear, feel)? What positive memories does this experience bring up? How does this compare to what I was doing before? If tuning in to your senses is difficult, you may choose to limit sensory input to just one source, e.g., close your eyes and listen to sounds of the trees and wind.

Process

1. Introduce topic and provide rationale.

2. Ask clients to reflect on a recent positive experience and identify those aspects of the experience that generated positive emotion.

3. Give each participant a piece of chocolate. Before they put it in their mouths, ask them to slow down and pay conscious attention to the experience of eating the chocolate. What sensations do they experience and pay attention to? What are they thinking about as they eat the chocolate? How do they feel?

4. Introduce content related to sensory perceptual sharpening and connect it to the experience of eating the chocolate.

5. Take participants on a walk through the grounds (or some other preferred activity) and ask them to be prepared to identify in a journal those aspects of the walk that generate positive emotion.

6. Debrief experience with a focus on how they have increased the amount of positive emotion experienced by just paying more attention to their experiences. Ask how this relates to future leisure choices and engagements.

In terms of program implementation, Dattilo (2008) provided a good overview of the preparation and implementation of a leisure education session. Generally, leisure education program processes include the following components:

Rationale for topic: Providing information about the importance of the topic and the benefits to participants of learning the topic sets the stage for full involvement in the session.

Self-awareness and personal reflection: Many educational philosophers suggest that learning is best accomplished when it is related to personal experience and incorporates a reflective component (Dewey, 1933). Thus is it is important for participants to reflect on their own capacities related to the experience and the relevance of the topic to their own desired goals.

Skills and knowledge development: This component of program implementation includes the introduction of new skills or knowledge that will support clients in achieving the goals of the session and the goals of the overall leisure education program. This may be accomplished through a variety of means, including traditional classroom-type instruction, guided discussions, or readings (Mundy, 1998).

Application of skills and knowledge. Learning is most effective when participants can practice or experience the skills or knowledge (Dewey, 1938). This may be accomplished through the use of learning activities, role-playing, homework, and other strategies (Dattilo, 2008; Mundy, 1998).

Reflection and debriefing: Once skills or knowledge have been acquired, it is important to foster transfer of learning (Gass, 1985). Processing or debriefing is a strategy used to facilitate awareness of the connection between what has just been learned and real-life situations (Priest & Gass, 1997). De-briefing is usually addressed through a series of questions designed to facilitate participants' under-standing of the meaning behind the session, skills, or information and to help them see the connection between the skills or knowledge learned and their own goals for their lives. A simple model of debrief-ing was outlined by Schoel, Prouty, and Radcliffe (1988) and involved three main questions: What? (What did we just do, learn, or experience?); So What? (What is the importance of this information to you?); and Now What? (How does the information learned connect to your life and how will you use this information?).

The skills needed by the RT professional to de-liver effective leisure education include general facilitation skills (active reflective listening, asking questions, etc.); group leadership skills; presentation and instructional skills; and knowledge of the leisure-related content (Dattilo, 2008; Mundy, 1998).

There are an additional set of facilitation skills that come from the counseling literature (Corey, 2001) that are also very helpful in leisure education and include such things as cognitive behavioral therapy, problem-solving therapy, social skills training, motivational interviewing, social network therapy, existential therapeutic approaches, and others. These skills support RT professionals' ability to bring about desired client change and typically focus on strategies related to changing thoughts (cognitive therapeutic approaches), behaviors (be-havioral therapies), and/or feelings (affective ap-proaches) (Hutchins & Vaught, 1997).

Most RT professionals use an eclectic approach, combining aspects of different counseling strategies based on the needs of the clients and the goals of leisure education intervention. The types of "learning activities" that can be used in leisure education are unlimited and include such things as games, sports, crafts, hobbies, worksheets, creative activities (drama, music, art), problem-solving activities, metaphorical activities, role-playing, homework, journaling, etc. (Dattilo, 2000; Mundy, 1998). The most important aspect to keep in mind when selecting learning activities is that the activity must illustrate or relate directly to the goals of the leisure education session.

Outcomes and Documentation

There have been a number of studies examining the effectiveness of leisure education interventions for a variety of client groups, including caregivers of adults with dementia and stroke, older adults, youth, individuals with mental illness, and individuals with intellectual disabilities. Generally leisure education programs have been found to increase a number of capacities associated with leisure involvement, including: knowledge of leisure (Charters & Murray, 2006); satisfaction with leisure, frequency of en-gagement in leisure experiences, perceptions of competence and self-determination in leisure, (Car-bonneau et al., 2011; Desrosiers et al., 2007; Hoge & Dattilo, 1999; Mitchell, 1998; Ryan et al., 2008); increased engagement in prosocial leisure; increased self-efficacy (Mitchell, 1998); increased decision making skills (Caldwell et al., 2004; Hoge & Dattilo, 1999); increased awareness of community resources

(Prvu, Navar, & Hagar, 1999); and improved social skills (Dattilo et al., 2003; Hoge & Dattilo, 1999). In addition, leisure education programs have resulted in the reduction of issues that compromise leisure involvement, including a reduction in perceived barriers to leisure (Desrosiers et al., 2007; Hoge & Dattilo, 1999; Mitchell, 1998; Ryan et al., 2008); and boredom (Caldwell, Baldwin et al., 2004; Finn, 2007). Finally, leisure education interventions have been shown to have positive effects on more distal or global outcomes, including: improved ability to cope with stress (Carruthers & Hood, 2002; Hood & Carruthers, 2002); reduction in anxiety (Aquadro et al., 2010); engagement in health promoting behaviors (Caldwell, Baldwin et al., 2004; Caldwell, Smith et al., 2004; Caldwell et al., 2010); reduced depression (Desrosiers et al., 2007); and improved quality of life (Carbonneau et al., 2011; Janssen, 2004).

While many leisure education outcome studies have focused on proximal or immediate goals, such as the impact of leisure education on leisure attitudes, behavior, and satisfaction, there is also a need to describe and test further the impact of leisure education programs on not only leisure-related outcomes, but the impact of changes in leisure behavior on other valued health and human service outcomes (Caldwell, 2003). Caldwell (2003) suggests using a logic model to delineate the causal pathways between what is done in RT practice and proximal, distal, and ultimate client outcomes. For example, the LWM suggests that leisure education programs will increase clients' mindful engagement in more authentic, meaningful leisure experiences that will, in turn, enhance their positive emotion and physical, cognitive, social, and emotional resources. This elevation of positive emotion and personal resources will lead to the ultimate intended outcome of RT services, well-being. While these links between leisure education, leisure behaviors, and desired well-being outcomes are theoretically based, outcome studies testing these relationships have not yet been conducted.

Documentation for interventions that involve leisure education should include changes in the ICF codes discussed in the Intervention section.

References

Anderson, L. & Heyne, L. (2012). *Therapeutic recreation practice: A strengths approach*. State College, PA: Venture.

Aquadro, M. A., Cunningham, P. H., Kang, M., & Slaughter-Ellis, C. (2010). Effect of a leisure education intervention on anxiety levels of individuals participating in a smoking cessation program. *Annual in Therapeutic Recreation, 18*, 53-65.

Biswas-Diener, R. (2008). *Invitation to positive psychology: Research and tools for the professional*. Retrieved June 7, 2011 from www.intentionalhappiness.com/workbooks.html.

Bedini, L. & Guinan, D. M. (1996). The leisure of caregivers of older adults: Implications for CTRSs in nontraditional settings. *Therapeutic Recreation Journal, 30*, 274-288.

Broach, E., Dattilo, J., & McKenney, A. (2007). Effects of aquatic therapy on perceived fun or enjoyment experiences of participants with multiple sclerosis. *Therapeutic Recreation Journal, 41*, 179-201.

Bryant, F. & Veroff, J. (2007). *Savoring: A new model of positive experience*. Mahwah, NJ: Erlbaum.

Caldwell, L. (2003). Basing outcomes on theory: Theories of intervention and explanation. In N. Stumbo (Ed.), *Client outcomes in therapeutic recreation services* (pp. 67-85). State College, PA: Venture Publishing.

Caldwell, L., Baldwin, C., Walls, T., & Smith, E. (2004). Preliminary effects of a leisure education program to promote healthy use of free time among middle school adolescents. *Journal of Leisure Research, 36*, 310-335.

Caldwell, L., Patrick, M., Smith, E., Palen, L., & Wegner, L. (2010). Influencing adolescent leisure motivation: Intervention effects of HealthWise South Africa. *Journal of Leisure Research, 42*, 203-220.

Caldwell, L., Smith, E., Flisher, A., Wegner, L., Vergnani, T., Mathews, C., & Mpofu, E. (2004). Health-wise South Africa: Development of a life skills curriculum for young adults. *World Leisure Journal, 3*, 4-17.

Carbonneau, H., Caron, C., & Desrosiers, J. (2011). Effects of an adapted leisure education program as a means of support for caregivers of people with dementia. *Archives of Gerontology and Geriatrics, 53*, 31-19.

Carbonneau, H., Martineau, E., Andre, M., & Dawson, D. (2011). Enhancing leisure experiences post traumatic brain injury: A pilot study. *Brain Impairment, 12*, 140-151.

Carruthers, C. & Hood, C. (2002). Coping skills program for individuals with alcoholism. *Therapeutic Recreation Journal, 36*, 154-171.

Carruthers, C. & Hood, C. (2007). Building a life of meaning through therapeutic recreation: The Leisure and Well-Being Model, part I. *Therapeutic Recreation Journal, 41*, 276-297.

Carter, M. J., Nezey, I. O., Wenzel, K., & Foret, C. (2001). Leisure education with caregiver support groups. *Activities, Adaptation and Aging, 24*(2), 67-81.

Charters, J. & Murray, S. (2006). Design and evaluation of a leisure education program for caregivers of institutionalized care recipients. *Topics in Geriatric Rehabilitation, 22*, 334-347.

Corey, G. (2001). *Theory and practice of counseling and psychotherapy*. Belmont, CA: Wadsworth.

Cory, L., Dattilo, J., & Williams, R. (2006). Effects of a leisure education program on social knowledge and skills of youth with cognitive disabilities. *Therapeutic Recreation Journal, 40*, 144-165.

Coyle, C., Shank, J., & Vliet, N. (2010). Leisure and rehabilitation. In L. Payne, B. Ainsworth, & G. Godbey (Eds.), *Leisure, health, and wellness* (pp. 263-277). State College, PA: Venture.

Dattilo, J. (2000). *Facilitation techniques in therapeutic recreation*. State College, PA: Venture.

Dattilo, J. (2002). Perceptions of a leisure education program by youth with mental retardation. *Annual in Therapeutic Recreation, 11*, 55-66.

Dattilo, J. (2008). *Leisure education program planning: A systematic approach* (3rd ed.). State College, PA: Venture.

Dattilo, J., Kleiber, D., & Williams, R. (1998). Self-determination and enjoyment enhancement: A psychologically based service delivery model for therapeutic recreation. *Therapeutic Recreation Journal, 32*, 258-271.

Dattilo, J., Williams, R., & Cory, L. (2003). Effects of computerized leisure education on knowledge of social skills of youth with intellectual disabilities. *Therapeutic Recreation Journal, 37*, 142-155.

Davidson, L., Shahar, G., Lawless, M., Sells, D., & Tondora, J. (2006). Play, pleasure, and other positive life events: "Non-specific" factors in recovery from mental illness? *Psychiatry, 69*, 151-163.

Desrosiers, J., Noreau, L., Rochette, A., Carbonneau, H., Fontaine, L., Viscogliosi, C., & Bravo, G. (2007). Effect of a home leisure education program after stroke: A randomized controlled trial. *Archives of Physical Medicine and Rehabilitation, 88*, 1095-1100.

Dewey, J. (1933). *How we think: A restatement of the relation of reflective thinking to the educative process*. Boston: D. C. Heath.

Dewey, J. (1938). *Experience and education*. New York: Collier Books.

Finch, K. (2006). Recreational therapy: Relieving pain in older adults with osteoarthritis. *American Journal of Recreation Therapy, 5*(1), 27-39.

Finn, P. R. (2007). An evaluation of the effects of a leisure education curriculum on delinquents' motivation, knowledge, and behavior changes related to boredom *Dissertation Abstracts International, A: The Humanities and Social Sciences, 67*, 4343.

Gass, M. (1985). Programming the transfer of learning in adventure education. *Journal of Experiential Education, 8*(3), 18-24.

Hoge, G. & Dattilo, J. (1999). Effects of a leisure education program on youth with mental retardation. *Education and Training in Mental Retardation and Developmental Disabilities, 34*, 20-34.

Hoge, G., Dattilo, J., & Williams, R. (1999). Effects of leisure education on perceived freedom in leisure of adolescents with mental retardation. *Therapeutic Recreation Journal, 33*, 320-333.

Hoge, G. & Wilhite, B. (1997). Integration and leisure education for older adults with developmental disabilities. *Activities, Adaptation, and Aging, 21*(3), 79-90.

Hood, C. (2003). Women in recovery from alcoholism: The place of leisure. *Leisure Sciences, 25*, 51-79.

Hood, C. & Carruthers, C. (2002). Coping skills theory as an underlying framework for therapeutic recreation services. *Therapeutic Recreation Journal, 36*, 137-153.

Hood, C. & Carruthers, C. (2007). Enhancing leisure experience and building resources: The Leisure and Well-Being Model, part II. *Therapeutic Recreation Journal, 41*, 298-325.

Hood, C. & Carruthers, C. (2013). Facilitating change through leisure: The leisure and well-being model of therapeutic recreation practice. In T. Friere (Ed.), *Positive Leisure Science: From Subjective experience to social contexts* (pp. 121-140). New York: Springer.

Hughes, S. & Keller, J. M. (1992). Leisure education: A coping strategy for family caregivers. *Journal of Gerontological Social Work, 19*, 115-128.

Hutchins, D. E. & Vaught, C. C. (1997). *Helping relationships and strategies*. Pacific Grove, CA: Brooks/Cole.

Hutchinson, S., Loy, D., Kleiber, D., & Dattilo, J. (2003). Leisure as a coping resource: Variations in coping with traumatic injury and illness. *Leisure Sciences, 25,* 143-161.

Janssen, M. (2004). The effects of leisure education on quality of life in older adults. *Therapeutic Recreation Journal, 38*, 275-288.

Lovell, T. A., Dattilo, J., & Jekubovich, N. (1996). Effects of leisure education on women aging with disabilities. *Activities, Adaptation and Aging, 21*(2), 37-58.

McDowell, C. F. (1983). *Leisure wellness: Concepts on helping strategies*. Eugene, OR: Sun Moon Press.

McKenney, A., Dattilo, J., Cory, L., & Williams, R. (2004). Effects of a computerized therapeutic recreation program on knowledge of social skills of male youth with emotional and behavioral disorders. *Annual in Therapeutic Recreation, 13*, 12-23.

McMahon, C. & Wardlaw, B. (2011). The psychosocial effects of a leisure education program on caregivers of aging adults. *Annual in Therapeutic Recreation, 19*, 12-27.

Mitchell, L. L. (1998). The effects of a leisure education program upon persons with chronic mental illnesses who reside in group homes. *Dissertation Abstracts International: Section B: The Sciences and Engineering, 59*(3-B), 1356.

Mueller, D. R. & Volker, R. (2005). Social skills training in recreational rehabilitation of schizophrenia patients. *American Journal of Recreation Therapy, 4*(3), 11-19.

Mundy, J. (1998). *Leisure education: Theory and practice*. Champaign, IL: Sagamore.

Priest, S. & Gass, M. (1997). *Effective leadership in adventure programming*. Champaign, IL: Human Kinetics.

Prvu, J., Navar, N., & Hagar, H. (1999). *The effects of leisure education on leisure satisfaction, leisure participation, and self-confidence for individuals with brain injury*. Paper presented at the Ninth Canadian Congress on Leisure Research, Acadia University, Wolfville, NS.

Ramella, K., Tennis, B., & Yoshioka, C. (2008). Making leisure choices using enabling switches. *Annual in Therapeutic Recreation, 17*, 73-82.

Robertson, B. J. (2001). The leisure education of incarcerated youth. *World Leisure Journal, 1*, 20-29.

Rogers, D., Lee, Y., & Yang, H. (2007). Adolescents with spinal cord injury: Indication and suggestions for recreation therapy practice. *American Journal of Recreation Therapy, 6*(1), 13-24.

Ryan, C. A., Stiell, K. M., Gailey, G. F., & Makinen, J. A. (2008). Evaluating a family centered approach to leisure education and community reintegration following a stroke. *Therapeutic Recreation Journal, 42*, 119-131.

Santiago, M. & Coyle, C. (2004). Leisure-time physical activity among women with mobility impairments: Implications for health promotion and leisure education. *Therapeutic Recreation Journal, 38*, 188-206.

Schoel, J., Prouty, R., & Radcliffe, P. (1988). *Islands of healing*. Project Adventure, Inc.

Seligman, M. E. P. (2002). *Authentic happiness*. New York: Free Press.

Shank, J. & Coyle, C. (2002). *Therapeutic recreation in health promotion and rehabilitation*. State College, PA: Venture.

Stumbo, N. & Peterson, C. A. (2008). *Therapeutic recreation program design: Principles and procedures* (5th ed.). New York: Benjamin Cummings.

Vuillerot, C., Hodgkinson, I., Bissery, A., Schott-Pethelaz, A., Iwaz, J., Ecochard, R., D'Anjou, M., Commare, M., & Berard, C. (2010). Self-perception of quality of life by adolescents with neuromuscular diseases. *Journal of Adolescent Health, 46*, 70-76.

32. Leisure Resource Awareness

Heather R. Porter

Recreational therapists assist clients in exploring and identifying leisure resources to maximize and optimize play, leisure, recreation, and community activity engagement. This chapter briefly reviews the process that recreational therapists typically follow to facilitate personal leisure resource awareness and community leisure resource awareness.

Personal Leisure Resource Awareness

Personal leisure resource awareness is the process of determining what resources are available in and around the client's home to engage in leisure.

The therapist explores the resources currently available to the client that will indirectly or directly influence his/her leisure involvement and choices. This list includes available equipment, space to do leisure, money and other ways to get leisure supplies, the availability of others to help with leisure activities, and the time available for leisure.

People tend to spend a significant amount of time in their homes. Although home leisure can be active (e.g., gardening, exercising, re-finishing large pieces of furniture), the majority of home leisure is passive or sedentary (television, computer, reading, talking on the phone, sewing, knitting). Passive leisure is a part of healthy leisure and many (but not all) of the choices need to be recognized for their cognitive and emotional health benefits (e.g., relaxation, learning, challenging cognition).

Before a therapist explores a healthy home leisure activity pattern for the client, the therapist needs to be aware of the resources available. The activities have to match the available resources. If resources are not available, the therapist needs assist the client in identifying ways to obtain resources so that activities can be successfully added to the client's activity pattern. For example, the client may need to raise funds to purchase a DVD player so the client can watch exercise DVDs or re-design the layout of the dining room to allow an area for making crafts.

Community Leisure Resource Awareness

Community leisure resource awareness is defined as identification of leisure participation resources available in the community, such as transportation, facilities, and programs. With this protocol the therapist can teach the client how to find leisure resources in the community that match his/her interests and allow greater participation.

Engaging in community leisure activities is recommended for health. Getting out of the house promotes exercise and socialization. Physical exercise and social support are vital components of good health (d570 Looking After One's Health, d7 Interpersonal Interactions and Relationships). Leisure in the community also exposes the client to new ideas and thoughts that can positively impact emotional and spiritual health (d930 Religion and Spirituality). Involvement in community activities may also provide the client with an opportunity to contribute to his/her community through volunteer work. Giving time to help others can boost self-esteem and self-worth. It can contribute to feelings of productivity and make the person feel needed and wanted. All of which contribute to finding meaning in one's life.

Indications

Therapists routinely explore home leisure activities and resources and community leisure activities as part of the initial evaluation process of all clients. Therapists must remember that a client's interests can change with disability and that prior areas of leisure involvement may no longer interest the client. For more information about exploring leisure choices, see the Activity Pattern Development chapter. If the client's involvement in home and community activities meets the health needs of the client and the client does not desire to become involved in any other home or community activities, then leisure resource awareness is not explored.

Therapists address leisure resource awareness if

- A client's leisure activities do not meet the client's health needs.
- A client desires to become involved in additional activities.
- A client is living in a new environment and is unaware of leisure resources, such as when s/he recently moved into a new area, home, or facility.
- There is a change in the client's abilities that will impact his/her ability to continue with prior leisure activities.

Contraindications

If significant cognitive impairments are evident, the therapist will need to talk with the client's family member, guardian, or caregiver (if permission is granted) to obtain information about the client's personal leisure resources. If the person is being transitioned to a residential facility, the therapist might also seek permission to talk with the director of the activities department to obtain a list of common activity offerings and provide the director with information about the client's interests. For clients who are unable to tell the therapist what they enjoy, the therapist may be able to learn more by exposing the client to various leisure activities and observing the client's reaction to each activity (behavior, level of participation, attitude, length of time engaged in the activity).

Clients who have significant cognitive impairments will most likely respond positively to simple, physically based, repetitive activities. Therapists must also remember that a client's interests can change with disability and that prior leisure involvement cannot be assumed to be a continued interest of the client. If there is a positive indication, leisure interest exploration will help determine the client's leisure attitudes, interests, and motivations to be able to match leisure desires to personal and community resources.

Protocols and Processes

Personal Leisure Resource Awareness

It typically takes 30 minutes or less to determine the personal leisure resources of the client. A quiet and non-distracting environment is best to promote attention and concentration. The therapist should have relevant materials, such as paper and pen to write down home leisure activities and leisure resources. The therapist explores the following areas:

Equipment and supplies: Things required for leisure activities. The therapist asks the client what activities s/he does at home. If the therapist is unfamiliar with the activity, the therapist asks the client to describe the activity (how is it done, equipment used). If the therapist is familiar with the activity, but suspects that the client uses adaptive equipment or techniques, the therapist gets a description of special equipment or techniques. If there are specific pieces of leisure equipment that the client does not mention and the therapist perceives the piece of equipment to be helpful in meeting the health needs of the client, the therapist asks if it is available (e.g., Do you have a computer? Do you have a bicycle?).

Home and neighborhood: Locations to engage in leisure activities. The therapist asks the client to describe his/her home to determine the amount of space for leisure and barriers to accessing areas (e.g., steps to enter the home; steps within the home; number and type of rooms; basement; whether rooms are packed tight with furniture or have a lot of open space; outdoor areas such as a garage, backyard, front yard, garden, pool, shed). The therapist also asks questions about the client's neighborhood (e.g., Do you have sidewalks? Is your neighborhood hilly? Are you on a busy road? Are there other kids on your block? Do you talk with you neighbor?). These questions help the therapist to be sure that adequate space is available for pursuing the client's leisure interests.

Finances: Ability to pay for leisure activities. If the client is an adult, the therapist asks the client if s/he is on a tight budget. This is a very general question that gives the therapist an idea of the client's finances. Activities have to fit within the client's budget or alternative funding sources need to be identified. If the client is a child or teenager, this question will be best directed to the parents. Other ways to obtain supplies for leisure activities should also be explored, such as the ability to get leisure supplies through donations and community programs where supplies are provided.

Assistance: Other people who are available to help the client with leisure activities. Find out who is available and the extent of their availability to help the client with leisure. Ask the client who lives with him/her and about other people the client spends time with. Relevant information includes their age, if they have any limitations in their ability to help him/her, whether they work, what hours they work, what they usually do for leisure, whether they have any common leisure interests with the client, whether they think they would have the time and desire to help the client with leisure activities, if needed. Finding out if there are common leisure interests and what the others enjoy is helpful, especially if the therapist perceives that assistance might be needed. Others are more likely to help if they enjoy the activity, too. This is not to say that others will only help a client engage in leisure activities if they like it, but it does make it more likely.

Time: Free time when enough energy is available to engage in leisure activities. Therapists ask clients to describe a typical workday and/or a typical non-work day. Therapists write this information down in the form of a timeline. This not only gives the therapist an idea of the amount time spent on leisure but also on the amount of leisure time available. It is also a good evaluation tool to determine the variety of leisure (physical, social, cognitive) and the value placed on leisure. Taking a timeline of daily tasks and activities also gives the therapist an opportunity to listen to how the client describes the day (Does it sound hectic to the client? Does it sound like the client is bored?). There are many other subtle cues that a therapist can pick up from this discussion, such as no one is around, the client is by himself most of the day, the client has too many things to do in a day, or the client is not adhering to the recommendations of his/her physician. A very brief example of a daily timeline looks like this:

8:00 A.M. wake-up, shower, dress

9:00 A.M. leave for work

9:30 A.M. work that entails ...

Noon lunch at my desk

6:00 P.M. leave work

6:30 P.M. home and eat dinner

7:30-11:00 P.M. watch television

Community Leisure Resource Awareness

It typically takes 30 minutes or less to determine the community leisure interests and resources of the client. A quiet and non-distracting environment is best to promote attention and concentration. The therapist should have relevant materials, such as paper and pen to write down community leisure activities and resources. The therapist explores the following areas:

Community leisure places: The therapist asks the client if s/he engages in any leisure activities in the community (e.g., YMCA, teenager hangout, the park, tennis courts at the recreation center).

Frequency: For each activity noted, the therapist asks the client how often s/he participates in the activity (e.g., every Tuesday and Thursday) and the times that s/he participates.

Accessibility of community leisure places: If the client's functional abilities have changed since his/her last involvement in the community activity, the therapist asks the client if s/he is familiar with the level of accessibility of the place in the community. Clients who are not experienced in living with a disability will not understand this question, so the therapist will need to guide them through the thought process. It might go like this for a person who is newly in a wheelchair: Is there a ramp or a level entrance to get in or are there steps? How many steps? Is there a railing? See the Disability Rights Education and Advocacy chapter for more information. Clients may not know the answers to these questions if they have never had to pay attention to them. In this case, therapists will need to teach the client about community accessibility and find out if the places that they like to go in the community meet their needs.

Finding new community leisure places that meet the needs of the client: If a client needs to find places in his/her community for leisure, the best place to start is by finding the leisure interests and motivations of the client and matching them with the health needs of the client. (See the Activity Pattern Development chapter for information on leisure interest testing and exploration.) Once the specific activity has been identified, the client and therapist explore places in the community that offer this activity, such as a recreation center, senior center, or dance studio. Start out by asking the client if s/he knows of a place in his/her community that offers this activity. If the client does not know, use search tool on the Internet or a phone book to find a place in the community. For example, click on a search tool, type in the client's home address, click on "find a business" (everything is called a business, even public recreation centers), and type in what you are looking for (e.g., recreation center, dance studio). A list of places will then appear in order of distance from the client's home. It provides you with the name of the facility, the address, the distance from the client's home, a link to the facility website (if available), and even directions on how to get there. It helps to print this list out and then cross them off one by one if they do not offer the activity or are unable to accommodate the needs of the client. Keep searching until you find a place where the client can engage in the activity. If you are unable to find the activity using this method, call organizations (e.g., call the Paralyzed Veterans Association or Special Olympics to help find an adaptive sporting program) and other recreational therapy professionals in the area who may be familiar with other programs that are not well advertised in the general community. If possible, a community integration session to the place in the community should be scheduled to do a full assessment of the facility and the program as described in the Community Participation: Transition, Inclusion, Integration, and Reintegration chapter.

Outcomes and Documentation

The recreational therapist documents the client's personal and community activities on the initial evaluation form along with any relevant information that the client is able to provide (e.g., "Client attends a seated senior exercise program three times a week at Live Well Senior Center. The client believes that the center is fully wheelchair accessible. Therapist will place a phone call to the center to clarify their level of accessibility."). The therapist can also evaluate the quality of the leisure participation with tools such as the *Activity Evaluation* form in Dehn's (1997) *Leisure Step Up*.

If a new home activity or community place for leisure is identified, it is documented along with its relevant information. Documentation may look like, "Identified a dance studio two miles from client's home that provides T'ai Chi. Client was set up with her local paratransit service through social services to take her back and forth to the program. The dance studio is fully wheelchair accessible and is able to accommodate the needs of the client — T'ai Chi from a seated position. Client plans to begin the program next month. Therapist to contact the client in three weeks to promote follow through, provide support and encouragement, and problem solve for any issues that have arisen."

Personal leisure resource awareness is an intervention that can be used for difficulties in many parts of d9 Community, Social, and Civic Life. If this protocol helps restore functionality to a particular activity, such as d9204 Hobbies, it may be documented in the chart notes as part of the treatment for that code. Community leisure resource awareness is an intervention that affects, among other things, the level of difficulty assigned to codes in many of the activities included in d9 Community, Social, and Civic Life.

References

Dehn, D. (1995). *Leisure Step Up*. Ravensdale, WA: Idyll Arbor.

33. Life Review

Yongho Lee and Elizabeth H. Weybright

The terms "life review" and "reminiscence" are often used interchangeably in the literature. Although there are many similarities, they are actually two different, distinct techniques. Reminiscence by definition is the simple recalling of the past through daydreaming, storytelling, or nostalgia by oneself or with others (Haber, 2006). (See the chapter on Reminiscence in this book for more information.) Recalling of the past usually includes positive past memories such as childhood play, accomplishments, early friendship, school, etc. (Lee, Tabourne, & Yoon, 2008). Life review, on the other hand, is a more structured form of reminiscence targeted at integrating both positive and negative memories by remembering, re-evaluating, and synthesizing to resolve conflicts (Webster & Haight, 1995). Life review has been found to be a highly effective and efficient therapeutic process that reduces behavioral problems, promotes self-control, and prevents further deterioration among older adults (Abramson & Mendis, 1990).

This chapter will look at two life review programs. One uses the Haight Life Review and Experiencing Form (LREF) that originated in the nursing literature. Its protocol specifies a one-to-one life review. The other is the Tabourne Life Review Program (LRP) developed for recreational therapists and implemented in a group format. Both are discussed in the Protocols section.

Indications

Life review therapy has primarily been used in long-term care facilities as a psychodynamic intervention technique for the elderly populations with emotional problems (b126 Temperament and Personality Functions, b152 Emotional Functions), especially those with Alzheimer's disease. One recent study found that a 40-minute life review session each week for six weeks was effective in decreasing depression among individuals living in a nursing home (Mastel-Smith et al., 2006).

The Life Review Program (LRP), developed by Tabourne (1991) was successfully used to address issues of frustration (b126 Temperament and Personality Functions, d240 Handling Stress and Other Psychological Demands), depression (b126 Temperament and Personality Functions, b130 Energy and Drive Functions), low self-esteem (b126 Temperament and Personality Functions), and psychological well-being (b126 Temperament and Personality Functions) (Tabourne, 1991, 1995; McKenzie, 2003). Tabourne (1995) found that the LRP had noticeable effects that included increased social interaction (d7 Interpersonal Interactions and Relationships) and decreased disorientation (b114 Orientation Functions) of individuals with Alzheimer's disease who lived in nursing homes.

While the LRP was implemented primarily with European-American elders in nursing homes, McKenzie (2003) and Lee, Tabourne, and Yoon (2008) replicated Tabourne's original LRP studies with African-American and Korean elders. McKenzie (2003) tested its applicability to African-American elders living in the community. McKenzie's Culturally Specific LRP demonstrated positive effects on the psychological well-being of African-American elders, though the results of the study were not statistically significant. A qualitative analysis, however, of participant interview data revealed positive effects of the intervention on participants' psychological well-being. While McKenzie (2003) addressed the need for a program for African-American elders, Lee, Tabourne, and Yoon (2008) addressed the need for incorporating more cultural aspects into the LRP to include Asian elders. Lee implemented the LRP with Korean elders with Alzheimer's disease. The study reported some significant effects on participants' emotional well-being in the areas of self-esteem, life satisfaction, and depression following the eight-week LRP intervention. This study was the first study that reported statistically significant results on the effects of the LRP intervention for elders.

Contraindications

Though life review rarely has a negative impact on clients, it may provoke negative memories of the past, which may cause uncomfortable feelings and psychological stress in elderly participants. Recreational therapists should be prepared to manage the situation as a therapeutic moment to resolve any psychological or emotional conflict that is caused by negative memories.

Clients with significant trauma in their lives and clients who have been involved in military action often do not want to share their experiences with anyone who has not had similar experiences. They should not be expected to participate in groups of non-peers (Newhouse, 2008).

Protocols

Burnside and Haight (1994) provide in-depth protocols for conducting one-to-one reminiscence, group reminiscence, and one-to-one life review. Although these protocols were developed by and target nurses, they can also serve to guide recreational therapy intervention. An abbreviated protocol for one-to-one life review is found in Table 16 using Haight's *Life Review and Experiencing Form* (LREF). For the complete protocol, see Burnside and Haight (1994).

Table 16: Haight's Life Review and Experiencing Form (LREF)

Pre-Intervention Session: Interview
Goals of session: Develop rapport, assess psychosocial status, share LREF with participant in preparation for life review.

Session 1: Childhood
Sample Questions:
What is the first thing you can remember in your life? Go as far back as you can.
Did you have any brothers or sisters? Tell me what each was like.

Session 2:

Adolescence
Sample Questions:
What other things stand out in your memory about being a teenager?
Do you remember your first attraction to another person?

Family and Home
Sample Questions:
What was the atmosphere in your home?
Who were you closest to in your family?

Session 3 and 4: Adulthood
Sample Questions:
What place did religion play in your life?
On the whole, would you say you had a happy or unhappy marriage?

Session 5 and 6: Summary and Evaluation
Sample Questions:
On the whole, what kind of life do you think you've had?
What are the best things about the age you are now?
What do you fear will happen to you as you grow older?

Termination Session
Goal of session: Final interview evaluation.

Note: Not all of the questions in the LREF are listed. See Burnside and Haight (1994) for the complete protocol. Reprinted with permission.

The questions included in the LREF are guidelines, not a set of interview questions that must be adhered to. Rather, the intent is to gather the feelings and experiences about the entire life span of the participant. This protocol spans eight sessions, although this is also a guideline. The length of sessions should be determined by the client and their satisfaction with each session. In the protocol, the first and last session serve as an assessment and evaluation session respectively. In between are six life review sessions covering: childhood (session 1); adolescence, family, and home (session 2); adulthood (sessions 3 and 4); and summarization of life review and evaluation of life (sessions 5 and 6).

One of the most common psychological symptoms among older adults, especially those with Alzheimer's disease, is a high prevalence of depressive symptoms (Lee, Tabourne, & Yoon, 2008).

Despite the fact that the prevalence of clinical depression is not as high as that of depressive symptoms among older adults, depressive symptoms in and of themselves among older adults can still lead to psychological distress, thus decreasing emotional well-being (Lee, Tabourne, & Yoon, 2008). It is important to address such depressive symptoms to improve the emotional state of individuals with Alzheimer's, a major issue among these individuals (Albert et al., 1996).

Individuals with Alzheimer's are commonly treated pharmacologically with antidepressant medications, which often produce unwanted or harmful side effects. As a result, it is necessary that non-pharmacological treatments be developed for and provided to this population. RT interventions are good alternatives to pharmacological treatment and can be provided in a non-threatening environment to treat depression as well as other emotional problems (Fitzsimmons & Buettner, 2002).

One such non-pharmacological RT intervention is the Life Review Program (LRP) developed by Tabourne (1991). It is a life review therapy technique that uses a review of the patient's life story as a therapeutic modality to mitigate emotional and psychological problems among older adults (Tabourne, 1991). Tabourne created and first introduced the LRP as an RT intervention for individuals with Alzheimer's disease and found that the LRP had marked, though not entirely significant, effects that included increased social interaction and decreased disorientation among individuals with Alzheimer's disease. The LRP successfully reduced disorientation, depression, and poor self-esteem of European-Americans with Alzheimer's disease (Tabourne, 1995). The LRP was later tested with community-dwelling African-American elders in the Midwest (McKenzie, 2003) and Korean elderly clients with Alzheimer's disease (Lee, Tabourne, & Yoon, 2008). Both studies verified positive effects of the LRP on psychological and emotional well-being of the elderly population living in different cultural contexts.

Processes

The LRP intervention is implemented as a group activity. The original LRP developed by Tabourne (1991), as well as the culturally specific LRP versions developed by McKenzie (2003) and Lee, Tabourne, and Yoon (2008), have themes for each session. Participants review their lives according to each theme. Each session is designed as a group activity and always begins with an introduction of the session for the day.

One concern about doing life review therapy in a group setting, rather than in the more common one-to-one setting, is that sensitive, personal experiences may be shared during the sessions. Participants in the group must be willing to share their experiences. It is also very important that therapists possess great levels of therapeutic communication skills and ensure an environment where all participants feel comfortable sharing their life experiences with other participants. One of the positive things about having group sessions is that it facilitates social networking and, as participants share their experiences, they find many things in common. This facilitates group cohesion. Generally five to seven participants are a good number to facilitate group discussion for a one-hour session.

A number of different activities are presented to the clients to facilitate the life review process such as singing songs, watching movies, playing childhood games, and performing skits. The general format for each session includes:

- a personalized welcome to each individual by name and confirmation of the time and location for the session.
- a reminder of the previous theme and an introduction to the current stage and corresponding theme of the session.
- a review of the contribution that each participant made in the previous session.
- content and procedures for the current topic and activity.
- debriefing.
- closure with information about the upcoming session.

Since LRP's target population is elders who may have cognitive dysfunctions, it is very important to begin with an introduction of each session followed by a review of the previous session to maintain the flow of the program. At the end of each session, debriefing will provide participants with an opportunity to reflect on the session they engaged in and what it really means to them. Besides just having fun, there are therapeutic effects of the program.

The progression of the LRP sessions mirror Erikson's developmental stages. The stages are used as themes for participants to reflect on each developmental life stage (see Table 17). For example, the first stage of Erikson's theory is infancy and its psychosocial crisis is basic trust versus basic mistrust. Even though the participants are not able to remember actual events from their infancy, an activity could be designed to evoke general memories surrounding infancy. Such was the case in the protocol used with South Korean elders with Alzheimer's disease (Lee, Tabourne, & Yoon, 2008). The protocol drew on a tradition in South Korea that when a new baby is born, people hang an object on their door to indicate whether it is a boy or girl. A series of pictures that show this tradition were presented to participants as a prompt for a discussion of their infancy.

Table 17: The Life Review Program

Session 1: Infancy
Describing parents' dream when having a baby.

Session 2: Early Childhood
Demonstrating memory of early childhood.

Session 3: Play age
Identifying what participants' worlds were like.

Session 4: School age
Reminiscing and reviewing school life.

Session 5: Adolescence
Demonstrating identity in adolescence.

Session 6: Young adulthood
Recalling the first intimate relationship.

Session 7: Adulthood
Demonstrating wisdom that can be passed on to next generation.

Session 8: Old age
Reviewing the entire life

Note: See Lee, Tabourne, and Yoon (2008) for complete protocol.
Reprinted with permission.

Facilitation Techniques

A variety of facilitation techniques are used in the LRP and the therapist is encouraged to adjust and utilize facilitation techniques to meet the specific characteristics, needs, and interests of the participants (Lee, Henningfeld, & Tabourne, 2012). For example, McKenzie (2003), who used Tabourne's LRP with African-American elders, utilized singing gospel music and dressing up with fancy hats for church, cooking many dishes to celebrate with large groups of people, and men's and women's social clubs to accent the prominent cultural components for older adults of African-American heritage. Below is a list of some common techniques. Two or more techniques can also be used simultaneously in an integrative approach to maximize outcomes.

Music: Music is a powerful tool to trigger memory and facilitate group cohesion. The use of music, especially songs that are familiar to participants, can facilitate recall of the past and help facilitate a fun, therapeutic environment.

Media: Pictures, movies, and art works that describe participants' past can help to recall the past.

Storytelling: Storytelling is the most common way of reviewing life in life review therapy. Therapists need to be skillful in creating a safe environment in which participants feel secure about telling their pasts.

Skit: Participants play their past as if they went back to the past. It is important that therapists help participants create a play that reflects their past and the things they could have done differently.

Outcomes and Documentation

Outcomes of the LRP can be measured and documented in several ways:

Quantitative measures: Psychological measures of emotional and psychological well-being for clients without Alzheimer's disease or with mild Alzheimer's disease can be helpful to measure the outcome of life review interventions. Possible tools include the *Rosenberg Self-Esteem Scale* (1989), *Center for Epidemiological Studies Depression Scale* (CES-D) (Redloff, 1977), and *Satisfaction with Life Scale* (SWLS) (Diener et al., 1985). Changes in scores for the ICF codes listed earlier can also be used to show the effects of the intervention.

Qualitative measures: Verbal interviews can be conducted with clients to facilitate the gathering of more in-depth information about clients' perceptions of life review.

- How did the program provide you an opportunity to review your life?
- How did you find meaning doing a life review?

- How could you identify who you were during the sessions?
- If you were to start your life all over again, would you repeat your life?
- How do you feel now (after the program)?
- What was the thing you will remember most about the program?
- While engaging in the program, could you find parts of yourself that would have otherwise been forgotten?

References

Albert, S. M., Del Castillo-Castaneda, C., Sano, M., Jacobs, D. M., Marder, K., Bell, K., Bylsma, F., Lafleche, G., Brandt, J., Albert, M., & Stern, Y. (1996). Quality of life in patients with Alzheimer's disease as reported by patient proxies. *Journal of the American Geriatrics Society, 44*, 1342-1347.

Abramson, T. & Mendis, K. (1990). The organizational logistics of running a dementia group in a SNF. *Clinical Gerontologist, 9*, 111-122.

Burnside, I. & Haight, B. (1994). Reminiscence and life review: Therapeutic interventions for older people. *Nurse Practitioner, 19*(4), 55-61.

Fitzsimmons, S. & Buettner, L. (2002). Therapeutic recreation interventions for need-driven dementia-compromised behaviours in community-dwelling elders. *American Journal of Alzheimer's Disease and Other Dementia, 17*(6), 367-81.

Diener, E. E., Emmons, R. A., Larsen, R. J., & Griffin, S. (1985). The satisfaction with life scale. *Journal of Personality Assessment, 49,* 71-75.

Haber, D. (2006). Life review: Implementation, theory, research, and therapy. *International Journal of Aging and Human Development, 63*(2), 153-171.

Lee, Y., Henningfeld, A. G., & Tabourne, C. E. S. (2012). Life review program as a therapeutic recreation modality. *Annual in Therapeutic Recreation, 20*, 59-67.

Lee, Y., Tabourne, C. E. S., & Yoon, J. (2008). Life Review Program as a therapeutic recreation intervention for Korean elderly with Alzheimer's disease: Qualitative analysis. *Annual in Therapeutic Recreation, 16*, 171-180.

Mastel-Smith, B., Binder, B., Malecha, A., Hersh, G., Symes, L., & McFarlane, J. (2006). Testing therapeutic life review offered by home care workers to decrease depression among home-dwelling older women. *Issues in Mental Health Nursing, 27*(10), 1037-1049.

McKenzie, S. E. (2003). The efficacy of a culturally relevant life review program: Effects on life satisfaction and psychological well-being of community-dwelling African American elders. Unpublished doctoral dissertation. University of Minnesota.

Newhouse, E. (2008). *Faces of Combat, PTSD & TBI*. Ravensdale, WA: Issues Press.

Redloff, L. S. (1977). The CES-D scale: A self-report depression scale for research in the general population. *Applied Psychology of Measurement, 1*, 385-401.

Rosenberg, M. (1989). *Society and the adolescent self-image*. Middletown, CT: Wesleyan University Press.

Tabourne, C. E. S. (1991). The effects of a life review recreation therapy program on confused nursing home residents. *Topics in Geriatric Rehabilitation, 7*(2), 13-21.

Tabourne, C. E. S. (1995). The effect of a life review program on disorientation, social interaction and self-esteem of nursing home residents. *International Journal of Aging and Human Development, 41*(1), 251-266.

Webster, J. D. & Haight, B. K. (1995). Memory lane milestones: Progress in reminiscence definition and classification. In B. K. Haight & J. D. Webster (Eds.). *The art and science of reminiscing: Theory, research, methods, and applications* (pp. 273-286). Washington, DC: Taylor & Francis.

34. Medical Play and Preparation

Heather R. Porter and Jennifer L. Sciolla

It is estimated that 50-75% of the four million children who undergo surgery in the United States develop significant fear and anxiety prior to surgery (Kain & Caldwell-Andrews, 2005). Children undergoing surgery and medical procedures are more vulnerable to stress than adults because they have limited cognitive capacities, less self-control, greater dependence on others, limited life experience, and less knowledge of the healthcare system (Li, Lopez, & Lee, 2007). In addition, a child's ability to cope with a medical procedure is influenced by other variables including age, developmental level, personality, ability to cope with new situations, prior healthcare experiences, knowledge about equipment and procedures, previous encounters with medical professionals, the child's diagnosis, the complexity and invasiveness of the upcoming procedure, the family composition, and the level of parental anxiety (Koller, 2007).

The inability to effectively cope with such stress (d240 Handling Stress and Other Psychological Demands) can cause frequent or exaggerated psychological symptoms, such as stress and anxiety, illness, eating and sleeping disturbances, social isolation, apathy, withdrawal, separation fears, post-traumatic stress, increased fears, decreased cooperative behavior, and other long-term manifestations from negative medical experiences that can magnify or complicate current health conditions (Rice, 2011; Koller, 2007). For example, Kain and Caldwell-Andrews (2005) conducted a literature review and found that children who experienced heightened anxiety prior to surgery had negative outcomes post surgery including delayed discharge from postoperative clinical recovery, increased nausea and vomiting, increased intravenous fluid requirements, emergence of delirium in the recovery room (shown by extreme agitation, crying, and thrashing), increased number of days the child had to stay at home, and increased postoperative pain and analgesic requirements. The authors also found that 40-55% of all children who undergo elective surgery exhibit new-onset maladaptive behaviors such as nightmares, separation anxiety, eating problems, and increased fear of doctors. Nineteen percent of the children still exhibit these behaviors at six months and six percent at one year after the surgery. Approximately 25% of children cry, scream, and try to avoid the anesthesia mask requiring forceful restraint resulting in the experience of a traumatic event.

Kain and Caldwell-Andrews (2005) identify specific risk factors for preoperative anxiety:

Age: Younger children have a higher risk of developing preoperative anxiety than older children. Children age one to five have the highest risk.

Temperament and baseline anxiety: Children who have high-trait anxiety, are shy or inhibited, and/or have a passive coping style shown by avoidance, withdrawal, or wishful thinking have a higher risk of developing preoperative anxiety.

Past medical encounters: The quality of the child's previous medical experiences (positive or negative) is more predictive of preoperative anxiety than the number of prior medical experiences.

Parents' level of anxiety: The parents' level of anxiety strongly influences the level of preoperative anxiety experienced by the child. Decreasing the parents' anxiety can help reduce the child's anxiety. Also, parents who are divorced or have a low educational level tend to rate themselves as more anxious preoperatively compared to parents who are married and have a higher educational level. Issues with parents' anxiety can be documented using ICF code e310 Immediate Family in e3 Support and Relationships.

Medical Play

Medical play is a common technique utilized by various health professionals, including recreational therapists, in pediatric settings to support the education and coping of children faced with a medical experience, such as surgery or another medical procedure. Its basis in psychoanalytic theory provides a means to reduce stress and anxiety. Its other basis in cognitive theory promotes intellectual growth through assimilation (taking new ideas, concepts, and points of view and incorporating them into one's own world views) and accommodation (adjusting one's perspective based on new ideas, concepts, and points of view), which can aid in coping (Hughes, 2009). Using play as a technique for education and coping provides the therapist with an opportunity to learn more about the child's understanding of a medical experience and assists the therapist in determining a care plan for how to best support the child during the medical episode.

In 1988, McCue defined medical play has having four specific characteristics and four specific types. Although these characteristics and types were defined over 25 years ago, they are still reflected in the literature today (Hart & Rollins, 2011).

Characteristics of Medical Play (McCue, 1988)

- Medical play is a form of play that contains medical themes and/or medical equipment.
- Medical play is offered and initiated by a therapist but is voluntarily maintained by the child.
- Medical play is usually enjoyable for the child and is often accompanied by laughter and relaxation, although the process of the play can sometimes be intense and aggressive.
- Medical play and psychological preparation are not synonymous. Education (not play) occurs when the therapist demonstrates a medical procedure or familiarizes a child with medical equipment. Play may follow such education if opportunities are made available.

Types of Medical Play (McCue, 1988)

Role rehearsal/role reversal medical play: The child takes on the role of the healthcare professional and reenacts medical events on dolls, puppets, and stuffed animals, such as giving a doll an injection. Real medical equipment is used when appropriate, along with commercially prepared toys. This type of play can be introduced as early as toddlerhood, when children are motivated by their sensory experiences and are intrigued by exploration. Toddlers enjoy using doctor kits and will sometimes mouth, bang, and experiment with the use of the items. Even if the child does not display the ability to use the equipment on a doll or stuffed animal, the exposure to the items in play is helpful for expression and familiarity. Young children do not have the vocabulary or cognitive capacity to process their experiences; therefore, the play allows them an outlet to communicate their feelings and knowledge. Depending on the child's developmental stage, their ability to independently explore equipment or to use verbal communication to support their play will vary.

Medical fantasy play: The child utilizes common play toys, such as blocks, dollhouses, and trucks, to simulate medical procedures and experiences. In this type of play, the child can avoid contact with feared objects, yet still play out topics of concern. The therapist can suggest certain themes during the play (e.g., "Was the car hurt? Where did it go?"), but the child must be allowed to direct the play in order to work on themes that are important to him/her.

Indirect medical play: The child engages in play with medical themes (e.g., sings "Old McDonald had a Hospital" as a substitute for "Old McDonald had a Farm," plays the board game "Operation," completes a jigsaw puzzle of a hospital room) and uses medical equipment in a nonmedical way (e.g., uses a syringe as a squirt gun; uses a bed pan as a drum). Indirect play can be helpful in desensitizing the child to medical themes and equipment. However opportunities for play with non-medical equipment and themes, such as singing songs that don't contain a medical theme, is also very important so the child is not overwhelmed with medical stimuli.

Medical art: The child uses art activities to express his/her understanding of, and reaction to, a medical experience. Medical equipment and supplies may or may not be used in creating the art. To the therapist, the artwork produced by the child may or may not directly relate to a medical experience. Consequently it is important for the therapist to ask exploratory questions to determine if a medical theme emerges for discussion, such as, "Tell me about your drawing" or "How do you feel about your painting?" Some ideas for art activities that use medical supplies include making puppets out of a medical glove, making a windsock out of an isolation gown, filling a syringe with paint and squirting it out on paper, gluing tongue depressors together to make a basket or house, and drawing faces on tongue depressors to make them into puppets.

Timing of Medical Play

Medical play is sometimes further described according to its timing. Medical play provided prior to a medical procedure is referred to as pre-operative medical play (or pre-procedural play) and medical play provided after a medical procedure is referred to as post-operative medical play (or post-procedural play).

Pre-operative medical play (or pre-procedural play) is provided prior to surgery or another medical procedure. It is defined as therapeutic play that is child-focused with the goal of assessing knowledge, exploring emotional responses, and decreasing impending stress and anxiety related to the medical experience that the child will undergo. Allowing time for this type of play prior to surgery or a medical procedure allows for rehearsal of coping strategies and identification of stress points. It can include materials that pertain directly to an impending medical experience or may serve as general exposure to medical themes and equipment. Children often have decreased anxiety and confusion when they have had the opportunity to explore medical equipment. Having opportunities to manipulate and freely engage in play with equipment provides a concrete reference of how to use the items and how the healthcare team refers to the items. After having the opportunity to play with medical equipment, many children have increased cooperation during surgeries and procedures. If a child has an impending surgery or procedure, the recreational therapist provides materials that relate directly to the medical event. For example, if a child will be going into the operating room, anesthesia masks, surgical hats, and gloves are offered as part of the child's play. See Appendix A in this chapter for a pre-operative medical play case study.

Post-operative medical play (or post-procedural play) is provided after a surgery or other medical procedure. It follows much the same process and function as pre-operative medical play. However, it is informed directly by how a child has processed a preceding medical event. Play continues to remain child-focused, while it revisits the rehearsal of coping strategies to evaluate their effectiveness, re-evaluates the identified stress points of the event and processes the steps or sequence of the surgery or medical procedure. The goal is to use play to increase mastery. Post-operative medical play also allows a child to freely express experiences without the use of words. Often children cannot verbally express the emotional content of an experience; therefore, it's important that a therapeutic play experience is offered after the medical event. This will allow a child to work through any lingering questions and will provide an outlet to retell the experience through play. In addition, it further offers a child the ability to develop mastery around the medical experience as s/he practices and processes the events that occurred. See Appendix A for a post-operative medical play case study.

Medical Procedure Preparation

In medical play (especially in pre-operative and pre-procedural medical play), therapists might incorporate medical procedure preparation. Medical procedure preparation is the formal process of educating the child and family about the specific procedure the child will undergo, such as the sequential steps of wound debridement. Education is provided through various modes, such as videos, pamphlets, pictures, discussion, demonstration, books, and orientation tours that include information related to all the senses. It is important to cover all that the child will hear, see, smell, feel, and taste. Medical procedure preparation might also use props such as medical equipment, dolls, and puppets. It may incorporate a medical play component to increase familiarity and further lessen anxiety, stress, and fear. The specific information presented to the child and family will vary depending on the procedure.

Efficacy

During medical play, children rarely adhere to only one type of play. For example, a child may engage in indirect medical play by using a syringe as a squirt gun and then, when she sees a doll in the corner of the room, switch to role rehearsal/role reversal medical play by giving the doll an injection with the water-filled syringe. This, along with lack of consistent terms used in studies, small sample sizes, and lack of clarity regarding the specific actions of the child and therapist in medical play sessions, can complicate the literature evaluation process. With that said, the literature does support the general value of medical play. For example, a review and synthesis of 29 studies by Koller (2007) showed that children who were prepared for medical experiences through a variety of venues including play, development of coping techniques, education, and familiarization with medical procedures had fewer negative symptoms compared to children who did not receive such preparation. To decrease needle phobia in children at a chemotherapy clinic, Kettwich and colleagues (2007) decorated syringes and winged needles with colorful images (e.g., flower and smiley face stickers on syringes, butterfly wings on conventional winged needles). Although the children in the study (n = 25, mean age 10.0 +/- 5.4 years) did not part take in decorating the needles, it was 76% effective in reducing aversion, anxiety, fear, and overall stress of injections. In a day surgery center, 203 children (7-12 year olds) were divided into a control group that received routine information preparation and an experimental group that participated in therapeutic play including a tour of the environment, a doll demonstration of anesthesia induction, exploration of medical equipment, and opportunities to reenact the procedure with a doll (Li & Lopez, 2008; Li, Lopez, & Lee, 2007). The children in the experimental group reported significantly lower anxiety scores in pre-and-post-operative periods and exhibited fewer negative emotions at induction of anesthesia than children in the control group.

Indications

As reviewed earlier, many children experience anxiety and fear surrounding surgery, medical procedures, and hospitalizations. ICF codes that suggest a need for medical play or preparation include b114 Orientation Functions, b126 Temperament and Personality Functions, b152 Emotional Functions, and d240 Handling Stress and Other Psychological Demands. Children who are hospitalized, children who are undergoing surgery or a medical procedure, and children who have experienced a surgery or medical procedure can benefit from Medical play unless contraindications discussed in the next section are present.

Contraindications

There are no formal contraindications in the literature for medical play and preparation. However, recreational therapists are attentive to each child's precautions and parameters to ensure they are not violated during the medical play and preparation sessions. For example, if a child has a latex allergy, the therapist would not choose activities that use latex gloves. If a child is on immunosuppressive therapy or has a compromised immune system, only new supplies should be used to avoid transmitting harmful organisms. Supplies and equipment must also meet general safety guidelines for children, such as using only non-toxic art supplies, no sharp objects, no small objects that could pose a choking hazard, etc. See Age-Appropriate Decisions later in the chapter for more information on toy and material choices. Medical equipment used in sessions must also be thoughtfully considered. For example, the therapist would not use a highly sensitive piece of medical equipment that would be damaged if dropped or have the potential to be misused by the child and cause harm. Children should not be allowed to reenact medical procedures on other children, as harm could be inflicted. If psychological distress is observed, such as severely heightened stress and anxiety, medical play and preparation should be stopped.

Protocols and Processes

Since medical play and preparation sessions are individually tailored, there is no specific protocol or process that is followed. There are guidelines however to assist the therapist in designing and facilitating medical play and preparation sessions.

Considerations

A review of the literature by Kain and Caldwell-Andrews (2005) recommends that prior to implementing a medical play and preparation session the therapist considers the following:

The child's age: Medical play and preparation must be individually tailored to the child's developmental age. For example, a program that is appropriate for a three year old might not be appropriate for a twelve year old.

The timing relative to the surgery or procedure: Participation in a medical play and preparation session or program more than five to seven days prior to surgery is the most beneficial for children six years and older. Having the session one day before surgery is the least beneficial. The longer interval between the preparation and surgery is needed for older children to adequately process the preparation information.

The child's previous hospitalization history: Children with previous hospitalizations respond best to programs that focus on coping skills training combined with actual practice. Also, one should not assume that previous coping skills training results in ability to implement the techniques in future medical procedures. During heightened periods of stress, children may have difficulty independently producing previously learned coping strategies and require memory cueing from a therapist or parent present during the procedure.

Parental involvement: Parents, particularly mothers, typically become very anxious when their children are undergoing surgery or medical procedures. Since parental anxiety influences the child's level of anxiety, parental education can be helpful. This may include videos, books, computerized multimedia, and interactive technology. Studies have also shown that parental involvement during medical procedures helps to reduce the child's anxiety and increase cooperation. However, therapists should consider providing training to the parents on how to best help their child during the procedure to maximize positive outcomes. Possible techniques include distracting the child through conversation or reading a story and providing reassuring touch and eye contact.

It is additionally recommended that each child's potential for experiencing stress in the hospital situation is assessed to determine needs. One way to do this is to rate the child's stress potential on a scale of one to five (Gaynard et al., 1990). One is the lowest where the child is medically stable with a good prognosis, has a well-functioning family support network, plays and interacts comfortably, and shows minimal signs of emotional distress. Five is the highest with imminent or recent experience in intensive care, challenging life situations, dysfunctional family, emotional needs not being met, and emotional overload. This type of scale is typically used by child life specialists to determine the extent of child life interventions needed, including medical play and preparation. Utilization of this scale by

recreational therapists in pediatric care (who are often dually certified as child life specialists) can be helpful in prioritizing children's needs for medical play and preparation.

Choosing a Specific Type of Medical Play

There are no formal guidelines to assist the therapist is choosing a specific type of medical play. The type of medical play chosen by the therapist will depend upon the assessed needs of the child, as well as the willingness of the child to engage. For example, medical art might be chosen to assist a child in processing a prior surgery. Indirect medical play or medical fantasy play might be chosen if a child exhibits extreme distress in the presence of medical equipment. Role reversal/role rehearsal medical play might be chosen to foster feelings of increased control during a procedure to decrease anxiety and stress.

Facilitating Medical Play and Preparation Sessions

This general outline of how to facilitate a medical play and preparation session is consolidated from multiple sources (Gaynard et al., 1990; Hart & Rollins, 2011; Rollins, Bolig, & Mahan, 2005), plus the clinical experiences of the chapter authors. Despite the sequential nature of the outline, it is recommended that therapists adapt the session or sessions to the child's unique needs. For example, the child may resist education about the procedure, but be willing to play with the stuffed animal and bandages.

Develop a supportive relationship: Medical play and preparation begins with the recreational therapist building a supportive relationship with the child. In a healthcare setting, there can be varying amounts of time available to build a trusting relationship. It is important to establish a connection as early as possible so that the child feels emotionally supported in play experiences. The therapist works to form a relationship where there is an environment for the child to feel safe in expressing feelings and emotions freely. It can begin with the basic assessment questions such as the child's age or favorite activities and should include a brief age-appropriate introduction to the recreational therapist's role on the child's healthcare team. If a child has a diagnosis or illness that prevents him from verbally engaging in conversation, or is a very young child, establishing rapport with a caregiver is essential. If a caregiver is not involved or available, the use of other healthcare team members can be helpful in establishing a plan to build the therapist's rapport with the child. As the child become comfortable in his/her environment and with the relationship, s/he will be more easily led into an expressive play experience. Often, the recreational therapist may enter a room or introduce herself to the child with an activity, play material, or other concrete object in hand. This sends a non-verbal message to the child that the therapist understands how important play is to the child and that the therapist is a friendly person.

Assess knowledge and understanding: Assess the child's knowledge and understanding of the procedure prior to deciding what information to share and what activity to employ.

Schedule the session: Prior to the session, the therapist schedules the length of the session. Allow for a minimum of twenty to thirty minutes for each session. The frequency of sessions offered to the child will vary depending on the child's needs and tolerance. Some children will enjoy this type of play and readily choose it often when given choices, while others may be less likely to independently participate.

Make age-appropriate decisions: Prior to the session, the therapist considers the child's developmental age to decide on language use and style of presentation. The therapist also chooses age-appropriate materials and supplies related to the session. Common medical supplies and equipment used in medical play and preparation sessions include stethoscopes, plastic syringes (used without the suction ring for safe play), Band-Aids, blood pressure cuffs, medicine cups, medical tape, and alcohol wipes. (See Appendix B for a comprehensive list.) For common procedures, the therapist might create specific kits, such as a needle kit. Dolls and stuffed animals are used to allow the child to reenact medical procedures and experiences in role reversal/role rehearsal medical play. When choosing toys and materials, heed the following recommendations adapted from Hart and Rollins (2011, p. xlv-xlvi & 335-336):

- Follow all age recommendations and information concerning the safe use of the toy. Adapt as necessary for children who are developmentally delayed.
- Do not use toys or other items with sharp edges, points, or small loose parts. Exceptions to this

might be made, such as one-on-one needle play with a child who has experienced repeated IV placements.

- Provide close supervision when using any objects that can be propelled.
- Be alert for toys with flexible joints that can catch a child's finger.
- Avoid small items that could cause a choking hazard.
- Only use toys, items, materials, or substances that are non-toxic. Toxic substances can be inhaled, ingested, or absorbed through the skin and cause medical issues.
- Consider whether the use of items with strong odors (e.g., scented markers) is beneficial (e.g., sensory stimulation) or harmful (e.g., invokes nausea after chemotherapy).
- Avoid glitter. The child could have it on his finger and rub his eye or ingest it.
- Children under the developmental age of seven should use blunt scissors only.
- Do not use balloons. They can pop and children can aspirate them.
- Do not use loud toys or other items because they can impair hearing or bother other children.
- Only use items that have a heating element or other electrical devices with children who are eight or older and only use low temperature glue guns.
- Consider the space requirements for use of the toys or other items. Avoid tight and crowded areas because they don't allow for full use or benefit of the toy or item and increase risk of accidents, such as spilling paint because there is not enough table space.
- Do not use solvents and solvent-containing products.
- Do not use powdered or dusty materials, such as chalk.
- Do not use aerosols and spray products.

See Appendix C for more information on the developmental needs, issues, responses, and preparation for hospitalized children.

Describe the procedure: If the session is preparation focused, the therapist describes the procedure (including the equipment, sequence, and duration) in terms of the anticipated sensory experience during the procedure. Dolls, drawings, photographs, and demonstrations are used. Preschool children commonly have misconceptions about medical equipment and subsequently use their imagination to invent uses for the equipment (McGrath & Huff, 2001). School-aged children and adolescents, on the other hand, typically ask questions and have a more abstract understanding of the healthcare setting. However, they don't usually know the function or proper name of equipment. Consequently, when discussing or using medical equipment in play or preparation sessions, it is important to educate the child or adolescent on its function and proper name so that during a medical episode or procedure the child or adolescent is able to readily apply that knowledge.

Present materials and allow for exploration: Allow the child to explore and play with the materials, equipment, and supplies. Facilitate interaction with materials, equipment, and supplies as needed. Non-medical play items should also be available in the session in case the child is fearful of the medical items and chooses to engage in medical fantasy play or medical art. Most children are familiar with how to use play as an outlet for communication and processing emotions. Therefore, a recreational therapist who is observing or facilitating medical play and preparation should be attentive to the play themes, verbal and non-verbal cues of the child, and the way in which materials are used and handled. These observations can assist in the interpretation of stress, confusion, and misconceptions around their upcoming procedures or past medical experiences. Children who have not had the opportunity to use play as an outlet for expression or coping may have a difficult time staying engaged in a medical play and preparation session that is unstructured. These children may do better when given fewer supplies or provided with specific requests from the therapist around the intent of the play. They also may have greater success when given suggestions by the therapist about the ways in which the materials provided could be used. Children who require physical support to independently engage in play, such as children with physical disabilities, may do best to verbally instruct the therapist and provide detailed descriptions around how to use the play materials on hand. For the school-aged population, having access to both pretend and real medical equipment is helpful. Some children may prefer to engage with the pretend medical equipment because it is less upsetting or stressful. The pretend

equipment, like those items found in doctor kits, is less scary and gives children a message that they are free to do with it what they please during play.

Adjust level of interjection and responsibility: In medical play and preparation sessions, the level of interjection and responsibility the recreational therapist assumes will vary. The role may range from supporting the child in their requests and strictly observing the play to extending and expanding upon the play of the child. Rollins, Bolig, and Mahan (2005) suggest that the most productive role lies in the middle, allowing the child to have control over the play experience while the therapist follows the events and themes of the play. This allows the child to maintain a sense of control as s/he expresses thoughts and emotions. With increased intervention by the recreational therapist, the child's play may change and his/her ability to freely express feelings may decrease. Therapists must be careful not to control the play session, ask ongoing questions, or make continued corrections. If this occurs, the child's control over play and the use of play themes can become stifled. Instead, the therapist should occasionally ask open-ended questions and use active listening techniques to best understand what is being observed. Active listening and leading techniques may be implemented as a way to explore an observed action, discern the intent of equipment usage, or comment on emotionally or physically intense play. For example, if the therapist observes a child using the blood pressure cuff on a doll's foot, the therapist might say, "I see that you are using the blood pressure cuff on the doll's foot; sometimes your nurse uses one of those on your arm." Likewise, as a child uses an exorbitant amount of tape or bandages on one area of the doll, the therapist might respond by saying, "You are using a lot of Band-Aids on the doll's leg. Could you tell me more about that?"

Identify coping techniques: Discuss and explore coping mechanisms for pain, fear, and stress anticipated to occur during the procedure and allow the child opportunities to practice the coping mechanisms before the procedure. Questions to ask include: What has worked and not worked in the past? What helps the child to relax? What does the child enjoy? Depending on the developmental age and abilities of the child, the therapist may need to implement the coping techniques without the child's input (e.g., hold and sing to an infant during an injection).

Allow for questions: The therapist encourages the child and family to ask questions.

Outcomes and Documentation

The use of medical play and preparation in a medical setting is an important tool for a child to increase coping and understanding while decreasing anxiety, stress, and confusion (b114 Orientation Functions, b126 Temperament and Personality Functions, b152 Emotional Functions, d240 Handling Stress and Other Psychological Demands). Documenting a child's experiences provides data about the child's ongoing learning and mastery of medical situations. In addition to documenting the day and time of the medical play and preparation sessions, the therapist typically documents observed developmental skills or stage, emotional functioning, ability to understand the medical experience, direct quotes made by the child, how the child identified each piece of equipment (e.g., "Here, dolly, this juice is for you. It will make you feel better." The child called the water in the medicine cup "juice."), if the child utilized equipment in non-traditional ways (e.g., swings the doll on the blood pressure cuff), and what routines and rituals the child establishes as part of the play (e.g., prior to initiating play the child is insistent that his stuffed bear is in the room). The summary of the process and events that occurred during the session help other medical professionals understand how to best support the child in future interactions. Attention to these things will help the therapist understand the child's knowledge, understanding, and beliefs, including fears, confusion, and misunderstandings. For a child who is hospitalized for an extended period of time, specific goals and objectives related to medical play and preparation might be set and tracked. Possible observations include the child's utilization of coping techniques, frequency and duration of negative reactions to procedures, or ability to identify and know the function of medical equipment. Changes in the parents' level of anxiety can be documented by noting a change in ICF code e310 Immediate Family.

Resources

Child Life Council
www.childlife.org
Organization that provides Child Life Certification and Child Life resources.

Medical Doll Pattern
www.craftingcomfort.org/documents/medicalplaydoll.pdf

Appendix A: Case Examples

Pre-operative medical play case study: An eight-year-old girl was admitted to the hospital and was awaiting a heart transplant. Common to these types of patients, her hospital stay was lengthy and the day of the procedure for which she and her family were awaiting, was unknown. During her admission, the child engaged in many activities and therapeutic interventions. Pre-operational medical play was introduced as a mechanism for her to explore medical equipment and process her hospital experience. As with many children of this age, she was given many choices around the types of materials she could use during her play. With each medical play session, her play became more complex and focused. Under the supervision of the therapist, she began to verbalize a desire to establish a routine around her play. She began by requesting the room be set up like an operating room. She would request a table and specific materials to enact what she would interpret as a heart transplant. In just a few sessions, the child had established a routine around how she set up the room, how she engaged with the doll, and the steps of the procedure she would conduct during her play. After the table and materials were displayed and placed in the appropriate ways, she would gather the instruments she needed. First, she would place to doll on the table. She would then use the "sterile" draping, cotton swabs, plastic syringes, and hemostats. Next, she would follow an established process of steps, which at times could consume up to two hours of time. This included setting the doll on the table, lining up plastic syringes in a row, placing the sterile draping on the chest of the doll, taking the cotton swab and "cleaning" around the dolls heart, using the hemostats to close the chest, and placing a Band-Aid on the doll's chest. When the child first engaged in medical play, each session was approximately one hour. As the child's play became more involved, her play scenario took up to two hours. This routine gave the impending procedure of the heart transplant boundaries and assisted the child in determining the steps that she would take as a patient someday. In this example the recreational therapist's role was to serve as an assistant to the patient. The therapist would hand the child needed items, would assist in the preparation of the room and furniture, and have a doll on hand. The recreational therapist also served as an observer, taking note of the repetitive nature of the play and working to clarify why the child was doing certain actions. Simple questions were used to move the play along.

Post-operative medical play case study: A four-year-old girl was admitted to the cardiac intensive care unit after an emergent cardiac event resulting in a breathing tube being inserted when she was unconscious. As her psychosocial needs were assessed, the recreational therapist determined that participating in medical play would be beneficial. It was determined that the goals of hospitalization would include the discovery of misconceptions around medical equipment and the enhancement of her age-appropriate coping skills. The child was non-verbal because of the tube and was otherwise developmentally appropriate. As the therapist introduced a doll with a similar breathing tube, the child was immediately focused on the tube and the way in which it was stabilized with medical tape. Each time they engaged in medical play, her play involved the process of removing the tape and re-taping the breathing tube around the doll's mouth. This process in the child's own medical routine was the most traumatic for her to endure. For the length of her admission, at least one time per week, the child used medical play to process, understand, and cope with her own stressors around the re-taping of her breathing tube. Her play served as her verbalization of the stress points in her care and allowed her to have control over the activity that caused her the most anxiety. After several weeks of play sessions, typically thirty to forty minutes in length, the child displayed decreased nervousness around the procedure and was able to recover to a baseline coping state more quickly afterwards.

Appendix B: Medical Play: Equipment and Materials

A doll or stuffed animal should be used during play to allow for the highest degree of freedom. There are several types of dolls that can be used. Blank cloth dolls are inexpensive and allow a child to create themselves or an alternate personality with markers. In most healthcare settings, children are allowed to keep these dolls. Teaching dolls are more expensive and can be ordered from many different companies to include specific equipment, organs, and entry sites (e.g., an opening for a PICC line insertion or a tracheostomy tube). If you are working with a child on isolation or any type of infection control and prevention precautions, the use of a blank cloth doll or a plastic baby doll is helpful. Plastic dolls can be cleaned properly via the guidelines and standards of the institution. To maintain a safe play environment, black suction rings should always be removed from syringes. The recreation therapist should know exactly how many syringes are available and account for them at the end of a session.

Suggested Supplies

Alcohol prep pads
Anesthesia mask
Arm boards
Band-Aids
Blood pressure cuff
Casting material
Cotton swabs/balls
Doll or stuffed animal
Gauze
ID bracelet
IV catheters/angiocath (adult supervision)
IV t-connectors (adult supervision)
Medical tape
Medicine cups
Ophthalmoscope
Oral syringes (varying sizes)
Preemie- or newborn-size blood pressure cuffs to use on dolls or animals
Stethoscope
Stickers for rewards
Surgical hat
Thermometer
Tongue depressors

Appendix C: Developmental Needs, Issues, Responses, and Preparation for the Hospitalized Child

Infant (0-1)

Erikson's stage of development: Trust vs. mistrust.

Needs: Security, protection, intimacy, consistency in caregiving, daily routine structure, interaction with parents (voice, touch, feel), quiet and soothing environment.

Hospitalization issues: Lack of stimulation, fear of pain, separation anxiety (first stage: protest — crying, screaming, kicking, refuses attention from others, looks for parents, lasts a few hours to weeks; second stage: despair — stops crying, appears depressed, develops hopelessness, withdrawn, quiet; third stage: detachment — after long period of parental absence, copes with pain by forming superficial attachment to others, becomes increasingly self-centered and more interested in material objects, when parents return has difficulty reattaching).

Possible responses if needs are not met: Failure to bond, failure to thrive, distrust, anxiety, delayed skills development, distress, decreased sense of control when there are no responses to cries or babbles.

Medical preparation education techniques: Presence of caregiver to offer comfort to infant when stressed; introduce self and explain procedure to caregiver; allow infant to explore related equipment as appropriate; orient caregiver to environment.

Toddler (1-3)

Erikson's stage of development: Autonomy vs. shame and doubt.

Needs: Parental presence; opportunities to explore, play, and socialize; daily routine structure; preparation for procedures; opportunities to develop autonomy (e.g., putting on one's own shirt, helping with tasks, making simple snack choice, etc.).

Hospitalization issues: Separation, distress with painful and non-painful medical procedures (fear of bodily injury and pain), frightening fantasies, immobility and restrictions that limit ability to play, explore, and socialize, and loss of routine and rituals.

Possible responses if needs are not met: Regression (including loss of newly learned skills), uncooperativeness, protest (verbal and physical), despair, negativism, temper tantrums, resistance.

Medical preparation education techniques: In addition to previous techniques, allow toddler to have mastery of things in the environment as able and appropriate (e.g., push button to open door, turn on light).

Preschoolers (3-6)

Erikson's stage of development: Initiative vs. guilt.

Needs: Requires concrete and hands-on experiences for preparation for procedures by using real equipment and having play opportunities for coping through medical play and expressive play that allows the therapist to detect fears, concerns, and misconceptions. Needs a safe area where medical procedures are never done, such as the playroom. The child's bed should not be used for procedures to decrease trouble sleeping. There should be opportunities to take on new roles and tasks without being punished for their initiative.

Hospitalization issues: Separation, fear of bodily injury and pain, physical restrictions, fear of loss of control, magical thinking (ability to wish things to happen), hospitalization is seen as punishment (did something wrong to get "sick").

Possible responses if needs are not met: Regression, anger toward primary caregiver, acting out, protest (less aggressive than toddler), despair and detachment, physical and verbal aggression, dependency, withdrawal.

Medical preparation education techniques: Introduce self to caregiver and child; explain what will happen during the session to decrease fears; orient caregiver and child to the procedures that will occur and the environment it will take place in; use dolls and medical equipment to demonstrate procedure; offer control whenever possible; explain the child's role (e.g., can't touch IV, have to drink juice) to increase a feeling of involvement; teach or provide coping strategies for pain and anxiety, such as distraction, singing, or playing; and provide rewards such as stickers.

School-age Children (6-12)

Erikson's stage of development: Industry vs. inferiority.

Needs: Parental presence and contact (phone, Skype); education about his/her illness or disability and what to expect (capable of cognitive reasoning); preparation for procedures; opportunities to play and engage in other activities such as journaling, games, drawing, crafts, and socialization to express feelings, master experiences by learning new skills, and cope with procedures and treatment (choose activities where success is likely to combat inferiority); hospital school program; structure and routine; peer interaction; opportunities to practice new skills and gain competence and confidence with physical changes from illness or surgery.

Hospitalization issues: Separation; fear of bodily injury, pain, or mutilation; fear of loss of control or mastery; fear of illness, disability, or death; distress when experiencing physical symptoms, such as nausea, pain, or dizziness; restricted activity; unfamiliar environment (e.g., wall cords that look like monsters at night, "mad" doctors, noisy roommates).

Possible responses if needs are not met: Regression, inability to complete some tasks, uncooperativeness, withdrawal, depression, displaced anger and hostility, frustration.

Medical preparation education techniques: Use techniques described for preschoolers, however introduce more complex coping strategies, such as visualization and inspirational music; allow the child to participate in the procedure as appropriate (e.g., hold the bandages) to increase cooperation and feeling of involvement; and allow child a say in the timing of the procedure if possible, for example to decrease conflict with other meaningful activities.

Adolescent (12-18)

Erikson's stage of development: Identity vs. role confusion.

Needs: Peer visitation and contact, as well as time to be alone; a special adolescent environment and policies to foster coping and cooperation; a hangout and activity room for teens only (e.g., video games, movies, computer, pool table, music, cooking, etc.) along with scheduled teen activities; liberal visiting policies; medical preparation education; staff who listen to concerns, answer questions, and involve teen in decision making; attention to privacy and confidentiality; opportunities for mobility and independence; opportunities to try out different identities without fear or judgment.

Hospitalization issues: Separation, fear of bodily injury or pain, dependence on adults, fear of loss of identity, body image and sexuality, concern about peer group status after hospitalization, anger and frustration due to loss of independence and control. Hospitalization is threatening because it separates adolescents from normal peer group activities, disrupts future plans, and increases insecurities about appearance, self-image, sexual functioning, and self-worth.

Possible responses if needs are not met: Uncooperativeness, withdrawal, anxiety, depression.

Medical preparation education techniques: Use techniques described for school-age children, but additionally encourage the adolescent to make a list of questions; show photographs of the procedure in addition to dolls and drawings; explore coping mechanisms with adolescent, especially using what has worked in other situations; talk about privacy issues such as who will examine the adolescent and where; encourage adolescent to bring own menstruation supplies (if preferred); and facilitate contact with peers if hospitalized through phones, Skype, and visits.

Adapted from: Pressley and McCormick (2007); Rollins, Bolig, and Mahan (2005); and Hart and Rollins (2011).

References

Gaynard, L., Wolfer, J. Goldberger, J., Thompson, R., Redbum, L., & Laidley, L. (1998). *Psychosocial care of children in hospitals: A clinical practice manual.* Rockville MD: Child Life Council.

Hart, R. & Rollins, J. (2011). *Therapeutic activities for children and teens coping with health issues.* John Wiley & Sons, Inc.: Hoboken, NJ.

Hughes, F. P. (2009). *Children, play, and development.* Thousand Oaks, CA: Sage.

Kain, Z. N. & Caldwell-Andrews, A. A. (2005). Preoperative psychological preparation of the child for surgery: An update. *Anesthesiology Clinics of North America, 23*, 597-614.

Kettwich, S., Sibbit, W., Brandt, J., Johnson, C., Wong, C., & Bankhurst, A. (2007). Needle phobia and stress-reducing medical devices in pediatric and adult chemotherapy patients. *Journal of Pediatric Oncology Nursing, 24*(1), 20-28.

Koller, D. (2007). Preparing children and adolescents for medical procedures. Child Life Council. Accessed via website www.childlife.org/files/EBPPreparationStatement-Complete.pdf.

Li, H. C. W. & Lopez, V. (2008). Effectiveness and appropriateness of therapeutic play intervention in preparing children for surgery: A randomized controlled trial study. *Journal for Specialists in Pediatric Nursing, 13*(2), 63-73.

Li, H. C. W., Lopez, V., & Lee, T. L. I. (2007). Effects of preoperative therapeutic play on outcomes of school-age children undergoing day surgery. *Research in Nursing & Health, 30*, 320-332.

McCue, K. (1988). Medical play: An expanded perspective. *Children's Health Care 16*(3), 157-161.

McGrath, P. & Huff, N. (2001). "What is it?" Findings on preschoolers' responses to play with medical equipment. *Child Care, Health and Development, 27*, 451-462.

Pressley, M. & McCormick, C. B. (2007). *Child and adolescent development for educators.* Guilford Press.

Rice, V. H. (2011). *Handbook of stress, coping, and health: Implications for nursing research, theory, and practice.* Thousand Oaks, CA: Sage.

Rollins, J., Bolig, R., Mahan, C. (2005). *Meeting children's psychosocial needs across the health-care continuum.* Austin, TX: Pro-Ed.

35. Mind-Body Interventions

Marieke Van Puymbroeck and Arlene A. Schmid

Mind-body medicine is one type of Complementary and Alternative Medicine (CAM), as identified by the National Center for Complementary and Alternative Medicine (NCCAM), a division of the National Institutes of Health. NCCAM defines mind and body practices as those that "…focus on the interactions among the brain, mind, body, and behavior, with the intent to use the mind to affect physical functioning and promote health."

Chinese medicine has promoted the idea that the mind is important in healing from illness for over 2,000 years (National Center for Complementary and Alternative Medicine, 2012). This is why, in typical mind and body practices or interventions, the practice includes physical movement or breathwork while focusing on the mind. Typical mind-body practices include meditation, yoga, and T'ai Chi, as well as others such as acupuncture and qi gong. Recreational therapists can use mind and body practices as therapeutic interventions with clients, but it is important to know that specialized training in some of the specific techniques (e.g., transcendental meditation, yoga, acupuncture) may be required.

Indications

Mind-body practices can be beneficial for most individuals, but are dependent on the specific technique. Carrington (1993) identified that the individuals who may benefit from meditation include those with: a need to increase self-reliance (e.g., b126 Temperament and Personality Functions, d177 Making Decisions, d210 Undertaking a Single Task, d220 Undertaking Multiple Tasks), separation anxiety (d760 Family Relationships), reduced productivity or creativity (e.g., b130 Energy and Drive Functions, d230 Carrying Out Daily Routine), anxiety or tension (b126 Temperament and Personality Functions, b152 Emotional Functions), alcohol or tobacco abuse (d570 Looking After One's Health), insomnia or hypersomnia (b134 Sleep Functions), mild depression (b126 Temperament and Personality Functions, b130 Energy and Drive Functions, b152 Emotional Functions), psychophysiological disorders, symptoms of chronic fatigue (b130 Energy and Drive Functions, b455 Exercise Tolerance Functions), submissive tendencies (b126 Temperament and Personality Functions, d710 Basic Interpersonal Interactions), low frustration tolerance (b126 Temperament and Personality Functions, d710 Basic Interpersonal Interactions), and/or excessive self-blame (b126 Temperament and Personality Functions). Freeman (2004) further identified that meditation is appropriate for individuals with low motivation (b130 Energy and Drive Functions), limited time, and moderate self-discipline. Meditation is also appropriate for healthy individuals seeking balance, calmness, and increased relaxation (National Center for Chronic Disease Prevention and Health Promotion, 2012).

McCall (2007) reported that yoga has been shown to address the following health conditions: alcoholism, drug abuse, and associated withdrawal; pregnancy (typical and atypical); psychological disorders (anxiety, depression, phobias); chronic diseases (asthma, cancer, carpal tunnel syndrome, chronic obstructive pulmonary disease, congestive heart failure, attention deficit hyperactivity disorder, diabetes, eating disorders, epilepsy, fibromyalgia, heart disease, hypertension, HIV/AIDS, multiple sclerosis, osteoarthritis, pain, pancreatitis, post-polio syndrome, rheumatoid arthritis); and acute illnesses, diseases, and disorders (infertility, insomnia, irritable bowel syndrome, menopause, migraine, pleural effusion, post-heart attack recovery, postoperative recovery, rhinitis sinusitis, urinary stress incontinence). Find appropriate ICF codes by studying the particular condition. Other health conditions that have been improved through yoga include chronic stroke (specifically increasing balance and reducing fear of falling) (b755 Involuntary Movement Reaction Functions, b235 Vestibular Functions) (Schmid, Van Puymbroeck, Altenburger, Schalk et al., 2012; Schmid, Van Puymbroeck, & Koceja, 2010), as well as increasing overall strength (b730 Muscle Power Functions) and flexibility (b710 Mobility of Joint Functions, b735 Muscle Tone Functions) among older adults and informal caregivers (Schmid, Van Puymbroeck, Altenburger, Dierks et al., 2012; Tatum, Bradley, & Igel, 2011; Van Puymbroeck et al., 2009; Van Puymbroeck, Hsieh, & Pernell, 2008; Van Puymbroeck, Payne, & Hsieh, 2007); a myriad of issues for breast cancer survivors (Culos-Reed et al., 2006; Moadel et al., 2007; Van Puymbroeck, Burk, Shinew, Kuhlenschmidt, & Schmid, 2013). Also, yoga has been shown to reduce leisure constraints (d920 Recreation and Leisure) in middle and older adults (Van Puymbroeck, Smith, & Schmid, 2011) and reduce body dissatisfaction (b180 Experience of Self and Time Functions) (Neumark-Sztainer et al., 2011). Finally, a recent systematic analysis of yoga for neuropsychiatric disorders found that for people with depression, yoga has been shown to be beneficial in mild depression, with or without medication, and yoga has been shown to be beneficial in individuals with schizophrenia when combined with medication. Further, the authors found that yoga is comparable to biofeedback and relaxation for youth with ADHD (Balasubramaniam, Telles, & Doraiswamy, 2013).

T'ai Chi has substantial research evidence to support its use with a variety of patient populations. A recent meta-analysis examined 40 studies of T'ai Chi on components of psychological well-being (Wang et al., 2010). The authors found that T'ai Chi was effective in the long and short term in increasing self-esteem, life satisfaction, and psychological well-being (b126 Temperament and Personality Functions) in individuals with and without chronic conditions. A number of studies have examined the use of T'ai Chi for older adults with positive outcomes. Li and colleagues found that T'ai Chi Ch'uan improved sleep duration and sleep quality (b134 Sleep Functions) and reduced risk of falls (b235 Vestibular Functions) (Li, Harmer, Fisher, & McAuley, 2004; Li et al., 2005; Li, Fisher, & Harmer, 2005). Wolf has reported reduced fear of falling (b126 Temperament and Personality Functions, b235 Vestibular Functions), reduced rate of falls, lower systolic blood pressure (b420 Blood Pressure Functions), and improved resting heart rate (b410 Heart Functions) (Wolf et al., 2001; Wolf et al., 1996; Wolf et al., 2003). T'ai Chi has been endorsed as a beneficial exercise for individuals with Parkinson's disease by the National Parkinson Foundation of the United States (National Parkinson Foundation, 2012) after a number of trials have demonstrated that T'ai Chi improved psychological and social factors (Lee, Lam, & Ernst, 2008).

Despite these benefits, in Western cultures there are many individuals who have specific concerns or misconceptions about what mind-body interventions using CAM and Eastern traditions include. Thus, it is important to clearly talk with your patients or clients about the specific technique and dispel any misperceptions at the initiation of the intervention.

Contraindications

Generally, mind-body techniques are safe and beneficial. However, techniques that require visualizing scenarios are contraindicated for individuals with diagnoses of psychosis, post-traumatic stress disorder, delusions, delirium, severe obsessive-compulsive disorder, and schizophrenia (Cooper & Stollings, 2009).

There are a few documented adverse events related to meditation. One study identified a woman who had brief periods of depressed mood (six and 10 years prior) and experienced an episode of mania characterized by a reduction in appetite, increased sleeplessness, talkativeness, and irritability following an intensive weekend retreat on Zen meditation (Yorston, 2001). Also, three individuals who had discontinued pharmacological treatment for schizophrenia were documented to have psychotic episodes following meditation (Walsh & Roche, 1979). Meditation is also contraindicated for individuals with a strong need for control (Freeman, 2004).

There are few reported adverse events related to participation in Hatha yoga. However, McCall (2007) reported that forward bends may cause problems for the low back and spine, particularly in the case of tight hamstrings. Further, he reported that neck injuries may be caused by shoulders and plow or headstand. Hamstring tears may be caused from standing forward folds, most likely due to insufficient warm ups or exhaustion, while shoulder injuries may be caused by reverse prayer pose, cow face pose, or chaturanga dandasana (McCall, 2007). Sacroiliac strains may be worsened through head-to-knee pose, cobbler's pose, wide-legged forward bends (seated or standing). Because the knees, ankles, and wrists are involved in so many postures, overuse or improper form may cause pain or discomfort. It is important that individuals avoid postures that cause pain in order to avoid injury.

According to the Mayo Clinic, individuals who have severe osteoporosis, a hernia, are pregnant, or have joint problems, back pain, or fractures should receive medical clearance prior to engaging in T'ai Chi (Mayo Clinic, 2012). Only one study has reported adverse events related to T'ai Chi, and these included sore knees, shoulders, and lower backs (Kirsteins, Dietz, & Hwang, 1991).

Other CAM techniques that require movement may be contraindicated based on the features of the specific disability or individual. Make sure to receive clearance before engaging clients in any physical activity. Note that many of the mind-body practices can be modified for individuals with all levels of ability.

Protocols and Processes

While there are many interventions in mind-body medicine, the following includes a brief description of the most common techniques that could be used by recreational therapists in practice. These techniques include meditation, yoga, and T'ai Chi. Because meditation, yoga, and T'ai Chi are three different mind-body techniques, each has information specific to it, which is described below.

Meditation

Meditation requires a quiet location, a comfortable posture, a focusing of attention, and an open attitude (National Center for Chronic Disease Prevention and Health Promotion, 2012). Depending on the type of meditation chosen, there are many resources on the internet that describe how to do it, as shown in the Resource section. Briefly, the eight types of meditation are mindfulness (a focus on being present), zazen (seated meditation, requires little instruction), Transcendental Meditation (seated, repeating a mantra), Kundalini (focus on breath

through energy centers), Qi gong (focus on breath and circulating energy), guided visualization (mental imagery of an event or environment), and heart rhythm meditation (focuses on breath and heartbeat) (Bair, 2010). Recreational therapists who choose to use meditation as an intervention with their patients or clients are encouraged to have personal experience with meditation, so that they can be a more effective facilitator.

Meditation has been increasingly accepted as a clinical intervention in the United States. The eight types of meditation described above can be divided into two families: concentrative techniques and nonconcentrative techniques (Freeman, 2004). In concentrative techniques, the individual concentrates on a specific stimulus, such as a sound. If during concentrative meditation, the individual's attention wanders, s/he is directed to gently bring the focus back to the stimulus. In nonconcentrative meditation, the individual observes nonjudgmentally the thoughts and feelings that s/he is experiencing (Freeman, 2004). An example of each family is described below.

Transcendental meditation (TM) is a concentrative technique in which the individual repeats a mantra that is appropriate for the individual's level of consciousness. The choice of mantra is essential to reach optimal consciousness. TM should be taught by an individual trained in TM. TM is recommended to be performed 20 minutes twice daily. A meta-analysis reported that there were clinically meaningful reductions in both systolic and diastolic blood pressure following regular participation in TM (Anderson, Liu, & Kryscio, 2008).

Mindfulness meditation (MM) is a nonconcentrative technique in which the individual observes his or her thoughts and mental activities without judgment. In MM, the focus is on the present, not the future or past. MM is recommended to be participated in three times per day for the first week, and then daily after that. A specific MM technique that has a lot of empirical support is Mindfulness-Based Stress Reduction (MBSR) (Kabat-Zinn, 1990). MBSR is an eight- to ten-week standardized intervention that patients engage in once per week for 2.5 hours, along with a 45-minute homework assignment six days per week. The MBSR intervention also requires one full-day intensive retreat during the training period. Individuals can be trained in the MBSR technique (required in order to teach it) by the

Center for Mindfulness in Medicine, Health Care, and Society at the University of Massachusetts Medical Center. A recent meta-analysis has shown that MBSR reduced stress, ruminative thinking, and trait anxiety in healthy individuals, as well as improved empathy and self-compassion (Chiesa & Serretti, 2009). A meta-analysis of MBSR for cancer patients found that MBSR was effective in improving mental health, specifically distress, quality of life, sleep, state of control, depression, anxiety, sense of coherence, mood, fatigue, post-traumatic growth, and spirituality (Ledesma & Kumano, 2008). Further, mindfulness-based therapy (MBSR and mindfulness-based cognitive therapy) has been shown to have a very strong effect on individuals with mood and anxiety symptoms, based on a meta-analysis by Hofmann et al. (2010).

Yoga

Yoga is a gentle physical activity that originated in India approximately 5000 years ago. The term yoga means "union" or "yoke," and refers to the emphasis of the practice on enhancing self-awareness. There are many types of yoga and the foundation of these is Hatha yoga. All yoga includes asanas (postures), a focus on breathing (pranayama), and meditation (dhyana). The major categories of asanas in Hatha yoga include relaxation, inversion, meditative, balance, standing, twists, backbends, forward bends, and side stretches (McCall, 2007). Many asanas can be modified based on ability level and can also be performed while seated. Sequences of asanas are typically developed to specifically target the needs of the group. For example, with breast cancer survivors, protocols such as those in Appendix A focus on increasing range of motion and stretching the chest area. Most research-based yoga protocols last for eight weeks and meet twice weekly for 60-75 minutes. Outside of research, most recommendations include engaging in yoga two to three times a week for gentle change, and four to six times a week for quicker changes (Corepower yoga, 2013).

T'ai Chi Ch'uan

T'ai Chi Ch'uan, more commonly known as T'ai Chi, is a martial art that originated in China over 600 years ago. Although it is referred to as a martial art, T'ai Chi consists of gentle, slow, flowing movements (Lan, Lai, & Chen, 2002). T'ai Chi differs from yoga as the focus in T'ai Chi is on the movement while in yoga the focus is on the breath during movement. T'ai Chi has several different types. Sun and Chen (1995) reported that simplified T'ai Chi has 24 sequential movements, while other styles have up to 85 movements. During the movements, participants are instructed to clear the mind and keep it calm, while relaxing the body and moving slowly and smoothly (Metzger & Zhou, 1996). Optimal dosing has not been identified for T'ai Chi, but general recommendations usually include practice two to three times per week (Weil, 2013).

Outcomes and Documentation

It is imperative, when documenting outcomes in recreational therapy practice, that the interventions were engaged in to meet specific goals or client needs that were identified in the initial assessment and that the outcome measures chosen address those goals or needs. Meditation, yoga, and T'ai Chi Ch'uan have been generally shown to improve psychological and physical functioning. Each intervention is tied to a specific aspect of the client's diagnosis. A large number of ICF codes were presented in the Indications section. Documentation of outcomes should include changes in any ICF codes cited as the purpose of the intervention.

Quality of participation measures are also included below, as recreational therapists often have goals to improve participation, and each of these mind-body techniques have been demonstrated to improve participation. Below are outcome measures that have been used in each category being used to measure the specific construct.

Psychological Functioning

- *Patient Health Questionnaire* (PHQ-9) (Kroenke, Spitzer, & Williams, 2001): Nine items, brief measure of depression severity, available online for free.
- *Perceived Stress Scale* (PSS) (Cohen, Kamarck, & Mermelstein, 1983): 14 items, measures self-perception of stress, available online for free.
- *Profile of Mood States* (POMS) (McNair, Lorr, & Droppelman, 1992): Six subscales (tension-anxiety, anger-hostility, fatigue-inertia, depression-dejection, vigor-activity, confusion-bewilderment), available for purchase at

www.mhs.com/product.aspx?gr=cli&prod=poms
&id=resources

Physical Functioning

- *Berg Balance Scale* (Berg, Wood-Dauphinee, &
  Gaytton, 1989; Berg, Wood-Dauphinee, & Williams, 1995): 14 items, measures static balance
  and fall risk in adults, available for free online.
- *Dynamic Gait Index* (Marchetti & Whitney,
  2006): Performance-based test for 20 feet walking, available for free online.
- *Timed Up and Go Test* (Podsiadlo & Richardson,
  1991): Performance-based test that includes
  standing up from a seated position and walking
  three meters, available for free online.

Participation

- *Medical Outcomes Study*, Short Form 36 (MOS
  SF-36) (Ware, Gandek, & IQOLA Project Group,
  1994): Extensively used, 36 items in eight subscales (physical functioning, role limitations due
  to physical problems, general health perceptions,
  vitality, social functioning, role limitations due to
  emotional problems, general mental health, and
  health transition), available for purchase from
  www.rand.org/health/surveys_tools/mos/mos_co
  re_36item.html
- *Nottingham Health Profile* (Hunt, McEwen, &
  McKenna, 1985): 45 items, assesses perceived
  health, available free online.

Resources

Transcendental Meditation Program
www.tm.org/
A comprehensive website that describes the evidence-based benefits, where to find a teacher, how to
become trained as an instructor, and much more.

Mindfulness Meditation
www.mindfulnessmeditation.org/
Learn more about Mindfulness Meditation at this
website and, if you join their mailing list, you can
receive the free e-book called *Medical Meditation —
How to Reduce Pain, Decrease Complications, and
Recover Faster From Surgery, Disease and Illness.*
Free Mindfulness Meditation podcasts are available
at http://marc.ucla.edu/body.cfm?id=22.

Yoga Journal
www.yogajournal.com/
The *Yoga Journal* offers a website that has updates of
yoga in the news, information on poses, a directory of
yoga teachers, lifestyle, and practice. There are also
videos available that provide sequences of postures
taught by master yoga teachers. The yoga journal also
offers conferences around the country.

Yoga.com
Yoga.com
Provides up-to-date articles about yoga, as well as
interviews with yogis and yoga teachers, in addition
to information about poses and workouts. They also
offer music recommendations for yoga practice.

The International Association of Yoga Therapists (IAYT)
www.iayt.org
Offers information on how to find yoga therapists,
information on yoga research, and conference information. IAYT also offers the Symposium on Yoga
Therapy (SYT) and Symposium on Yoga Research
(SYR) every two years.

T'ai Chi
www.egreenway.com/taichichuan/short.htm.
A large collection of T'ai Chi information, including
videos, information, and extended history of T'ai Chi.

International Magazine of T'ai Chi Ch'uan
www.tai-chi.com/
Offers information for the novice to the advanced
practitioner, including information on where to find a
T'ai Chi teacher.

Appendix A: Yoga Protocol for Breast Cancer Survivors

Originally published in Van Puymbroeck,
Schmid, Shinew, and Hsieh (2011). Prepared and
executed by Jennifer Cameron Juday, Certified Yoga
Teacher.

The postures were selected from the traditions of
B. K. S. Iyengar and Sri K. Pattabhi Jois and works
by Tias Little and Surya Little. All postures were
modified for the individual needs of participants,
including eliminating a posture if contraindications
existed. The eight-week intervention began with
simple postures and progressed in terms of complexity during the intervention period.

Breathing Techniques

Three-Part Breathing (full puraka and rechaka/inhalation and exhalation)

Ujjayi (Victory Breath, with and without kumbhaka/retention)

Nadi Sodhana (Alternate Nostril Breathing)

Kapalabhati (Skull-Shining Breath)

Postures

Standing/Kneeling

Samasthiti/Tadasana (Equal Standing/Mountain)

Cat/Cow (On All Fours)

Adho Mukha Svanasana (Downward-Facing Dog)

Padangusthasana (Hand-to-Toe Forward Bend)

Parighasana (Kneeling Gate Pose)

Virabhadrasana II (Warrior 2)

Parsvakonasana (Extended Side Angle)

Parsvottanasana (Pyramid)

Padottanasana (Wide-Leg Forward Bend)

Trikonasana (Triangle)

Chaturanga Dandasana (Modified Plank)

Virabhadrasana I (Warrior 1)

Garudhasana (Eagle) (arms only)

Arm-to-Wall Stretch

Virasana (Hero)

Prone

Balasana (Child's Pose)

Bhujangasana (Cobra)

Shalabhasana (Locust)

Balancing

Vrksasana (Tree)

Virabhadrasana III (Modified Warrior 3) Seated

Paschimottanasana (Seated Forward Bend)

Purvottanasana I (Reverse Table Top)

Janu Sirsasana (Seated Head-to-Knee Pose)

Marichyasana III (Modified Seated Twist)

Supine

Supta Gomukhasana (Cow-Face Pose, modified to supine position)

Supta Padangusthasana (Supine Hand-to-Toe)

Setubandhasana Sarvangasana (Bridge)

Jathara Parivartanasana I (Reclining Twist)

Viparita Karani (Legs Up Wall Restorative Inversion)

Savasana (Corpse/Relaxation Pose, both supported and unsupported variations)

Possible advanced poses depending on practitioners

Surya Namaskar A (Sun Salutation A)

Parivrtta Parsvakonasana (Revolved Side Angle)

Parivrtta Trikonasana (Revolved Triangle)

Halasana (Plow)

Salamba Sarvangasana (Shoulder Stand)

Dhanurasana (Bow)

References

Anderson, J. W., Liu, C., & Kryscio, R. J. (2008). Blood pressure response to transcendental meditation: A meta-analysis. *American Journal of Hypertension, 21*(3), 310-316.

Bair, A. (2010). 8 basic kinds of meditation (and why you should meditate on your heart). Retrieved February 15, 2013, from www.iam-u.org/index.php/8-basic-kinds-of-meditation-and-why-you-should-meditate-on-your-heart.

Balasubramaniam, M., Telles, S., & Doraiswamy, P. M. (2013). Yoga for the mind: A systematic review of randomized controlled trials. *Frontiers in Psychiatry, 1*, 0.

Berg, K., Wood-Dauphinee, S., & Gaytton, D. (1989). Measuring balance in the elderly: Preliminary development of an instrument. *Physiotherapy Canada, 41*, 304-311.

Berg, K., Wood-Dauphinee, S., & Williams, J. I. (1995). The Balance Scale: Reliability assessment with elderly residents and patients with an acute stroke. *Scandinavian Journal of Rehabilitation Medicine, 27*(1), 27-36.

Carrington, P. (1993). Modern forms of meditation. In P. M. Lehrer (Ed.), *Principles and practice of stress management.* New York: Guilford Press.

Chiesa, A. & Serretti, A. (2009). Mindfulness-based stress reduction for stress management in healthy people: A review and meta-analysis. *The Journal of Alternative and Complementary Medicine, 15*(5), 593-600.

Cohen, S., Kamarck, T., & Mermelstein, R. (1983). A global measure of perceived stress. *Journal of Health and Social Behavior, 24*(4), 385-396.

Cooper, K. & Stollings, S. (2009). Guided imagery for anxiety. *Fast Facts and Concepts, 211.* www.eperc.mcw.edu/fastfact/ff_211.htm.

Corepower yoga. (2013). Yoga tips, yoga help, and yoga class preparation. Retrieved January 23, 2013, from www.corepoweryoga.com/information/yoga-beginners/first-yoga-class-preparation-How_often.

Culos-Reed, S. N., Carlson, L. E., Daroux, L. M., & Hately-Aldous, S. (2006). A pilot study of yoga for breast cancer survivors: Physical and psychological benefits. *Psychooncology, 15*(10), 891-897.

Freeman, L. (2004). Meditation. In *Complementary & Alternative Medicine: A Research-Based Approach* (2nd ed.). St. Louis: Mosby.

Hofmann, S. G., Sawyer, A. T., Witt, A. A., & Oh, D. (2010). The effect of mindfulness-based therapy on anxiety and depression: A meta-analytic review. *Journal of Consulting and Clinical Psychology, 78*(2), 169.

Hunt, S. M., McEwen, J., & McKenna, S. P. (1985). Measuring health status: A new tool for clinicians and epidemiologists. *The Journal of the Royal College of General Practitioners, 35*(273), 185.

Kabat-Zinn, J. (1990). *Full catastrophe living: Using the wisdom of your body and mind to face stress, pain and illness.* New York, NY: Delacorte.

Kirsteins, A. E., Dietz, F., & Hwang, S. M. (1991). Evaluating the safety and potential use of a weight-bearing exercise, T'ai-Chi Ch'uan, for rheumatoid arthritis patients. *American Journal of Physical Medicine and Rehabilitation, 70*, 136-141.

Kroenke, K., Spitzer, R. L., & Williams, J. B. (2001). The PHQ-9: validity of a brief depression severity measure. (0884-8734 (Print)). doi: D - NLM: PMC1495268 EDAT- 2001/09/15

10:00 MHDA- 2001/10/26 10:01 CRDT- 2001/09/15 10:00
AID - jgi01114 [pii] PST - ppublish.

Lan, C., Lai, J. S., & Chen, S. Y. (2002). T'ai Chi Ch'uan: An ancient wisdom on exercise and health promotion. *Sports Medicine, 32*(4), 217-224.

Ledesma, D. & Kumano, H. (2008). Mindfulness-based stress reduction and cancer: A meta-analysis. *Psychooncology, 18*(6), 571-579.

Lee, M. S., Lam, P., & Ernst, E. (2008). Effectiveness of T'ai Chi for Parkinson's disease: A critical review. *Parkinsonism & Related Disorders, 14*(8), 589.

Li, F., Harmer, P., Fisher, K. J., & McAuley, E. (2004). T'ai Chi: Improving functional balance and predicting subsequent falls in older persons. *Medicine and Science in Sports and Exercise, 36*(12), 2046-2052.

Li, F, Harmer, P., Fisher, K. J., McAuley, E., Chaumeton, N., Eckstrom, E., & Wilson, N. L. (2005). T'ai Chi and fall reductions in older adults: A randomized controlled trial. *The Journals of Gerontology Series A: Biological Sciences and Medical Sciences, 60*(2), 187-194.

Li, F., Fisher, K. J., & Harmer, P. (2005). Improving physical function and blood pressure in older adults through cobblestone mat walking: A randomized trial. *J Am Geriatr Soc, 53*(8), 1305-1312.

Marchetti, G. F. & Whitney, S. L. (2006). Construction and validation of the 4-item dynamic gait index. *Physical Therapy, 86*(12), 1651-1660. doi: 10.2522/ptj.20050402.

Mayo Clinic. (2012). T'ai Chi: A gentle way to fight stress. Retrieved December 28, 2012, from www.mayoclinic.com/health/tai-chi/SA00087.

McCall, T. (2007). *Yoga as medicine. The yogic prescription for health and healing.* New York: Bantam Dell.

McNair, D. M., Lorr, M., & Droppelman, L. F. (1992). EdiTS manual for the profile of mood states. San Diego, California: Education and Industrial Testing Service.

Metzger, W. & Zhou, P. (1996). *T'ai Chi Ch'uan and Qigong: Techniques and training.* New York: Sterling Publishing.

Moadel, A. B., Shah, C., Wylie-Rosett, J., Harris, M. S., Patel, S. R., Hall, C. B., & Sparano, J. A. (2007). Randomized controlled trial of yoga among a multiethnic sample of breast cancer patients: Effects on quality of life. *J Clin Oncol, 25*(28), 4387-4395. doi: JCO.2006.06.6027 [pii]10.1200/JCO.2006.06.6027.

National Center for Chronic Disease Prevention and Health Promotion. (2012). Meditation and health. www.cdc.gov/features/meditation/

National Center for Complementary and Alternative Medicine. (2012). What is complementary and alternative medicine? Retrieved February 1, 2013, from http://nccam.nih.gov/health/whatiscam.

National Parkinson Foundation. (2012). With T'ai Chi, seniors cope with Parkinson's. Retrieved January 10, 2013, from http://parkinson.org/About-Us/Press-Room/NPF-In-The-News/2012/March/With-tai-chi,-seniors-cope-with-Parkinson-s.

Neumark-Sztainer, D., Eisenberg, M. E., Wall, M., & Loth, K. A. (2011). Yoga and Pilates: Associations with body image and disordered-eating behaviors in a population-based sample of young adults. *The International Journal of Eating Disorders, 44*(3), 276-280. doi: 10.1002/eat.20858.

Podsiadlo, D. & Richardson, S. (1991). The timed "Up & Go": a test of basic functional mobility for frail elderly persons. (0002-8614 (Print)).

Schmid, A. A., Van Puymbroeck, M., Altenburger, P. A., Dierks, T. A., Miller, K. K., Damush, T. M., & Williams, L. S. (2012). Balance and balance self-efficacy are associated with activity and participation after stroke: A cross-sectional study in people with chronic stroke. *Archives of Physical Medicine and Rehabilitation, 93*(6), 1101-1107. doi: 10.1016/j.apmr.2012.01.020.

Schmid, A. A., Van Puymbroeck, M., Altenburger, P. A., Schalk, N. L., Dierks, T. A., Miller, K. K., … & Williams, L. S. (2012). Poststroke balance improves with yoga: A pilot study. *Stroke; a Journal of Cerebral Circulation, 43*(9), 2402-2407. doi: 10.1161/STROKEAHA.112.658211.

Schmid, A. A., Van Puymbroeck, M., & Koceja, D. M. (2010). Effect of a 12-week yoga intervention on fear of falling and balance in older adults: A pilot study. *Archives of Physical Medicine and Rehabilitation, 91*(4), 576-583. doi: 10.1016/j.apmr.2009.12.018.

Sun, W. Y. & Chen, W. (1995). *T'ai Chi Ch'uan: The gentle workout for mind & body.* New York: Sterling Publishing.

Tatum, N. G., Bradley, R. C., & Igel, C. (2011). Therapeutic yoga to improve balance and floor transfer in older adults. *Topics in Geriatric Rehabilitation, 27*(2), 134-141. doi: Doi 10.1097/Tgr.0b013e31821bff1d.

Van Puymbroeck, M., Burk, B. N., Shinew, K. J., Kuhlenschmidt, M. C., & Schmid, A. A. (2013). Perceived health benefits from yoga among breast cancer survivors. *American Journal of Health Promotion: AJHP.* doi: 10.4278/ajhp.110316-QUAL-119.

Van Puymbroeck, M., Gleckler, W., Schmid, A. A., Hsieh, P. C., Wang, C., & Koceja, D. (2009). The effects of a 12-week yoga program on the fear of falling in older adults. *International Journal of Yoga Therapy, Supplement 2009,* 53.

Van Puymbroeck, M., Hsieh, P.C., & Pernell, D. (2008). Comparison of two physical activity interventions on the physical fitness for informal caregivers. *American Journal of Recreation Therapy, 7*(1), 35-41.

Van Puymbroeck, M., Payne, L. L., & Hsieh, P. C. (2007). A phase I feasibility study of yoga on the physical health and coping of informal caregivers. *Evidence Based Complementary and Alternative Medicine, 4*(4), 519-529.

Van Puymbroeck, M., Schmid, A., Shinew, K. J., & Hsieh, P. C. (2011). Influence of Hatha yoga on physical activity constraints, physical fitness, and body image of breast cancer survivors: A pilot study. *International Journal of Yoga Therapy 21,* 49-60.

Van Puymbroeck, M., Smith, R., & Schmid, A. (2011). Yoga as a means to negotiate physical activity constraints in middle aged and older adults. *International Journal of Aging and Human Development, 10*(2), 117-121.

Walsh, R. & Roche, L. (1979). Precipitation of acute psychotic episodes by intensive meditation in individuals with a history of schizophrenia. *American Journal of Psychiatry, 136*(8), 1085-1086.

Wang, C. C., Bannuru, R., Ramel, J., Kupelnick, B., Scott, T., & Schmid, C. H. (2010). T'ai Chi on psychological well-being: systematic review and meta-analysis. *Bmc Complementary and Alternative Medicine, 10.* doi: Artn 23 Doi 10.1186/1472-6882-10-23.

Ware, J. E., Gandek, B., & IQOLA Project Group. (1994). The SF-36 health survey: Development and use in mental health research and the IQOLA project. *International Journal of Mental Health, 23*(2), 49-73.

Weil, R. (2013). T'ai Chi. *MedicineNet.com.* from www.medicinenet.com/tai_chi/article.htm.

Wolf, S. L., Sattin, R. W., O'Grady, M., Freret, N., Ricci, L., Greenspan, A. I., … Kutner, M. (2001). A study design to investigate the effect of intense T'ai Chi in reducing falls among older adults transitioning to frailty. *Controlled Clinical Trials, 22*(6), 689-704.

Wolf, S. L., Barnhart, H. X., Kutner, N. G., McNeely, E., Coogler, C., & Xu, T. (1996). Reducing frailty and falls in older persons: An investigation of T'ai Chi and computerized balance training. Atlanta FICSIT Group. Frailty and Injuries: Cooperative Studies of Intervention Techniques. *Journal of the American Geriatrics Society, 44*(5), 489.

Wolf, S. L., Sattin, R. W., Kutner, M., O'Grady, M., Greenspan, A. I., & Gregor, R. J. (2003). Intense T'ai Chi exercise training and fall occurrences in older, transitionally frail adults: A randomized, controlled trial. *Journal of the American Geriatrics Society, 51*(12), 1693-1701.

Yorston, G. A. (2001). Mania precipitated by meditation: A case report and literature review. *Mental Health, Religious Culture, 4*(2), 209.

36. Montessori Method

Genee Bower and Heather R. Porter

The Montessori Method was first developed by Dr. Maria Montessori as a method for educating young children in a slum outside of Rome, Italy. Dr. Montessori created a Casa dei Bambini or House of Children in which everything in the environment, including the furnishings and learning materials, was designed to be both inviting to children (encouraging exploration) and familiar to the child (utilizing practical, everyday materials and tasks for learning) (Montessori, 1914). Montessori (1914) believed "the spirit must take from its environment the nourishment which it needs to develop according to its own 'laws of growth'" (p. 4). To this end, Dr. Montessori provided children with materials and tasks that broke learning into a step-by-step process, which built upon itself. Activities not only broke tasks down into steps, but also had increasingly complex progressions built into them, allowing for continued challenge and mastery. In this way, Montessori learning activities were highly adaptable to the ever-changing skill levels of each child, allowing each child to learn at his/her own pace. Additionally, materials offered multisensory cues, including tactile cues, such as texture or weight, and visual cues, such as color and size. When given instruction, children were shown a step-by-step demonstration with as little verbal instruction as possible. The success achieved by the children in the Casa dei Bambini astonished Dr. Montessori and the world, launching a new philosophy in the education of the young child. In recent years, the Montessori Method has gained new attention in the field of healthcare as a therapeutic intervention, especially when working with clients with dementia.

A search was conducted in the EBSCOhost databases, Academic Search Premier, AgeLine, CINAHL, ERIC, Hospitality and Tourism Complete, MEDLINE, PsycARTICLES, Psychology and Behavioral Sciences Collection, PsycINFO, Social Work Abstracts, and SPORTDiscus with Full Text. The search utilized the search terms Montessori as well as filters for peer reviewed journal articles written in English and published between January 1, 2007, and March 16, 2013. This search yielded 116 results. Of these results, 21 articles were irrelevant, 71 were related to education or early childhood education, and 24 were related to utilizing the Montessori Method as an intervention for people with dementia. No other populations were identified. The focus of this article is on utilizing the Montessori Method for dementia. To gather further information, reference lists and available "cited by" indices were also searched for relevant materials.

Dementia

Dementia is a "chronic, global, usually irreversible deterioration of cognition" which impairs an individual's ability to independently complete activities of daily living (Merck, 2007). Dementia occurs in five percent of those between the ages of 65 and 74 and 40% of the population above the age of 85 (Merck, 2007). Worldwide, 35.6 million cases are reported, with 5.6 million of those cases in the United States (Desai, Schwartz, & Grossberg, 2012). Dementia accounts for over half of new patients admitted to nursing homes (Merck, 2007).

Although symptoms vary both across specific types of dementia and individual cases, dementia can generally be divided into three stages: early, intermediate, and late stage. Symptoms will generally, but not always, progress gradually, with deterioration in short- and long-term memory (b144 Memory Functions), language skills (b167 Mental Functions of Language), cognitive skills (b1 Mental Functions), and the ability to learn or recall new information (d1 Learning and Applying Knowledge) (Merck, 2007).

Dementia eventually erodes a person's ability to manage life and self-care activities independently (Merck, 2007). The combination of cognitive deterioration and loss of independence often leads to frustration, irritability, and other behavioral symptoms (b126 Temperament and Personality Functions, b152 Emotional Functions, d240 Handling Stress and Other Psychological Demands, d710 Basic Interpersonal Interactions, d720 Complex Interpersonal Interactions) (Merck, 2007).

Psychiatric or behavioral symptoms arise in 90% of cases of dementia (Fung, Tsang, & Chung, 2012). While some behaviors are directly attributable to cognitive losses, such as short-term memory deficits, Kovach and colleagues (2005) described the Model of Consequences (C-NDB) which connects many behaviors to needs which remain unmet. In this model, behavioral symptoms are seen as a communication from the person with dementia about some type of need. These behavioral symptoms can be categorized into aggressive behaviors, including physical and verbal aggression; physical behaviors such as pacing, wandering, and perseverative motions; and vocal behaviors, which may include asking questions repetitively (b180 Experience of Self and Time Functions, b164 Higher-Level Cognitive Functions, d710 Basic Interpersonal Interactions, d720 Complex Interpersonal Interactions) (Cohen-Mansfield et al., 2010).

Hancock and colleagues (2005) explored the diverse needs of individuals with dementia, identifying whether those needs were met or unmet for each individual. The findings indicated one in five people surveyed had seven or more unmet needs, and 94% had at least one unmet need (Hancock et al., 2005). The three most common unmet needs were for stimulating daytime activity (e.g., d9 Community, Social, and Civic Life, d570 Looking After One's Health), resolution of psychological distress (b152 Emotional Functions, d240 Handling Stress and Other Psychological Demands), and company (e.g., d7 Interpersonal Interactions and Relationships; d9 Community, Social, and Civic Life) (Hancock, et al., 2005). Hancock et al. (2005) also found unmet needs were associated with depression (b126 Temperament and Personality Functions, b130 Energy and Drive Functions, b152 Emotional Functions, d240 Handling Stress and Other Psychological Demands), anxiety (b126 Temperament and Personality

Functions, b152 Emotional Functions), and increased behavioral symptoms (d7202 Regulating Behaviors within Interactions).

Schölzel-Dorenbos, Meeuwsen, and Rikkert (2010) further developed this work into a Hierarchy Model of Needs in Dementia, dividing identified needs into five levels, based on Maslow's Hierarchy of Needs, and again emphasized the connection between unmet needs and behavioral symptoms. Schölzel-Dorenbos et al. (2010) identified consequences of unmet needs; including behavioral symptoms, increased caregiver burden, decreased health related quality of life (HRQoL), and institutionalization. Schölzel-Dorenbos et al. (2010) point out:

> Professionals should be aware that in dementia care often only the basic levels of needs are partially met, that many needs remain unmet and that much can be done to improve HRQoL. The first goal is to address the simplest goals, but the ultimate goal is to also meet more complex (e.g., emotional and social) unmet needs in such a way that this improves HRQoL. (p. 117)

Utilizing the Montessori Method has been shown to be effective in meeting these types of needs in a variety of studies. Some of the positive outcomes of these studies include:

- decreasing agitation (b126 Temperament and Personality Functions, b152 Emotional Functions, d240 Handling Stress and Other Psychological Demands) (Lin et al., 2009; Giroux, Robichaud, & Paradis, 2010)
- increasing engagement (b130 Energy and Drive Functions, b140 Attention Functions, d9 Community, Social, and Civic Life) (Jarrott, Gozali, & Gigliotti, 2008; Lin et al., 2009)
- improvements in aggressive and nonaggressive behaviors (b152 Emotional Functions, d710 Basic Interpersonal Interactions, d720 Complex Interpersonal Interactions) (Lin et al., 2009)
- decrease in anomia (b144 Memory Functions, b167 Mental Functions of Language, d330 Speaking) (Albrecht, 2010)
- increased participation, including increased active participation, greater periods of participation, decreased time in passive or non-participation, and lower levels of cueing or stimulation required by staff for participation as compared to

regular programming of a non-Montessori nature (d7 Interpersonal Interactions and Relationships, d9 Community, Social, and Civic Life) (Giroux, et al., 2010)

- greater positive affect (b126 Temperament and Personality Functions, b152 Emotional Functions) (Giroux, et al, 2010)
- greater independence in eating ability (d550 Eating) (Lin et al., 2011; Lin et al., 2010; Nightingale, 2011)

Indications

The Montessori Method can be used with all stages of dementia (Mahendra et al., 2011). Mahendra et al. (2011) point out that while individuals with dementia display deficits in memory function (b144 Memory Functions), certain memory functions actually remain fairly intact, including the ability to attend to pleasurable stimuli and procedural memory. By tapping into these spared abilities, interventions such as Montessori-based programming can provide opportunities for success, achievement, and even improvement in behaviors, affect, and functional abilities. The Montessori Method may be particularly useful when clients with dementia are showing signs of boredom or restlessness, or exhibiting some of the behavioral symptoms which may indicate these conditions (Brenner, 2012).

Contraindications

Although the Montessori Method is designed to be adaptable for all levels of development and skill, certain precautions should be considered with clients with dementia. Depending on the stage of dementia, certain Montessori materials, such as small manipulatives or sorting and pouring items may not be appropriate because clients may place these items in their mouths. Activities can be adapted by replacing these items with something that is safe to eat or something larger. Also, if a client has difficulty with fine motor skills (d440 Fine Hand Use) due to lost dexterity or pain from secondary conditions, such as arthritis, activities that focus on fine motor skills may need to be adapted (e.g., utilizing adaptive grips, building up grips with foam tubing, or using materials which are easier to grasp). The key to success with the Montessori Method is to adapt the activity to the client in such a way as to ensure success while still presenting a challenge (Brenner, 2012).

Protocols and Processes

The Montessori Method is not so much a set prescription for a narrow group of clients as it is a philosophy of care which can be adapted to a wide variety of clients. One of the strengths of the Montessori Method, its adaptability and flexibility, can also be a potential challenge when utilizing the theory to design and implement treatment sessions or programming. Just how does one know the program they are implementing is truly Montessori based? Does the application of one of the Montessori ideas, such as brightly colored materials, make an activity Montessori? To provide guidance, a list of foundational principles gleaned from Montessori's work (1912) as well as that of Brenner (2012) and Elliot (2007) follows. These specific principles are applied throughout the APIE process, including when choosing materials, choosing activities, designing progressions, and implementing leadership. A sample activity which was conducted successfully (Albrecht, 2010), accompanies each principle as an illustration of putting these principles into practice.

Principle 1: Choosing Materials

When choosing materials, ensure they are familiar, pleasing, and easy to sense (see, hear, read, grasp, etc.).

When Dr. Montessori (1912) prepared the environment in her children's house, she insured that every element was designed for the accessibility and engagement of her young pupils, including furniture sized for the young child, blocks, learning materials, and even brooms and dustpans sized for little hands to easily manipulate. She used brightly colored, aesthetically pleasing materials. In adapting this concept for the client with dementia, one can follow Dr. Montessori's lead by combining elements which please the senses with elements which take into consideration the population's particular needs, such as sensory loss or memory deficits.

Example: Albrecht (2010) successfully utilized an activity involving silk flowers in one case study to assist a client with anomia due to dementia. The activity used silk versions of four common (*familiar, pleasing, easy to sense*) types of flowers (rose, daffodil, daisy, and sunflower) and a poster board on which to sort them. The poster board had four holes through which the stems of the flowers could be placed. Under each hole there were four round stickers and four square stickers. Additional cueing material included four circles to match the round stickers (*familiar, easy to sense*) on the board, and four squares to match the square stickers. Each circle contained a picture of one of the types of flowers, and each square contained the typed name of one of the four flowers.

Principle 2: Choosing Activities

When choosing activities, ensure they are self-correcting, able to be broken down into steps, easily adapted to an appropriate level of challenge, and meaningful for clients.

Choosing activities that hold meaning for the client not only increases the likelihood of their participation in the activity, it also magnifies the benefits received from the activity (Brenner, 2012; Elliot, 2007). For example, Brenner (2012) writes of a woman who loved flowers. This woman was exhibiting behavioral symptoms which were causing her caregivers and family distress. When presented with fresh flowers and supplies for flower arranging, she immediately became engrossed in the activity and created arrangements for each table in the dining room. Not only was the client no longer engaged in destructive behaviors, she was fully engaged in an activity she enjoyed that held meaning for her, while also contributing to her community.

In addition to choosing activities based on interest, finding activities that are congruent with abilities also requires consideration. To give some guidance to the practitioner in choosing appropriate activities for the three stages of dementia, Mahendra et al. (2011) compiled information from Camp (1999) and Vance and Johns (2002) to create a chart which divides Montessori activities into categories and describes which stage of dementia each category may be most appropriate for. The activity categories which fall under each stage are as follows:

- *Mild dementia*: Matching activities, including sorting; care of the person, including folding and hanging clothes; care of the environment, including plant care, flower arranging, and setting tables; fine motor activities, including stringing beads, lacing, and painting; and squeezing activities including using a hole punch, tongs, or garlic press.
- *Moderate dementia*: All of the above activities and seriation activities (arranging items in a spe-

cific order such as smallest to largest); pouring activities such as pouring drinks; and scooping activities utilizing spoons, scoops, or bowls.
- *Late stage dementia*: Scooping activities utilizing spoons, scoops, or bowls; and sensory discrimination activities such as sounds, colors, weights, temperature, or smell.

Lastly, recreational therapists may want to consider the utilization of intergenerational activities. Lee, Camp, and Malone (2007) conducted a study on the effects of intergenerational Montessori-based programming and found that by creating dyads of one adult with one child, residents had periods of constructive engagement that averaged five times longer and had lower levels of passive or non-active engagement when compared with regularly scheduled, non-Montessori programming. The study emphasizes the need for carefully planned activities that match the skill levels of the participants (Lee et al., 2007).

Example: The utilization by Albrecht (2010) of squares and circles described above is one example of a *self-correcting* element. By providing the shapes as additional cues to where each item can be placed, the client is able to self-assess and correct when an error is made. This enhances the client's chances of success. The activity was *broken down into steps* with each level of matching, from the typed word to the photograph and the three-dimensional representation in the form of the silk flower. This activity could be *adapted* for greater difficulty by removing the additional cue of the shapes described earlier, or it could be made easier by adding color cues for each type of flower. Additionally, a completed sample board could be given to the client when first beginning the activity. Finally, as mentioned previously, it is important that the activity hold *meaning* for the client. The choice of flowers was appropriate for this client. Perhaps a choice of model cars would hold more meaning for a different client.

Principle 3: Progressions

Ensure progressions move from simple to complex, concrete to abstract, and, where applicable, top to bottom and left to right.

Dr. Montessori (1912) utilized progressions as a foundation for her method. This element of the Montessori Method is particularly important for use with clients with dementia, as it provides the adaptability required to match a client's skill level to an appropriate progression of an activity. By choosing the appropriate progression level of an activity a client is able to experience success (Brenner, 2012) and build on the strengths which created that success (Elliot, 2007).

Example: In the example activity, Albrecht (2010) began by inviting the client to read the names of each of the flowers on the cards and then place that card on the board. Then the client was invited to place each picture on the board above the name which it matched. Finally the client was given the artificial flowers to place above the pictures and names. In this case, Albrecht was assessing the client's ability to move from the abstract to the concrete, which is why the items were ordered in this way. One could use the same materials, and utilizing the above principles of progression, begin with placing the *simple, concrete* silk flowers at the top, then progress to the more *complex, abstract* picture, and finally to the most *abstract* representation, the typed word.

Principle 4: Leading

When leading activities, whenever possible, use demonstration rather than verbal instruction; utilize visual and/or sensory cues; maximize the chances of success, while still presenting adequate challenge; utilize preserved skills and strengths as much as possible; emphasize the process, rather than the outcome; build on strengths; and work to minimize barriers.

Mahendra, Scullion, and Hammerschlag (2011) identify five key elements of leading a successful intervention for clients with dementia. Each of these elements is a hallmark of the Montessori Method.

- Provide repeated presentation of target information.
- Incorporate learning by doing and requiring active generation of target responses.
- Reduce the possibility of errors during initial learning.
- Tap into relatively spared sustained attention and minimize distractions.
- Use rich, tangible sensory stimuli and meaningful cues to support retrieval.

Example: Albrecht (2010) utilized visual cues in the form of the flowers themselves, the photos, and the circle and square shapes in order to *maximize her*

client's chances of success. When the client had difficulty, Albrecht (2010) gave verbal cues, as necessary, which also increased the client's chances of success and emphasized the client's *process* of working through the challenge, rather than focusing on an outcome of a correct answer with no cueing necessary. By providing multiple cues and easily read print, Albrecht (2010) also *minimized barriers*. In repeating the exercise with the client, Albrecht (2010) tapped into procedural memory, an *often-preserved ability* in clients with dementia, and was able to *build* on the client's earlier successes. Although it is not stated by Albrecht, it would certainly be possible to *demonstrate* the activity prior to inviting the client to participate.

Outcomes and Documentation

Various measures and tools have been used in studies to document the effectiveness of the Montessori Method for clients with dementia. Tracking the client with ICF assessments to connect the intervention with the diagnosis is always a useful plan. The following information details some of the other tools and how they were utilized in studies. The use of appropriate tools to measure the effectiveness of Montessori interventions is crucial to the continued efforts to explore how this method can best be utilized to effectively treat clients with dementia.

Cohen-Mansfield Agitation Inventory (CMAI)
Frequency of agitated behaviors
Lin et al., 2009

Ease-of-Care Inventory
To obtain a picture of agitation from the staff point of view
Lin et al., 2009

Philadelphia Geriatric Center Affect Rating Scale (ARS)
Affect
Giroux, Robichaud, and Paradis, 2010

Apparent Affect Rating Scale (AARS)
Affect
Jarrott et al., 2008; Lin et al., 2009

Menorah Park Engagement Scale
Level of active participation and engagement
Jarrott et al., 2008; Van der Ploeg and O'Connor, 2010

Edinburgh Feeding Evaluation in Dementia (EdFED)
Independent eating ability
Lin et al., 2010, 2011

Eating Behavior Scale (EBS)
Independent eating ability
Lin et al., 2010, 2011

*Myers-Menorah Park Montessori Based Assessment System (MMP/MAS) *currently being developed*
Preserved skills and strengths that can be built on (Camp and Malone, 2007). Utilizes:

- Hand washing.
- Short story.
- Depth perception and color intensity booklet.
- Category sorting, fine motor skills, and color matching.
- Dressing vest.

Resources

Brenner Pathways Alzheimer's Memory Support

www.brennerpathways.org/about/

This website hosted by Tom and Karen Brenner provides an overview of the Montessori Method for clients with dementia, as well as a blog with activity ideas and inspirational and anecdotal entries.

The Myers Research Institute

www.myersresearch.org/home.html

Multiple studies on Montessori-based dementia programming have been conducted by the Myers Research Institute. Their website provides access to their newsletter, as well as Montessori materials including games and manuals.

Center for Applied Research in Dementia

www.cen4ard.com/Home.php

This organization conducts research and offers publications related to Montessori-based interventions for dementia, as well as a recommended reading list, and training in the Montessori Method for clients with dementia.

References

Albrecht, S. (2010). Activity development in dementia due to Alzheimer's disease. *Activities Directors' Quarterly for Alzheimer's & Other Dementia Patients, 11*(1), 27-34.

Brenner, T. (2012). The Montessori method in dementia care. *Journal of Dementia Care, 20*(4), 18-19.

Camp, C. J. (1999). *Montessori-based activities for persons with dementia: Volume 1.* Beachwood, OH: Menorah Park Center for Senior Living.

Cohen-Mansfield, J., Dakheel-Ali, M., Jensen, B., Marx, M. S., & Thein, K. (2012). An analysis of the relationships among

engagement, agitated behavior, and affect in nursing home residents with dementia. *International Psychogeriatrics / IPA, 24*(5), 742-11.

Desai, A. K., Schwartz, L., & Grossberg, G. T. (2012). Behavioral disturbance in dementia. *Current Psychiatry Reports, 14*(4), 298-309.

Elliot, G. (2007). A focus on Montessori-based dementia programming. *Canadian Nursing Home, 19*(1), 35-49.

Fung, J. K. M, Tsang, H. W. H., & Chung, R. C. K. (2012). A systematic review of the use of aromatherapy in treatment of behavioral problems in dementia. *Geriatrics & Gerontology International, 12*(3), 372-382.

Giroux, D., Robichaud, L., & Paradis, M. (2010) Using the Montessori approach for a clientele with cognitive impairments: A quasi-experimental study design. *International Journal Aging and Human Development, 71*(1), 23-41.

Hancock, G. A., Woods, B., Challis, D., & Orrell, M. (2006). The needs of older people with dementia in residential care. *International Journal of Geriatric Psychiatry, 21,* 43-49.

Jarrott, S. E., Gozali, T., & Gigliotti, C. M. (2008) Montessori programming for persons with dementia in the group setting. *Dementia, 7*(1), 109-125.

Kovach, C. R., Noonan, P. E., Schlidt, A. M., & Wells, T. (2005). A model of consequences of need-driven, dementia-compromised behavior. *Journal of Nursing Scholarship, 37*(2), 134-140.

Lee, M. M., Camp, C. J., & Malone, M. L. (2007). Effects of intergenerational Montessori-based activities programming on engagement of nursing home residents with dementia. *Clinical Interventions in Aging, 2*(3), 477-483.

Lin, L., Huang, Y., Su, S., Watson, R., Tsai, B. W., & Wu, S. (2010). Using spaced retrieval and Montessori-based activities in improving eating ability for residents with dementia. *International Journal of Geriatric Psychiatry, 25,* 953-959.

Lin, L., Huang, Y., Watson, R., Wu, S., & Lee, Y. (2011). Using a Montessori Method to increase eating ability for institutionalized residents with dementia: A crossover design. *Journal of Clinical Nursing, 20,* 3092-3101.

Lin, L., Yang, M., Kao, C., Wu, S., Tang, S., & Lin, J. (2009). Using acupressure and Montessori-based activities to decrease agitation for residents with dementia: A crossover trial. *The American Geriatrics Society, 57,* 1022-1029.

Mahendra, N., Scullion, A., & Hammerschlag, C. (2011). Cognitive-linguistic interventions for persons with dementia: A practitioner's guide to 3 evidence-based techniques. *Topics in Geriatric Rehabilitation, 27*(4), 278-288.

Merck Manual; 2007; Retrieved September 16, 2012 www.merckmanuals.com/professional/neurologic_disorders/delirium_and_dementia/dementia.html.

Montessori, M. (1912). A critical consideration of the new pedagogy in its relation to modern science. The Montessori Method: Scientific pedagogy as applied to child education in "The Children's Houses" with additions and revisions by the author. (pp. 1-24) (A. E. George, Trans.). New York: Frederick A. Stokes Company. (Original work published 1909). Retrieved from http://digital.library.upenn.edu/women/montessori/method/method.html.

Montessori, M. (1914). *Dr. Montessori's own handbook.* (pp. 1-68) New York: Frederick A. Stokes Company.

Nightingale, D. (2011). Montessori success for people living with dementia. *Journal of Dementia Care, 19*(2), 36-38.

Schölzel-Dorenbos, C. J., Meeuwsen, E. J., & Olde Rikkert, M. G,. (2010). Integrating unmet needs into dementia health-related quality of life research and care: Introduction of the Hierarchy Model of Needs in Dementia. *Aging and Mental Health, 14*(1), 113-119.

Skrajner, M. J., Malone, M. L., Camp, C. J., McGowan, A., & Gorzelle, G. J. (2007). Research in practice I: Montessori-based dementia programming. *Alzheimer's Care Quarterly, 8*(1), 53-64.

Vance, D. E. & Johns, R. N. (2002). Montessori improved cognitive domains in adults with Alzheimer's disease. *Phys. Occup. Ther. Geriatr., 20*(3, 4), 19-36.

Van der Ploeg, E. S. & O'Connor, D. W. (2010). Evaluation of personalised, one-to-one interaction using Montessori-type activities as a treatment of challenging behaviours in people with dementia: The study protocol of a crossover trial. *BMC Geriatrics, 10*(3).

37. Motor Learning and Training Strategies

Heather R. Porter

A motor skill is a coordinated voluntary motor sequence that is purposeful and goal oriented, such as throwing a ball. Types of motor skills include (O'Sullivan & Schmitz, 2010):

Gross motor skills: Involve the use of large muscle groups where precision of movement is not important to the successful execution of the skill (e.g., running, jumping, throwing).

Fine motor skills: Utilization of small muscle groups where precision of movement is important to the successful execution of the skill (e.g., painting, writing, typing).

Closed motor skills: Skills that are performed in a stable and predictable environment (e.g., walking in a quiet therapy gym).

Open motor skills: Skills that are performed in a variable and unpredictable environment (e.g., walking at a busy shopping mall).

Discrete motor skills: Skills that have a clear beginning and end point as defined by the task (e.g., opening a milk carton).

Serial motor skills: Discrete motor skills that are chained together in a sequential pattern (e.g., performing the sequential motor skills to paint a picture — open a bottle of paint, pour the paint in a cup, pick up a paint brush, dip the paint brush in the paint, manipulate the brush on the paper, and so on).

Continuous motor skills: Skills that have beginning and end points that are defined by the individual or an external factor (e.g., swimming, bicycling).

Simple motor skills: Skills that involve a single motor action (e.g., kicking a ball).

Complex motor skills: Skills that involve multiple motor actions to produce a coordinated movement (e.g., running and kicking a soccer ball during a game).

Dual-task motor skills: Skills that require the integration of multiple motor actions (e.g., walking and carrying shopping bags).

Criterion skills: Skills being monitored to assess the success or failure of the client in performing an action. A single criterion skill may be made up of a large set of other skills.

Precursor skills: The set of skills that need to be available before a criterion skill can be accomplished.

Impairments in motor control, defined as the underlying neuromuscular system processes that activate motor skills, are addressed though a variety of motor learning techniques to aid in motor recovery or development. Motor control is typically divided into two types: reactive motor control (motor responses that are a reaction to an outside stimulus, such as putting one's hand out to stop a fall) and proactive or anticipatory motor control (motor responses that are planned in preparation for the task at hand, such as getting into position to effectively launch the basketball into the hoop) (O'Sullivan & Schmitz, 2010).

Indications

Clients may have impairments with motor skills (b760 Control of Voluntary Movement Functions) as a result of injury (e.g., car accident, stroke) or delayed development. Motor skills might also be impaired as a result of the aging process from a decline in CNS function, changes in body weight or shape, and lower levels of physical activity causing a loss of muscle strength or flexibility and range of motion (b710 Mobility of Joint Functions, b730 Muscle Power Functions, b735 Muscle Tone Functions, b740 Muscle Endurance Functions) (O'Sullivan & Schmitz, 2010). Motor skill impairments may also be diagnosed with codes in d4 Mobility.

Motor recovery is highly variable and full recovery may not be achievable. It is more likely that the therapist will be able to assist the client in attaining modified motor skills, such as using the torso and legs to propel a ball if throwing is no longer possible. In some instances, motor recovery does not happen and the therapist will need to utilize a compensation approach to adapt the activity for abilities and limitations.

Some clients may exhibit spontaneous recovery from the initial neural repair process of the body unrelated to intervention, whereas others may show function-induced recovery in response to therapeutic interventions designed to stimulate the neural connections. Despite the course of motor recovery, stimulation of motor recovery should be initiated early in the rehabilitation process to combat learned non-use (O'Sullivan & Schmitz, 2010).

Contraindications

When working on motor recovery, utilizing the specific activity (e.g., throwing a baseball) as the criterion skill can be contraindicated. For example, in order to throw a baseball from a seated position, the client must first have good static and dynamic sitting balance, trunk control, and trunk rotation and flexion. The client will also need sufficient active range of motion in the arm that will be throwing the baseball, as well as the ability to grasp and release the ball. These lead-up skills are often referred to as precursor skills. It is also important to note that integrating all of these components into a whole (throwing the baseball) is a skill in and of itself that requires training.

Having a client engage in a criterion skill in a situation where the client lacks adequate precursor skills may facilitate bad motor habits (e.g., compensating for deficits by utilizing other muscle groups and movements) and also induce feelings of fear, increase risk of injury or harm, and reduce self-efficacy and self-worth. In this situation, the therapist begins by working on the precursor skills required for the criterion skill. As precursor skills are accomplished, the therapist can then introduce the client to more complex movements that integrate precursor skills into a whole. For example, if the client demonstrates good trunk stability, along with sufficient shoulder, elbow, and wrist active range of motion, but is unable to open and close his fist, the therapist

might work on having the client bat a balloon, integrating all of the precursor skills into a single task. Keep in mind, however, that therapy sessions are not fully linear. For example, although the therapist may integrate several precursor skills into a whole as the client's skills progress (e.g., batting a balloon), the therapist can also continue to work on single precursor skills that are still needed to perform the criterion skill, in this example that would be working on tasks that facilitate the ability to open and close the fist. These precursor skills are integrated as the skills are achieved.

It is also important to remember that prolonged practice of precursor skills without accompanying practice of the criterion skill can lead to limited transfer of precursor skills into a criterion skill resulting in "splinter skills" (single skills that do not relate to an ability to complete a functional task) (O'Sullivan & Schmitz, 2010). Additionally, clients who experience severe impairments, such as severe stroke or traumatic brain injury, may be more prone to develop splinter skills due to severe CNS dysfunction impairing the ability to integrate and transfer precursor skills into a whole.

Protocols and Processes

Prior to implementing a treatment plan aimed at motor recovery, the therapist first conducts a comprehensive assessment to determine baseline levels of physical functioning (strength, endurance, active range of motion), along with cognitive, social, and emotional functioning that can influence motor behavior. This may include memory, attention, level of caregiver involvement, stress, delusions, and many other areas of functioning. The therapist also assesses personal and environmental contextual factors that influence or have the potential to influence motor behavior and function, such as personality and environmental challenges.

O'Sullivan and Schmitz (2010) additionally discuss the importance of assessing information about the skills being observed. Therapists should assess the client's "anticipation timing" (the ability of the client to time movements related to a target, such as swinging a bat to hit a baseball) and to consider "regulatory conditions" (things in the environment that require the individual to mold his/her movements in order to be successful, such as stepping onto an escalator).

Therapists should note if the movement is a closed skill being performed in a standardized environment or an open skill being performed in a variable and changing environment. They should also note if the movements are a self-paced skill initiated, controlled, and modified by the individual, such as a walk in the park, or if they are an externally paced skill dictated by the environment, such as crossing a busy street. All of this information is then integrated to form an individualized treatment plan to improve motor recovery in the context of personally meaningful activity.

Clients who lack the ability to complete part or all of a motor task often need to have the task broken down into discrete steps. There are two intertwined processes used to teach motor skills to clients. The first process is to conduct a task analysis of the activity so that both the client and the therapist are familiar with the discrete steps required to complete the activity. The second process is using information on how people learn to maximize skill development. Both of these are combined with knowledge of sequential motor return to best identify and stimulate the client's progress. The following can be used as a rule of thumb for the common order of motor return (O'Sullivan & Schmitz, 1988, p. 271):

- Gross motor control precedes the development of fine motor control.
- Return of function tends to occur in cephalocaudal order (head to toe).
- Return of function tends to occur in proximal-distal directions (center of body to peripherals of body; shoulder to hand).
- Flexion and extension before rotation.
- Isometric movements (holding a posture) before isotonic control (moving in a posture).
- Symmetrical movement patterns before asymmetrical movement patterns.
- Discrete movements before continuous movements.
- Static control before dynamic control of posture.

O'Sullivan and Schmitz (2010, 2007) outline a three-phase process that clients go through as they learn new motor skills. The three phases are the cognitive phase, the associative phase, and the autonomous phase.

Cognitive Phase of Motor Learning

The first step in learning a new motor skill is to develop an understanding of the task. To understand the task the client must be able to do four things: know the specific steps and demands of the task, compare his/her abilities against the skills required, develop strategies to compensate for missing skills, and organize his/her thought process to learn and complete elements of the task. Training strategies at this phase include:

Demonstrating the task at the ideal performance speed.

Providing clear and concise verbal instructions on how to perform the skill to prepare the client for movement and reduce uncertainty and anxiety. Verbal instructions and cues might be given for timing of movements, what movement to perform, how to perform the movement. Asking the client to verbalize the components of the task will give the therapist feedback on how well the task is understood.

Teaching individual components of the task and then the task as a whole. This may involve stringing together a series of movements to perform an entire task, such as completing a transfer or putting together a set of precursor tasks such as those involved in throwing a baseball.

Manually guiding the client through the desired movement. This consists of hands-on assistance to guide the client's movements, enhance the client's understanding of the movement sequence, and allow the client to learn the sensation of the movement. The therapist only provides the amount of assistance needed with the goal of decreasing guided movements.

Giving added attention to important elements of the task. The client should concentrate on each component of the movement and look closely at how each movement affects the task.

Reinforcing the importance of performing a slow and controlled movement.

Using visual feedback, for example a long mirror, as a direct modality for feedback.

Repeating movement in a quiet and distraction-free environment to enhance learning and attention.

Identifying consistent movement errors and intervening on only those movements. Do not overstimulate or frustrate the client by commenting on errors that are not consistent.

Intervening if safety concerns arise.

Allowing adequate rest periods.

Associative Phase of Motor Learning

The second phase is called the associative phase. At this phase the client practices movement patterns learned in the first phase. Through practice, skills become more refined and errors decrease. Visual and verbal cues become less important and proprioceptive cues become very important. Training strategies at this stage include:

Having organized and consistent practice sessions that allow for trial and error learning, limiting corrections to consistently observed errors. Feedback should reinforce good habits and movements while pointing out consistent poor habits and movements. Clients with motor dysfunction may not be receiving full sensory feedback due to CNS dysfunction and therefore need verbal instructions to modify movements, but the goal in this stage is to move to proprioceptive feedback.

Encouraging the client to feel the movement. The client should learn to listen to proprioceptive cues and decrease reliance on visual cues and hands-on guidance from the therapist.

Encouraging client to self-assess performance, recognize intrinsic feedback, and modify movements accordingly. The client should be taking a more active decision-making role.

Practicing movements in a more real-life environment, such as walking in the hallways with other people instead of in the clinic, and gradually progressing to practicing movement patterns in an environment that is less predictable, such as walking outdoors.

Autonomous Phase of Motor Learning

The third phase is called the autonomous phase. The client continues to refine his/her movement pattern skills, and the need for cues from the therapist decreases. Movements are more automatic, error-free, and can be performed in any environment. Training strategies include:

Continuing practice sessions that are organized and consistent.

Encouraging the client to strive for consistent performance.

Promoting development of movement pattern skills in real-life environments that have fewer controls.

Designing and causing distractions that challenge divided attention so the client can work on maintaining focus on movement patterns when challenged with simultaneously occurring tasks (e.g., holding a conversation while walking or carrying an item while walking).

Outcomes and Documentation

Motor learning can be measured by changes in performance throughout the period of training, retention (ability to perform the skill after an extended time period of no training), generalizability (ability to generalize and adapt the motor skill to another task), and resistance to contextual change (ability to perform the skill in different environments) (O'Sullivan & Schmitz, 2010). Changes in ICF codes discussed in the Indications section also document the efficacy of the treatment interventions.

Measuring performance changes during rehabilitation is the most common, although it should not be the sole source of measurement. Therapists need to be aware that many variables can influence performance such as fatigue, medication, motivation, and mood. Consequently, when measuring performance changes, these variables should also be recorded.

References

O'Sullivan, S. & Schmitz, T. (2010). *Improving functional outcomes in physical rehabilitation*. Philadelphia, PA: F. A. Davis Company.

O'Sullivan, S. & Schmitz, T. (2007). *Physical rehabilitation* (5th ed.). Philadelphia, PA: F. A. Davis Company.

O'Sullivan, S. & Schmitz, T. (1988). *Physical rehabilitation: Assessment and treatment*. Philadelphia, PA: F. A. Davis Company.

38. Neuro-Developmental Treatment

Kathryn D. Elokdah

The 1940s brought a new treatment for children with cerebral palsy through the work of Berta Bobath, a physiotherapist, and her husband Karel, a physician. For almost 50 years they developed and refined their belief that movement is not learned, but rather that experiencing the sensations of movement are what enable individuals to learn how to move effectively (Keser et al., 2013). Their body of work is known and utilized worldwide as Neuro-Developmental Treatment (NDT) or the Bobath Approach. NDT focuses on improving motor control and motor output to improve functional skills (NDTA, 2005).

There has been a long history of neurophysiological approaches promoting development or recovery from motor impairment. They have gone by several names as the field has developed. The Muscle Re-education Approach was used in the 1920s. The techniques were called a Neurodevelopmental Approach from the 1940s to 1970s. Specific names during that period included the Sensorimotor Approach developed by Rood in the 1940s, the Movement Therapy Approach developed by Brunnstrom in the 1950s, the Neuro-Developmental Treatment or Bobath Approach developed by Bobath in the 1960s to 1970s, and the Proprioceptive Neuromuscular Facilitation (PNF) Approach developed by Knot and Voss, also in the 1960s to 1970s.

In the 1980s the Motor Relearning Program for Stroke was developed and the Contemporary Task-Oriented Approach was developed in the 1990s (MacWalter, n.d.; Pollock et al., 2007). The 2000s and 2010s produced many more approaches for motor recovery. Electric stimulation, including transcutaneous electrical nerve stimulation, functional electrical stimulation, neuromuscular electrical stimulation, and electromyographic biofeedback, has been used with some success for several different

clinical purposes including motor recovery (Van Peppen et al., 2004).

Robotic-aided systems developed almost simultaneously and divided into upper (Volpe et al., 2000) and lower limb training robots (Visintin et al., 1998). Robotic systems continue to be designed and some provide partial body-weight-supported treadmill training (Nilsson et al., 2001). The 2000s and 2010s have seen virtual reality systems developed as a standalone approach (Riva et al., 1997) and used in combination with robotic-aided systems (Walker et al., 2010).

Constraint-Induced Movement Therapy was developed in the 2000s. It continues to show positive outcomes, alone and combined with other approaches (Veerbeek et al., 2014). See the Constraint-Induced Movement Therapy chapter for more information.

Thermal Stimulation (Chen, Liang, & Shaw, 2005) rounds out a not-all-inclusive list of approaches started in 2000s and 2010s. Other approaches currently being investigated include motor imagery (Dodakian, Stewart, & Cramer, 2014), mirror therapy (Thieme et al., 2012) and neural stem cell transplantation (Wang & Zhang, 2014). Clinicians and researchers continue to investigate novel approaches to optimize the development and recovery of motor impairment.

This chapter will discuss one of the major approaches currently utilized to rehabilitate clients — NDT (Edwards, 2002; Lennon, Ashburn, & Baxter, 2006; Szklut & Philibert, 2007).

Indications

The NDT Approach was developed for the treatment of individuals with pathophysiology of the central nervous system (CNS), primarily children with cerebral palsy (CP) (Bobath & Bobath, 1964; Szklut & Philibert, 2007). It was then extended to include adults with impaired neurological conditions including cerebral vascular accident (CVA) (Bobath, 1990; Tyson et al., 2009). This approach continues to evolve over time and the founders, Berta and Karel Bobath, encouraged integration of new neuro-scientific evidence, keeping NDT dynamic (Bobath, 1980; Szklut & Philibert, 2007).

Clinicians and researchers implement NDT alone and integrated with other techniques to develop or recover motor function beyond the diagnoses of CP and CVA. The Bobath Centre in London, United Kingdom, states that they provide service for the treatment of neuro-developmental conditions such as CP and treatment of people with acquired neurological conditions caused, for example, by strokes or head injury, multiple sclerosis, incomplete spinal cord injury, and Parkinson's (Bobath Centre, 2013). Multiple research studies (Czupryna & Nowotny, 2012; Kiebzak et al., 2012; Yue et al., 2012) utilize or acknowledge NDT interventions as "standard of care" in the treatment of clients throughout the world. Reports are available from the United States (Natarajan et al., 2008), the United Kingdom (Tyson et al., 2009), Poland (Kim et al., 2012), China (Yue et al., 2012), Korea (Kim et al., 2012), Turkey (Huseyinsinoglu, Ozdincler, & Krespi, 2012), Australia (Brock et al., 2011), Japan (Anttila et al., 2008), India (Arya et al., 2012), Croatia (Jelica et al., 2011), Canada (Levin & Panturin, 2011), Norway (Anttila et al., 2008), and elsewhere.

When a client presents with motor impairments of CNS pathophysiology origins, treatment with NDT should be considered. Successful implementation of NDT includes reduced impairment and improved functional ability via normalized movement patterns. Research implemented with adults post-stroke shows significant changes in several aspects: normalization of upper limb muscle tone (b735 Muscle Tone Functions) in individuals post ischemic stroke on the *Ashworth Scale for Grading Spasticity* (Mikolajewska, 2012), faster return of the ability to perform ADLs (e.g., d230 Carrying Out Daily Routine, d5 Self-Care), improvement in functional condition and regression of pareses when combined with PNF treatment as assessed with the *International Scale of Muscle Weakness* (ISMW), *Barthel Index*, and modified *Rankin Scale* (Brzuszkiewicz-Kuzmicka, Kuzmicki, & Domaniecki, 2012).

Constraint-Induced Movement Therapy and the Bobath Concept (NDT) have similar efficiencies in improving functional ability, speed, and quality of movement in the paretic arm among individuals who sustained a stroke with a high level of function (b7 Neuromusculoskeletal and Movement-Related Functions) (Huseyinsinoglu et al., 2012). They also are effective for recovering walking velocity (d450 Walking) (Brock et al., 2011), more normal movement patterns (e.g., b770 Gait Pattern Functions), functional ability (Lennon, 2001), leg function (e.g., b760 Control of Voluntary Movement Functions), balance (b755 Involuntary Movement Reaction Functions, d415 Maintaining a Body Position), transfer (d420 Transferring Oneself), walking (d450 Walking), and stair climbing (d4551 Climbing). Measures improved on the Motor Relearning Programme (MRP) during rehabilitation of individuals who sustained a stroke as assessed with *Motor Assessment Scale, Sødring Motor Evaluation Scale, Nottingham Health Profile*, and the *Barthel Index* (Langhammer & Stanghelle, 2011). Shoulder pain (b2801 Pain in Body Part) was reduced and tone increased (b735 Muscle Tone Functions) (Luke, Dodd, & Brock, 2004).

Adults with CP had improved gait patterns with enhanced stability of gait and posture (b147 Psychomotor Functions, b770 Gait Pattern Functions, d415 Maintaining a Body Position), as well as pelvic-limb dissociation (Kim et al., 2012).

Children with CP have had positive outcomes with NDT as well. A small study looked at 44 children with a central coordination disorder (CCD) in early life who were treated according to Vojta's Method (VM) with elements of sensory integration (SI) and NDT. The researchers measured the effect on the development of visual perception later in life. As adolescents, original subjects were tested with a visual perception IQ test. The conclusions showed early treatment of children with CCD with VM, SI, and NDT affords a possibility of normalizing their psychomotor development (b147 Psychomotor Functions) early enough to prevent consequences in the form of cognitive impairments in later life (Kiebzak et al., 2012). Additional research implemented on children with CP shows improvement in the following areas: foot and knee behavior during gait (b710 Mobility of Joint Functions, b760 Control of Voluntary Movement Functions, b770 Gait Pattern Functions) (Czupryna & Nowotny, 2012); functional speech skills (e.g., b320 Articulation Functions, b330 Fluency and Rhythm of Speech Functions) (Puyuelo & Rondal, 2005); motor function (b760 Control of Voluntary Movement Functions, b147 Psychomotor Functions), and self-care skills (d5 Self-Care) as tested with the *Gross Motor Function Measure* and *Pediatric Evaluation of Disability Inventory* (Knox & Evans, 2002). When NDT was done in conjunction with surgery on the cervical dorsal root, improvement was found in upper limb motor function (b760 Control of Voluntary Movement Functions; d445 Hand and Arm Use) (Zhang et al., 2009).

In addition, there have been research studies proving the effectiveness of NDT with other neurological diseases such as muscular dystrophy (Oygard, Haestad, & Jorgensen, 2011) and multiple sclerosis (Smedal et al., 2006). In 2013, Keser et al. concluded, "although trunk exercises based on the Bobath concept are rarely applied in MS rehabilitation, the results of this study show that they are as effective as routine neurorehabilitation exercises" (p. 133).

The outcomes expected from implementation of NDT are improved normal movement patterns, which facilitate improvement in an individual's functional ability (Bobath, 1990; Bobath, 1980). The theory and applied learning of treatment techniques to promote normal movement are provided in post-graduate NDT education.

Contraindications

No evidence-based research of NDT effectiveness exists for treatment of other causes beyond pathophysiology of the CNS. Spina bifida, for example, does not involve damage to the brain and the Bobath Centre in Britain does not provide treatment to these individuals (Centre, 2013). There is also no current research that use of NDT for other causes is contraindicated. Broadly, NDT, along with all treatment approaches, continues to be challenged for validity and effectiveness in the treatment of diseases and disabilities. Contraindications will be formulated from future evidence.

Despite more than 50 years of clinical use, NDT's effectiveness remains questionable (Paci, 2003). A systematic review of interventions for children with CP was completed in 2013 by Novak, et al., with the aim of describing the best available

intervention evidence. It concluded with the recommendation to not utilize NDT (passive handling and guidance to optimize function) for attaining three intervention outcomes: normalized movement; preventing contracture development; and enhanced social, emotional, and cognitive skills (p. 900). There also was a recommendation to cautiously use NDT only with a sufficiently sensitive outcome measure to attain the intervention outcome of improved function.

Tempering this recommendation is a systematic review and meta-analysis from 2014 by Veerbeek, et al., that concludes, "Contrary to previous reviews which concluded that neurological treatment approaches (NDT/Bobath) were not superior by Van Peppen et al., and Kollen et al., the present review demonstrates that neurological treatment approaches are less effective when compared to focused interventions such as modified CIMT, bilateral arm training, or strengthening when applied in a task-specific way. Research on the effectiveness of NDT continues. It began as an oral tradition and purposefully developed as a 'living' approach incorporating new knowledge." It continues with many explanations as to why a technique so widely used for more than 50 years by thousands of therapists thrives. It has had few randomized control trials and at present controversy remains (Brock et al., 2011; Mikolajewska, 2013).

NDT still is a treatment approach that is applied worldwide. As stated by Szklut and Philibert (2007), in neurological rehabilitation, therapy approaches for remediation of motor deficits

> are not mutually exclusive, and each requires a level of training and practice for competence as well as experience in normal development. Most therapists synthesize information from different intervention technique and use an eclectic approach, pulling relevant pieces from a variety of intervention modalities to best meet the needs of each child (or adult patient). (p. 441)

Protocols and Processes

NDT is defined as a clinical reasoning approach (Kollen et al., 2009). Recreational therapy interventions that are cognizant of NDT principles utilize normal patterns of movement in sessions to reduce impairment and increase functional performance. To apply NDT principles, recreational therapists begin each session by observing the client at rest and in motion. They look for normal range of motion, posture, limb tone, movement patterns, timing and sequencing as part of coordination patterns, balance, symmetry and integration of both sides of the body, and ability to hold a posture (Bobath, 1990). When an impairment is identified, a recreational therapist utilizes physical handling and inhibition techniques to facilitate attaining and sustaining normal body positions and movements with recreational tasks as treatment modalities.

Principles of treatment include avoiding activities and exercises that increase abnormal tone or strengthen abnormal movement responses and using treatment techniques to suppress or eliminate these patterns (Vining Radomski & Trombly Latham, 2008). A recreational therapist does not select tasks where objects are manipulated or handled on the client's lap, which encourages posterior pelvic, trunk, and neck flexion and internal rotation of hips and shoulders when unsupported sitting is impaired. When hemiparesis of the arm is noted, the recreational therapist helps the client use shoulder flexion for reaching upward rather than allowing the abnormal movement pattern of shoulder elevation with trunk rotation and flexion.

A recreational therapist should select and configure treatment activities that encourage or strengthen normal movement patterns in the client's trunk and extremities (Bobath, 1990). While playing darts, a recreational therapist can assist the client to position the hemiparetic arm with intact pain sensation against a dartboard and assist the client to stabilize it with trunk body weight pressure, as the client removes the darts with the other, intact hand. When assisting the client to transfer from sitting to standing to play basketball, the configuration should require both feet to be on the floor, shoulder width apart, with heels back as far as space allows, strengthening normal ascension muscles and facilitating normal movement patterns.

When indicated, the recreational therapist should help the client use existing motor control on the hemiplegic side for recreational performance. If the client is working on sitting balance, a recreational therapist can use intermittent unsupported sitting and reaching during a game of cards by placing the cards slightly toward the affected side.

To help a client who lacks adequate strength and control of the affected arm and leg for normal recreational performance, the therapist should develop compensations and adaptations that encourage use of the affected side and decrease the development of abnormal movements and asymmetrical postures.

Throwing and catching games can be easily adapted. Activities and games can be played with intermittent standing. Weak arms can be integrated into the task by standing at a table or counter during the game. Objects can be selected that are lighter weight and easier to grasp. Beanbag toss can be played underhanded while seated with both feet on the floor shoulder width apart and trunk elongated. As the bag is thrown to a target, the throwing shoulder is flexed forward with the forearm supinated, elbow extended, palm up, fingers open, and the thumb away from the index finger.

NDT Interventions

A survey of experienced working therapists report that NDT interventions include mobilizations, facilitated movements, practicing components of activities, and practicing activities (Tyson et al., 2009).

Mobilizations happen when a therapist uses touch to guide a client's body into a desired position or through a movement pattern. Mobilizations are accompanied by stabilizations and are done when a client is unable to move a desired body part independently. Mobilization of an impaired shoulder girdle is common post-CVA. A trained recreational therapist can mobilize the client's shoulder and facilitate active use while bowling to engage the affected arm while compensating for any co-occurring trunk weakness.

Facilitated movements are a less invasive level of intervention, although they also require direct touching and guiding of the client as movement occurs. They can include pelvic tilts, weight transfers, selective movements of body parts, reaching, and bridging. Many can be applied while sitting or standing in applied recreational therapy practice. When working with a client presenting with a posterior pelvic tilt, a recreational therapist could use a gross motor task such as shooting a basketball or throwing horseshoes after pre-positioning the client in unsupported sitting with the client's back not touching the chair and feet shoulder width apart on the floor. The therapist then has the client perform an anterior pelvic tilt by rising to a tall sit and leaning forward at the hips as the ball or horseshoe is released.

When working with a client presenting with one-sided leg weakness and impaired ability to perform bilateral weight bearing, a recreational therapist could use a gross motor task such as throwing a baseball or swinging a racquet after pre-positioning the client in supported or unsupported standing position with feet on the floor. The therapist then has the client perform a weight shift toward the weak side of the body as the ball is released or the racquet is swung toward the target placed in the hemispheric space across midline.

When working with a client presenting with arm weakness and impaired ability to perform functional movements following stroke, it is important to note whether the client is able to elevate the shoulder and recognize and report pain. If the client can, a recreational therapist could use tabletop tasks such as board games or painting. After pre-positioning the pelvis in neutral, placing the feet shoulder width apart on the floor, performing shoulder girdle mobilization, and pre-positioning the affected arm to weight bear safely, the therapist has the client use the intact limb to manipulate game pieces or art supplies that have been placed in the hemispheric space across midline.

Practicing components of activities follows as a natural step after facilitating movements. The surveyed therapists reported practicing components of activities with NDT interventions that involved rolling, sitting, transferring, standing, and walking. Each activity is dissected into components in what is sometimes referred to as activity analysis. Clients are assessed for performance of all of the components and practice occurs for any deficits. On a related note, it is common practice when a client is not independent in performing a desired recreational activity to begin with practicing components. NDT utilizes the same framework.

Recreational activities can be used as a modality to practice components of activities and thereby build skill components for more complex and challenging activities. Sitting unsupported for brief periods can be gradually increased in duration and with less assistance from the therapist while playing games or creating art. Playing an electronic portable keyboard can be used to increase the range a client can abduct a shoulder or the range fingers can flex and extend.

Either can be used to work toward independence in performance of those tasks or as pre-recreation skill development for sitting on a standard piano bench while playing independently.

Practicing activities themselves is the final NDT intervention reported. Due to the nature of the population, reaching activities while sitting and standing were listed as an additional area that receives practice. A recreational therapist may think of these as general functional skills for generic recreation task performance. Some recreational therapy interventions that can be used to facilitate motor development or recovery via normal body movement include:

Reaching activities in sitting or standing positions while doing games (board games, air hockey, billiards, bowling, darts, horseshoes, ping pong, shuffleboard, Wii Fit, Wii Sports), jigsaw puzzles, arts and crafts, gardening, performing music, sports (badminton, baseball, basketball, casting and fishing, football, golf, hockey, soccer, tennis, volleyball), martial arts, aerobics, and dance.

Walking while gardening, doing sports, shopping, eating out, and dancing.

Rolling and lie-to-sit transfers in yoga and Pilates.

Sit-to-stand transfers to and from a piano bench, bus seat, car seat, restaurant seat, public restroom, locker room bench, exercise machines, pool deck, sandy beach, ground in the garden, and water craft.

Physical Handling Techniques

Physical handling techniques through key points of control on the body are central to the application of NDT (Szklut & Philibert, 2007). How, when, where, and why a therapist touches and guides a client's movements are all part of the clinical evaluation and decision making a recreational therapist does as the NDT approach is brought to life in a treatment session (Stammer, 2006).

Some of the techniques a therapist will learn in an NDT workshop include how they can observe the client's body and feel the body with their hands. The therapist will learn about starting postures and several techniques to control movements to other positions and to increase the client's function. Therapists need to attend workshops with an NDT instructor before they try to apply NDT principles.

These principles can be applied via simple adjustments during treatment sessions or more comprehensively following advanced training in complex neuromuscular facilitation techniques. One universal adjustment a recreational therapist may implement during treatment of clients with asymmetry due to a physical disability is to select treatment modalities that utilize hemiparetic limbs. This may seem obvious, but clients receiving treatment in acute physical rehabilitation settings are often focused on one-sided compensatory strategies and skill development (Geyer & Gomez, 2009). This focus ensures that clients become increasingly proficient at using the unaffected limb. Acute physical rehabilitation can be more about the shortsighted goal of "getting the client up and walking regardless of the quality of movement" versus "getting the client up and walking with an optimal repertoire of balanced and symmetrical movements to facilitate long-term safety and health." Clinicians are challenged to carefully assess the balance between the restoration of neurologic control and a focus on functional independence with compensatory techniques (Harvey et al., 2011).

Integration of NDT at an elementary level can only benefit an individual by normalizing body positions and mechanics. These positioning adjustments are effective regardless of the physical task performed. The alignment of a base of support impacts all structures above that base. While seated, this translates to the position of the pelvis, which impacts the movement of the person's trunk, arms, neck, and head. The position of the feet during standing impacts the movement of the entire body. In practice, a person's functional arm movements are impacted by the position of the pelvis and trunk. When a pelvis is posteriorly tilted, a resulting trunk flexion occurs. This, in turn, causes an inward rotation of the shoulder and arm with reduced functional range of motion.

Clients who are moving the playing pieces of a board game will perform better if they are sitting upright with their hips, knees, and ankles in 90 degrees of flexion and with their feet flat on the floor. A recreational therapist cognizant of NDT principles will realize the connection between pelvis, trunk, and arms. They will comprehensively guide the client's body to optimize physical outcomes of the treatment intervention.

Individuals with CNS pathophysiology have dysfunction in posture and movement that cause func-tional activity limitations (Bobath, 1990; Butler & Darrah, 2001; Szklut & Philibert, 2007). NDT aims to inhibit spasticity and synergies using inhibitory postures and movements and to facilitate normal autonomic responses that are involved in voluntary movement (Bakhtiary & Fatemy, 2008; Lennon et al., 2006). The general aims of treatment are to normalize tone, to determine which abnormal patterns need to be inhibited, and to decide which normal movement components need to be facilitated.

The therapist prepares the client for functional skills by focusing on the components of normal movement essential to functional activity (Luke et al., 2004). The current framework for learning the theory and skills required to utilize and apply the NDT approach to an individual with CNS pathophysiology is to receive post-graduate education. There is currently a U.S. national organization, Neuro-Developmental Treatment Association (NDTA) that provides coursework, seminars, conferences, and certification. There are also other international organizations, such as the International Bobath Instructors Training Association, that are good contacts for training and educational opportunities. Most organizations formally seek professional audience members from the fields of physical therapy, occupational therapy, and speech language pathology. Recreational therapists have attended and received advanced training at NDT workshops. The stated purpose of the NDTA is to promote the unique qualities of the NDT approach by providing specialized clinical training to healthcare professionals; supporting clinical research; and supporting clients' and families with education, resources, and information (NDTA, 2011).

Outcomes and Documentation

Expected outcomes from application of NDT by a recreational therapist include reduction of motor and physical impairments and increased functional performance in recreation. Common areas evaluated and rehabilitated are range of motion or distance a limb can move, strength or force generation, speed or rate of movement, endurance or sustainability, coordination or precision, balance, and skill or task performance. Each of these discrete variables are observed, measured, and recorded in the evaluation documentation. Impairments are considered in the development of a corresponding treatment plan. A variety of standardized assessment tools exist for motor and physical performance and all can be used in conjunction with the NDT approach.

Please see the chapter on Activity and Task Analysis for a sample of applicable ICF codes. The most important ones will be part of b4 Functions of the Cardiovascular, Hematological, Immunological, and Respiratory Systems; b7 Neuromusculoskeletal and Movement-Related Functions; and d4 Mobility. These can be used to document physical domain performance. ICF qualifiers can be used to document the magnitude or severity of the problem in question. They are used in combination with the ICF code (World Health Organization, 2013):

ICF Generic Qualifier Scale

0 = NO problem (none, absent, negligible) 0-4%

1 = MILD problem (slight, low…) 2-24%

2 = MODERATE (medium, fair) 25-49%

3 = SEVERE (high, extreme…) 50-95%

4 = COMPLETE (total…) 96-100%

An example of an abbreviated evaluation and treatment plan using ICF terminology, for a 30-year-old female post-CVA who uses a wheelchair for mobility, is

Client Goal: Regain independence getting to and from a restaurant seat and a wheelchair

ICF classification: d4200 Transferring Oneself While Sitting

ICF category definition: Moving from a sitting position on one seat to another on the same or a different level.

ICF category with qualifier — prior function: d4200._ _ _ 0 Transferring oneself while sitting, no participation restriction (no difficulty transferring in a real-life community environment).

ICF category with qualifier — current function: d4200._ _ _ 2 Transferring oneself while sitting, moderate participation restriction (moderate difficulty transferring in a real-life community environment).

RT Goal: Wheelchair to restaurant seat transfers with modified independence due to increased time with safe technique that includes weight bearing through bilateral lower extremities (d4200._ _ _ 0).

Conclusion

Many neurophysiological approaches promoting the development and recovery of motor impairment have proven effective. In the Western world, the Bobath Concept or neurodevelopmental treatment (NDT) is the most popular treatment approach used in stroke rehabilitation, yet the relative effectiveness of the Bobath Concept has not been established (Kollen et al., 2009). NDT is one approach a recreational therapist with the necessary advanced training can utilize when providing treatment for clients with CNS pathophysiology and subsequent dysfunction of movement.

Acknowledgments: Thanks is extended to Brigit Sullivan, NIH Library Writing Center, for editorial assistance.

Resources

Neuro-Developmental Treatment Association (NDTA)

www.ndta.org

1540 S. Coast Highway, Ste 203

Laguna Beach, CA 92651

800-869-9295

info@ndta.org

A resource for NDT continuing education courses, research, and certification in NDT/Bobath approach for adults and children. Recreational therapists have attended professional educational opportunities.

References

Anttila, H., Autti-Ramo, I., Suoranta, J., Makela, M., & Malmivaara, A. (2008). Effectiveness of physical therapy interventions for children with cerebral palsy: A systematic review. *BMC Pediatr, 8*(14), 1471-2431.

Arya, K. N., Verma, R., Garg, R. K., Sharma, V. P., Agarwal, M., & Aggarwal, G. G. (2012). Meaningful task-specific training (MTST) for stroke rehabilitation: A randomized controlled trial. *Top Stroke Rehabil, 19*(3), 193-211.

Bakhtiary, A. H. & Fatemy, E. (2008). Does electrical stimulation reduce spasticity after stroke? A randomized controlled study. *Clin Rehabil, 22*(5), 418-425.

Bobath, B. (1990). *Adult hemiplegia: Evaluation and treatment* (3rd ed.). Oxford, England: Heinemann.

Bobath, K. (1980). *A neurophysiological basis for the treatment of cerebral palsy*. Oxford: Mac Keith Press.

Bobath, K., & Bobath, B. (1964). The facilitation of normal postural reactions and movements in the treatment of cerebral palsy. *Physiotherapy, 50*, 246-262.

Bobath Centre. (2013). Who would benefit from Bobath Treatment? The Bobath Approach. Retrieved January 4, 2013, from www.bobath.org.uk/TheBobathApproach.html.

Brock, K., Haase, G., Rothacher, G., & Cotton, S. (2011). Does physiotherapy based on the Bobath concept, in conjunction with a task practice, achieve greater improvement in walking ability in people with stroke compared to physiotherapy focused on structured task practice alone?: A pilot randomized controlled trial. *Clin Rehabil, 25*(10), 903-912.

Brzuszkiewicz-Kuzmicka, G., Kuzmicki, S., & Domaniecki, J. (2012). Relationships between kinesiotherapy methods used in rehabilitation and the course of lost function recovery following surgical treatment of cranio-cerebral trauma. *Brain Inj, 26*(12), 1431-1438.

Butler, C., & Darrah, J. (2001). Effects of neurodevelopmental treatment (NDT) for cerebral palsy: An AACPDM evidence report. *Dev Med Child Neurol, 43*(11), 778-790.

Chen, J. C., Liang, C. C., & Shaw, F. Z. (2005). Facilitation of sensory and motor recovery by thermal intervention for the hemiplegic upper limb in acute stroke patients: A single-blind randomized clinical trial. *Stroke, 36*(12), 2665-2669. doi: 10.1161/01.STR.0000189992.06654.ab.

Czupryna, K., & Nowotny, J. (2012). Foot and knee behaviour during gait in response to the use of additional means of treatment in cerebral palsied children. *Ortop Traumatol Rehabil, 14*(5), 453-465.

Dodakian, L., Stewart, J. C., & Cramer, S. C. (2014). Motor imagery during movement activates the brain more than movement alone after stroke: A pilot study. *J Rehabil Med, 46*(9), 843-848. doi: 10.2340/16501977-1844.

Edwards, S. (2002). *Neurological physiotherapy*. Edinburgh: Churchill Livingstone.

Geyer, J. D. & Gomez, C. R. (2009). *Stroke: A practical approach*. Philadelphia, PA: Wolters Kluwer Health/Lippincott Williams and Wilkins.

Harvey, R. L., Roth, E. J., Yu, D. T., & Celnik, P. (2011). Stroke syndromes. In R. L. Braddom (Ed.). *Physical Medicine & Rehabilitation* (4th ed.) (p. 1177). Philadelphia: Elsevier Saunders.

Huseyinsinoglu, B. E., Ozdincler, A. R., & Krespi, Y. (2012). Bobath concept versus constraint-induced movement therapy to improve arm functional recovery in stroke patients: A randomized controlled trial. *Clin Rehabil, 26*(8), 705-715.

Jelica, S., Seper, V., Davidovic, E., & Bujisic, G. (2011). Optimizing the function of upstanding activities in adult patients with acquired lesions of the central nervous system by using the Bobath concept approach: A case report. *Coll Antropol, 1*, 309-311.

Keser, I., Kirdi, N., Meric, A., Kurne, A. T., & Karabudak, R. (2013). Comparing routine neurorehabilitation program with trunk exercises based on Bobath concept in multiple sclerosis: pilot study. *J Rehabil Res Dev, 50*(1), 133-140.

Kiebzak, W., Kowalski, I. M., Domagalska, M., Szopa, A., Dwornik, M., Kujawa, J., ... Sliwinski, Z. (2012). Assessment of visual perception in adolescents with a history of central coordination disorder in early life: 15-year follow-up study. *Arch Med Sci, 8*(5), 879-885.

Kim, S. J., Kwak, E. E., Park, E. S., & Cho, S. R. (2012). Differential effects of rhythmic auditory stimulation and neurodevelopmental treatment/Bobath on gait patterns in adults with cerebral palsy: A randomized controlled trial. *Clin Rehabil, 26*(10), 904-914.

Knox, V. & Evans, A. L. (2002). Evaluation of the functional effects of a course of Bobath therapy in children with cerebral palsy: A preliminary study. *Dev Med Child Neurol, 44*(7), 447-460.

Kollen, B. J., Lennon, S., Lyons, B., Wheatley-Smith, L., Scheper, M., Buurke, J. H., ... Kwakkel, G. (2009). The effectiveness of the Bobath concept in stroke rehabilitation: What is the evidence? *Stroke, 40*(4), 29.

Langhammer, B. & Stanghelle, J. K. (2011). Can physiotherapy after stroke based on the Bobath concept result in improved quality of movement compared to the motor relearning programme? *Physiother Res Int, 16*(2), 69-80.

Lennon, S. (2001). Gait re-education based on the Bobath concept in two patients with hemiplegia following stroke. *Phys Ther, 81*(3), 924-935.

Lennon, S., Ashburn, A., & Baxter, D. (2006). Gait outcome following outpatient physiotherapy based on the Bobath concept in people post stroke. *Disabil Rehabil, 28*(13-14), 873-881.

Levin, M. F. & Panturin, E. (2011). Sensorimotor integration for functional recovery and the Bobath approach. *Motor Control, 15*(2), 285-301.

Luke, C., Dodd, K. J., & Brock, K. (2004). Outcomes of the Bobath concept on upper limb recovery following stroke. *Clin Rehabil, 18*(8), 888-898.

MacWalter, R. E. Y. (n.d.). Medical treatment and rehabilitation in stroke. Retrieved February 22, 2011, from www.dundee.ac.uk/medther/StrokeSSM/Rehab/tsld001.htm.

Mikolajewska, E. (2012). NDT-Bobath method in normalization of muscle tone in post-stroke patients. *Adv Clin Exp Med, 21*(4), 513-517.

Mikolajewska, E. (2013). Associations between results of post-stroke NDT-Bobath rehabilitation in gait parameters, ADL and hand functions. *Adv Clin Exp Med, 22*(5), 731-738.

Natarajan, P., Oelschlager, A., Agah, A., Pohl, P. S., Ahmad, S. O., & Liu, W. (2008). Current clinical practices in stroke rehabilitation: Regional pilot survey. *J Rehabil Res Dev, 45*(6), 841-849.

NDTA. (2005). *Advances in practice* (Vol. 12(2)): NDTA worldwide.

NDTA. (2011). Organization home webpage information. from www.ndta.org.

Nilsson, L., Carlsson, J., Danielsson, A., Fugl-Meyer, A., Hellstrom, K., Kristensen, L., ... Grimby, G. (2001). Walking training of patients with hemiparesis at an early stage after stroke: A comparison of walking training on a treadmill with body weight support and walking training on the ground. *Clin Rehabil, 15*(5), 515-527.

Novak, I., McIntyre, S., Morgan, C., Campbell, L., Dark, L., Morton, N., Stumbles, E., Wilson, S. A., & Goldsmith, S. (2013). A systematic review of interventions for children with cerebral palsy: State of the evidence. *Dev Med Child Neurol, 55*(10), 885-910.

Oygard, K., Haestad, H., & Jorgensen, L. (2011). Physiotherapy, based on the Bobath concept, may influence the gait pattern in persons with limb-girdle muscle dystrophy: a multiple case series study. *Physiother Res Int, 16*(1), 20-31.

Paci, M. (2003). Physiotherapy based on the Bobath concept for adults with post-stroke hemiplegia: A review of effectiveness studies. *J Rehabil Med, 35*(1), 2-7.

Pollock, A., Baer, G., Langhorne, P., & Pomeroy, V. (2007). Physiotherapy treatment approaches for the recovery of postural control and lower limb function following stroke: A systematic review. *Clin Rehabil, 21*(5), 395-410.

Puyuelo, M. & Rondal, J. A. (2005). Speech rehabilitation in 10 Spanish-speaking children with severe cerebral palsy: A 4-year longitudinal study. *Pediatr Rehabil, 8*(2), 113-116.

Riva, G., Bolzoni, M., Carella, F., Galimberti, C., Griffin, M. J., Lewis, C. H., ... Wann, J. (1997). Virtual reality environments for psycho-neuro-physiological assessment and rehabilitation. *Stud Health Technol Inform, 39*, 34-45.

Smedal, T., Lygren, H., Myhr, K. M., Moe-Nilssen, R., Gjelsvik, B., Gjelsvik, O., & Strand, L. I. (2006). Balance and gait improved in patients with MS after physiotherapy based on the Bobath concept. *Physiother Res Int, 11*(2), 104-116.

Stammer, M. (2006). "So is NDT just everything, then?" *NDTA Newsletter* (May-June ed., Vol. 13).

Szklut, S. E. & Philibert, D. B. (2007). Management of functional problems and movement disorders. In D. A. Umphred (Ed.), *Neurological Rehabilitation* (5th ed.) (pp. 418-461). St. Louis: Mosby Elsevier.

Thieme, H., Mehrholz, J., Pohl, M., Behrens, J., & Dohle, C. (2012). Mirror therapy for improving motor function after stroke. Cochrane Database Syst Rev, 3, CD008449. doi: 10.1002/14651858.CD008449.pub2.

Tyson, S. F., Connell, L. A., Busse, M. E., & Lennon, S. (2009). What is Bobath? A survey of UK stroke physiotherapists' perceptions of the content of the Bobath concept to treat postural control and mobility problems after stroke. *Disabil Rehabil, 31*(6), 448-457.

Van Peppen, R. P., Kwakkel, G., Wood-Dauphinee, S., Hendriks, H. J., Van der Wees, P. J., & Dekker, J. (2004). The impact of physical therapy on functional outcomes after stroke: what's the evidence? *Clin Rehabil, 18*(8), 833-862.

Veerbeek, J. M., van Wegen, E., van Peppen, R., van der Wees, P. J., Hendriks, E., Rietberg, M., & Kwakkel, G. (2014). What is the evidence for physical therapy poststroke? A systematic review and meta-analysis. *PLoS One, 9*(2), e87987. doi: 10.1371/journal.pone.0087987.

Vining Radomski, M. & Trombly Latham, C. A. (Eds.). (2008). *Occupational therapy for physical dysfunction* (6th ed.). Philadelphia: Lippincott Williams and Wilkins.

Visintin, M., Barbeau, H., Korner-Bitensky, N., & Mayo, N. E. (1998). A new approach to retrain gait in stroke patients through body weight support and treadmill stimulation. *Stroke, 29*(6), 1122-1128.

Volpe, B. T., Krebs, H. I., Hogan, N., Edelstein, O. L., Diels, C., & Aisen, M. (2000). A novel approach to stroke rehabilitation: Robot-aided sensorimotor stimulation. *Neurology, 54*(10), 1938-1944.

Walker, M. L., Ringleb, S. I., Maihafer, G. C., Walker, R., Crouch, J. R., Van Lunen, B., & Morrison, S. (2010). Virtual reality-enhanced partial body weight-supported treadmill training poststroke: Feasibility and effectiveness in 6 subjects. *Arch Phys Med Rehabil, 91*(1), 115-122. doi: 10.1016/j.apmr.2009.09.009.

Wang, D. & Zhang, J. (2014). Effects of hypothermia combined with neural stem cell transplantation on recovery of neurological function in rats with spinal cord injury. *Mol Med Rep.* doi: 10.3892/mmr.2014.2905.

World Health Organization. (2013). How to use the ICF: A practical manual for using the International Classification of Functioning, Disability, and Health (ICF). Exposure draft for comment. (pp. 17). Geneva: World Health Organization.

Yue, Z. H., Li, L., Chang, X. R., Jiang, J. M., Chen, L. L., & Zhu, X. S. (2012). [Comparative study on effects between electroacupuncture and acupuncture for spastic paralysis after stroke]. *Zhongguo Zhen Jiu, 32*(7), 582-586.

Zhang, P., Hu, W., Cao, X., Xu, S. G., Li, D. K., & Xu, L. (2009). [Selective cervical dorsal root cutting off part of the vertebral lateral mass fixation combined with exercise therapy for treating spastic cerebral paralysis of the upper limbs caused by cerebral palsy]. *Zhongguo Gu Shang, 22*(10), 763-764.

39. Physical Activity

Heather R. Porter

Regular physical activity is vital for health. According to the Physical Activity Guidelines for Americans (U.S. Department of Health and Human Services, 2008), there is strong to moderate evidence to support the value of regular engagement in 150 minutes of moderate intensity aerobic activity per week. For children and adolescents, regular physical activity is associated with improved cardiorespiratory and muscular fitness, improved bone health, improved cardiovascular and metabolic health biomarkers, favorable body composition, and reduced symptoms of depression. For adults and older adults, regular physical activity is associated with lower risk of early death, lower risk of coronary heart disease, lower risk of stroke, lower risk of high blood pressure, lower risk of adverse blood lipid profile, lower risk of type 2 diabetes, lower risk of metabolic syndrome, lower risk of cancer (colon, breast cancer, lung cancer, endometrial), prevention of weight gain, weight loss, weight maintenance after weight loss, improved cardiorespiratory and muscular fitness, prevention of falls, reduced depression, better cognitive function, better functional health, reduced abdominal obesity, lower risk of hip fracture, increased bone density, and improved sleep.

Unfortunately, less than half (48%) of American adults, and only 25% of individuals with disabilities, meet the 2008 Physical Activity Guidelines for Americans (Centers for Disease Control and Prevention [CDC], 2014), putting them at risk for the previously mentioned health conditions. Only one in three children are physically active every day, partly because they spend more than 7.5 hours a day in front of a computer, video game, or smart phone screen (President's Council on Fitness, Sports, and Nutrition, 2014) and only about 27% of high school students participate in 60 minutes of daily physical activity (CDC, 2014).

This behavior has resulted in physical inactivity becoming the fourth leading risk factor for mortality, causing an estimated 3.2 million deaths annually throughout the world (World Health Organization [WHO], 2014). People who are insufficiently active have a 20-30% increased risk of death compared to people who engage in at least 30 minutes of moderately intensity physical activity on most days of the week (WHO, 2014). The drop in physical activity is predominantly due to sedentary leisure, home, and work behavior; passive modes of transportation, such as using cars instead of bicycles; and urban issues including fear of violence and crime in outdoor areas, high-density traffic with few sidewalks, low air quality, lack of parks or sports and recreation facilities (WHO, 2014). All of these problems affect individuals with disabilities more.

On the positive side, physical activity is a modifiable risk factor. It is something that can be changed. This is a good thing because "there is irrefutable evidence of the effectiveness of regular physical activity in the primary and secondary prevention of … chronic diseases [including] cardiovascular disease, diabetes, cancer, hypertension, obesity, depression, and osteoporosis, [as well as] premature death" (Warburton, et al., 2006).

Regular physical activity has additional health-related outcomes for individuals with disabilities and health conditions. For example, regular physical activity can have a protective effect on dopamine neurons in individuals who have Parkinson's disease (Farley et al., 2008), can decrease pain and the number of tender points in individuals who have fibromyalgia (Kelly & Loy, 2008), and may reverse type 2 diabetes if weight loss also occurs (National Diabetes Information Clearinghouse, 2013). Depending on the other variables associated with physical activity, even more benefits can be obtained.

For example, if physical activity takes place in a group or team setting, the added benefit of social support might be obtained. If the form of physical activity is only slightly above the client's abilities, the experience of flow might be obtained. If the person masters the particular form of physical activity, a sense of accomplishment and mastery may develop. All of these can spill into and affect other aspects of life.

Indications

Maintaining, improving, or developing the following are common therapeutic reasons for engaging in physical activity. Also listed are the related ICF codes that may show up during diagnosis. When these ICF codes are seen, the therapist should consider physical activity as one of the treatment modalities.

- exercise tolerance (b455 Exercise Tolerance Functions)
- immune system (b435 Immunological System Functions)
- pain management (b280 Sensation of Pain)
- cognition (b1 Mental Functions, d1 Learning and Applying Knowledge)
- cardiovascular system (b410 - b429 Functions of the Cardiovascular System)
- respiratory system (b440 - b449 Functions of the Respiratory System)
- mobility and movement functions (b147 Psychomotor Functions, b260 Proprioceptive Function, b7 Neuromusculoskeletal and Movement-Related Functions, d4 Mobility)
- body weight and appetite (d570 Looking After One's Health, b530 Weight Maintenance Functions)
- stress management (d240 Handling Stress and Other Psychological Demands)
- psychological and emotional health (b126 Temperament and Personality Functions, b180 Experience of Self and Time Functions)
- sleep functions (b134 Sleep Functions)
- metabolism (b540 General Metabolic Functions)
- self-care, overall health maintenance, prevention of secondary conditions and complications (d570 Looking After One's Health)
- leisure time physical activity (d920 Recreation and Leisure)

Contraindications

Prior to having a client engage in physical activity, clearance must be obtained from the client's physician indicating (1) type of exercise permitted such as aerobic, stretching and flexibility, or strength and resistance training; (2) engagement recommendations, such as time, intensity, and frequency; (3) any precautions that need to be followed or parameters that need to be monitored (e.g., heart rate, blood pressure, oxygen saturation levels, falls, glucose levels); and (4) any type of movement or exercise that should not be done, such as restricted movements after a total hip replacement, limits on the amount of weight to be lifted, or other limitations caused by the client's medical condition, such as immunological deficiencies. Depending on the setting, the client may ask the physician directly for clearance (e.g., a client who desires to participate in a community exercise program) or the therapist may seek clearance for the client (e.g., therapist who is working with a client in an inpatient physical rehabilitation setting).

Protocols and Processes

Prior to implementing a physical activity protocol, it is important to understand the differences between physical activity, exercise, leisure time physical activity (LTPA), and active living.

Physical activity is defined as any bodily movement produced by the skeletal muscles resulting in increased energy expenditure.

Exercise is a type of physical activity that is planned, structured, and repetitive for the purpose of improvement and maintenance of physical fitness, such as going for a 30-minute brisk walk three times a week (Caspersen, et al., 1985).

Like exercise, LTPA is a type of physical activity. It is "an activity undertaken in the individual's discretionary time that increases the total daily energy expenditure" and is chosen based on personal needs, interests, and motivations (Bouchard et al., 2006, p. 12).

Active living is a way of life that integrates physical activity into everyday activity, such as riding a bike to work and taking the stairs, and puts ownership on multiple professionals (e.g., city planners, public recreation) to design policies and environments that promote active living, such as more green space or bike lanes. The concept of active living, although starting out with a focus on only physical activity, has grown into a much broader concept of being "actively engaged in living all aspects of one's life both personally and in families and communities in a meaningful and enriching way … [in which] physical activity and exercise is undeniably a core component" (Iwasaki, Coyle, & Shank, 2010, p. 484). As recreational therapists we actively promote and assist clients in attaining regular physical activity through structured exercise, LTPA, and active living components.

Preparing for Physical Activity

Obtain Clearance from the Physician

For the typically healthy individual, it is recommended that clearance is obtained from a physician prior to engagement in physical activity, as the individual might not be aware that a current health condition requires modifications or avoiding some types of physical activity. For individuals who have health conditions, clearance from a physician is required prior to physical activity to ensure safety, reduce chances of experiencing adverse effects, and maximize potential positive outcomes.

Educate the Client and/or Caregiver

The extent of education, content taught, and specific people educated will vary depending upon the client's functioning and abilities. Education includes, but is not limited to:

- The relation of physical activity to the client's recovery and health promotion.
- The specific precautions, parameters, and restrictions set by the physician.
- Contraindications for particular forms of physical exercise (e.g., running is contraindicated after a total joint replacement).
- How to monitor vital signs.
- Adaptations including equipment and techniques to assist the client in maintaining precautions, parameters, and recommendations.
- Adaptations to maximize performance in physical activity, such as color-coded play and stop buttons to help a client with cognitive difficulties use an exercise video.
- Recommendations for the amount of time, frequency, and intensity of physical activity.

Although education to increase knowledge and skills is often in behavior change theories, having knowledge and skills does not always equal action.

Just because someone knows the benefits of physical activity and knows how to engage in physical activity safely, doesn't mean that the person will do it. Getting people to engage in physical activity regularly is easier said than done, as there is a wide array of contextual factors including motivation, self-efficacy, knowledge, resources, transportation, social support, access, and skills that influence engagement. Given the complexity of the issue, a multi-system and collaborative approach that addresses intrapersonal, interpersonal, and structural constraints and facilitators is needed. In this system recreational therapy plays an important role. See the Theories, Models, and Concepts chapter to learn about health behavior change theories.

Choose Specific Forms of Physical Activity

Once recommendations and specific orders from the physician are obtained, appropriate forms of physical activity that meet the physician's recommendations or orders are identified and chosen in collaboration with the client. When choosing forms of physical activity consider the following:

Functional baselines: What are the client's current functional baselines in all domains? Look at abilities, skills, and limitations in the physical, cognitive, and social domains. To maximize success, forms of physical activity must match the client's abilities. This relates to the concept of "flow." Physical activities that are below the client's abilities can induce feelings of boredom and disinterest, physical activities that are far above the client's abilities can induce feelings of anxiety and avoidance, but physical activities that meet and are slightly above the client's abilities will induce a sense of achievable challenge where the activity itself motivates continued participation. Functional baselines are also needed to begin thinking about possible physical activity modifications and adaptations.

Needs: What are the primary outcomes from physical activity engagement that are desired for the client in all health domains? What form of physical activity is needed to attain the desired outcomes?

Interests and motivations: What are the client's leisure interests? What does the client consider to be enjoyable? How can the client's interests be integrated into specific forms of physical activity to aid in initiation and sustained engagement in physical activity? Research has shown that the experience of enjoyment during physical activity is a mediator to initiation and sustained engagement in physical activity (DiLorenzo et al., 1998; Johnson & Heller, 1998; Lindgren & Fridlund, 1999; Tsai, 2005; Dishman et al., 2005; Williams et al., 2006). Research has also shown that enjoyment is an outcome of personally meaningful experiences (Porter, et al., 2012; Porter, et al., 2011). In other words, "when a person engages in an activity that produces something that is personally meaningful (e.g., a feeling of connection with a loved one), the positive emotion of enjoyment is felt" (Porter et al., 2012, p. 205-206). Consequently, the therapist's quest is to not only find out what interests the client, but also to determine the underlying personal meanings that may be gained from such experiences. For example a client might enjoy doing arts and crafts with her daughter because it has the personal meaning of spending quality time with the daughter. It is the personal meaning that can then be worked into forms of physical activity to motivate engagement, such as going for walks with the daughter. It is also important to note that not all clients have a healthy leisure lifestyle that allows for the discovery of desired personal meanings. For example, a client might desire to escape from a stressful life, yet not engage in forms of leisure that allow for this. Consequently, when exploring interests with a client who has limited leisure experiences, it might be more advantageous to start out by discussing what s/he desires in life. The goal is to identify the underlying personal meanings that the client desires to experience. These can subsequently be worked into forms of physical activity. When exploring personal meanings, keep in mind that people typically search for six types of meanings in leisure activities (including LTPD) (Porter et al., 2012): (1) a sense of connection and belonging within the self, with individuals and groups, with animals or nature, with a higher power or spirit, and with one's culture or history; (2) internal balance; (3) reflection and expression of one's identity, building one's identity, and transforming one's identity; (4) freedom and autonomy; (5) control or power over oneself and things and control and power reflected to others; and (6) competence/mastery.

Facilitators and barriers: To maximize the likelihood of engagement in physical activity, therapists identify the facilitators that are currently present in the client's life, such as people and things that foster, encourage, and promote engagement in physical activity. The goal is to identify, strengthen, and maintain these facilitators. Examples of facilitators include supportive and encouraging family members, a nearby park trail, an hour of protected "me-time" in the morning after the kids go to school, and a completed registration for an upcoming 5K run/walk. Barriers, including people and things that discourage or hinder engagement in physical activity, are also explored. The goal is to identify, minimize, or extinguish these barriers. Examples of barriers include tight finances, inaccessible gym facilities, lack of time, and difficulty using transportation.

Resources: The client's resources related to physical activity engagement needs to be explored. Time and money are the overall resources. Specific resources, such as clothes, shoes, equipment, space, videos, memberships, etc., should also be explored.

Engaging in Physical Exercise

The therapist assesses the client's understanding of the information previously presented and establishes goals with the client (as appropriate) related to the physical exercise. Some possible goals for an independent client include: Client is able to independently locate, palpate, and count pulse rate. Client can adapt exercise movements to stay within movement restrictions set by physician with minimal verbal cues.

Most clients will have a target heart rate set by their physician. The usual calculation for a person's target heart rate sets it at 50-70% of his/her maximum heart rate (Centers for Disease Control and Prevention, 2011). To calculate the client's maximum heart rate subtract the person's age from 220. To calculate the client's target heart multiply the client's maximum heart rate by 50% and 70% to find the target zone. For a 50-year-old client the maximum rate would be $220 - 50 = 170$. The target rate should be at least the lower value of $170 \times .50 = 85$ bpm and not exceed $170 \times .70 = 119$ bpm. Some medications affect heart rate, so target heart rates are not appropriate measures for all clients.

Warm-up

Vital signs are taken before exercising to determine a resting baseline and to make sure that the client is within his/her precautions and parameters prior to engaging in physical activity. If appropriate, ask the client to measure his/her vital signs and check the client's accuracy. If the therapist assessed pulse at

77 beats per minute and client assessed pulse at 89 beats per minute, the therapist may need to re-teach the client alternative monitoring techniques. One adaptation commonly used for taking a pulse is to hold the ears shut with the fingers and take an apical pulse by listening to the number of heartbeats while looking at the second hand on a wall clock.

If precautions and parameters are within the client's limits, a warm-up is initiated. This is usually five to ten minutes of light activity to increase heart and lung function and warm up muscles to prevent injury. Standard warm-up activities are light walking and range of motion exercises with the intent of lubricating joints and moving, but not stretching, ligaments and tendons. The latest recommendations are to postpone stretching exercises where the client is trying to significantly increase the length of muscles until after warm-ups and usually after aerobic exercise.

Following the warm-up, vital signs are re-assessed to determine a post warm-up baseline and the safety of the client in maintaining precautions and parameters.

Cardiovascular Activity

After the warm-up, increased cardiovascular activity is initiated. The amount of time that cardiovascular activity is sustained will vary based on the client's exercise functions, willingness to participate, and cognitive ability to sustain participation. For healthy adults, it is recommended that aerobic activity within their target heart rate be maintained for 20 minutes. People who have particular health conditions, however, may not be able to sustain 20 minutes of cardiovascular activity, and it may not be safe for an individual to perform at the target heart rate level or maintain aerobic activity for such a prolonged period of time. Depending on the client's medical condition, the physician may state a specific period of time that the client is allowed to participate in cardiovascular activity. Physical measures other than heart rate may be required for assessing the safety of the physical activity. These can include blood pressure, respiration, and oxygen saturation level.

When the client is engaged in cardiovascular activity, the therapist closely monitors the client. Vital signs are taken every five to ten minutes. If vital signs become close to the client's limits or an unexpected change in vital signs is noted (e.g., irregular heart rhythm), the cool down portion of the exercise program should be initiated to bring the cardiorespiratory system back to a resting state. No further exercise should be done before the situation is reported to the medical team and the client's needs are re-evaluated. In addition to vital signs, therapists monitor outward signs of fatigue including:

Shortness of breath: This can be monitored with the talk test, which is making sure the client has enough breath to carry on a conversation while exercising.

Inability to perform exercise movements correctly: When the client can no longer perform movements that were performed correctly earlier, it may be an indication of fatigue in the muscles being used.

Inability to maintain good posture: A change in posture may indicate fatigue.

Difficulty maintaining intensity: Reduced numbers of repetitions or decreases in the movement range, speed, or focus are indications of fatigue.

Difficulty maintaining prior level of balance: Requiring increased assistance to maintain balance relative to the start of the activity or reductions in the range of motion in the activity to help maintain balance can result from fatigue.

Strength Exercises

Strength exercises may be done before or after the cardiovascular exercises. Generally after is preferred because the body has a chance to warm up more. As with cardiovascular activity, the amount of effort put into approved strength exercises will depend on the client's willingness to participate and cognitive ability to sustain participation. One important consideration during strength exercises is the concept of sets and repetitions. Strength exercises are done in sets for a reason. A particular number of repetitions are required for the most efficient building of muscle tissue. Typically, six to twelve repetitions are used in a set. Because the muscles are being stressed by the strength exercise, they need a chance to recover slightly between sets for maximum benefit. Make sure the client pauses between sets to allow the muscles to relax slightly and to allow blood to restore the oxygen and nutrient levels in the muscles.

Strength training, resistance training, and weight lifting all refer to exercises that build muscle. Strength training helps the client to build muscle or to regain strength following an injury or surgery. Weight lifting is a typical way to build strength, but some clients may have conditions where weights are not appropriate. This should be covered in the physician's recommendations. If it is not, make sure you understand the client's limitations before you make a plan.

There are several important aspects of strength training that the therapist must consider when devising a program. Balance between muscle pairs must be maintained. Do not exercise one muscle (such as the quadriceps) without also exercising the other muscle in the pair (the hamstring) unless there are specific recommendations from the physician. Muscle strength is important, but studies have shown that the balance between muscle pairs is slightly more important for proper muscle function in regards to balance and the most efficient physical movements (Johnston, 1992; Rosenstein, 2008; Whitney et al., 2000). Regular strength training is important, especially in adulthood, because lean muscle mass is gradually lost through the aging process. Muscle also burns fat at a higher rate during aerobic activity, thus contributing to weight loss.

The therapist continues to closely monitor the client during these exercises. Vital signs are again taken every five to ten minutes. If vital signs become close to the client's limits or an unexpected change in vital signs is noted (e.g., irregular heart rhythm), the cool down portion of the exercise program is initiated to bring the cardiorespiratory system back to a resting state. Again, the therapist must report the conditions that limited the planned activity to the medical team before more exercise sessions are planned. In addition to vital signs, therapists again monitor outward signs of fatigue including:

- shortness of breath.
- inability to perform exercise movements.
- inability to maintain good posture.
- difficulty maintaining the same number of repetitions.
- difficulty maintaining balance.

Cool-Down

Once the client's tolerance or allowance for cardiovascular exercise is exhausted, the cool-down portion of the exercise program is initiated. The purpose of the cool-down is to bring the body back to a resting state and reduce the stress on the body. It consists of light cardiovascular activity, range of motion exercises, breathing exercises, and stretching exercises.

Outcomes and Documentation

The therapist is responsible for documenting the physical activity the client accomplished in a way that the rest of the medical team can evaluate. It is also important for the documentation to be in a form that allows the client to see his/her progress in increasing fitness and ability. The documentation should include:

- Amount of time engaged in cardiovascular activity.
- The intensity of the cardiovascular activity. Objective measures should be recorded if possible such as exact distance walked in a stated amount of time or the number of repetitions of an exercise that are done during the aerobic activity.
- Exact amounts of weight and numbers of repetitions for every strength exercise.
- The client's ability to self-monitor vital signs and outward signs of fatigue.
- The client's ability to adapt exercises to meet needs including range and intensity restrictions.
- The client's ability to perform the exercises correctly and safely.
- The client's reaction to participation in the exercise program.
- Vital sign measurements.
- Progress in resolving problems discussed in the Indications section.

Changes in ICF codes used as the basis for treatment, from those listed in the Indications section, can be documented to show improvement in health and function.

In the literature, there appears to be a paradigm shift from measuring aerobic fitness to musculoskeletal fitness. Muscle strength and flexibility are joining endurance because "improvements in indicators of health status can occur as a result of increasing physical activity levels in the absence of changes in aerobic fitness. This is particularly evident in elderly populations, where regular physical activity can lead to reductions in risk factors for chronic disease and disability without markedly changing traditional physiological performance markers (e.g., cardiac output and oxidative potential)" (Warburton, et al., 2006, p. 805).

Resources

Alberta Centre for Active Living

www.centre4activeliving.ca

Evidence-based physical activity information for practitioners and decision-makers. Includes a Physical Activity Counseling Toolkit with handouts for practitioners to use when counseling clients on starting and maintaining a physically active lifestyle.

Physical Activity Guidelines for Americans

www.health.gov/paguidelines/

Developed by the Office of Disease Prevention and Health Promotion

Provides guidelines and resources related to physical activity engagement. Be sure to look at the "Related Resources" link for a variety of toolkits, programs, trainings, assessment, and tracking resources.

References

Bouchard, C., Blair, S. N., & Haskell, W. (2006). *Physical activity and health* (2nd ed.). Champaign, IL: Human Kinetics.

Caspersen, C. J., Powell, K. E., & Christenson, G. M. (1985). Physical activity, exercise, and physical fitness: Definitions and distinctions for health-related research. *Public Health Rep, 100*(2), 126-131.

Centers for Disease Control and Prevention. (2014). Facts about physical activity. Accessed via www.cdc.gov/physicalactivity/data/facts.html.

Centers for Disease Control and Prevention. (2011). Target heart rate and estimated maximum heart rate. Accessed via www.cdc.gov/physicalactivity/everyone/measuring/heartrate.html.

DiLorenzo, T. M., Stucky-Ropp, R. C., Vander Wal, J. S., & Gotham, H. J. (1998). Determinants of children's physical activity. *Preventive Medicine, 27*, 470-477.

Dishman, R. K., Motl, R. W., Saunders, R., Felton, G., Ward, D. S., Dowda, M., & Pate, R. R. (2005). Enjoyment mediates effects of a school-based physical-activity intervention. *Medical Science of Sports Exercise, 37*(3), 478-487.

Farley, B. G., Fox, C. M., Ramig, L. O., & McFarland, D. H. (2008). Intensive amplitude-specific therapeutic approaches for Parkinson's disease: Toward a neuroplasticity-principled rehabilitation model. *Topics in Geriatric Rehabilitation, 24*(2), 99-114.

Iwasaki, Y., Coyle, C., & Shank, J. (2010). Leisure as a context for active living, recovery, health, and quality of life for persons with mental illness in a global context. *Health Promotion International, 25*(4), 483-494.

Lindgren, E. & Fridlund, B. (1999). Influencing exercise adherence in physically non-active young women: Suggestion for a model. *Women in Sport & Physical Activity Journal, 8*(2), 17-44.

Johnson, N. & Heller, R. (1998). Prediction of patient non-adherence with home-based exercise for cardiac rehabilitation: The role of perceived barriers and perceived benefits. *Preventive Medicine, 27*, 56-64.

Johnston, K. (1992). *The effects of exercise on standing balance, pain, and coping resources maintenance: A comparison of land and water exercise for arthritis patients.* Dissertation. Georgia State University, Atlanta, GA.

Kelley, C. & Loy, D. P. (2008). Comparing the effects of aquatic and land-based exercise on the physiological stress response of women with fibromyalgia. *Therapeutic Recreation Journal, XLII*(2), 103-118.

National Diabetes Information Clearinghouse. (2013). Diabetes overview. Retrieved from www.diabetes.niddk.nih.gov/dm/pubs/overview/index.aspx.

Porter, H., Iwasaki, Y., & Shank, J. (2011). Conceptualizing meaning-making through leisure experiences. *Society & Leisure, 33*(2), 167-194.

Porter, H., Shank, J., & Iwasaki, Y. (2012). Promoting a collaborative approach with recreational therapy to improve physical activity engagement in type 2 diabetes. *Therapeutic Recreation Journal, XLVI*(3), 202-217.

President's Council on Fitness, Sports, and Nutrition. (2014). Physical activity. Accessed via www.cdc.gov/physicalactivity/data/facts.html.

Rosenstein, A. (2008). *Water exercises for Parkinson's: Maintaining endurance, strength, flexibility, and balance* (revised ed.). Enumclaw, WA: Idyll Arbor, Inc.

Tsai, E. (2005). A cross-cultural study of the influence of perceived positive outcomes on participation in regular active recreation: Hong Kong and Australian university students. *Leisure Sciences, 27*, 385-404.

U.S. Department of Health and Human Services. (2008). *2008 physical activity guidelines for Americans.* Accessed via www.health.gov/paguidelines/pdf/paguide.pdf.

Warburton, D., Nicol, C., & Bredin, S. (2006). Health benefits of physical activity: The evidence. *CMAJ, 174*(6), 801-809.

Whitney, L., Deel, D., Marple, J., Metzger, S., Wilder, M., & Harrison, A. (2000). Balance, fear of falling, and quality of life in arthritic elders participating in an aquatic exercise program. *Physical Therapy, 80*, S36.

Williams, D. M., Papandonatos, G. D., Napolitano, M. A., Lewis, B. A., Whiteley, J. A., & Marcus, B. H. (2006). Perceived enjoyment moderates the efficacy of an individually tailored physical activity intervention. *Journal of Sport and Exercise Psychology, 28*(3), 300-309.

World Health Organization. (2014). Physical activity. Accessed via www.who.int/topics/physical_activity/en/.

40. Reality Orientation

Robert M. Beland

Reality orientation (RO) programs have been part of treatment protocols in long-term care facilities, physical rehabilitation, and psychiatric treatment facilities for many years. In recent years, some practitioners refer to reality orientation as part of the general modality of Cognitive Stimulation Therapy (Spector, Woods, &, Orrell, 2008). The primary treatment goals are aimed at improving a person's orientation to self, place, and time. In addition to specific programs for RO, many facilities designed for individuals with Alzheimer's, such as Memory Care Units, have been established (O'Connell et al., 2007; Reimer et al., 2004).

Although research regarding RO's effectiveness is mixed, it still remains an integral part of many rehab programs conducted not only by recreational therapists (RT), but also by activity professionals, occupational therapists, physical therapists, psychologists, social workers, nurses, nursing assistants (CNA), and even support staff. Common RO equipment includes a RO board, signs, and radios or televisions (Knapp et al., 2006).

Indications

RO is a primary treatment for individuals who have symptoms of disorientation to person (self and others), place, and/or time (b114 Orientation Functions). It may also be useful to individuals who experience symptoms of general confusion, non-recognition of others, or a lack of sense of direction or relationship with their surroundings (Spector et al., 2003), such as those with mild to severe Alzheimer's, dementia, or organic brain syndrome (Akanuma et al., 2011; Spector et al., 2001). In practice, RO is commonly an integral component of the milieu treatment environment (Scanland & Emershaw, 1993) and is also seen as an alternative to physical restraint. Since physical aggression is often caused by stress

(d240 Handling Stress and Other Psychological Demands) and anxiety (b152 Emotional Functions) in the treatment setting, RO may offer the client the opportunity to calm down (McCloskey, 2004). This can be done by reducing the confusion in the client's environment, whether it is mental confusion or confusion in their physical environment. One of the goals of RO is to develop a daily routine (d230 Carrying Out Daily Routine). McCloskey (2004) emphasizes that keeping a daily routine minimizes the stress of the client, which consequently reduces emotional outbursts (b1304 Impulse Control, b152 Emotional Functions, d720 Complex Interpersonal Interactions).

Some say that RO is a management tool that should be integrated in the total rehabilitation process including programming, evaluation, quality improvement, and tracking systems for long-term care (Moyle et al., 2008). Reality orientation, since it is conducted on a daily basis, additionally provides routine and assists with basic day structuring (Lancioni et al., 2009).

Contraindications

Contraindications to RO are assessed on an individual basis. Current medical practice warns of avoiding RO if it leads to increased frustration (b152 Emotional Functions) for the individual (Rayner, O'Brien, & Shoenbachler, 2006). For example, it would not be in the best interest of the person with severe Alzheimer's disease to be continually reminded that his wife has died resulting in the experience of recurrent psychological distress (Sarne-Fleischmann & Tractinsky, 2008). There is also evidence that RO may not be useful with acute traumatic brain injury. In a study by De Guise et al. (2005), a regular RO program was administered to clients suffering from traumatic brain injury (TBI).

There was no statistical difference between this group and a control group for the duration of post-traumatic amnesia. As with any treatment program, it should not be assumed that RO is for everyone. It is the responsibility of the therapist to evaluate the need and potential for benefit or harm to the individual.

Protocols

The specific RO protocol may vary depending on individual needs. Evidence-based practice regarding RO entails establishing "what works for whom," rather than a standard approach. This may require readiness to adopt a more empirical approach, using simple single-case designs, with the person as their own control. The current state of research indicates a diverse portrayal of how RO may or may not work for various disabilities. Since there is enough evidence to show that RO may be effective, it should be included among the various modalities that recreational therapists and other healthcare professionals practice (Knapp et al., 2006). This represents an area for future research.

However, since the goal of RO is to facilitate a person's awareness of person, place, and/or time, it is critical that daily monitoring be done. Orientation is perpetuated through (1) structured individual and/or group sessions, (2) unstructured individual encounters, and (3) orientation materials in the environment (Spector, Woods, & Orrell, 2008). In most cases, RO is administered by the recreational therapist daily in an individual or group format and incorporated by all staff as part of the therapeutic milieu, such as a nurse orienting the person to the correct name of the facility when the wrong facility name is verbalized. RO group sessions are typically held every morning for approximately 30 minutes and the length of individual sessions will vary depending on the needs and tolerance of the participants (Spector, Woods, & Orrell, 2008).

Processes

Prior to implementing RO, the recreational therapist needs to ascertain the client's level of orientation. In addition to asking the individual direct orientation questions, the therapist can observe the person's behavioral responses to assess orientation, especially for individuals who are unable to speak or whose speech is impaired. Useful questions may include: Does the client seem to be aware of being a separate individual? Does the client get lost easily when walking around the hospital floor? Is the client unable to find his/her room? Does the client attempt to put on a heavy coat when it is 80°F outside? Does the client's facial expression look puzzled or fearful when someone in his/her immediate family is standing in front of him/her?

Orientation to self is the most basic function. Orientation to person seems to come back before orientation to place. And orientation to place seems to come back before orientation to time. Orientation to person is a retrograde memory function, (client's ability to remember information that occurred before the injury) while orientation to place and time require the client to learn, retain, and recall new information. Problems with retrograde memory may resolve due to the normal healing process of the brain, whereas the ability to learn, retain, and recall new information includes more complex skills that take longer to recover.

The therapist challenges the person with an orientation task in each sphere (person, place, and time) by posing questions. Appropriate multi-modal cueing (e.g., verbal cues, visual cues, gestural cues) is provided to assist the person in identifying the correct answer (Spector et al., 2007). The therapist must already know the answers to the questions to be able to determine the accuracy of the client's answers. Sample questions include:

Person (orientation to self): What is your name? How old are you? Are you a boy or a girl? Are you a grandfather (social roles)? (Patton, 2006a; Thomas et al., 2003).

Person (orientation to others): Do you have any brothers, sisters, or children? What are their names? How old are they? Who is your nurse for the day? Who is your recreational therapist? A therapist can show the person pictures of people and ask the person to tell the therapist who they are (Kasl-Godley & Gatz, 2000; Patton, 2006a).

Place: What city and state are we in? What is the name of this facility? What floor are you on? What is your room number? Topographical orientation (also known as spatial orientation) is a form of orientation to place covered in the ICF as part of b1800 Experience of Self, being aware of "one's position in the reality of the environment around oneself." It is a common form of orientation that is assessed and addressed in a rehabilitation setting. Topographical orientation is the mental function that produces awareness of where one is in relation to the environment using both visual and non-visual input to understand the layout of one's world. For example, if a client is standing in front of the hospital cafeteria, she should be able to form a "mental map" of where she is in relation to her room. A topographical orientation question might be "How do we get to the activity room from here?" (Patton, 2006b; Thomas et al., 2003; Saddichha & Pandey, 2008).

Time: What time of day is it? Which meal did you just eat? What activity are you going to next? What day of the week is it? What month is it? What season is it? What is the year? (Malone, 2012; Olsson et al., 2000).

Besides orienting a client to person, place, and time, it is critical that other areas are equally supported. Staff (e355 Health Professionals) and family (e310 Immediate Family) involvement in all aspects of the client's daily life ensure that reality orientation efforts have a chance of succeeding. The following techniques are useful since they address the person's everyday environment and routine while offering staff and family members practical ways to assist in the orientation of the person.

Developing and adhering to a daily routine for the client. A structured and consistent routine will help to orient the client because it will be predictable and repetitive. For example, the client always goes to speech therapy at nine in the morning, followed by recreational therapy at ten in the morning. As a result of this schedule, the client may begin to associate therapy with a specific time, thus increasing the client's attention to time. In addition, the client will travel the same route, the client's room to the speech clinic, the speech clinic to the recreational therapy clinic, the recreational therapy clinic back to the client's room. A consistent travel pattern will assist the client in remembering the environmental layout, including topographical orientation. The environment can be confusing if you are always coming and going from different places and from different directions (Camp, Zeisel, & Antenucci, 2011; Meuser, 2011).

Organizing the client's personal environment so that it consistently enhances orientation (e.g., shoes are always inside the closet on the floor, orientation materials are always kept in a binder on the side of the wheelchair) (Day, Higgins, & Keatinge, 2011).

Making and posting clear signage for specific locations (e.g., a big arrow and a picture of a toilet that points to where the bathroom is located and then a big picture of a toilet on the outside of the bathroom door) (Hulme et al., 2010; Qizilbash et al., 2002).

Teaching the client to look for landmarks (e.g., notice the large painting of the night sky on the wall, notice the lobby area, notice the pool) (Malone, 2012).

Using orientation materials such as a calendar on the wall in the client's room (have the client cross off the day after dinner), maps (e.g., a simple map of the client's unit, a map of the client's neighborhood), pictures with labels (e.g., pictures of each family member with the name written beneath each picture). Other ideas include making sure the client has and uses a watch or a clock and using a memory book (also called a log book) (Farina & Villanelli, 2008).

Using a daily orientation group that focuses on cognitive remediation techniques for orientation. Many facilities run a reality orientation group first thing in the morning (either before or after breakfast) to orient clients to the day and to help them prepare their orientation materials for the day (e.g., review each client's therapy schedule and make sure it is put in the memory book, check the correctness of the calendar inside the memory book) (Manepalli, Desai, & Sharma, 2009; Zanetti et al., 2002).

Using cognitive remediation techniques to orient the client at the beginning of each treatment session. For example, ask the client what his/her name is, what therapy s/he is now attending, what is typically done at this therapy, what the name of the hospital is, what time of day it is, etc.

If a client does not fully recover orientation functions, the therapist will have to adapt or modify the client's environment and tasks (e1 Products and Technology) to maximize functioning. The therapist shifts from a restorative approach to an adaptation approach. In addition, the therapist will need to educate the client's caregivers on how to promote further recovery of orientation after discharge. While further recovery does not happen with dementia, it is very likely for a client with a traumatic brain injury being discharged from an inpatient rehabilitation center. Adaptation and modification of the client's environment are very important for the client's safety, functioning, and emotional health (Boccardi & Frisoni, 2006; Woods et al., 2012). If the client is not properly oriented, injury could result. For example, the client could become lost. Another consideration is that of functioning. If a client is not properly oriented to time, then the client's sleep cycle could become disturbed and activities might be initiated at inappropriate times (e.g., client thinks that it is morning when it is evening and attempts to get ready for work). Finally, disorientation can affect the emotional health of clients. Being told, "No, you're wrong. That's not right." can take a toll on the client's temperament (b126 Temperament and Personality Functions), possibly leading to depression.

Compensatory strategies for disorientation are not very different from what a therapist uses to enhance the skills of orientation. Compensatory strategies used during treatment are kept and carried over into the client's daily routine outside of the hospital setting. The therapist is responsible to assess assimilation of the compensatory strategies into the client's "real life" and make changes as necessary to promote best functioning. Changes should be as minimal as possible. For example, a client may have used a large binder to hold reference papers for orientation in the hospital setting, but now finds it difficult to constantly carry around the large binder for community tasks such as grocery shopping, hiking with the kids, and bike riding. The therapist may suggest using a backpack to carry the binder so that the client's hands are free for activity. If the client is able to alter the shape and content of the memory book, without additional disorientation, to a smaller date book organizer, then it would fit in a waist pack, back pants pocket, or pocket book. It is not unusual for a client to have a large binder in the home environment and a small date book organizer in the community environment.

In recent years, technology has provided an additional resource for RO programming. Gowans et al. (2007) have demonstrated the value of technology and computer use to help people with dementia improve their overall quality of life including RO. Astell et al. (2010) have indicated that the use of touch screen technology has improved the daily lives not only of clients but of staff and caregivers as well. Wherton and Monk (2008) demonstrated how a digital clock can be very useful in an RO program for time and how a portable compass can assist in place and location orientation. Sixsmith et al. (2012) also point out how technology can improve the quality of

life for people with disabilities such as orientation to place in their home environments. Such technology may include ambient assisted living. Ambient assisted living refers to any technology that improves the daily lives of a home's residents. Everything from voice-activated controls, panic alarms, remote control of windows or doors, and temperature control devices are part of the growing industry of ambient design.

Kuwahara et al. (2010) have demonstrated the value of using reminiscence videos to improve the stress levels of persons with dementia living at home. Even the use of digital photo diaries, which can be used in an RO context, has been shown to increase (or improve) autonomy and independence for persons with dementia (Harrefors et al., 2012). Consequently, healthcare professionals would be wise to keep current of the latest technological gadgets and how they might be used in RO programming.

Outcomes and Documentation

The first consideration to measuring outcomes is to understand the meaningfulness of the outcomes. For example, a therapist may be able to say that in one month a client improved his orientation to self (he knew his name) by 100%. However, if in June he knew his name only once and in July he knew his name twice, it should not be considered meaningful. The various goals of RO are that the client has regular, daily improvement. Responses to orientation may be recorded in a client's treatment record, progress notes, or discharge summary, if appropriate.

The ICF is a framework that promotes a more holistic model of client care with the focus on enabling clients to participate in society, in contrast to the previous focus on pathology and impairments. ICF codes related to RO techniques include b114 Orientation Functions, d135 Rehearsing, b144 Memory Functions, and other ICF codes that were identified previously in the chapter.

The most common method of measuring orientation is the scale called *orientation x3*. As burlingame and Blaschko (2010) point out, the protocols for determining orientation x3 are not well developed, so the scores should always be taken as a general measurement of orientation and not as specific orientation. Similarly to consciousness, variability in orientation is seen throughout the day. In addition to noting the time of day that the therapist is measuring orientation, the therapist should measure the client's response in the following ways. Possible chart notes are shown.

Terms of sphere: "Client is oriented to person without cueing, but is not oriented to time." "Client is alert and oriented x3 [oriented in all three spheres]." If a client is not alert, it is very hard for him/her to be oriented.

Percentage of orientation: "Client is oriented to place at 50%" — this means that the client was able to answer only 50% of the orientation questions about place or that the client was observed being disoriented to place about half the time through behavioral observation.

Level of assistance needed: "Client requires moderate verbal cues to orient to place."

Relation to task dysfunction: "Client requires moderate verbal cues to locate the cafeteria secondary to poor topographical orientation."

Other standardized measures may include the *Mini-Mental State Examination*. Because these scores are thought to decline by an average of four points per year for dementia, the benefits of RO might equate to a six-month delay in the usual cognitive deterioration (Dodds, 2009). Whether such a delay is of functional benefit to an individual client would necessarily vary. Other assessment instruments include the *Wechsler Memory Scale* and the Self-Care Functioning subscale of the *Monitoring of Side Effects Scale* (MOSES).

Resources

National Council of Certified Dementia Practitioners
www.nccdp.org
This organization provides several resources related to recreational therapy, activity therapy, Alzheimer's disease, and reality orientation with directions to links and resources categories.

Nursing Home Activity Resources
www.nursinghomeactivitiesresource.com/index.shtml
This web site provides practical ideas for activities with older adults and persons with Alzheimer's, along with reality orientation activities.

References

Akanuma, K., Meguro, K., Meguro, M., Sasaki, E., Chiba, K., Ishii, H., & Tanaka, N. (2011). Improved social interaction and increased anterior cingulate metabolism after group reminiscence with reality orientation approach for vascular dementia. *Psychiatry Research, 192*(3), 183-7.

Astell, A., Ellis, M., Bernardi, L., Alm, N., Dye, R., Gowans, G., & Campbell, J. (2010). Using a touch screen computer to support relationships between people with dementia and caregivers. *Interacting with Computers, 22*(4), 267-275.

Boccardi, M. & Frisoni, G. (2006). Cognitive rehabilitation for severe dementia: Critical observations for better use of existing knowledge. *Mechanisms of Ageing and Development, 127,* 166-172.

burlingame, j. & Blaschko, T. (2010). *Assessment tools for recreational therapy and related fields* (4th ed.). Enumclaw, WA: Idyll Arbor.

Camp, C. J., Zeisel, J., & Antenucci, V. (2011). Implementing the "I'm Still Here Approach": Montessori methods for engaging persons with dementia. In P. E. Hartman-Stein & A. La Rue (Eds.) *Enhancing cognitive fitness in adults*, (pp. 401-417). New York: Springer.

Day J., Higgins I., & Keatinge, D. (2011). Orientation strategies during delirium: Are they helpful? *Journal of Clinical Nursing, 20*(23-24), 3285-94.

de Guise E., LeBlanc J., Feyz M., & Lamoureux J. (2005). Prediction of the level of cognitive functional independence following traumatic brain injury in acute care setting. *Brain Injury, 19*, 1085-1093.

Dodds, J. (2009*). A pilot study investigating the effectiveness of cognitive rehabilitation therapy with patients with schizophrenia with a forensic history.* Edinburgh: University of Edinburgh.

Farina, E. & Villanelli, F. (2008). Cognitive rehabilitation in middle-aged Alzheimer patients. In Sil Jeong, H. (Ed.), *Alzheimer's disease in the middle-aged* (pp 97-116). New York: Nova Science.

Gowans, G., Dye, R., Alm, N., Vaughan, P., Astell, A., & Ellis, M. (2007). Designing the interface between dementia patients, caregivers and computer-based intervention. *The Design Journal, 10*(1) 12-23.

Harrefors, C., Sävenstedt, S. Lundquist, A. Lundquist, B., & Axelsson K. (2012). Professional caregivers' perceptions on how persons with mild dementia might experience the usage of a digital photo diary. *The Open Nursing Journal, 6*, 20-29.

Hulme, C., Wright, J., Crocker, T., Oluboyede, Y., & House, A. (2010). Non-pharmacological approaches for dementia that informal carers might try or access: A systematic review. *International Journal of Geriatric Psychiatry*, 25(7), 756-763.

Kasl-Godley, J. & Gatz, M. (2000). Psychosocial interventions for individuals with dementia: An integration of theory, therapy, and a clinical understanding of dementia. *Clinical Psychology Review, 20*, 755-782.

Knapp, M., Thorgrimsen, L., Patel, A., Spector, A., Hallam, A., Woods, B., & Orrell, M., (2006). Cognitive stimulation therapy for people with dementia: Cost-effectiveness analysis. *The British Journal of Psychiatry, 188*, 574-580.

Kuwahara, N., Yasuda, K., Tetsutani, N., & Morimoto, K. (2010). Remote assistance for people with dementia at home using reminiscence systems and a schedule prompter. *International Journal of Computers in Healthcare, 1*(2) 126-143.

Lancioni, G., Pinto, K., La Martire, M., Tota, A., Rigante, V., Tatulli, E., et al. (2009). Helping persons with mild or moderate Alzheimer disease recapture basic daily activities through the use of an instruction strategy. *Disability and Rehabilitation, 31*(3), 211-219.

Malone, M. (2012). Interventions for treating persons with dementia. Presented at the annual convention of the Ohio Speech Language and Hearing Association.

Manepalli, J., Desai, A., & Sharma, P. (2009). Psychosocial-environmental treatments for Alzheimer's disease. *Primary Psychiatry, 16*(6), 39.

Mathew, G. (1987). Use of computer for reality-orientation in a man with cognitive deficits. *Journal of the British Institute of Mental Handicap, 15*(3), 122-123.

McCloskey, R. (2004). Caring for patients with dementia in an acute care environment. *Geriatric Nursing, 25*(3), 139-144.

Meuser, T. (2011). Oral life review in older adults: Principles for the social service professional. In P. E. Hartman-Stein & A. La Rue (Eds.) *Enhancing cognitive fitness in adults,* (pp. 183-198). New York: Springer.

Moyle, W., Olorenshaw, R., Wallis, M., & Borbasi, S. (2008). Best practice for the management of older people with dementia in the acute care setting: A review of the literature. *International Journal of Older People Nursing, 3*(2), 121-130.

O'Connell, B., Gardner, A., Takase, M., Hawkins, M., Ostaszkiewicz, J., Ski, C., & Josipovic, P. (2007). Clinical usefulness and feasibility of using reality orientation with patients who have dementia in acute care settings. *International Journal of Nursing Practice, 13*, 182-192.

Olsson, R., Greinger, L., Kucharewski, R., Bahmer, W., Gilbert, M., & Eichner, H. (2000). A reliability analysis of a clock test for patients diagnosed with Alzheimer's disease: Implications for kinesiology. *Clinical Kinesiology, 54(*2), 44-47.

Patton, D. (2006a). Reality orientation: Its use and effectiveness within older person mental health care. *Journal of Clinical Nursing, 15*(11), 1440-9.

Patton D. (2006b). The value of reality orientation with older adults who are mentally ill: A study from the Republic of Ireland. *Gerontological Nursing, 32*(12), 6-13.

Qizilbash, M., Schneider, L., Chui, H., Tariot, P., Brodaty, H., Kaye, J., & Erkinjutti, T. (eds.) (2002) *Evidence-based dementia practice.* Malden, MA: Blackwell Publishing.

Rayner, A., O'Brien, J., & Shoenbachler, B. (2006). Behavior disorders of dementia: Recognition and treatment. *American Family Physician, 73,* 647- 654.

Reimer, M., Slaughter, S., Donaldson, C., Currie, G., & Eliasziw, M. (2004). Special care facility compared with traditional environments for dementia care: A longitudinal study of quality of life. *Journal of the American Geriatrics Society, 52*(7), 1085-1092.

Saddichha, S. & Pandey, V. (2008). Alzheimer's and non-Alzheimer's dementia: A critical review of pharmacological and nonpharmacological strategies. *American Journal of Alzheimer's Disease and Other Dementias, 23*(2), 150-161.

Sarne-Fleischmann, V. & Tractinsky, N. (2008). Development and evaluation of a personalised multimedia system for reminiscence therapy in Alzheimer's patients. *International Journal of Social and Humanistic Computing, 1*(1), 81-96.

Scanland, S. & Emershaw, L. (1993, June). Reality orientation and validation therapy — Dementia, depression and functional status. *Journal of Gerontological Nursing,* 7-11.

Sixsmith, A., Woolrych, R., Bierhoff, I., Mueller, S., & Byrne, P. (2012). Ambient assisted living: From concept to implementation. In A. Glascock & D. Kutzik (Eds.), *Essential lessons for the success of telehomecare* (pp. 259-286). IOS Press: Amsterdam, Netherlands.

Spector, A., Woods, B., & Orrell, M. (2008). Cognitive stimulation for the treatment of Alzheimer's disease. *Expert Review of Neurotherapeutics, 8*(5), 751-757.

Spector, A., Orrell, M., Davies, S., & Woods, B. (2007). Withdrawn: Reality orientation for dementia. *Cochrane Database of Systematic Reviews, 18*(3), CD001119.

Spector, A., Thorgrimsen, L., Woods, B., Royan, L., Davies, S., Butterworth, M., & Orrell, M. (2003). Efficacy of evidence-based cognitive stimulation therapy programme for people with dementia. *The British Journal of Psychiatry, 183,* 248-254.

Spector, A., Orrell, M., Davies, S., & Woods, B. (2001). Can reality orientation be rehabilitated? Development and piloting of an evidence-based programme of cognition-based therapies for people with dementia. *Neuropsychological Rehabilitation, 11*(3/4) 377-397.

Thomas, H., Feyz, M., LeBlanc, J., Brosseau, J., Champoux, M., Christopher, A., et al. (2003). North Star Project: Reality orientation in an acute setting for patients with traumatic brain injuries. *Journal of Head Trauma Rehabilitation, 18*(3) 292-302.

Wherton, J. & Monk, A. (2008). Technological opportunities for supporting people with dementia who are living at home. *International Journal of Human-Computer Studies, 66*(8), 571-586.

Woods, B., Aguirre, E., Spector, A., & Orrell, M. (2012). Cognitive stimulation to improve cognitive functioning in people with dementia. Cochrane Database of Systematic Reviews.

World Health Organization. (2001). International Classification of Functioning, Disability and Health. Endorsed by the 54th World Health Assembly on May 22, 2001.

Zanetti, O., Oriani, M., Geroldi, C., Binetti, G., Frisoni, G., Di Giovani, G., & De Vreese, L. (2002). Predictors of cognitive improvement after reality orientation in Alzheimer's disease. *Age and Ageing, 31,* 193-196.

41. Reminiscence

Elizabeth H. Weybright and Heather R. Porter

Reminiscence, introduced as a therapeutic tool by Robert Butler in 1963, is a technique used to review and evaluate past life events, often with the goal of facilitating self-acceptance and enhancing psychological well-being (Pinquart & Forstmeier, 2012). It is defined as a "process of thinking or telling someone about past experiences that are personally significant" and is believed to be a central task in the aging process (Pinquart & Forstmeier, 2012, p. 541).

Although participation in reminiscence generally leads to positive outcomes, this may differ by the function of reminiscence. Taxonomies have been developed which separate reminiscence based on the functions they serve (Webster, 1993, 1997). Watt and Wong (1991) developed one such taxonomy using data collected from semi-structured interviews with 460 individuals ranging in age from 65 to 95 years old. Transcripts were analyzed for thematic content, guided by theory and prior empirical findings. Six types or categories of reminiscence were identified (adapted from Wong, 1995 and Dattilo & McKenney, 2011):

Integrative reminiscence: Integrative reminiscence works to combine the past with the present and facilitate self-acceptance to "achieve a sense of meaning, coherence, and reconciliation with regard to one's past" (Watt & Wong, 1991, p. 44). This type of reminiscence is most similar to Butler's Life Review and its adaptive qualities come from the integration of past and current life events (Watt & Wong, 1991). (See the chapter on Life Review in this book for other techniques of life review.) The recreational therapist can incorporate integrative reminiscence by asking clients to share meaningful experiences from their lifetime and discuss their major accomplishments. Watt and Wong suggest therapists can also aid clients in accepting their current life situation and

abilities by helping "clarify or redefine life goals so that the client may learn to accept his/her limitations" (1991; p. 53). Integrative reminiscence is associated with successful aging.

Instrumental reminiscence: Instrumental reminiscence is a type of problem-focused coping, shown to buffer against stressful situations, where individuals use their past experiences and how they coped with those difficulties to help solve current problems. It contributes to subjective perceptions of competence and continuity through recollection of past plans, how one coped with past difficulties, attained goals, and successfully solved problems. It may enhance a personal sense of mastery (Wong & Watt, 1991). For this type, the recreational therapist may ask the clients to talk about a time in which they faced a challenging situation and how they overcame it. This recollection may aide the client in solving a current problem while enhancing feelings of autonomy and control, which are associated with positive feelings such as life satisfaction. Instrumental reminiscence is associated with successful aging.

Transmissive reminiscence: Similar to oral history, transmissive reminiscence involves sharing life events with the intention of instilling values and ideas important to the individual. It involves passing cultural heritage and personal legacy (Watt & Wong, 1991) on to others through storytelling, moral instruction, sharing traditional values, and sharing personal wisdom or lessons learned in the past. To facilitate transmissive reminiscence, the recreational therapist can ask clients about family or cultural traditions, and ask about the culture and practices they experienced growing up. Recreational therapists could also work with clients in small groups or individually to document culture and tradition to pass along to family members. Transmissive reminiscence is associated with successful aging.

Narrative reminiscence: Narrative reminiscence is most similar to storytelling and sharing descriptive or factual information from one's past. When reminiscence cannot be categorized elsewhere, it is considered narrative reminiscence (Wong & Watt, 1991). It includes statements of autobiographical facts, such as a simple autobiographical sketch or anecdotes from the past in the absence of psychological evaluations present in other categories of reminiscence. This type of reminiscence may be prompted by questions asking clients to share about specific life events (e.g., birthdays, holidays). Narrative reminiscence has a neutral effect on successful aging.

Obsessive reminiscence: Obsessive reminiscence is characterized by a focus on unpleasant past events and feelings such as shame or guilt. It includes statements of guilt, bitterness, disappointment, and despair regarding the past, including persistent or repeated rumination on unpleasant past events. Such rumination can be associated with internalizing disorders including anxiety and depression (Watt & Wong, 1991). When an individual engages excessively in obsessive reminiscence, a referral for psychiatric services may be indicated. Obsessive reminiscence can inhibit successful aging.

Escapist reminiscence: Escapist reminiscence focuses on positive past experiences from a fantasy or daydreaming perspective as a means to escape an individual's current situation. It includes statements that "glorify the past and deprecate (or belittle) the present," such as boasting exaggeratedly about past achievements or exaggerating the pleasant aspects of the past and desiring to return to "the good old days" (Watt & Wong, 1991, p. 273). While daydreaming can encourage creativity and provide a temporary reprieve from an unpleasant environment, being preoccupied with the past may prevent an individual from addressing day-to-day needs and be indicative of mental health concerns such as depression. When an individual engages excessively in escapist reminiscence, a referral for psychiatric services may be indicated. Escapist reminiscence can be detrimental to successful aging.

Research Findings

Research related to types of reminiscence has identified positive outcomes for older adults with depression or depressive symptoms. For example, Karimi and colleagues (2010) conducted a study of 29 older adults in long-term residential care reporting depressive symptoms. The participants were assigned to an integrative reminiscence group, an instrumental reminiscence group, or a control group (a social discussion group). Each group had six weekly sessions lasting 90 minutes each. The integrative reminiscence group focused on self-worth, including disconfirmation of negative beliefs about the self and the future; alternatives to self-blame; internal guidelines for the evaluation of self-worth; and renewed sources of self-worth. The instrumental reminiscence group focused on coping, including coping resources, primary and secondary appraisal strategies, and problem- and emotion-focused coping responses. The social discussion group talked about concerns related to older adults, including changes in family relationships, supportive organizations for older adults, etc. Following the intervention, depressive symptoms in the integrative reminiscence group were significantly lower than those in the social-discussion control group, while no significant difference was found in depressive symptoms between the instrumental group and the control group.

In a study by Shellman, Mokel, and Hewitt (2009), 56 community dwelling urban African-American older adults were randomized into an integrative reminiscence group, an attention control group focusing on health education, and a control group with no active intervention. Each group was held for 45 minutes once a week for eight weeks. In the integrative reminiscence group, the participants reflected on childhood memories, holiday traditions, and work and family life. The facilitator probed and validated experiences with the goals of identifying and shifting thinking that might lead to depression by reframing thinking about the past, identifying coping strategies, and emphasizing competence. Following the interventions, the integrative reminiscence group had significantly lower depressive symptoms compared to the other two groups.

Integrative reminiscence has also shown positive effects outside of reducing depressive symptoms. In a study of 108 older adults with mild to moderate depression, participation in an integrative/narrative reminiscence group called "The Story of Your Life" yielded not only a reduction in depressive symptoms, but also higher feelings of mastery. The effects were maintained in a follow-up three months after the intervention. In this study, four participants were paired with one facilitator for eight two-hour sessions with the following themes: introduction and meeting, youth, work and care, difficult times, social relations, turning points metaphors, meaning, and future (Bohlmeijer et al., 2009).

Wu (2010) studied 74 older adult veterans participating in an integrative reminiscence group held once a week for 12 weeks. Following the intervention, participants exhibited improved self-esteem, life satisfaction, sense of positive self-value, and sense of belonging to the institution, in addition to reduced depressive symptoms. In a previous study involving the same author (Chao et al., 2006), 12 older adults in long-term residential care who received nine weekly one-hour reminiscence sessions also experienced positive changes in self-esteem.

As a final example, a review of the reminiscence literature related to dementia by Cotelli, Manenti, and Zanetti (2012) found evidence that reminiscence interventions (when combined with other common older adult interventions such as reality orientation and sensory stimulation) may be helpful in improving mood (e.g., well-being, reduced agitated behavior), cognitive function (e.g., autobiographical memory), social communication, activity level, and brain function (e.g., increase in cerebral metabolism in the anterior cingulate).

Outside of individual studies, meta-analyses have also been conducted on reminiscence interventions and have yielded interesting findings. For example, an evaluation of 128 reminiscence studies on nine outcome variables by Pinquart and Forstmeier (2012) found moderate outcomes regarding ego-integrity, death preparation, mastery, mental health symptoms, positive well-being, social integration, and cognitive performance. Most of the outcomes were maintained at follow up. They also found that reminiscence interventions for individuals who were depressed or had chronic disease had larger effects related to depressive symptoms, and those who received a more structured, evaluative reminiscence intervention benefited more from the intervention than those who received a less structured, narrative reminiscence intervention. The authors additionally postulated a preventive effect from participation in reminiscence interventions. Another meta-analysis of 15 controlled trials related to reminiscence interventions also indicated beneficial effects on happiness and depression (Chin, 2007).

In a meta-analysis, the structure of reminiscence sessions was found to impact outcomes. For example, according to Webster, Bohlmeijer, and Westerhof (2010), studies generally concluded that people with higher levels of depression benefit more from reminiscence interventions than people with low or moderate levels of depression. The studies also showed that the effects of structured, evaluative reminiscence interventions are stronger than the effects of unstructured, simple reminiscence interventions. The authors concluded that unstructured, simple reminiscence still can be beneficial for less distressed persons, but structured, evaluative reminiscence interventions would better serve persons with higher levels of distress.

Lastly, in current healthcare practice, non-pharmacological approaches are gaining increased attention. In relation to reminiscence, a meta-analysis of 20 controlled outcome studies conducted by Bohlmeijer, Smit, and Cuijpers (2003) found that reminiscence and life review significantly reduced depressive symptoms in older adults and may offer "a valuable alternative to psychotherapy or pharmacotherapy" (p. 1088).

Indications

If clients show deficits in any of the areas covered in the Research Findings section, they may be candidates for reminiscence interventions. These include diagnoses with concerns about identity formation, self-esteem, life satisfaction, social interaction, social skills, isolation, anxiety, depression, other mental health symptoms, and overall well-being. Relevant ICF codes include b126 Temperament and Personality Functions, b130 Energy and Drive Functions, b152 Emotional Functions, b180 Experience of Self and Time Functions, and d7 Interpersonal Interactions and Relationships.

Contraindications

The use of reminiscence is contraindicated for individuals who have experienced previous traumatic life experiences or who have a diagnosis of post-traumatic stress disorder, unless conducted by a counselor in a psychotherapeutic setting. Although discussing topics unrelated to traumatic experiences is often safe, access to mental health services may be needed. This is especially important to keep in mind when discussing sensitive topics with older adults who may have current physical limitations, including weakened cardiovascular systems, as vividly recalling traumatic events can result in physiological reactions which could exacerbate previous health conditions (Cook, Ruzek, & Cassidy, 2003).

Protocols

Reminiscence, as previously reviewed, can be applied as an evaluative, structured intervention or as a simple, unstructured intervention. It can occur in a variety of contexts including group or individual settings. To best understand the possible contexts available to recreational therapists, Bornat and colleagues (1998) identified five formats of reminiscence that are typically found in residential settings, such as assisted living facilities and skilled nursing facilities. Listed in order from the most structured to the least structured, they include:

Formal group: Most commonly used form of reminiscence with structured, regularly scheduled meeting times. Discussion is focused on pre-planned themes.

Formal individual: The same as formal group but instead of a group setting, it is done with one participant individually.

Informal (intimate) individual: An unstructured, unscheduled type of reminiscence, often taking the form of a casual or informal conversation, conducted while providing care, such as dressing or feeding.

Informal ad hoc (groups and individual): Informal conversations or "small talk" between staff members and participants either individually or as a collective where memories are discussed.

Reminiscence-related activities: An activity where reminiscence is not the main goal (e.g., singing songs, traveling), but where memory and/or experience sharing occurs. For example, during a music group, specific songs bring up memories and experiences that a client shares with the group.

Research shows that there are no differences in outcomes between group and individual formats (Bohlmeijer, Smit, & Cuijpers, 2010; Hsieh & Wang, 2003; Pinquart & Forstmeier, 2012). Consequently, the format chosen by the therapist will depend on factors such as the needs, abilities, and goals of the client. For example, individuals with dementia may have difficulty interacting in a group situation and may be more engaged in a one-to-one or small group setting (Woolf et al., 2002). As reviewed in the

Indications section above, however, the majority of reminiscence research validates the use of group reminiscence interventions and advocates for the utilization of integrative reminiscence and structured, evaluative reminiscence, as this results in overall stronger effects compared to simple, unstructured reminiscence interventions.

A protocol for an evidence-based, structured reminiscence group with older adults developed by Stinson (2009) is provided in Table 18. This protocol has been evaluated twice (Stinson, 2009; Stinson & Kirk, 2006) and found to reduce depression between pre- and post-intervention measures. Stinson's protocol specifies that reminiscence groups meet for one hour twice a week for six weeks. Although this protocol targets nurses as group leaders, it is appropriate for use by recreational therapists. Stinson's protocol provides themes and activities for each bi-weekly session. When planning individual or group reminiscence interventions, the Stinson protocols can provide a structured framework. For example, the Stinson protocols specifically mention dates from the 1920s to the 1960s. Recreational therapists should adjust those dates so that they are relevant to the members of each group. Baby Boomers, who were born after 1945, for example, will probably not have many memories of events 20 years before they were born. For additional protocols see Burnside and Haight, 1994.

Table 18: Stinson's Protocol for Structured Reminiscence

Week One, Session One
Introducing leaders and members.
Concentrate on personal background.
Encourage members to bring a picture of an animal
　　or a stuffed animal that represents them.
Have members introduce themselves and tell why the
　　animal reminds them of themselves.
Have extra stuffed animals available.

Week One, Session Two
Remembering the past through songs from the 1920s
　　to 1960s.
Play different songs in chronological order.
See if members recognize songs and discuss any
　　special memories associated with the songs.
Have members talk about a song that might have
　　special meaning to them and explain why it has
　　special meaning.

Encourage clapping and singing.

Week Two, Session Three
Sharing photographs.
Have a show-and-tell session about personal memorabilia.
Give members time to explain the attachment associated with pictures.
Discuss families.
Discuss friends.
Talk about fun times.

Week Two, Session Four
Discussing work, home life, volunteer activities, and first job.
Pass around picture cards showing specific occupations.
Discuss children and volunteer activities from the 1920s to 1960s.
Specifically ask questions to get people to talk about "paths not taken."
Encourage participants to bring memorabilia from their career or occupation (badges, pictures, etc.).

Week Three, Session Five
Remembering a favorite holiday.
Discuss holidays.
Bring scents and cues associated with the past.
Sing songs about holidays.
Talk about foods associated with holidays.
Talk about clothes worn on holidays.
Talk about traditions associated with holidays.

Week Three, Session Six
Remembering school days.
Discuss the first day of school.
Have participants talk about school days.
Show pictures of schools from the 1920s to 1960s.
Discuss teachers and clothing styles.

Week Four, Session Seven
Remembering toys from childhood.
Bring toys from the past.
Discuss first toys.
Discuss unusual toys.
Discuss favorite toys.
Discuss toys made at home.
Show pictures of toys.

Week Four, Session Eight
Remembering first date, spouse, wedding, marriage.
Discuss first dates.
Discuss proposals.

Discuss weddings.
Discuss marriages.
Play songs from the past.
Show a short clip of an old movie that includes "courting."
Have members bring wedding pictures.

Week Five, Session Nine
Remembering family and pets.
Discuss children, pets, and family.
Encourage members to show pictures of their family and pets.

Week Five, Session Ten
Remembering foods.
Discuss favorite foods of childhood, favorite foods at holidays, and favorite smells.
Discuss recipes.
Have participants bring recipes and discuss memories associated with recipes.

Week Six, Session Eleven
Remembering friends.
Talk about friends.
Encourage participants to bring pictures of friends.
Describe the friends in the pictures.
Discuss fun times with friends.
Discuss fun memories.
Discuss friends in the assisted living facility.

Week Six, Session Twelve
Closure.
Have participants talk about their experiences in the group.
Share any last thoughts about the topics discussed previously.
Serve refreshments.
Give certificates.

Reprinted with permission from Stinson, C. K. (2009). Structured group reminiscence: An intervention for older adults. *Journal of Continuing Education in Nursing, 40*(11), 521-528.

Processes

While the processes are dependent on the structure of the session, the recreational therapist should consider specific issues including client assessment, planning for the reminiscence intervention, and implementation. A review of each of these issues follows.

Assessment

Prior to initiating a reminiscence intervention, identify potential clients and assess for the following:

Current level of cognitive functioning: Not all participants may be appropriate for a group setting. Participants with moderate to severe dementia may be better suited for a one-to-one intervention or a small-group intervention (Stinson, 2009; Woolf et al., 2002). Such individuals may require a higher level of supervision than the therapist of a large group may be able to provide. In addition, it is important to acknowledge the contributions of an individual with a cognitive impairment. This may mean adapting to off-topic responses and moods (Tolson & Schofield, 2012).

Sensory limitations, specifically the ability to communicate with others: Participants suitable for large groups should be able to actively listen and respond appropriately to other group members (Stinson, 2009).

Planning

When planning a reminiscence group, consider the following:

Group size: Group size is dependent on the cognitive functioning level of the participants, the comfort level of participants in the group, the topic of discussion, and the degree of group structure. When participants are alert and able to articulate feelings and respond appropriately to each other's contributions, then eight to twelve participants are appropriate. This would most likely be in a community or independent living setting. When participants have impaired cognitive functioning, such as an assisted living setting, six to eight participants are appropriate (Martinez-Cox, Dattilo, & Sheldon, 2011; Woolf et al., 2002). Both of these groups would be considered in the large group category. Small groups of two to five clients and one-on-one activities should also be considered when there are more severe impairments.

Recreational therapist: While there should be at least one therapist present that is experienced with conducting reminiscence groups, therapy ratios are also dependent upon facility, state, and federal staffing regulations.

Structure of sessions (length, setting, topics, etc.): When planning a structured group reminiscence intervention, the format or structure of the sessions is developed by the recreational therapist. When par-

ticipants have mild to no cognitive impairments, a typical session should last between 45 and 60 minutes and be held in the same location each week for consistency. Participants with cognitive impairments should be evaluated to determine whether they are appropriate for an individual or group session, as they may need additional assistance. The room should comfortably hold all participants and be located in a quiet area to reduce participant distractions (Martinez-Cox, Dattilo, & Sheldon, 2011; Stinson, 2009).

Dealing with sad and traumatic memories: Reminiscence can trigger both positive and negative memories, and while it can serve as a means of coping with the negative memories, the recreational therapist should be prepared to provide support to any participant who becomes seriously distressed. This support can come in a variety of forms, including helping the client debrief after a particularly difficult session and/or providing referrals to counseling or psychotherapy (Woolf, Rosefield, Stanton, & Gordon, 2002). For individuals with mood disorders, such as depression, or where there is the possibility of post-traumatic stress disorder, the therapist should discuss the intervention with the client's psychiatrist or physician prior to implementation.

Implementation

During implementation, consider the following (Burnside & Haight, 1994; Stinson, 2009):

Providing group reminders: Providing reminders about when and where the session will be held prior to the start of each group prevents participants from forgetting or dropping out and gives them time to reflect on the topic being discussed.

Themes: While it is important to hold the intervention in the same location each session for consistency, at times it may be appropriate to take a "field trip" to facilitate the recall of life experiences or to fit with a session theme. For example, the recreational therapist may take participants to a kitchen or cooking area to discuss themes related to food. Session themes facilitate discussion and recollection between participants and can include a variety of topics including major life events (e.g., marriage, children, graduation), regularly occurring events (e.g., holidays, birthdays), or focused topics (e.g., a specific city, clothing, transportation).

The use of props (multi-sensory triggers): In addition to themes, props also facilitate recollection and interaction. To stimulate memory, multi-sensory props can be used, such as music, photographs, and aromas. For example, a cooking theme could include the touch, sight, and sound of cooking utensils and the taste and smell of actual food.

Outcomes and Documentation

A variety of outcomes have been commonly targeted in reminiscence (Bohlmeijer et al., 2003; Burnside & Haight, 1994; Stinson, 2009). These can be documented related to the treatment objectives. They include:

- self-esteem, life satisfaction, and overall well-being (b126 Temperament and Personality Functions, b130 Energy and Drive Functions)
- social interaction, social skills, and isolation (d7 Interpersonal Interactions and Relationships)
- identity formation (b180 Experience of Self and Time Functions)
- anxiety, depression, and mental health symptoms (b126 Temperament and Personality Functions, b152 Emotional Functions)

Behavioral outcomes from reminiscence can also be measured through direct observation of social interactions and social skills as part of d7 Interpersonal Interactions and Relationships.

Recreational therapists who desire to measure or research outcomes related to reminiscence interventions are encouraged to consider the *Reminiscence Functions Scale* (RFS; Webster, 1993). The RFS is used to identify how a participant uses reminiscence in his/her life and if it is serving as an adaptive or maladaptive method. The scale has demonstrated reliability and validity for use with older adults (Robitaille et al., 2010). The types of reminiscence outlined in the RFS correspond well to Watt and Wong's (1991) six types of reminiscence described earlier in the chapter. The RFS has also been found to associate with health outcomes when paired with other scales concerned with the following constructs

- Anxiety: *State-Trait Anxiety Inventory* (STAI) (Spielberger, Gorsuch, & Lushene, 1970)
- Depression: *Beck Depression Inventory*, revised (BDI-II) (Beck, Steer, & Brown, 1996)
- Life satisfaction: *Satisfaction with Life Scale* (SWLS) (Diener et al., 1985)
- Well-being: *General Health Questionnaire* (GHQ) (Goldberg, 1978)

Resources

The International Institute for Reminiscence and Life Review (IIRLR)
www.reminiscenceandlifereview.org
The IIRLR brings together participants to further define reminiscence and life review as an interdisciplinary field of study in the areas of practice, research, education, volunteer, and individual application.

Reminiscence Magazine
www.reminisce.com/
A bi-monthly magazine with pictures, stories, and events from the 1920s through the 1950s.

Books
Gibson, F. (2004). *The past in the present: Using reminiscence in health and social care.* Baltimore, MD: Health Professions Press.
Provides a guide to forming reminiscence groups, examples of specific triggers to use, and assessment forms for use with reminiscence groups.

Schweitzer, P. & Bruce, E. (2008). *Remembering yesterday, caring today: Reminiscence in dementia care, a guide to good practice.* Philadelphia, PA: Jessica Kingsley.
Provides a detailed guide to using reminiscence work with older adults who have dementia.

References

Beck, A. T., Steer, R. A., & Brown, G. K. (1996). *Beck Depression Inventory: Second edition manual.* San Antonio: TX: Psychological Corporation.

Bohlmeijer, E., Kramer, J., Smit, F., Onrust, S., & van Marwijk, H. (2009). The effects of integrative reminiscence on depressive symptomatology and mastery of older adults. *Community Mental Health Journal, 45*, 476-484. doi: 10.1007/s10597-009-9246-z.

Bohlmeijer, R., Smit, F., & Cuijpers, P. (2003). Effects of reminiscence and life review on late-life depression: A meta-analysis. *International Journal of Geriatric Psychiatry, 18*(12), 1088-1094. doi: 10.1002/gps.1018.

Bornat, J., Chamerlayne, P., Chant, L., & Pavey, S. (1998). *Redefining reminiscence in care settings.* London, University of East London, Centre for Biography in Social Policy.

Burnside, I. & Haight, B. (1994). Reminiscence and life review: Therapeutic interventions for older people. *Nurse Practitioner, 19*(4), 55-61.

Butler, R. N. (1963). The life review: An interpretation of reminiscence in the aged. *Psychiatry, 26*(1), 65-76.

Chao, S. Y., Liu, H. Y., Wu, C. Y., Jun, S. F., Chu, T. L., Huang, T. S., & Clark, M. J. (2006). The effects of group reminiscence therapy on depression, self esteem, and life satisfaction of elderly nursing home residents. *Journal of Nursing Research, 14*(1), 36-45.

Chin, A. M. H. (2007). Clinical effects of reminiscence therapy in older adults: A meta-analysis of controlled trials. *Hong Kong Journal of Occupational Therapy, 17*(1), 10-22.

Cook, J. M., Ruzek, J. I., & Cassidy, E. (2003). Possible association of posttraumatic stress disorder with cognitive impairment among older adults. *Psychiatric Services, 54*(9), 1223-1225.

Cotelli, M., Manenti, R., & Zanetti, O. (2012). Reminiscence therapy in dementia: A review. *Maturitas, 72*(3), 203-205. doi: 10.1016/j.maturitas.2012.04.008.

Dattilo, J. & McKenney, A. (2011). *Facilitation techniques in therapeutic recreation.* State College, PA: Venture Publishing.

Diener, E., Emmons, R. A., Larsen, R. J., & Griffin, S. (1985). The Satisfaction with Life Scale. *Journal of Personality Assessment, 49*(1), 71-75.

Gibson, F. (2004). *The past in the present: Using reminiscence in health and social care.* Baltimore, MD: Health Professions Press.

Goldberg, D. (1978). *Manual for the General Health Questionnaire.* Oxford: Oxford University Press.

Hsieh, H. F. & Wang, J. J. (2003). Effect of reminiscence therapy on depression in older adults: A systematic review. *International Journal of Nursing Studies, 40*(4), 335-345. Doi: 10.1016/S0020-7489(02)00101-3.

Karimi, H., Dolatshahee, B., Momeni, K., Khodabakhshi, A., Rezaei, M., & Kamrani, A. A. (2010). Effectiveness of integrative and instrumental reminiscence therapies on depression symptoms reduction in institutionalized older adults: An empirical study. *Aging and Mental Health, 14*(7), 881-887.

Martinez-Cox, L., Dattilo, J., & Sheldon, K. (2011). Therapeutic reminiscence. In J. Dattilo & A. McKenney, *Facilitation techniques in therapeutic recreation.* State College, PA: Venture.

Pinquart, M. & Forstmeier, S. (2012). Effects of reminiscence interventions on psychosocial outcomes: A meta-analysis. *Aging & Mental Health, 16*(5), 541-558. doi:10.1080/13607863.2011.651434.

Robitaille, A., Cappeliez, P., Coulombe, D., & Webster, J. D. (2010). Factorial structure and psychometric properties of the Reminiscence Functions Scale. *Aging & Mental Health, 14*(2), 184-192.

Shellman, J. M., Mokel, M., & Hewitt, N. (2009). The effects of integrative reminiscence on depressive symptoms in older African Americans. *Western Journal of Nursing Research, 31*(6), 772-786.

Spielberger, C. D., Gorsuch, R. L., & Lushene, R. E. (1970). *Manual for the State-Trait Anxiety Inventory.* Palo Alto, CA: Consulting Psychologists Press.

Stinson, C. K. (2009). Structured group reminiscence: An intervention for older adults. *Journal of Continuing Education in Nursing, 40*(11), 521-528.

Stinson, C. K. & Kirk, E. (2006). Structured reminiscence: An intervention to decrease depression and increase self-transcendence in older women. *Journal of Clinical Nursing, 15*(2), 208-218. doi: 10.1111/j.1365-2702.2006.01292.x.

Tolson, D. & Schofield, I. (2012). Football reminiscence for men with dementia: Lessons from a realistic evaluation. *Nursing Inquiry, 19*(1), 63-70. doi: 10.1111/j.1440-1800.2011.00581.x.

Watt, L. M. & Wong, P. T. P. (1991). A taxonomy of reminiscence and therapeutic implications. *Journal of Gerontological Social Work, 6*(1 & 2), 37-57.

Webster, J. D. (1993). Construction and validation of the Reminiscence Functions Scale. *Journal of Gerontology: Psychological Sciences, 48*(5), 256-262.

Webster, J. D. (1997). The reminiscence functions scale: A replication. *International Journal of Aging and Human Development, 44*, 137-148.

Webster, J. D., Bohlmeijer, E. T., & Westerhof, G. J. (2010). Mapping the future of reminiscence: A conceptual guide for research and practice. *Research on Aging, 32*(4), 527-564. doi: 10.1177/0164027510364122.

Wong, P. T. P. (1995). The process of adaptive reminiscence. In B. K. Haight & J. D. Webster (Eds.). *The art and science of reminiscing: Theory, research, methods, and applications* (pp. 23-35). Washington, DC: Taylor & Francis.

Wong, P. T. P. & Watt, L. M. (1991). What types of reminiscence are associated with successful aging? *Psychology and Aging, 6*(2), 272-279.

Woolf, V., Rosefield, J., Stanton, P., & Gordon, S. (2002). *Capturing memories: The art of reminiscing.* Portland, OR: Vallentine Mitchell.

Wu, L. (2011). Group integrative reminiscence therapy on self-esteem, life satisfaction and depressive symptoms in institutionalised older veterans. *Journal of Clinical Nursing, 20*, 2195-2203. doi: 10.1111/j.1365-2702.2011.03699.x.

42. Sensory Interventions

Heather R. Porter

Humans are multisensory beings requiring stimulation of the sensory systems, including gustatory, tactile, visual, auditory, and olfactory systems, as well as the proprioceptive and vestibular systems. Sensory stimulation is necessary for survival, development, health, learning, functioning, safety, security, reproduction, nourishment, and quality of life (Pagliano, 2012).

The Senses

The human body has hundreds of millions of sense receptors that "convert energy in the environment into electrical activity in the nerves" (Pagliano, 2012, p. 12). The sensory receptors send information to the spinal cord, which sends it to the brain where the information is integrated and interpreted. There are at least six receptor types in the body (Pagliano, 2012):

- Chemoreceptors respond to chemical stimuli (e.g., smell, taste)
- Mechanoreceptors respond to mechanical stress or strain to detect changes in pressure, position, or acceleration (e.g., stretch, touch, hearing, equilibrium)
- Nociceptors respond to tissue damage and produce sensations of pain
- Photoreceptors respond to light (e.g., vision)
- Proprioceptors respond to position
- Thermoreceptors respond to temperature

Senses can be divided into two primary types (Pagliano, 2012): interoception senses and exteroception senses.

Interoception Senses

Interoception senses access stimuli from inside the body. They include:

Proprioception: Proprioceptors in the muscles and tendons provide information about the body's position, tension, and movement of body parts. They provide information about the location of body parts, our relation to gravity, and where we are in space. Muscle spindles, a type of proprioceptor in muscles, have both motor and sensory components that are thought to play a major role in sensorimotor development. Sensorimotor development takes place when sensory experiences are coordinated with motor activity. For example, touching your nose with your index finger requires the use of proprioception to know where your arm and nose are in space, as well as the movement of the arm.

Vestibular: Vestibular sense receptors are located in the inner ear. They allow us to perceive acceleration, keep our head in proper position (which is also essential for vision), maintain an upright posture in relation to the external environment, and coordinate body movements during running, walking, and movements of the head (e.g., performing a cartwheel).

Other internal senses: We have a variety of additional receptors in the body that provide us with information. For example, receptors in the stomach signal hunger and thirst, and receptors in the bladder and rectum signal the need for emptying.

Exteroception Senses

Exteroception senses access stimuli from outside the body. They can be further broken down into "near" exteroception senses and "distant" exteroception senses. Near senses, such as taste, touch, and cutaneous senses that register pressure, pain, and temperature, tell us about our immediate world. Distant senses, such as vision and hearing, tell us about the world that is beyond our body. In order for exteroception senses to access information, they need to have a context, which is supplied from the interoception senses of proprioception and the vestibular sense. Our senses work together, so all our perceptions are multisensory to some degree. The exteroception senses include:

Olfactory: There are about 40 million olfactory receptors in the nose that can distinguish up to 10,000 odors. Through experiences, we learn that certain odors, such as smoke and gas, signal danger and others, such as the smell of breast milk cueing the infant to eat or the smell of apple pie reminding the individual of his grandmother, signal familiarity. The interconnection of smell and memory are very strong.

Gustatory: Taste buds are found on the tongue, the inside of the mouth, and in the lungs. They consist of sweet, salt, sour, bitter, and meaty taste receptors. Receptors in the mouth also provide information about texture and temperature, and, in combination with the olfactory sense, determine flavor. Taste aids in the development of eating, chewing, and swallowing skills, which strengthen muscle tone (a prerequisite for speech).

Visual: There are about 130 million photoreceptors in the retina that help us determine shape, see in dim light, and distinguish up to 10 million shades of color.

Tactile and cutaneous: These are also known as the somatic senses or somatosensory system. The somatic senses inform us about touch, pressure, temperature, and pain. There are three different types of touch. *Passive touch* is quickly desensitized, such as the sensation of wearing clothing. *Active touch* or *haptic perception* involves the integration of the somatosensory system and proprioception, along with activation of the motor and sensorimotor functions to recognize objects. *Functional touch* is the use of touch that contributes to our experience, enjoyment, and learning. Touching things allows us to learn about the object and discriminate among textures, density, state, surface to depth, size, temperature, vibration, and shape. Each thing that is learned about an object through touch is linked together with other information we have learned about the object through the use of other senses, such as its color or taste, to form an overall impression of the object. Touch lets us understand the world around us (e.g., the carpet is soft so when I fall on it I don't experience much pain, however the sidewalk is hard and rough so when I fall on it I experience a greater amount of pain).

Through the exploration process, other higher order functions, such as memory, spatial ability, scanning, gross and fine motor function, are also challenged.

Auditory: The receptors in the ear allow us to perceive the frequencies and loudness of sounds. The sound waves travel from the outer ear to the middle ear and then into the inner ear where sound waves are converted into nerve impulses for transmission to the auditory cortex. Having two ears creates a bilateral auditory system that also provides valuable information about where the sound is coming from. This enables us to estimate its distance and location.

Sensory Processing and Integration

Individual sense receptors fire when they are stimulated, nothing more. Sensory processing is the ability of the brain to perceive and interpret the incoming stimuli. Sensory processing is a complex process. The sense receptors first have to be stimulated to a *detection threshold* in order for them to fire. Once the receptors fire, the information travels to the brain where it has to be perceived or recognized. This is called the *recognition threshold*. The information is then compared and contrasted to previous knowledge and experiences in order to form meaning and resultant thought and action, requiring the use of memory and higher-level cognitive processes. When thought about an action occur, the sensory process has reached the *differential threshold*. For example, consider a person who steps into a stream to engage in fly-fishing and his foot begins to slip on a slimy rock in the streambed. The proprioceptors in the foot muscles reach the detection threshold and send signals of imbalance to the brain. The person also "sees," "feels," and "hears" a strong current in the water causing other sense receptors to meet the detection threshold. All of the firings are sent to the spinal cord, which sends them to the brain where they meet the recognition threshold. The brain quickly integrates all of the sensory input, along with past experiences of stepping into a stream, to form an interpretation of what is happening and resultant actions. The recognition that the foot is slipping and that the whole body needs to be repositioned meets the differential threshold. However, what if the person is an older adult who has dementia, and whose proprioceptors in the feet are not as sensitive due to the aging process? The proprioceptors might not fire because they do not meet the detection threshold, or they might not fire at a strong enough intensity to alert the brain to the stimuli and fail to meet the recognition threshold. The detection threshold may also not be met if there are competing stimuli such as trying to figure out if the person he sees further down the bank is someone he knows. If there are problems with impaired memory or higher level cognitive processing, despite sufficient firing of the sensory receptors to meet the recognition threshold, the person might have difficulty finding meaning in the sensory signals, which means they don't reach the differential threshold. As illustrated in this example, there are a series of thresholds in sensory processing. Breakdowns that impair the ability to fully process and integrate sensory information can occur in any of them and have a rippling impairment effect that could negatively impact functioning, safety, development, learning, etc. Consequently, sensory functioning warrants considerable attention during the assessment process, and therapists should be careful to not make the assumption that a fully operational sense means the brain is able to integrate it and use it in a meaningful way.

Sensory Deprivation

Utilizing our senses is commonly taken for granted, as it is mostly an automatic process. Normally the world around us, being a multisensory world, provides the stimulation we need to grow and enhance our well-being. It's when our senses become impaired, or our environment lacks the stimulation we need, that we begin to realize the magnitude of sensory deprivation on holistic health and functioning.

As children, sensory play, which engages one or more senses, comes naturally and is a vital component of development. With each sensory experience, new neural connections are made and strengthened, which in turn strengthens learning, thought, and creativity. The neuroplasticity of the brain constantly integrates bits and pieces of information to form meaning and a cohesive understanding of the world. Some children, however, have impairments that limit their ability to engage in sensory play; live in environments, such as abusive situations, poor quality foster homes, or institutions, where sensory experiences are limited; and/or have a lack of support to foster engagement in sensory play because of, for example, poor parenting or lack of caring adults in

their lives. Some children may also have impairments in processing sensory information, tolerating sensory stimuli, or over-fixating on a particular stimulus limiting their engagement in other forms of sensory stimuli resulting from autism, sensory processing disorder, intellectual disability, or other problems. They may have impaired utilization of senses due to sensory impairments, cognitive impairments, or physical impairments. Prolonged sensory deprivation in young children is a major concern, as it "results in severe disturbances in physical development, social and emotional functioning, behavior and communication, learning and even compromises the very survival of the child" (Pagliano, 2012, p. 8). For example, Perry and Pollard (1997) found that a brain scan of a child who was subjected to extreme sensory deprivation had significant cortical atrophy and a smaller head, compared to a child who was not sensory deprived.

In addition to sensory deprivation being a major concern during the developmental years, it is also a major concern throughout life, as it can occur in any person at any age for a multitude of reasons. When it occurs, it impacts the quantity or quality of sensory stimulation. Some of the causes include:

Aging process: During the aging process, senses deteriorate. Visual acuity, depth perception, hearing, peripheral field, sensitivity to low spatial frequencies, and skin sensitivity all decrease with age (Rogers, 2012).

Mental health conditions: Individuals with mental health conditions may withdraw from society as a whole, particular environments, and/or other people as a result of, or to cope with, diagnostic-related symptoms, such as depression and anxiety. Likewise, sensory deprivation may induce mental health symptoms. "When people are not receiving sufficient sensory stimulation to generate such pleasure they go into a state of (dis)ease, which is akin to depression. They become agitated. When they are in this state for prolonged periods of time, they may resort to self-stimulation and close off from the outside world of sensory stimulation" (Pagliano, 2012, p. 30).

Sensory impairments: The lack of a sense (e.g., blindness, deafness) or reduction of a sense (e.g., poor vision or hearing) decreases quantity and quality of sensory experiences.

Physical, cognitive, and neurological impairment: Physical and cognitive impairments may limit a person's ability to access and participate in stimulating activities and environments. Cognitive and neurological impairments may also hinder the ability to recognize, process, interpret, and integrate sensory stimuli.

Environment: Environments may lack sufficiently varied sensory stimulation. Plain white walls, lack of social interaction, and being confined to a room or hospital unit are all recipes for sensory deprivation. Additionally, over time, exteroception senses experience fatigue. For example, the first time a room freshener is plugged into an outlet it fills the room with a wonderful scent, but over time it is hardly noticeable to the people who are in the room, although someone entering the room might notice it right away. Consequently, individuals who live in an unchanging environment are more likely to become less stimulated by that environment as time goes on (Pagliano, 2012). A changing environment is required to avoid sensory deprivation.

Caregivers: Caregivers might lack adequate training, motivation, or initiation to assist those who need help in accessing and participating in sensory experiences.

Meaningful and appropriate sensory experiences: Sensory experiences presented, available, or accessible might not be personally meaningful, developmentally appropriate, or adapted and modified to meet the individual's needs, thus limiting interest, motivation, and/or ability to participate. To be effective the experiences need to meet the differential threshold.

Lack of sensory experiences can have severe consequences (Pagliano, 2012):

> Without multisensory stimulation we are cut off from ourselves and from the outside world. We are starved of our own humanity. This is because sensory stimulation is the source of all human meaning and enjoyment — our purpose and our rewards. Our relationship with our senses is what makes life worth living. Over time the way we perceive sensory stimulation becomes our own perception of our selves. Multisensory stimulation therefore supplies the very building blocks of who we are and who we become (p. 6).

As lack of engagement with the environment continues, sensory deprivation grows, engaging such individuals with their environments becomes more challenging, and severe disturbances in physical development, social and emotional functioning, behavior, and communication occur. The resulting symptoms of panic, hallucinations, psychological distress, anxiety, bizarre thoughts, antisocial behavior, and disorientation commonly result in the prescription of medication to combat the adverse behaviors, which in turn further exacerbates the sensory deprivation (Pagliano, 2012; American Heritage Stedman's Medical Dictionary, 2002; American Heritage New Dictionary of Cultural Literacy, 2005; Random House Dictionary, 2014). The behaviors and functional losses can also have a negative effect, further compounding the problems. For example, embarrassment about functional loss may lead to decreased participation and withdrawal, which further decreases sensory experiences and increases functional losses.

Due to the impact of sensory deprivation on the mind and body, sensory deprivation may be mistakenly diagnosed as a neurological impairment or dementia and not adequately treated. Sensory deprivation has been found to speed up degenerative changes related to aging (Oster, 1976) and alter physiological changes in the body, such as decreased reflex response, metabolic changes, circulatory changes, a lower level of consciousness, decreased respiratory rate, increased heart rate, and lower blood pressure (Kemp, 1984). These changes result in psychophysiological maladaptive behaviors, such as decreased learning, inability to deal with stress, submissiveness, dependence, low sociability, low intellect, decreased conceptual ability, lower attention span, hallucinations, and delusions (Oster, 1976). Since these symptoms mimic other health conditions, it can be easily understood why individuals might be misdiagnosed. For older adults who have a confirmed diagnosis of dementia, sensory deprivation has been found to additionally cause unhappiness, annoyance, agitation, depression, and behavioral problems (Baker et al., 2001; Milev et al., 2008; Ward-Smith, Llanque, & Curran, 2009).

Effects of sensory deprivation have also been seen in young healthy people (Siebens, 1990). After three hours of experimental bed rest, verbal fluency, color discrimination, orientation to time, and reversible figures detection deteriorated. Some subjects additionally reported hallucinatory-like experiences and psychological or emotional discomfort, such as feeling lonely.

Research has shown, however, that reversal of sensory deprivation is possible. For example, Koluchova (1972, 1976) reported on identical twin boys who were subjected to horrific neglect from the ages of two to seven. They were kept in a dark cellar, physically abused, and malnourished resulting in rickets, social anxiety, fear of people, and profound physical and intellectual impairments. At the age of seven, when they were found, the boys were adopted by an educator and enrolled in a special school for children with disabilities. By the age of 14, the boys had caught up developmentally with their non-disabled peers and went on to have stable and productive lives. They both married, had children, and held responsible jobs. Although the brain progresses through critical developmental stages during specific time frames, this story challenges the notion that the brain can't recover function when developmental stages are missed.

In more recent research, a systematic review of 40 studies by Seitz and colleagues (2012) found that non-pharmacological interventions consisting of exercise, recreational activities, music therapy, and other forms of sensory stimulation significantly improved dementia-related neuropsychiatric symptoms.

Indications

Sensory-based interventions are utilized with a variety of populations for behavior management in dementia and developmental or intellectual disability; development of new sensory-related cortical maps in autism spectrum disorders, sensory processing disorder, stroke, and traumatic brain injury; and remediation of symptoms related to sensory deprivation.

ICF codes may indicate a need for sensory-based interventions either because of a fundamental deficit or because sensory issues cause other difficulties. Therapists should consider these interventions when there are deficits in b126 Temperament and Personality Functions, b147 Psychomotor Functions, b156 Perceptual Functions, b2 Sensory Functions and Pain, especially b270 Sensory Functions Related to Temperature and Other Stimuli and b280 Sensation

of Pain, d110 - d129 Purposeful Sensory Experiences, including d110 Watching, d115 Listening, d120 Other Purposeful Sensing, d130 Copying, d230 Carrying Out Daily Routine, d710 Basic Interpersonal Interactions, and d720 Complex Interpersonal Interactions.

Contraindications

Since sensory interventions are utilized with people of all ages with varying degrees of abilities and limitations, precautions need to be taken when choosing sensory-based activities and materials so adverse effects from secondary health conditions do not occur. For example, don't use items that could be used to self-harm, small non-food items that could be a choking hazard, unstable play equipment, or stimuli that invoke agitation and aggression.

Protocols and Processes

Sensory Stimulation

Sensory stimulation, the therapeutic process of stimulating one or more senses, is most commonly utilized with individuals who have sensory deprivation to restore functioning and improve associated losses; reduce negative behaviors such as outbursts, agitation, or aggressive behaviors; and measure progression from Rancho Los Amigos Level 1 (coma stage) to Rancho Los Amigos Level 2 (low arousal stage) in those who sustained a traumatic brain injury. The activities and stimuli for sensory stimulation have these characteristics:

Carefully chosen for therapeutic value

Activities are chosen to stimulate particular senses that increase the likelihood of obtaining the desired outcome (e.g., alertness, behavior change, verbalizations, relaxation) based upon assessments and clinical interviews. Although activities have inherent characteristics that guide clinical decisions, a full assessment of the client's behaviors and reactions to stimuli is needed. For example, a client with dementia who is typically non-verbal might begin to sing when music from his adolescent years is played, while another client might become agitated and attempt to stop the music.

There will be individual differences, but research has shown that some activities are especially helpful for certain dementia-related behaviors or conditions as described here.

Agitated behavior: rhythmical music, slow tempo instrumental activities, singing, glockenspiel or bells activities, and new age or pseudo-classical music. The activities must be adjusted to functional level and incorporate personal styles or interest (Lin et al., 2001, Kolanowski et al., 2011; Baker et al., 2003).

Anxiety: muffs and squeezies (Buettner, 1999).

Difficulty making needs known: message magnets (Buettner, 1999).

Lethargy or passivity: electronic busy box, home decorator books, picture dominos (Buettner, 1999).

Restlessness and repetitive behaviors: an activity apron or pillow, a fishing box, flower arranging, hanging laundry, looking inside a purse or wallet, sewing cards, a table cloth with activities, squeeze balls, tether balls, expanding spheres, building blocks, fabric books, and wave machines (Buettner, 1999; Cohen-Mansfield et al., 2010).

Verbal aggression: latch-box doors, tetherball game, polar fleece hot water bottle, stuffed animal (Buettner, 1999).

Wandering: table ball game, looking inside purse, and hanging the laundry (Buettner, 1999).

For individuals with dementia, the stimulation of multiple senses instead of single senses through activity has also been shown to aid in behavior management. For example, multi-sensory stimulation was found to increase spontaneous speech, increase better relations with others, improve initiation, decrease boredom and inactivity, increase positive emotions, and improve level of activity and alertness (Baker et al., 2001; Baker et al., 2003). When multi-sensory motor stimulation using kinetic stimuli along with visual, auditory, olfactory, gustatory, and tactile stimuli was used with individuals who had dementia and agitation, they demonstrated less physical and verbal agitation and increased activity participation (Buettner, 1999; Cohen-Mansfield et al., 2010).

Able to be manipulated and experienced by the individual

To foster active engagement with the stimulus activity, the individual must be able to manipulate and experience the materials. For example, using a pinecone to stimulate tactile sensation and processing would not be appropriate for an individual who lacks the hand function to grasp and manipulate the pinecone or doesn't have upper extremity tactile sensation (e.g., prosthetic limb). An exception to this is made

when working with clients who sustained a traumatic brain injury to monitor progression from Rancho Los Amigos Level 1 (coma stage) to Rancho Los Amigos Level 2 (low arousal stage). In this case the therapist presents or applies various stimuli to the client instead of it being manipulated by the client. Although not supported by research, it is believed that sensory stimulation might help in progressing the client from the coma stage to the low arousal stage or, at the very least, serves as a useful way to monitor level progression (Lombardi et al., 2002). Gustatory stimulation would be contraindicated for individuals at a Rancho Los Amigos Level 1 because a comatose client can't take food or drink by mouth, but other senses can be stimulated, such as auditory (e.g., playing music), tactile (e.g., applying a cool washcloth to the client's forehead or neck, massaging the client's hand, positioning a fan to blow air on the client), visual (e.g., turning the lights on and off), and olfactory (e.g., spraying a room freshener, bringing food with a strong scent in the room).

Reflective of the client's personality

Clients often have long-standing dispositions to gratify needs in a particular manner. For example, for a client who exhibits fidgeting behaviors, handheld stimuli might be well received. A client who has an impulse to wander might respond better to movement-based sensory activities. For individuals with dementia, tailoring activities to the client's interest and functional level have been shown to increase engagement, alertness, and attentiveness (Kolanowski et al., 2011).

Personally meaningful

Therapists consider the intrinsic personal meaning of the activity to the client. "Even though a sense organ may have the sense acuity to access a particular type of stimulation, the person will not engage with that stimulation unless it is powerful enough to capture their attention" (Pagliano, 2012, p. 23). The sensory experience must not only be strong enough to pass the detection threshold. It must also pass through the recognition threshold and differential threshold. Consequently, stimuli must be meaningful to the person in order to capture a person's attention. If the stimuli also generate pleasure, continued engagement occurs. When continued engagement occurs, neural connections are strengthened and functional changes are observed. If the activity isn't interesting to the client, initial engagement in the activity, as well as continued engagement in the activity in other settings, will be unlikely.

Keep in mind that the goal is not only to promote engagement in activities in structured therapy sessions, but to also design activity experiences that motivate the client to continue activity engagement in other settings. Continued activity engagement outside of therapy sessions with appropriate support from trained families or caregivers provides additional therapeutic stimulation to strengthen outcomes and carry over skills.

In regards to individuals with dementia, when poorly selected activities are chosen, negative outcomes may occur and the individual may become disengaged from the activity (Buettner, 1999; Cohen-Mansfield et al., 2010; Kolanowski et al., 2011; Lin et al., 2011; Milev et al., 2011). Carefully crafting personally meaningful experiences in an environment that highlights a person's strengths and minimizes challenges allows the client to experience success, control, and flow, and seek continued sensory stimulation. If failures are routinely experienced, learned helplessness (the belief that failure is unavoidable and permanent) can ensue and purposeful use of the client's senses can diminish.

To increase meaningfulness of the activity or stimulus, therapists might present additional themed stimuli and that revolve around a particular place, activity, holiday, event, time in life, or season to stimulate a personal connection with the stimuli and encourage reminiscence. For example, a beach theme might include sunscreen lotion for olfactory, tactile, and visual stimulation; a small plastic bucket and shovel for tactile and visual stimulation; a large conch shell for auditory, tactile, and visual stimulation; sounds of waves and seagulls for auditory stimulation; etc. The therapist typically passes around the items, provides assistance manipulating and experiencing the stimuli, as needed, and facilitates reminiscence related to the theme.

Provided in a non-directive approach

Therapists allow the individual to be in control of stimuli with no intellectual or intentional demands (Baker et al., 2001). Stimuli and sensory activities are presented in a manner that allows the client to control how s/he interacts with the stimuli. For example, when presented with a drum, one client might turn it upside down and hit it with his knee, while another

client might roll the drum up and down her lap. If objects are being used in an unsafe manner, the therapist intervenes.

Provided in an appropriate environment

Sensory stimulation might occur in a specially designed room (e.g., Snoezelen room) that includes sensory stimulation equipment, in a quiet non-distracting environment that fosters increased attention to the particular stimulus, or in a real-life activity setting, such as a greenhouse. The chosen environment is determined based on the needs, abilities, and goals of the client. For example, if sensory stimulation is being used as a break to induce a sense of calmness, a sensory room might be appropriate. However, if the goal is for the client to practice implementing learned sensory stimulation techniques to induce a sense of calmness in a group activity, the use of an activity-specific environment might be better. For individuals with developmental or intellectual disabilities Snoezelen rooms have been found to reduce anxiety (Carter & Stephenson, 2012), reduce stereotyped behaviors (Hill et al., 2012), reduce maladaptive behavior (Carter & Stephenson, 2012; Kaplan et al., 2006; Patterson, 2004), increase relaxation (Chan et al., 2005), and increase positive emotions (Chan et al., 2005).

Provided individually, in dyads, or small groups

Sensory stimulation is most often delivered through individual sessions, dyads, or small groups depending upon the needs and abilities of the clients. Individuals with dementia tend to benefit the most from structured one-to-one sensory stimulation sessions (Baker et al., 2001).

Provided daily

Structured sensory stimulation sessions typically occur on a daily basis and range in length from 10 minutes to 30 minutes depending upon the needs, abilities, and tolerance of the client. In long-term residential care, sessions are often best delivered in the morning prior to dementia sundowning and fatigue. In addition to the provision of structured sensory stimulation sessions, it is recommended that sensory stimulation be integrated routinely into daily activities (Baker et al., 2001; Kolanowski et al., 2011; Lin et al., 2011).

When sensory stimulation sessions stop, negative withdrawal effects can occur and result in poor outcomes (Baker et al., 2001; Kolanowski et al.,

2011). Consequently, family and caregivers who interact with the client should also be trained to incorporate sensory stimulation into daily routines to promote and reinforce desired outcomes (Buettner, 1999).

Sensory Integration and Processing

In autism spectrum disorder (ASD), abnormal responses to sensory stimuli called sensory modulation are common. These lead to functional impairment (Hazen et al., 2014). Sensory modulation occurs in approximately 69-95% of individuals with ASD (Hazen et al., 2014). There are three categories of sensory modulation (Hazen et al., 2014):

Sensory over-responsivity (SOR): the experience of distress or display of exaggerated negative response to sensory input, often leading to avoidance and hypervigilance related to the stimulus. For example, a child might be especially sensitive to the feel of clothing tags and may therefore refuse to wear such clothing or become anxious and upset when wearing such clothing, resulting in outbursts.

Under-responsivity (UR): slowness to respond to or unawareness of a stimulus that would normally elicit a response. For example, a child might be unresponsive to pain, such as continually touching a prickly plant or banging his head against a wall.

Sensory seeking (SS): an unusual craving for, or preoccupation with, certain sensory experiences. For example, a child might repeatedly rub a soft cloth against his face.

Sensory integration (SI) is a framework described by A. Jean Ayres in the 1970s. As summarized by Zimmer and Desch (2012), Ayres theorized that the sensory system, much like other body systems, develops and matures over time to effectively integrate sensory input. During this developmental period, deficits in the firing or functioning of sensory neurons may occur, resulting in sensory integration dysfunction. This, in turn, can cause additional developmental, learning, and/or emotional regulation dysfunction, which can be seen not only in ASD, but also in other developmental and intellectual disabilities. To improve SI dysfunction, the sensory system is challenged in a therapeutic manner to reorganize associated cortical maps. Essential components of SI to improve sensory processing include the following considerations (Parham et al., 2007, as cited in Hazen et al., 2014; Roley et al., 2007).

Equipment used in sessions, as well as the surrounding environment, must ensure client safety. Use of a matted floor, secure swings, foam blocks, and other safe equipment is required.

Intervention is family centered and based on sensory processing patterns.

Activities provide enriched sensory experiences, especially vestibular, tactile, and proprioceptive sensation, with opportunities to integrate the sensory experiences with other sensations. All activities are designed to maintain appropriate arousal level and alertness to promote attention and learning. They challenge postural, oral-motor, ocular-motor, and bilateral motor control, promote praxis, and challenge independent organization of activities, and are collaborative with the child. The creative engagement in play is not directed by the therapist. Challenges in the activities are tailored to present that "just right challenge" to promote neuroplasticity, challenge the child to make adaptive responses to changing and increasingly complex environmental demands, facilitate success, and tap into the child's intrinsic motivation to play and interact.

To promote continued engagement in sensory experiences in an effort to develop new sensory-related cortical maps, active participation is necessary. To encourage active and sustained participation, activities must induce a sense of flow with a challenge that matches or is slightly above the client's ability. In the flow state, the client feels totally absorbed in the activity and loses awareness of time. If the activity is too simple or too complex, engagement will be unlikely and either boredom or anxiety will ensue, prompting the client to cease engagement. Consequently, sensory-based activities must be individually tailored and modified to meet the abilities and needs of the client, while providing minimal sensory challenges.

It is also important to note that "children with sensory processing issues appear to have a delayed level of play, particularly in the complexity of their social play, and a decreased duration of time engaging with toys and objects, and they prefer toys that satisfy a sensory need … [and] that children's play preferences can be influenced by the play and sensory preferences of the parent" (Watts, Stagnitti, & Brown, 2014, p. e43). Consequently, during sensory-based play interventions, therapists should additionally be attentive to social interactions in the play, complexity of play, duration of play, and play preferences with sub-goals of fostering developmental play growth.

In regards to effectiveness of SI, research is mixed. For example, a systematic review of 25 studies on SI interventions for individuals with ASD found three studies with positive results, although there were methodological flaws, eight with mixed results, and 14 reporting no benefits (Lang et al., 2012). SI interventions are a common intervention for ASD. They should be provided, but more research to support their value is required (Hazen et al., 2014).

Sensory Diet

A sensory diet is typically developed for individuals who have ASD or other forms of development or intellectual disability. It consists of a regimen of regularly scheduled, sensory-based activities provided throughout the day so that the child's sensory needs are met in a safe, controlled, and socially appropriate manner (Hazen et al., 2014). This approach can be especially effective with children who are "sensory seekers," who often seek out movement, visual, tactile, or proprioceptive input in ways that interfere with or disrupt daily routines, or that compromise personal safety or the safety of those around them.

Sensory experiences might be embedded into the child's daily routine, such as sitting on a ball while engaging in tabletop tasks or playing ball toss with a vibrating ball. They may also be used as breaks from the daily routine to induce a sense of calm, increase attention, and/or decrease outbursts, disruptions, or impulsive behavior. The specific sensory strategies and activities depend on the sensory needs of the child. Examples of sensory experiences might include listening to music or nature sounds; looking at pictures or watching a television program; chewing gum; munching on crunchy, chewy, salty, or sour snacks; swinging, bouncing, or jumping; activities that load muscles such as dragging, pushing, or carrying heavy items; and deep pressure massage. Enjoyable sensory experiences are also commonly utilized as part of Applied Behavioral Analysis as a reward for positive behaviors. Clients are further taught and encouraged, if they are able, to understand their needs for stimuli, identify their responses to stimuli, increase self-control over impulses, increase tolerance, and identify and initiate coping responses.

Environmental Adaptation and Positive Behavioral Support

Positive Behavioral Support (PBS) is the process of anticipating and planning for the needs of a client to minimize challenges, optimize functioning, and maximize participation through the use of environmental adaptation. For example, during a family holiday dinner with lots of people, having a quiet room available for a child with ASD to escape to when feeling overstimulated could be helpful in decreasing behavioral outbursts, as well as strengthening the child's internal locus of control.

Children with ASD who are overresponsive might benefit from calm, predictable, and organized environments with natural light, along with selecting items that the child can tolerate to maximize engagement with the environment. Children with ASD who are underresponsive to sensory stimuli might benefit from music with a faster beat, stronger stimuli, and frequent changes in position to keep them engaged with the environment (Hazen et al., 2014). When children with ASD become fixated on particular sensory stimuli and have difficulty transitioning to a new activity, the use of external strategies in the environment to assist with transitions can be helpful. Examples include a picture schedule on the wall and a timer to indicate how much time is left prior to transitioning to a new activity.

Environmental Enrichment

Environmental Enrichment (EE) "is a noninvasive strategy that has been seen to improve learning and memory performance. While EE has no true definition, it usually consists of the addition or implementation of sensory, cognitive, and motor stimuli in a subject's environment" (Patel, 2012, p. 492). Much of the research in this area is conducted on mice. In mouse models, mice with induced neurodegenerative disorders that were provided with EE were found to have improved memory formation. For example, in Alzheimer's disease (AD), the hippocampus and cortex decreases in size and weight, along with loss of functioning neurons and synapses. In mice that were induced with AD, EE was shown to reduce AD-like neurodegenerative characteristics (Patel, 2012). In mice that were induced with Huntington's disease (HD), which is characterized by degeneration of the cerebral cortex resulting in dementia and movement disorder, EE was shown to delay motor and cognitive deficits, ameliorate reduced adult neurogenesis in the dentate gyrus and hippocampus, reduce neuronal loss, increase motor function, and extend survival (Patel, 2012). In mice that were induced with Parkinson's disease (PD), which is characterized by motor impairment along with dementia in the late stages, exposure to EE improved motor function (Patel, 2012).

In an attempt to translate EE research to humans, Woo and Leon (2013) conducted a randomized controlled trial of 28 male children with ASD aged three to twelve years. The study did not indicate if the children were SOR, UR, or SS types. The children were assigned to either a sensorimotor enrichment group or a control group. The children received interventions in their home. The children in the sensorimotor enrichment group received daily exposure to multiple sensorimotor stimuli distributed throughout the day. The parents were briefly educated and provided with a kit that contained the sensorimotor supplies needed to facilitate 34 different sensorimotor activities. The parents were instructed to engage their children in four to seven sensorimotor activities, twice a day, for a total of 15-30 minutes a day for six months and to change the sensorimotor activities every two weeks to something more challenging. See Woo and Leon (2013) for a full list of supplies and activity descriptions. At the start of the experiment and after six months, the cognitive performance and autism severity of the children were measured. At the end of six months, the children in the sensorimotor group, compared to the control group, exhibited a significant decrease in severity of autism, as measured by the *Childhood Autism Rating Scale*, and improved cognition. They scored an average of 11.3 points higher than the control group as measured by the *Leiter-R Visualization and Reasoning Battery*. Additionally, 69% of the parents in the sensorimotor group, compared to 31% of the parents in the control group, reported improvement in their children over the six-month study.

Unlike the mice studies described by Patel (2012), where sensory stimuli were added to the environment, the Woo and Leon study utilized a parent to facilitate sensorimotor activities. Although the study was referred to as EE (enriching the home environment of the children), it could have also been labeled as sensory stimulation, since sensory stimulation is purposeful and often facilitated exposure to sensory stimuli. Despite questions about the classification of Woo and Leon's study, this is a prime area for research in recreational therapy. Possible studies include comparing a long-term residential facility with low EE to one with high EE for the effects on cognitive and motor function among residents with neurodegenerative diseases or comparing autism severity and cognitive skills of children with ASD who engage in different levels of sensory-rich leisure and play experiences.

Therapists additionally recognize that the sensory environment that passively surrounds an individual can also have a profound impact on health and behaviors. For example, exposure to bright light, either natural or artificial, can reduce depression and agitation, improve sleep, regularize circadian rest-activity rhythms, and shorten hospital stays for clients with dementia and seasonal affective disorders (Ulrich & Zimring, 2004). Brief encounters with real or simulated nature settings in a hospital setting have been found to elicit significant recovery from stress (Parsons & Hartig, 2000; Ulrich, 1999), increased tolerance for pain (Tse et al., 2002), reduced anxiety (Miller, Hickman, & Lemasters, 1992), and decreased agitated-aggressive behavior in late-stage dementia (Whall et al., 1997). Art in hospital settings was found to have mixed results, especially on psychiatric units where it could be misinterpreted (Ulrich, 1991). The use of aromatherapy with individuals who have dementia has also been found to be effective on measures of agitation and neuropsychiatric symptoms (Holt et al., 2009). Hospital gardens were found to reduce stress, foster access to social support, provide opportunities for positive escape, and increase sense of control (Cooper-Marcus & Barnes, 1995; Ulrich, 1999). Carpet, compared to vinyl flooring, seems to substantially increase length of visitation time in rehabilitation hospitals (Harris, 2000). Colored walls with full-color, three-spectrum lighting in elementary classrooms reduced students' blood pressure and reduced off-task behaviors by 22% resulting in improved academic performance with fewer errors and increased speed (Grube, 2013). Elementary school children with and without attention problems who engaged in physical movement, such as doodling, bouncing on a yoga ball, or physical activity, before or during academic tasks improved comprehension, test scores, and on task behavior (Suneeta & Devender, 2012).

As therapists, it is vitally important that attention is paid to the surrounding environment to provide an environment that optimizes functioning and health. As reviewed previously, for some, including individuals with autism, this might entail reducing certain sensory stimuli that induce adverse behavior. For others, including individuals with Alzheimer's disease, a sensory-enriched environment might be desired to combat loss of functioning due to neurodegenerative disease. The breadth of literature on this topic is more than can be thoroughly reviewed in this chapter. Consequently, therapists are encouraged to conduct their own literature review about how environmental enrichment and modifications affect specific behaviors and populations they are working with.

Outcomes and Documentation

There are a variety of standardized assessment tools related to sensory-based functioning. For individuals with ASD and other developmental or intellectual disabilities, therapists should consider:

Sensory Processing Measure (SPM) and SPM-P: Provides a complete picture of children's sensory processing difficulties at school and at home. SPM: ages 5-12, SPM-P: ages 2-5. Available at www.wpspublish.com.

Test of Sensory Functions in Infants (TSFI): Offers an objective way to determine whether (and to what extent) an infant has sensory processing deficits. Ages four to 18 months. Available at www.wpspublish.com.

Sensory Profile: Determines how children process information in everyday situations. Ages three to ten years. Available at www.pearsonclinical.com.

Sensory Profile 2: Standardized forms completed by caregivers and teachers to assess children's sensory processing patterns. Ages birth to 14 years. Available at www.pearsonclinical.com.

Infant/Toddler Sensory Profile: Examines patterns in young children who are at risk related to sensory processing. Available at www.pearsonclinical.com.

Adolescent/Adult Sensory Profile: Identifies sensory processing patterns and effects on functional performance. Ages 11 and up. Available at www.pearsonclinical.com.

Therapists who are utilizing sensory-based interventions to combat sensory deprivation or manage behaviors should consider tools that measure the specific behavior they want to change. Potential sources for measures that cover behaviors such as agitation, mood, cognition, motor activity, etc., include:

Dementia Outcomes Measurement Suite (DOMS): DOMS is a federal initiative to help address the issues related to a rapidly growing population with dementia or Alzheimer's disease. To address this, one of the major requirements is to create a common assessment language for use by all professionals. This site provides access to a variety of assessment tools, such as the *Cohen-Mansfield Agitation Inventory*, which assesses the frequency of agitated behaviors in older adults, covering aggressive behavior, physically nonaggressive behavior, and verbally agitated behavior. Go to www.dementia-assessment.com.

Rehabilitation Measures Database (RMD): A comprehensive database of rehabilitation-related assessment tools, such as the *Berg Balance Scale* and *Geriatric Depression Scale*. Many are free. The website contains links to the assessment tools and manuals. Go to www.rehabmeasures.org.

Therapists can additionally use ICF codes to indicate the level of impairment a client has with specific sensory-based functions, such as b156 Perceptual Functions, b2 Sensory Functions and Pain, especially b270 Sensory Functions Related to Temperature and Other Stimuli and b280 Sensation of Pain, d110 - d129 Purposeful Sensory Experiences, including d110 Watching, d115 Listening, d120 Other Purposeful Sensing, and d130 Copying.

Therapists might also use ICF codes to indicate the level of impairment or difficulty a client has with sensory-based behaviors, such as b126 Temperament and Personality Functions, b147 Psychomotor Functions, d230 Carrying Out Daily Routine, d710 Basic Interpersonal Interactions, and d720 Complex Interpersonal Interactions.

In discipline-specific documentation, therapists commonly document stimuli presented and how they were experienced; behavioral responses to stimuli; patterns of behavior related to particular stimuli (e.g., sensory triggers and facilitators related to engagement and behavior); ability to detect stimuli, accurately perceive stimuli, and integrate stimuli into a complex whole; sensory preferences; self-stimulating behaviors; length of sensory-based sessions;

tolerance level of particular stimuli; functional improvements from sensory-based interventions; specific sensory experiences incorporated into daily activities to improve the sensory diet; and environmental adaptations made to facilitate functioning and maximum participation.

Resources

The Ultimate Guide of Sensory Play Activities from the PLAY Group

www.oneperfectdayblog.net/2013/02/22/the-ultimate-guide-of-sensory-play-activities/

Recipes for Sensory Fun

www.kidpartners.net/Assets/Recipes_for_Sensory_E xperiences__1_.pdf

Sensory Fun: Loads of Play Ideas to Stimulate the Senses

www.clickspecialednz.com/doc/approach/03_sensor/r es/Sensory%20play.pdf

101 Sensory Activities

www.myteacherpages.com/webpages/schynoweth/fil es/101sensoryactivities-lindagoddard.pdf

References

American Heritage New Dictionary of Cultural Literacy (3rd ed.). (2005). *Sensory deprivation.* Retrieved from http://dictionary.reference.com/browse/sensory+deprivation.

American Heritage Stedman's Medical Dictionary. (2002). *Sensory deprivation.* Retrieved from http://dictionary.reference.com/browse/sensory+deprivation.

Baker, R., Bell, S., Baker, E., Gibson, S., Holloway, J., Pearce, R., Dowling, Z., Thomas, P., Assey, J., & Wareing, L. A. (2001). A randomized controlled trial of the effects of multi-sensory stimulation (MSS) for people with dementia. *British Journal of Clinical Psychology, 40,* 81–96.

Baker, R., Holloway, J., Holtkamp, C. C. M , Larsson, A., Hartman, L. C., Pearce, R., Scherman, B., Johansson, S., Thomas, P. W., Wareing, L. A., & Owens M. (2003). Effects of multi- sensory stimulation for people with dementia. *Journal of Advanced Nursing, 43*(5), 465–477.

Buettner L. L. (1999). Simple Pleasures: A multilevel sensorimotor activity program for nursing home residents with dementia. *Am J Alzheimer's Dis Other Demen, 14,* 41-52.

Carter, M. & Stephenson, J. (2012). The use of multi-sensory environments in schools servicing children with severe disabilities. *Journal of Developmental and Physical Disabilities, 24*(1), 95-109.

Chan, S., Fung, M. Y., Tong, C. W., & Thompson, D. (2005). The clinical effectiveness of a multisensory therapy on clients with developmental disability. *Research in Developmental Disabilities, 26*(2), 131-142.

Cohen-Mansfield, J., Marx, M. S., Dakheel-Ali, M., Regier, N. G., Thein, K., & Freedman, L. (2010). Can agitated behavior of nursing home residents with dementia be prevented with the use of standardized stimuli? *The American Geriatrics Society, 58,* 1459-1464.

Cooper-Marcus, C. & Barnes, M. (1995). *Gardens in healthcare facilities: Uses, therapeutic benefits, and design recommendations.* Martinez, CA: Center for Health Design.

Grube, K. (2013). The color on the wall. *American School and University, 86*(3), 219.

Harris, D. (2000). Environmental quality and healing environments: A study of flooring materials in a healthcare telemetry unit. *Doctoral dissertation,* Texas A&M University, College Station.

Hazen, E. P., Stornelli, J. L., O'Rourke, J. A., Koesterer, K., McDougle, C. J. (2014). Sensory symptoms in autism spectrum disorders. *Harvard Review of Psychiatry, 22*(2), 112-124.

Hill, L., Trusler, K., Furniss, F., & Lancioni, G. (2012). Effects of multisensory environments on stereotyped behaviours assessed as maintained by automatic reinforcement. *Journal of Applied Research in Intellectual Disabilities, 25*(6), 509-521.

Hiroto, D. S. & Seligman, M. E. (1975). Generality of learned helplessness in man. *Journal of Personality and Social Psychology, 31*(2), 311-327.

Holt, F. E., Birks, T., Thorgrimsen, L. M., Spector, A. E., Wiles, A., & Orrell, M. (2009). Aroma therapy for dementia. *The Cochrane Collaboration of Systematic Reviews.*

Kaplan, H., Clopton, M., Kaplan, M., Messbauer, L., & McPherson, K. (2006). Snoezelen multi-sensory environments: Task engagement and generalization. *Research in Developmental Disabilities, 27,* 443-455.

Kemp, B. (1984). *Fundamentals of nursing: A framework for practice.* Boston, MA: Little, Brown, and Company.

Kolanowski, A., Litaker, M., Buettner, L., Moeller, J., & Costa, P. T. (2011). A randomized clinical trial of theory-based activities for the behavioral symptoms of dementia in nursing home residents. *The American Geriatrics Society, 59,* 1032-1041.

Koluchova, J. (1972). Severe deprivation in twins: A case study. *Journal of Child Psychology and Psychiatry, 13,* 107-114.

Koluchova, J. (1976). The further development of twins after severe and prolonged deprivation: A second report. *Journal of Child Psychology and Psychiatry, 17,* 181-188.

Lang, R., O'Reilly, M., Healy, O., Rispoli, M., Lydon, H., Streusand, W., Davis, T., Kang, S., Sigafoos, J., Lancion, G., Didden, R., & Giesbers, S. (2012). Sensory integration therapy for autism spectrum disorders. A systematic review. *Research in Autism Spectrum Disorders, 6*(3), 1004-1018.

Lin, Y., Chu, H., Yang, C. Y., Chen, C. H., Chen, S. G., Chang, H. J., Hsieh, C. J., & Chou, K. R. (2010). Effectiveness of group music intervention against agitated behavior in elderly persons with dementia. *Int J Geriatr Psychiatry, 26,* 670-678.

Lombardi, F., Taricco, M., De, T., Telaro, A. E., & Liberati, A. (2002). Sensory stimulation for brain injured individuals in coma or vegetative state. *Cochrane Database of Systematic Reviews.*

Milev, R. V., Kellar, T., McLean, M., Mileva, V., Luthra, V., Thompson, S., & Peevar, L. (2008). Multisensory stimulation for elderly with dementia: A 24-week single-blind randomized controlled pilot study. *Am J Alzheimer's Dis Other Demen, 23,* 372-376.

Miller, A. C., Hickman, L. C., & Lemasters, G. K. (1992). A distraction technique for control of burn pain. *Journal of Burn Care and Rehabilitation, 13*(5), 576-580.

Oster, C. (1976). Sensory deprivation in geriatric patients. *Journal of the American Geriatrics Society, 24,* 461-463.

Pagliano, P. (2012). *The multisensory handbook: A guide for children and adults with sensory learning disabilities.* New York, NY: Routledge.

Parham, L. D., Cohn, E. S., Spitzer, S., et al. (2007). Fidelity in sensory integration intervention research. *American Journal of Occupational Therapy, 61,* 216-627.

Parsons, R. & Hartig, T. (2000). Environmental psychophysiology. In J. T. Cacioppo & L. G. Tassinary (Eds.), *Handbook of psychophysiology* (2nd ed.) (pp. 815-846). New York, NY: Cambridge University Press.

Patel, T. R. (2012). Environmental enrichment: Aging and memory. *Yale Journal of Biology and Medicine, 85*, 491-500.

Patterson, I. (2004). Snoezelen as a casual leisure activity for people with a developmental disability. *Therapeutic Recreation Journal, 38*(3), 289-300.

Perry, B. D. & Pollard, R. (1997). Altered brain development following global neglect in early childhood. *Proceedings from the Society for Neuroscience Annual Meeting*. New Orleans: The Society for Neuroscience.

Random House Dictionary. (2014). *Sensory deprivation*. Retrieved from http://dictionary.reference.com/browse/sensory+deprivation.

Rogers, M. E. (2012). Balance and falls preventions. Retrieved from www.acsm.org/access-public-information/articles/2012/01/10/balance-and-fall-prevention.

Roley, S., Mailloux, Z., Miller-Kuhaneck, H., & Gennon, T. (2007). Understanding Ayres sensory integration. *OT Practice, 12*(17), CE1-8.

Seitz, D. P., Brisbin, S., Hermann, N., Rapoport, M. J., Wilson, K., Gill, S. S., Rines, J., Le Cair, K., & Conn, D. (2012). Efficacy and feasibility of nonpharmacological interventions for neuropsychiatric symptoms of dementia in long term care: A systematic review. *Journal of American Medical Directors Association, 13*(6), 503-506.

Siebens, H. (1990). Deconditioning. In Kemp, B., Brummel-Smith, K., & Ramsdell, J. (Eds.). *Geriatric rehabilitation*. Boston, MA: College-Hill Publication.

Suneeta, K. & Devender, R. (2012). The effects of added physical activity performance during listening comprehensive task for students with and without attention problems. *Educational Studies, 13*(1), 19-32.

Tse, M. M. Y., Ng, J. K. F., Chung, J. W. Y., & Wong, T. K. S. (2002). The effect of visual stimuli on pain threshold and tolerance. *Journal of Clinical Nursing, 11*(4), 462-469.

Ulrich, R. S. (1991). Effects of interior design on wellness: Theory and recent scientific research. *Journal of Health Care Interior Design, 3*(1), 97-109.

Ulrich, R. S. (1999). Effects of gardens on health outcomes: Theory and research. In C. Cooper Marcus & M. Barnes (Eds.). *Healing gardens* (pp. 27-86). New York, NY: Wiley.

Ulrich, R. & Zimring, C. (2004). *The role of the physical environment in the hospital of the 21st century: A once-in-a-lifetime opportunity*. Robert Wood Johnson Foundation Report. Accessed via www.healthdesign.org/sites/default/files/Role%20Physical%20Environ%20in%20the%2021st%20Century%20Hospital_0.pdf.

Ward-Smith, P., Langues, S. M., & Curran, D. (2009). The effect of multisensory stimulation on persons reading in an extended care facility. *Am J Alzheimer's Dis Other Demen, 24*, 450-455.

Watts, T., Stagnitti, K., & Brown, T. (2014). Relationship between play and sensory processing: A systematic review. *The American Journal of Occupational Therapy, 68*(2), e37-e46.

Whall, A. L., Black, M. E., Groh, C. J., Yankou, D. J., Kupferschmid, B. J., & Foster, N. L. (1997). The effect of natural environments upon agitation and aggression in late stage dementia patients. *American Journal of Alzheimer's Disease and Other Dementias*, September-October, 216-220.

Woo, C. C. & Leon, M. (2013). Environmental enrichment as an effective treatment for autism: A randomized controlled trial. *Behavioral Neuroscience, 127*(4), 487-497.

Zimmer, M. & Desch, L. (2012). Sensory integration therapies for children with developmental and behavioral disorders. *American Academy of Pediatrics, 129*(6), 1186-1189.

43. Sexual Well-Being

Heather R. Porter

Sexuality is a basic human need and right, and has therefore been steadily gaining attention in healthcare across all disciplines. Various terms have been used to classify this topic, including sexual health, sexual activity, and sexual well-being. The term "sexual well-being" has been steadily gaining popularity, as it reflects the multi-faceted nature and holistic view of sexuality (Taylor & Davis, 2007). Sexuality is not merely the engagement in sexual activity. It also includes psychological and sociological aspects, such as self-concept, self-esteem, body image, religious and cultural values, social roles, sexual expression, communication of sexual feelings, sexual attitudes, sexual beliefs, sexual behavior, sexual orientation, and the development and maintenance of social and intimate relationships (Davis & Taylor, 2006).

The World Health Organization (WHO, 2010) notes that although more research is needed to explore the various dimensions of the term "sexual well-being," it is likely to be culturally and contextually specific; could be linked to aspects such as sexual identity, sexual preference, and sexual behavior; could include expressions of sexuality by people living with physical and intellectual disabilities or illness; and would most likely be assessed using a self-perceived measure to capture both positive and negative elements of sexual health, such as comfort, satisfaction, and motivation.

A few of the issues related to sexual well-being for individuals with acquired disability or chronic illness, include low self-esteem due to role changes and feelings of loss of control, sexual activity difficulties due to impairments, feeling unloved or unattractive, difficulties communicating with partners about feelings, and difficulties establishing or maintaining an intimate or sexual relationship (Taylor & Davis, 2007).

Indications

Since sexuality is a basic human need and right, and the role of healthcare practitioners is to maximize the client's potential, the topic of sexuality is a common component of practice. It is rare that specific assessment tools are utilized outside of research studies to identify sexuality issues or concerns. Issues and concerns are predominately identified during the "Permission" level as described in the Protocols and Processes section below. Issues related to sexuality may also surface in routine quality of life measures, such as the World Health Organization's *Quality of Life BREF* (WHO-QOL-BREF). The items related to sexuality in quality of life measures are typically broad and few. For example, there is only one item in the WHO-QOL-BREF, which asks, "How satisfied are you with your sex life?" Therapists need to pay attention to the questions that are there because they may point out the need to broach the topic with the client.

In regards to adolescents, clinicians often have their own personal values about the age when engaging in sexual activity is appropriate. Regardless of personal opinions, data suggests that permission to talk about sexuality should be extended to adolescents as well. In the U.S., the average age of first intercourse is 16 for males and 17 for females; 25% of males and 26% of females have had sexual intercourse by age 15; 15% of high school students have had sexual intercourse with four or more partners; approximately six percent of boys and girls have had sexual intercourse before the age of 13; and 10% of women between the ages of 15 and 19 become pregnant every year (The Kinsey Institute, 2012; Centers for Disease Control and Prevention, 2013). Adolescence is a time of finding identity, including sexual identity. General sexual interest can lead to actively seeking information about sexuality through internet sites, videos, and pictures. Clients experiment sexually with themselves and others. Because youth lack the cognitive and emotional maturity to make wise and healthy decisions about sexuality, they are ill prepared to process their experiences and cope with consequences of sexual activity (Zupanick, 2014). Couple all of this with a health condition and adolescents are bound to have questions.

ICF codes related to sexuality include b640 Sexual Functions, b670 Sensations Associated with Genital and Reproductive Functions, d570 Looking After One's Health, and d770 Intimate Relationships.

Contraindications

Although the topic of sexuality is typically not appropriate to discuss with children, we unfortunately live in a world where some children experience sexual abuse or are exposed to sexual activity. Consequently, a child may initiate a conversation about sexuality or exhibit signs of sexual abuse. The therapist must be attentive to visible, as well as nonvisible signs of sexual abuse, inquire about observations as appropriate, and report suspected abuse.

In regards to adolescents, adults, and older adults, therapists should be attentive to the client's wishes and not continue a conversation about sexual well-being if the individual finds it offensive or uncomfortable.

The utilization of the PLISSIT and Ex-PLISSIT model, as reviewed below, assumes that the client is cognitively intact, possesses a basic understanding of sexuality, and is able to initiate and sustain conversation. Consequently, depending upon the severity of the client's deficits, conversation about sexuality may be contraindicated. Even if conversation is contraindicated, healthcare professional must recognize that sexuality is still a basic human need and expressions of sexuality and related difficulties might be observed and need to be addressed. For example, in a long-term care facility an individual with dementia may develop an intimate relationship with another resident. The family member who is the guardian of the individual may disagree with this relationship and demand that it be terminated claiming that it is harmful to the resident. The resident, on the other hand, is an adult and has adult sexual needs. The ethics surrounding such issues are complex and there isn't always a clear answer.

In other situations, the client may not have received sexual education due to cultural issues, religious beliefs, or ignorance on the part of an educator or caregiver. A common example is "Although Sam is 17 years old, he functions at a 10-year-old level, so he doesn't have the capacity to understand what sex is about. There's no need to talk with him about this." Clients at age 17 usually feel sexual drives regardless of their mental functioning. They need instruction that they can understand before the therapist provides sexuality information related to impairments or injuries or specific suggestions to problem solve for difficulties.

Protocols and Processes

PLISSIT Model

About 40 years ago, Annon (1976) developed the PLISSIT model, which has been widely used by a variety of healthcare practitioners to address sexuality with clients. The PLISSIT model is a four-step process that helps practitioners "identify their role in the assessment and evaluation of an individual's sexual wellbeing needs" (Taylor & Davis, 2007, p. 136).

PLISSIT is an acronym that stands for four progressive levels of intervention: Permission (P), Limited Information (LI), Specific Suggestions (SS), and Intensive Therapy (IT). Practitioners have varying levels of comfort and knowledge related to sexuality and the specific issues of the client, therefore the practitioner begins with Permission (P) and then either continues to the next step in the process or refers the client to others who are able to address it.

Permission (P)

Talking about sexuality can be uncomfortable for clients. Some may find it embarrassing or inappropriate, while others may have questions they are apprehensive to ask due to the sensitive nature of the topic. Lack of inquiry on the part of the client should not be interpreted as lack of concern about sexuality. Hence the therapist is responsible for opening the door for the conversation by giving the client permission to talk about the subject.

The manner that the therapist approaches the subject will vary depending on the client. However, it is always done with respect and sincerity. A possible example of starting the conversation is, "In addition to the goals that we set for your stay here I was wondering if you would like information on issues related to sexuality. It is common for people to have questions about sexuality after having heart surgery. Would you like to talk about it with me or someone else on your team?" Notice in the example provided that the therapist normalizes sexuality by saying that "many people have questions." This helps to lessen client anxiety. Other comments that can help to lessen anxiety include those that validate how the client is feeling, such as, "I know this must be an awkward conversation that you probably didn't expect to have" or "I sense that this topic makes you uncomfortable. Would you like to change the subject? Just know that if you change your mind, we can talk about it or, if you prefer, I can give you some information in a sealed envelop that you can read on your own."

Therapists should also be aware that clients may bring up issues related to sexuality in indirect ways, such as making sexual jokes or making sexual advances towards the therapist to test out attractiveness, or making statements such as, "No one is ever going to want to date me." Indirect statements provide the therapist with an opportunity to approach the subject and give the client permission to talk about it. For example, in response to a sexual joke the therapist might respond by saying, "Jokes aside, has anyone talked with you about sexuality after having an amputation? It's normal to have questions. Is this something you would like to talk about with me or someone else?" Being attentive to indirect statements from clients and normalizing the conversation about sexuality opens the door to discussion about sexual well-being.

Although permission to talk about sexuality should be given by all healthcare providers, clients tend to gravitate to healthcare providers where they feel a sense of comfort and understanding. In recreational therapy practice, a strong therapeutic relationship is formed and therapy outcomes directly relate to engagement in meaningful activities related to social recreation, leisure, and community activities. Consequently, it is not uncommon for topics related to sexuality to emerge (e.g., "I feel uncomfortable going to the school dances because no one is going to be attracted to a guy in a wheelchair" or "We like to go to a bed and breakfast in Pennsylvania during autumn because the changing colors of the leaves is so romantic; but I don't feel very romantic lately.") and

for recreational therapists to provide education and counseling related to sexuality.

Limited Information (LI)

Once a question is raised or an issue is identified, limited information is provided. For example, if a male client who had a complete spinal cord injury is concerned about not being able to achieve an erection, the therapist might respond by saying, "It's not uncommon to have this concern. There are different devices, as well as medication, that can help achieve an erection." If a female client doesn't feel sexually attractive because of her injury and is therefore apprehensive of being intimate with her partner, the therapist might respond by saying, "Some people find it helpful to talk with their partner about how they feel. Despite how well people know each other, it can be difficult for partners to truly understand how the other person feels."

The goal is to provide a small amount of information that addresses the expressed concern. Providing the client with limited information often prompts the client to discuss the issue in greater depth, or the therapist may find that the limited information is sufficient to meet the current needs of the client. If the therapist doesn't know the answer to the question, the therapist should offer to find out the information for the client, while maintaining the agreed upon confidentiality. The therapist might also ask the client if s/he is willing to talk to another healthcare provider who is knowledgeable of the topic.

Specific Suggestions (SS)

Should the conversation progress, the client may be interested in discussing specific suggestions related to sexuality (e.g., what is the specific external device that helps in achieving an erection, how to begin a talk with a partner about feelings). Other specific suggestions might revolve around the use and/or manipulation of equipment, such as issues related to wearing a colostomy bag, catheter, oxygen, or prosthesis; sexual positions that improve performance and comfort and decrease risks of secondary problems, such as trouble breathing; and problem solving for specific issues including loss of bowel control during sexual activity, lack of lubrication, inability to ejaculate, difficulty with speech, or fatigue. Therapists might also refer clients to specific resources where they can access specific suggestions, such as the "Sexuality for the Woman with Cancer" discussion on the American Cancer Society website.

Due to the sensitivity of the topic, many clients want assurances that the discussion is not documented or discussed with other people. The therapist should inform the client that s/he will not discuss the specifics of the conversation with others. However, if specific questions need to be answered, such as clearance from a physician to engage in sexual activity, the therapist will need to divulge the client's name. If it is determined that further information is needed or that the client could benefit from additional conversations with other staff, the therapist will check with the client before making these arrangements. The therapist also informs the client that documentation will reflect the specific information provided, but the details of the conversation will not be part of the medical chart.

Intensive Therapy (IT)

Healthcare professionals recommend intensive therapy when the first three levels of intervention have not satisfactorily met the needs of the client. Intensive therapy is provided by mental health professionals, such as licensed sex therapists, who are specifically trained in sexual practices and techniques to promote healthy and satisfying sexual and intimate relationships.

Ex-PLISSIT Model

The PLISSIT model, as just described, is a linear model. The healthcare provider begins at the first level of permission and then moves forward through the remaining levels. Rarely, however, does the process of addressing sexuality follow this format. For example, the therapist can't make the assumption that giving permission during one session guarantees that the client feels permission to bring up a different concern about sexuality during another session. As a result, the Extended PLISSIT model, referred to as the Ex-PLISSIT model, was devised. It is an extension of the PLISSIT model. It suggests that all four levels of the PLISSIT Model are interconnected and that any of the levels can be addressed at any time. Giving permission was changed from a one-time event to giving permission to discuss sexuality on a regular basis, not just during the healthcare stay. Sexuality is a dynamic concept where issues change in response to functional changes and social or psychological circumstances. Also in the Ex-PLISSIT

model, the therapist and client engage in reflection to review and challenge client assumptions in order to develop knowledge and self-awareness as part of each of the levels of interventions (Davis & Taylor, 2006; Taylor & Davis, 2007; Taylor & Davis, 2006).

Outcomes and Documentation

The therapist documents that permission to discuss sexuality was given, the limited information and/or specific suggestions provided, the client's self-report about the ability to apply the information learned, referrals made, and resource given. Changes in the ICF codes related to sexuality should be documented. The ICF codes include b640 Sexual Functions, b670 Sensations Associated with Genital and Reproductive Functions, d570 Looking After One's Health, and d770 Intimate Relationships.

Resources

Online resources related to disability and sexuality.

Burns
www.phoenix-society.org/downloads/resources/sex_and_intimacy_guidlines_20110613_115355_4.pdf
Addressing Sexuality with Adult Burn Survivors

Cancer
www.cancer.org/treatment/treatmentsandsideeffects/physicalsideeffects/sexualsideeffectsinwomen/sexualityforthewoman/sexuality-for-the-woman-with-cancer-toc
Sexuality for the Woman with Cancer

www.cancer.org/treatment/treatmentsandsideeffects/physicalsideeffects/sexualsideeffectsinmen/sexualityfortheman/index
Sexuality for the Man with Cancer

Dementia
www.ilcuk.org.uk/index.php/publications/publication_details/the_last_taboo_a_guide_to_dementia_sexuality_intimacy_and_sexual_behaviour
The Last Taboo: A Guide to Dementia, Sexuality, Intimacy, and Sexual Behaviour in Care Homes

Intellectual Disability
www.craconferences.com/resources/cra/Sexuality%20in%20People%20Who%20Have%20ID%20-%20Rights,%20Behaviors,%20Responses%20and%20Professionalism.pdf

Sexuality in People Who Have Intellectual Disability

Mental Illness

www.mifa.org.au/sites/www.mifa.org.au/files/docum
ents/My_sexual_health_matters.pdf

My Sexual Health Matters: Information for People
with a Mental Illness

Multiple Sclerosis

www.msif.org/includes/documents/cm_docs/msinfoc
usissue6en.pdf?f=1

Intimacy and Sexuality in Multiple Sclerosis

Spinal Cord Injury

https://www.craighospital.org/repository/documents/
HeathInfo/PDFs/785.MenandSexafterSCI.pdf

Sexual Function for Men after Spinal Cord Injury

https://www.craighospital.org/repository/documents/
HeathInfo/PDFs/786.WomenandSexafteraSpinalCord
Injury.pdf

Sexual Function for Women after Spinal Cord Injury

Stroke

http://strokefoundation.com.au/site/media/FS02_Sexr
elationship_web.pdf

Sex and Relationship after Stroke

Traumatic Brain Injury

www.tbicommunity.org/resources/publications/Sexua
l_Functioning_after_TBI.pdf

Sexual Functioning and Satisfaction after Traumatic
Brain Injury: An Educational Manual

References

Annon, J. (1976). The PLISSIT model: A proposed conceptual
scheme for the behavioural treatment of sexual problems.
Journal of Sex Education and Therapy, 2(1), 1-15.

Centers for Disease Control and Prevention. (2013). Sexual risk
behavior data and statistics. Retrieved from
www.cdc.gov/healthyyouth/sexualbehaviors/data.htm.

Davis, S. & Taylor, B. (2006). From PLISSIT to Ex-PLISSIT. In
S. Davis (Ed.), *Rehabilitation: The use of theories and
models in practice* (pp 101-129). Elsevier Health Sciences.

Taylor, B. & Davis, S. (2007). The extended PLISSIT model for
addressing the sexual wellbeing of individuals with an
acquired disability or chronic illness. *Sexuality & Disability,
25*, 135-139.

Taylor, B. & Davis, S. (2006). Using the extended PLISSIT model
to address sexual healthcare needs. *Nursing Standard,
21*(11), 35-40.

The Kinsey Institute. (2012). Frequently asked sexuality questions
to The Kinsey Institute. Retrieved from
www.iub.edu/~kinsey/resources/FAQ.html.

World Health Organization. (2010). Measuring sexual health:
Conceptual and practical considerations and related
indicators. Retrieved from
http://whqlibdoc.who.int/hq/2010/who_rhr_10.12_eng.pdf.

Zupanick, C. E. (2014). The development of adolescent sexuality.
Retrieved from
www.sevencounties.org/poc/view_doc.php?type=doc&id=41
180&cn=1310.

44. Social Skills Training

Katelynn Ropars and Heather R. Porter

Social interactions with each other and the external world are part of our human make-up. Consequently, lack of social interaction, whether by choice, dysfunction, or withholding, can have a profound effect on human development and behavior leading to depression, attachment problems from lack of bonding, and many other issues (Hari & Kujala, 2009). In a recent Gallup Poll of over 17,000 U.S. adults, the researchers found that five to six hours a day of socializing with others was needed to have more happy moments, fewer stressful moments, and a thriving sense of well-being (Rath & Harter, 2010). Social interaction with others also fosters the development of social support, which can have far-reaching health effects. For example, Hartman's (2013) review and synthesis of the literature related to social support and spinal cord injury found that social support correlated with (1) better mental health (reduced depression, drug and alcohol abuse, feelings of helplessness, negative thinking, and suicidal ideation); (2) fewer secondary health conditions (reduced urinary tract infections, decubitus ulcers, contractures, circulation problems, fatigue, stomach and bowel problems, muscle spasms, pain, and injuries, and improved weight management); (3) better functioning and participation (improved community integration, mobility, productivity, independence, and interest in leisure activities); and (4) higher life satisfaction, coping, and quality of life (shown by a fighting spirit, hope, a sense of humor, positive cognitive appraisals, self-efficacy, life satisfaction, and well-being).

Impairments with social skills are one of the many factors that can impair social interactions. Social skills can generally be understood as "the personal skills needed for successful social communication and integration" (Dictionary.com's 21st Century Lexicon, 2013). The details are not as clear.

While there are numerous definitions and measures of social skills, there is "no universally agreed upon set of behaviors (taxonomy) that are known as social skills" (Matson, 2009, p. 62). Table 19 provides a sampling of behaviors that are generally called social skills.

Table 19: Sampling of Social Skills

Beginning Social Skills
Initiating and maintaining eye contact
Joint reference (shift gaze during conversation between speaker and object)
Listening
Active listening
Empathetic listening
Acknowledging presence of others
Ceasing activity to attend to communication
Greeting others
Using the right voice, nice voice
Initiating interaction
Identifying appropriate moments to initiate a conversation
Answering
Taking turns talking
Nonverbal turn taking
Asking a question
Saying thank you
Introducing yourself
Introducing others
Using proper tone of voice
Using appropriate voice volume
Using appropriate rate of speech
Clarity of speech
Attention to task
Orientation to social stimuli
Reaction to name

Conversation Skills

Starting a conversation
Maintaining a conversation
Terminating a conversation
Interrupting appropriately
Knowing what to ask in conversations

Dealing with Stress and Feelings of Aggression
Dealing with teasing
Dealing with fear
Dealing with bossiness
Dealing with bullying
Dealing with fighting
Dealing with intolerance
Dealing with violent play
Dealing with disrespect for others and public
    property
Dealing with over-competitiveness
Dealing with feeling mad
Deciding if it's fair
Accepting consequences
Asking permission
Negotiating
Helping others
Using self-control
Standing up for your rights
Avoiding trouble with others
Keeping out of fights
Ignoring when appropriate
Seeking help from others
Dealing with frustration
Responding appropriately when someone says "no"
Saying "no"
Accepting "no"
Responding appropriately when someone tries to hurt
    you
Responding appropriately when someone asks you to
    do something you can't or don't want to do
Responding appropriately when things don't go right
Relaxing
Trying when it's hard
Dealing with mistakes
Being honest
Knowing when to tell
Dealing with losing
Wanting to be first
Deciding what to do
Making a complaint
Answering a complaint
Showing sportsmanship after the game
Dealing with embarrassment

Dealing with being left out
Standing up for a friend
Responding to peer pressure and persuasion
Responding to failure
Dealing with contradictory messages
Dealing with an accusation
Getting ready for a difficult conversation
Dealing with group pressure
Dealing with disappointment
Giving and accepting criticism
Coping with transitions
Giving negative feedback
Accepting negative feedback

*Decision-Making, Planning, and Problem Solving
Skills*
Deciding on something to do
Deciding what caused a problem
Setting a goal
Attaining a goal
Gathering information
Arranging problems by importance
Making a decision
Concentrating on a task
Anticipating a difficult situation
Identifying a problem
Identifying solutions
Predicting and understanding consequences
Deciding on a solution
Convincing others
Prioritizing
Avoiding being victimized
Knowing when to tell
Moral reasoning
Awareness of choices
Identifying alternatives
Time management

Feelings Skills
Knowing your feelings
Awareness of feelings
Expressing your feelings appropriately
Understanding feelings
Identifying feelings
Using "I" statements
Understanding the feelings of others
Dealing with someone else's feelings
Expressing affection
Rewarding yourself
Feeling left out

Asking to talk

Showing affection

Dealing with boredom

Being honest

Expressing caring and admiration

Appropriate emotional response

Empathy towards others in distress

Sharing affective experiences

Appropriate touching, hugging, and kissing

Help Seeking Skills

Asking for help

Asking for a favor

Asking a question

Interrupting

Asking for and giving information

Making Friends and Social Relationship Skills

Reading/interpreting peer body language

Reading/interpreting facial expressions

Reading/interpreting verbal tone

Using body language to communicate

Assuming other social perspectives

Understanding vocal inflection

Using vocal inflection effectively

Recognizing and choosing a communication style

Joining in

Waiting your turn

Sharing

Offering help

Asking someone to play

Playing a game

Apologizing

Smiling

Touching the right way

Giving and receiving compliments

Introducing yourself

Respecting personal space

Recognizing social limits based on relationships

Responding appropriately to situations

Increasing frequency of interaction

Talking to strangers

Private behaviors and public places

Cooperation

Self-disclosure

Choosing friends

Making positive statements about others

Using courtesy words

Sustaining social interaction

Increasing play interactions

Waiting your turn

Appreciating individual strength

Rules, Laws, and Classroom Skills

Knowing rules and directions

Following rules and directions

Questioning rules

Using adults as resources

Interacting with authority

Completing assignments

Using time wisely

Taking risks

Obeying laws

Self-Care Skills

Appropriate dress

Good hygiene and grooming

Appropriate eating and drinking

Adapted from: Special School District (n.d.), McGinnis and Goldstein (1990), Stumbo and Wardlaw (2011), and behaviors noted in the literature review conducted by the authors.

Indications

Social skills training is indicated when a social skills deficit is recognized. Social skills can occur because of cognitive impairments, motor impairments, sensory impairments, developmental disability, and mental illness, as well as personality, adjustment, learned behavior, and culture (Hari & Kujala, 2009; Stumbo & Wardlaw, 2011). Some conditions that commonly affect social skills include traumatic brain injury, stroke, cerebral palsy, blindness, deafness, mutism, autism spectrum disorder, attention-deficit hyperactivity disorder, dyslexia, learning disabilities, schizophrenia, bipolar disorder, conduct disorder, oppositional defiant disorder, and social anxiety.

Many ICF codes relate to social skills. Any of these may be an indication that social skills training is a treatment option.

b114 Orientation Functions

b126 Temperament and Personality Functions

b130 Energy and Drive Functions

b140 Attention Functions

b152 Emotional Functions

b156 Perceptual Functions

b160 Thought Functions

b164 Higher-Level Cognitive Functions

b167 Mental Functions of Language

b180 Experience of Self and Time Functions

d110 Watching

d115 Listening

d120 Other Purposeful Sensing

d130 Copying

d135 Rehearsing

d155 Acquiring Skills

d160 Focusing Attention

d163 Thinking

d166 Reading

d170 Writing

d172 Calculation Functions

d210 Undertaking a Single Task

d220 Undertaking Multiple Tasks

d230 Carrying Out Daily Routine

d240 Handling Stress and Other Psychological Demands

d310 Communication with — Receiving — Spoken Messages

d315 Communicating with — Receiving — Nonverbal Messages

d325 Communicating with — Receiving — Written Messages

d330 Speaking

d335 Producing Nonverbal Messages

d345 Writing Messages

d350 Conversation

d355 Discussion

d360 Using Communication Devices and Techniques

d510 Washing Oneself

d520 Caring for Body Parts

d530 Toileting

d540 Dressing

d550 Eating

d560 Drinking

d570 Looking After One's Health

d710 Basic Interpersonal Interactions

d720 Complex Interpersonal Interactions

d730 Relating with Strangers

d740 Formal Relationships

d750 Informal Social Relationships

d760 Family Relationships

d770 Intimate Relationships

d815 Preschool Education

d820 School Education

d910 Community Life

d920 Recreation and Leisure

Contraindications

There is no universal contraindication in the literature for social skills training. An individualized, comprehensive clinical assessment is necessary to determine the needs, abilities, and underlying causes of social skill deficits to determine any contraindications to social skills training or a particular social skills training technique (Riley, 2013). Several types of clients may not be appropriate for group social skills training or may benefit more from individual or carefully client-matched social skills training sessions. These include those who don't have the ability to initiate or sustain social interactions, are not ready to grasp social causality, and/or have significant language impairment. They may be very young or have a severe developmental disability. Others who should be seen individually include clients with a history of significant peer rejection. Individuals who are currently experiencing a psychotic episode, severe depression, or high social anxiety should also not be part of a group until the acute problem is resolved (Palmer & Dryden, 1994; Riley, 2013).

Protocols and Processes

Selecting and Teaching Social Skills

Stumbo and Wardlaw (2011), after an extensive review of the social skills training literature, recommend that recreational therapists consider using a blended model, which the authors adapted from Nelson (1988), Stephens (1978), and Strain, Odom, and McConnell (1994), for selecting and teaching social skills.

The model outlines an eight-step process that can be used with all populations for selecting and teaching social skills in a group. In this model, the therapist begins by selecting a particular group of individuals (e.g., early adolescents with autism) and then identifies social skill impairments that are common for that particular population to subsequently measure and address. Although not reflected in this model, recreational therapists may take a different initial approach, especially when conducting individual work. Instead of starting out by identifying social skill impairments that are common to a particular diagnosis, the therapist might opt to observe the individual and/or utilize a standardized assessment tool to identify specific social skill deficits. Outside of individual work, this alternative approach could also be used to determine individual abilities and needs and place individuals with similar needs together in dyads or small groups. An outline of the eight-step group process recommended by Stumbo and Wardlaw (2011) is provided below along with the alternative steps suggested by the authors of this chapter.

Step 1

Stumbo and Wardlaw: Select individuals and groups to target based on diagnoses.

Ropars and Porter: Select an individual based on observations and/or standardized assessments.

Step 2

Stumbo and Wardlaw: Select target behaviors for social skills instruction that can be acquired or learned in a reasonable period of time, will be effective in gaining positive responses from peers and family, reduce negative behaviors, are group-entry or group-approach behaviors, increase the person's social acceptance, are similar to those of peers without disabilities, are considered important to the "hopeful friend," can be maintained after intervention is terminated, can generalize across settings, co-vary with specific social behaviors of peers in different situations, and are socially acceptable behaviors. No deviant behaviors should be taught. It is also recommended that therapists consider additional factors when choosing a target behavior including the adaptive developmental level of the individual, primary and secondary disability problems, and magnitude and type of social skills problems. Behaviors should usually be appropriate to clients' peer group, clients' culture, socioeconomic or social class, gender, and physical environment. They should match the orientation of the instructional setting and lead to reinforcement from peers.

Ropars and Porter: Observe the individual and/or utilize standardized assessments to determine target behaviors. Observation should take place in the client's real-life situations and environments whenever possible. The therapist should be familiar with social skill deficits that are common to the client's diagnosis so that appropriate standardized assessment tools that measure commonly anticipated social skill deficit behaviors can be chosen. Select the target behavior based on identified deficits and needs from the observation and testing, as well as considerations outlined by Stumbo and Wardlaw.

Step 3

Both: Task analyze the selected behavior to determine the specific component tasks of the behavior to be taught and determine the criterion level needed to master the social skill.

Step 4

Stumbo and Wardlaw: Assess skill level in a natural and contrived setting. If the skill is adequate, the training moves to the next skill and starts again at Step 1.

Ropars and Porter: Assessment of skill in real-life settings was already determined in Step 2. Skip this step.

Step 5

Both: Select a teaching strategy, such as direct instruction, social modeling, social reinforcement, contingency contracting, demonstration, or role-playing.

Step 6

Both: Implement the teaching strategy.

Step 7

Stumbo and Wardlaw: Reassess skill achievement.

Ropars and Porter: If a standardized assessment tool was used, re-administer the tool to determine new baselines.

Step 8

Both: If the client shows sufficient competence related to the skill, move to the next skill starting at Step 2. If the client is not competent or has not mastered the skill, select another teaching strategy and repeat Steps 5 through 8.

Social Skills Training for Children and Adolescents with Developmental Disabilities

To provide further guidance for recreational therapists, a literature review from 2006-2012 was conducted on children and adolescents with developmental disabilities and social skills training using six databases (SPORTSDiscus, Academic File One, Ebschohost, PubMed, Social Sciences Citation Index, Science Citation Index), Google Scholar, and searching the *American Therapeutic Recreation Association Annual* and the *American Journal of Recreation Therapy* (Ropars, 2013). Keywords included children, adolescents, cerebral palsy, mental retardation, learning disabilities, intellectual disabilities, autism, social skills, social skills training, and social skills interventions. A total of 39 relevant journal articles were identified and subsequently synthesized to yield the following findings and recommendations:

Frequency, duration, and length of sessions: In the literature the frequency of social skills training sessions and the length of social skills training programs varied tremendously. There were also no significant relationships observed between the number of intervention sessions, hours of intervention, or total days from the beginning to the end of the intervention with treatment outcomes. It is recommended in the literature that social skills interventions should be implemented more intensely and frequently then the level presently delivered to children with social skill deficits (Gresham, Sugai, & Hornes, 2001 as cited in Bellini et al., 2007).

Setting: According to the literature review, the use of community-based, real-life environments, such as classrooms and playgroups, were chosen most often for social skills training because they produce higher maintenance effects and higher generalization effects across participants, settings, and play stimuli (Bellini et al., 2007; Canney & Byrne, 2006). Table 20 shows where different types of settings have been beneficial based on client diagnosis. Recreational therapists should use environments that have proven to be beneficial for their client's diagnosis whenever possible. The following key is utilized in the tables that follow: Learning Disability = LD, Intellectual Disability = ID, Mental Retardation = MR, Autism Spectrum Disorder = ASD.

Table 20: Social Skills Training Setting

Group based, clinical: ASD; Source: Tse et al. (2007).

Group based, community: LD, ID, MR, and ASD; Sources: Bellini et al. (2007); Canney and Byrne (2006); Cetin and Avcioğlu (2010); Cotugno (2009); DeRosier et al. (2011); Epp (2008); Gooding (2011); Hopkins et al. (2011); Kasari et al. (2012); Kokina and Kern (2010); Kroeger, Schultz, and Newsom (2007); Leaf et al. (2010); Lopata et al. (2008); Licciardello, Harchik, and Luiselli (2008); MacKay, Knott, and Dunlop (2007); Mazurik-Charles and Stefanou (2010); Minihan, Kinsella, and Honan (2011); Sheridan et al. (2011).

Individual based, clinical: MR and ASD; Sources: Castorina and Negri (2011); Hagopian, Kuhn, and Strother (2009); Laugeson et al. (2009); Tetreault and Lerman (2010).

Individual based, community: MR and ASD; Sources: Avcioğlu (2012); Banda, Hart, and Liu-Gitz (2010); Bellini et al. (2007); Bock (2007); Crawford, Gray, and Woolhiser (2012); Delano and Snell (2006); Deitchman et al. (2010); Frankel et al. (2010); Harper, Symon, and Frea (2008); Kasari et al. (2012); Koegel, Vernon, and Koegel (2009); Laushey et al. (2009); Mitchell, Parsons, and Leonard (2007); Ratto et al. (2011); Scattone, Tingstrom, and Wilczynski (2006); Stanton-Chapman and Snell (2011); Tekinarslan and Sucuoğlu (2007).

Teaching methods and interventions: Fifteen types of interventions were used in the studies. A brief description of each intervention and the diagnoses for which the intervention was used are provided below. Although interventions should be chosen based on multiple factors including client's abilities and needs, individual vs. group, real-life vs. clinical setting, time limits, and so forth, it is hoped this guide will assist recreational therapists who work with a particular population to key in on common interventions.

Table 21: Teaching Methods and Interventions

Cognitive-behavioral interventions: Problem-solving approach (used with ID, MR, and ASD). Sources: Canney and Byrne (2006); Cotugno (2009); DeRosier et al. (2011); Epp, (2008); Gooding (2011); Tekinarslan and Sucuoğlu (2007).

Concept mastery: An interactive process in which the therapist and the clients co-construct the necessary elements of a concept in order to promote clients' understanding. The necessary elements of the concept include definitions, characteristics, and examples of the concept (used with ASD). Source: Laushey et al. (2009).

Direct instruction: The use of a therapist to teach appropriate and inappropriate social skills (used with ID, MR, and ASD). Sources: Avcioğlu (2012); Banda, Hart, and Liu-Gitz (2010); Bellini et al. (2007); Cotugno, (2009); Crawford, Gray, and Woolhiser (2012); Deitchman et al. (2010); DeRosier et al. (2011); Frankel et al. (2010); Gooding (2011); Hagopian, Kuhn, and Strother (2009); Kasari et al.

(2012); Kokina and Kern (2010); Kroeger, Schultz, and Newsom (2007); Laugeson et al. (2009); Laushey et al. (2009); Leaf et al. (2010); Lopata et al. (2008); Minihan, Kinsella, and Honan (2011); Stanton-Chapman and Snell (2011); Tekinarslan and Sucuoğlu (2007).

Discussion: Conversation about appropriate social skills in a language appropriate for the client (used with ID and ASD). Sources: Castorina and Negri (2011); Cotugno, (2009); Delano and Snell (2006); Epp (2008); MacKay, Knott, and Dunlop (2007); Minihan, Kinsella, and Honan (2011); Stanton-Chapman and Snell (2011).

Environmental modification: Modifications made to the social and physical environment that promote social interaction (used with MR and ASD). Source: Bellini et al. (2007).

Family based interactions: Inclusion of family members to help reinforce skills outside of training setting (used with ASD). Sources: Castorina and Negri (2011); DeRosier et al. (2011); Frankel et al. (2010); Kokina and Kern (2010); Laugeson et al. (2009).

Modeling appropriate behavior: Clients are given a sheet outlining the steps of the skill, which are then explained and modeled by the therapist (used with MR and ASD). Sources: Banda, Hart, and Liu-Gitz (2010); Castorina and Negri (2011); DeRosier et al. (2011); Frankel et al. (2010); Gooding (2011); Kasari et al. (2012); Kokina and Kern (2010); Kroeger, Schultz, and Newsom (2007); Laugeson et al. (2009); Laushey et al. (2009); Lopata et al. (2008); MacKay, Knott, and Dunlop (2007); Minihan, Kinsella, and Honan (2011); Tekinarslan and Sucuoğlu (2007); Tetreault and Lerman (2010).

Peer/interventionist training: The use of peers (also referred to as interventionists) to teach appropriate and inappropriate social skills (used with LD, ID, and ASD). Sources: Avcioğlu (2012); Banda, Hart, and Liu-Gitz (2010); Bellini et al. (2007); Bock (2007); Cetin and Avcioğlu (2010); Cotugno, (2009); Crawford, Gray, and Woolhiser (2012); Delano and Snell (2006); DeRosier et al. (2011); Frankel et al. (2010); Gooding (2011); Harper, Symon, and Frea (2008); Kasari et al. (2012); Kokina and Kern (2010); Kroeger, Schultz, and Newsom (2007); Laugeson et al. (2009); Laushey et al. (2009); Leaf et al. (2010); Lopata et al. (2008); Licciardello, Harchik, and Luiselli (2008); MacKay, Knott, and Dunlop (2007);

Minihan, Kinsella, and Honan (2011); Ratto et al. (2011); Sheridan et al. (2011); Stanton-Chapman and Snell (2011); Tse et al. (2007).

Performance, feedback, and reinforcement: Verbally enforcing correct responses (used with ID, MR, and ASD). Sources: Avcioğlu (2012); Deitchman et al. (2010); Frankel et al. (2010); Gooding (2011); Kasari et al. (2012); Hagopian, Kuhn, and Strother (2009); Koegel, Vernon, and Koegel (2009); Kroeger, Schultz, and Newsom (2007); Laugeson et al. (2009); Licciardello, Harchik, and Luiselli (2008); Lopata et al. (2008); Minihan, Kinsella, and Honan (2011); Tetreault and Lerman (2010).

Pivotal response treatment: Based in Applied Behavioral Analysis and incorporating motivational procedures to improve responding (used with ASD). Sources: Harper, Symon, and Frea (2008); Koegel, Vernon, and Koegel (2009).

Role-play: Acting out social situations (used with LD, MR, and ASD). Sources: Castorina and Negri (2011); DeRosier et al. (2011); Gooding (2011); Laugeson et al. (2009); Laushey et al. (2009); Leaf et al. (2010); Lopata et al. (2008); MacKay, Knott, and Dunlop (2007); Mazurik-Charles and Stefanou (2010); Minihan, Kinsella, and Honan (2011); Ratto et al. (2011); Sheridan et al. (2011); Stanton-Chapman and Snell (2011); Tekinarslan and Sucuoğlu (2007); Tse et al. (2007).

Self-management: Alternative strategies based on self-control such as presenting anger without harming others (used with ID, MR, and ASD). Sources: Avcioğlu (2012); Cotugno, (2009); Deitchman et al. (2010).

Social-behavioral learning theory: Learning behavior through observation of others (used with LD and ASD). Sources: Bock (2007); Cotugno, (2009); DeRosier et al. (2011); Sheridan et al. (2011).

Social stories: A method of teaching children with autism how to "read" social situations. Uses a short story that describes the salient aspects of a specific social situation that a child may find challenging, explains the likely reactions of others in the situation, and provides information about appropriate social responses (used with ASD). Sources: Delano and Snell, (2006); Kokina and Kern (2010); Kroeger, Schultz, and Newsom (2007); Scattone, Tingstrom, and Wilczynski (2006).

Technology: Use of computers (avatars, virtual environments) or video cameras (watching social skills) (used with ASD). Sources: Deitchman et al. (2010); Hopkins et al. (2011); Mitchell, Parsons, and Leonard (2007); Tetreault and Lerman (2010).

Activities in interventions: In the literature review, two types of activities were predominantly used in the interventions: creative arts and free-time play activities. Overall, selecting tasks and materials that require participants to use frequent social exchanges was found to be the most helpful. The conclusion was that the recreational therapist should choose materials for the group rather than the individual creating opportunities to use and develop social skills (Cetin & Avcioğlu, 2010; Hagopian, Kuhn, & Strother, 2009).

Outcomes and Documentation

Given the lack of a taxonomy of social skills, the multitude of social skills training strategies and protocols, and the utilization of social skills training with diverse populations, it is difficult to identify all possible outcomes. However, in the literature review on social skills training for children and adolescents with developmental disabilities, improvements were identified in the areas discussed below.

Intellectual Disability

Presenting anger without harming others and solving dissimilarities by talking and solving conflicts without fighting (Avcioğlu, 2012).

Self-awareness, awareness of and respect for others, sitting attentively, listening to people's opinions, and contributing to the group (Canney & Byrne, 2006).

Basic social skills, basic and advanced communication skills, initiating and maintaining interactions, working as a group, emotional skills, self-control skills, dealing with aggressive behaviors, accepting consequences, giving directions, and cognitive skills (Cetin & Avcioğlu, 2010).

Learning Disability

Listening, following directions, problem solving, and knowing when to tell, as well as in ratings of overall social ability (Sheridan et al., 2011).

Mental Retardation

Recruiting attention and interacting with others in an appropriate manner (Hagopian, Kuhn, & Strother, 2009).

Apologizing, coping with teasing, and avoiding inappropriate touching (Tekinarslan & Sucuoğlu, 2007).

Autism Spectrum Disorders

Social initiations and responses (Banda, Hart, & Liu-Gitz, 2010).

Play skills, joint attention, language skills, social interactions, social responses, and duration of interaction (Bellini et al., 2007).

Increase in the percentage of time spent participating in cooperative learning activities during social studies, playing organized sport games during noon recess, and visiting with peers during lunch (Bock, 2007).

Identification of discrete skills and non-verbal social cues such as eye contact, body language, tone of voice, and facial expression (Castorina & Negri, 2011).

Teacher-preferred social behavior, peer-preferred social behavior, and social adjustment behavior (Cotugno, 2009).

Conversation skills, non-verbal skills, leisure education, friendship skills, boundaries and personal space, handling bullying, and assertiveness (Crawford, Gray, & Woolhiser, 2012).

Frequency of social initiation (Deitchman et al., 2010).

Duration and appropriateness of social engagement during play sessions, seeking attention, initiating comments, initiating requests, and making contingent responses (Delano & Snell, 2006).

Self-efficacy, social awareness, motivation for social interaction, social communication skills, and improvement in unusual mannerisms (DeRosier et al., 2011).

Knowledge of rules of social etiquette relevant to making and keeping friends, frequency of hosted get-togethers, and better quality of friendships (Laugeson et al., 2009).

Assertiveness, cooperation, responsibility, self-control, internalizing behavior, external behavior, and reduced hyperactivity (Epp, 2008).

Hosted play dates and social skill and play date behavior (Frankel et al., 2010).

Social competence and increased self-initiated on-task behavior (Gooding, 2011).

Social contact with typical peers and social initiations (Harper, Symon, & Frea, 2008).

Eye gaze, expression matching, face recognition, emotion recognition, and social interactions (Hopkins et al., 2011).

Friendship nominations, classroom social skills, and reduced playground isolation (Kasari et al., 2012).

Initiations of social engagement during communication, nonverbal dyadic orienting, and overall affect (Koegel, Vernon, & Koegel, 2009).

Appropriate behavior, academic and functional skills, transitions, and reduced anxiety (Kokina & Kern, 2010).

Initiation behaviors, responding behaviors, and interacting behaviors (Kroeger, Schultz, & Newsom, 2007).

Frequency of hosted get-togethers, better quality of friendships, and overall level of social skills (Laugeson et al., 2009).

Responding appropriately to a peer's question, appropriately initiating interactions with a peer, and reading a peer's facial expression and responding according to the expression (Laushey et al., 2009).

Social interactions (Leaf et al., 2010).

Social skills and problem behavior (Lopata et al., 2008).

Social initiations and social responses (Licciardello, Harchik, & Luiselli, 2008).

Social and emotional perspective taking, conversation skills, and friendship skills (MacKay, 2007).

Social awareness, social cognition, and social responsiveness (Mazurik-Charles & Stefanou, 2010).

Non-verbal communication and relationship skills (Minihan, Kinsella, & Honan, 2011).

Judgments and reasoning about where to sit in videos of real cafes and buses (Mitchell, Parsons, & Leonard, 2007).

Asking questions, topic change, and quality of rapport (Ratto et al., 2011).

Social interactions (Scattone, Tingstrom, & Wilczynski, 2006).

Rate of initiations with an immediate peer response and turn-taking skills (Stanton-Chapman & Snell, 2011).

Reductions in irritability, lethargy, withdrawal, stereotypic behavior, hyperactivity, inappropriate speech, conduct problems, over-sensitivity, self-isolating and ritualistic behavior, self-injury, stereotypic behavior, insecurity, and anxiousness (Tse et al., 2007).

Getting attention, requesting attention, and sharing a toy (Tetreault & Lerman, 2010).

Measurement Tools

Outcomes can be measured by observing the client's ability to perform target skills. It is strongly recommended that recreational therapists also include the use of standardized assessment tools to increase objective measurement and use the ICF codes when documenting behavioral changes. Measuring outcomes is essential to increase the documentation of efficacy for particular social skills training interventions. Some standardized tools include:

Aberrant Behavior Checklist (ABC): Measures problem behaviors of people with developmental disabilities.

Achieved Learning Questionnaire (ALQ): A parent report used to assess children's learned social skills.

Behavior Assessment System for Children Parent/Teacher Rating Scales (BASC-PRS, BASC-TRS): A rating scale that quantifies parent and teacher perceptions of children's behavior and skills.

Benton Facial Recognition Test (Short Form): Measures the children's facial recognition skills.

Child and Adolescent Social Perception Measure (CASP): Measures social perception using non-verbal and situational cues.

Child Behavior Checklist (CBCL): Designed to obtain data on behavioral and emotional problems and competencies.

Contextual Assessment of Social Skills (CASS): A role-play measure of social skill for individuals with high-functioning autism.

Conversation Rating Scale (CRS): A questionnaire that rates the participant's interest in the conversation.

Diagnostic Analysis of Nonverbal Accuracy 2 (DANVA2): A computer-based research instrument that assesses the ability to accurately identify four basic emotions (i.e., happy, sad, angry, and fearful) through facial expressions or spoken language cues.

Friendship Qualities Scale (FQS): An adolescent self-report measure that assesses the quality of best friendships.

Home and Community Social Behavior Scales (HCSBS): Measures student's social behavior in the school and home settings.

MGH YouthCare Social Competence/Social Skill Development Scale (SCDS): Social competency and social skill development for children with ASD, including cognitive aspects, social interpersonal skills, and self-awareness.

Nisonger Child Behavior Rating Form (N-CBRF): Measures emotional and behavioral problems of children and adolescents with developmental disabilities.

Peer Language and Behavior Code (PLBC): Measures verbal and nonverbal interactions between children.

Piers-Harris Self-Concept Scale (PHS): Self-report measure of self-concept.

Pupil Evaluation Inventory — Teacher (PEI): Assesses peer ratings of the behavior of male and female children in grades one through nine.

Quality of Play Questionnaire (QPQ): Measures frequency of get-togethers with peers over the previous month and the level of conflict during these get-togethers.

Skillstreaming Survey (SS): Measures social skills and social behaviors.

Social Competence with Peers Questionnaire — Parents (SCPQ-P): Measures whether particular social skills and competencies are fully, partly, or not at all established.

Social Competence with Peers Questionnaire — Pupils (SCPQPU): Assesses whether particular skills and competencies are fully, partly, or not at all established.

Social Interaction Observation Code: Measures the frequency, duration, and nature (positive or negative) of the videotaped social interactions.

Social Responsiveness Scale (SRS): Measures severity and types of social impairments that are characteristic of autistic spectrum conditions in children and adolescents.

Social Self-Efficacy Scale: Measures children's perceived self-efficacy for social tasks.

Social Skills Assessment — Elementary Age: Measures how children typically think, behave, or handle situations.

Social Skills Assessment Scale: Uses teachers to assess students' social skills.

Social Skills Questionnaire — Parents (SSQ-P): Measures a parent's perception of their child's social skills.

Social Skills Questionnaire — Pupils (SSQ-PU): Assesses whether particular skills and competencies are fully, partly, or not at all established.

Social Skills Rating Scale (SSRS): Measures a wide range of social skills including the broad domains of cooperation, assertion, responsibility, and self-control.

Teacher Perception of Social Skills (TPSS): Measures teacher's perceptions of students' social skills.

Test of Adolescent Social Skills Knowledge (TASSK): Measures adolescents' knowledge about the specific social skills taught during the intervention.

The Awareness of Social Inference Test (TASIT): Measures emotion recognition, the ability to understand when conversational inference such as sarcasm is being made, and the ability to differentiate between different kinds of counterfactual comments (lies and sarcasm).

Vineland Adaptive Behavior Scales, Survey Form (VABS): Objectively measures adaptive functioning and social skills in autism and other developmental disabilities.

Walker-McConnell Scale of Social Competence and Social Adjustment (WMS): Measures constructs of social competence and school adjustment related to social functioning.

ICF codes: The ICF codes listed in the Indications section are related to social skills training. These should be used to measure changes resulting from treatment. The list includes the three-digit codes to consider. Documentation should include the four- and five-digit details of these codes.

References

Avcioğlu, H. (2012). The effectiveness of the instructional programs based on self-management strategies in acquisition of social skills by the children with intellectual disabilities. *Educational Sciences: Theory & Practice, 12*(1), 345-351.

Banda, D. R., Hart, S. L., & Liu-Gitz, L. (2010). Impact of training peers and children with autism on social skills during center time activities in inclusive classrooms. *Research in Autism Spectrum Disorders, 4*(4), 619-625.

Bellini, S., Peters, J. Benner, L., & Hopf, A. (2007). A meta-analysis of school-based social skills interventions for children with autism spectrum disorders. *Remedial & Special Education, 28*(3), 153-162.

Bock, M. A. (2007). The impact of social-behavioral learning strategy training on the social interaction skills of four students with Asperger syndrome. *Focus on Autism & Other Developmental Disabilities, 22*(2), 88-95.

Canney, C. & Byrne, A. (2006). Evaluating circle time as a support to social skills development: Reflections on a journey in school-based research. *British Journal of Special Education, 33*(1), 19-24.

Castorina, L. L. & Negri, L. M. (2011). The inclusion of siblings in social skills training groups for boys with Asperger syndrome. *Journal of Autism & Developmental Disorders, 41*(1), 73-81.

Centers for Disease Control. (2012). Data and Statistics for Cerebral Palsy. Retrieved from www.cdc.gov/ncbddd/cp/data.html.

Cetin, M. E. & Avcioğlu, H. (2010). Investigation of the effectiveness of social skills training program prepared through drama technique for mentally disabled students. *International Online Journal of Educational Sciences, 2*(3), 792-817.

Cotugno, A. J. (2009). Social competence and social skills training and intervention for children with autism spectrum disorders. *Journal of Autism and Developmental Disorders, 39*(9), 1268-77.

Crawford, M. E., Gray, C., & Woolhiser, J. (2012). Design and delivery of a public school social skills training program for youth with autism spectrum disorders: A five year retrospective of the school/community/home (SCH) model of social skills development. *Annual in Therapeutic Recreation, 20,* 17-35.

Deitchman, C. R., Reeve, S. A., Reeve, K. F., & Progar, P. (2010). Incorporating video feedback into self-management training to promote generalization of social initiations by children with autism. *Education & Treatment of Children (West Virginia University Press)*, 475-488.

Delano, M. & Snell, M. E. (2006). The effects of social stories on the social engagement of children with autism. *Journal of Positive Behavior Interventions, 8*(1), 29-42.

DeRosier, M. E., Swick, D. C., Davis, N. O., McMillen, J. S., & Matthews, R. (2011). The efficacy of a social skills group intervention for improving social behaviors in children with high functioning autism spectrum disorders. *Journal of Autism and Developmental Disorders, 41*(8), 1033-1043.

Dictionary.com's 21st Century Lexicon. (2013). *Social skills.* Accessed via website http://dictionary.reference.com/browse/social+skills.

Encyclopedia of Mental Disorders. (2012). Social Skills Training. Retrieved from www.minddisorders.com/Py-Z/Social-skills-training.html.

Epp, K. (2008). Outcome-based evaluation of a social skills program using art therapy and group therapy for children on the autism spectrum. *Children & Schools, 30*(1), 27-36.

Frankel, F., Myatt, R., Sugar, C., Whitham, C., Gorospe, C. M., & Laugeson, E. (2010). A randomized controlled study of parent-assisted children's friendship training with children having autism spectrum disorders. *Journal of Autism and Developmental Disorders, 40*(7), 827-842.

Gooding, L F. (2011). The effect of a music therapy social skills training program on improving social competence in children and adolescents with social skills deficits. *Journal of Music Therapy, 48*(4), 440-462.

Gresham, F. M., Sugai, G., & Hornes, R. H. (2001). Interpreting outcomes of social skills training for students with high incidence disabilities. *Teaching Exceptional Children, 67,* 331-334.

Hagopian, L. P., Kuhn, D. E., & Strother, G. E. (2009). Targeting social skills deficits in an adolescent with pervasive developmental disorder. *Journal of Applied Behavior Analysis, 42*(4), 907-911.

Hari, R. & Kujala, M. V. (2009). Brain basis of human social interaction: From concepts to brain imaging. *Physiol Rev, 89,* 453-479.

Harper, C. B., Symon, J. B. G., & Frea, W. D. (2008). Recess is time-in: Using peers to improve social skills of children with

autism. *Journal of Autism and Developmental Disorders, 38*(5), 815-826.

Hartman, K. (2013). Benefits of social support for individuals with spinal cord injury. Accessed via website www.rtwiseowls.com.

Hopkins, I. M., Gower, M. W., Perez, T. A., Smith, D. S., Amthor, F. R., Wimsatt, F. C., & Biasini, F. J. (2011). Avatar assistant: Improving social skills in students with an ASD through a computer-based intervention. *Journal of Autism and Developmental Disorders, 41*(11), 1543-1555.

Kasari, C., Rotheram-Fuller, E., Locke, J., & Gulsrud, A. (2012). Making the connection: Randomized controlled trial of social skills at school for children with autism spectrum disorders. *Journal of Child Psychology and Psychiatry, and Allied Disciplines, 53*(4), 431-439.

Koegel, R. L., Vernon, T. W., & Koegel, L. K. (2009). Improving social initiations in young children with autism using reinforcers with embedded social interactions. *Journal of Autism and Developmental Disorders, 39*(9), 1240-1251.

Kokina, A. & Kern, L. (2010). Social story interventions for students with autism spectrum disorders: A meta-analysis. *Journal of Autism and Developmental Disorders, 40*(7), 812-826.

Kroeger, K. A., Schultz, J. R., & Newsom, C. A. (2007). Comparison of two group-delivered social skills programs for young children with autism. *Journal of Autism and Developmental Disorders, 37,* 808-817.

Laugeson, E. A., Frankel, F., Mogil, C., & Dillon, A. R. (2009). Parent-assisted social skills training to improve friendships in teens with autism spectrum disorders. *Journal of Autism and Developmental Disorders, 39*(4), 596-606.

Laushey, K. M., Heflin, L. J., Shippen, M., Alberto, P. A., & Fredrick, L. (2009). Concept mastery routines to teach social skills to elementary children with high functioning autism. *Journal of Autism and Developmental Disorders, 39*(10), 1435-1448.

Leaf, J. B., Dotson, W. H., Oppeneheim, M. L., Sheldon, J. B., & Sherman, J. A. (2010). The effectiveness of a group teaching interaction procedure for teaching social skills to young children with a pervasive developmental disorder. *Research in Autism Spectrum Disorders, 4*(2), 186-198.

Lopata, C., Thomeer, M. L., Volker, M. A., Nida, R. E., & Lee, G. K. (2008). Effectiveness of a manualized summer social treatment program for high-functioning children with autism spectrum disorders. *Journal of Autism and Developmental Disorders, 38*(5), 890-904.

Licciardello, C. C., Harchik, A. E., & Luiselli, J. K. (2008). Social skills intervention for children with autism during interactive play at a public elementary school. *Education & Treatment of Children (West Virginia University Press),* 27-37.

MacKay, T., Knott, F., & Dunlop, A. (2007). Developing social interaction and understanding in individuals with autism spectrum disorder: A groupwork intervention. *Journal of Intellectual & Developmental Disability, 32*(4), 279-279.

Matson, J. L. (2009). *Social behavior and skills in children.* Springer.

Mazurik-Charles, R., & Stefanou, C. (2010). Using paraprofessionals to teach social skills to children with autism spectrum disorders in the general education classroom. *Journal of Instructional Psychology, 37*(2), 161-169.

McGinnis, E. & Goldstein, A. P. (1990). Skillstreaming in early adulthood. Teaching prosocial skills to the preschool and kindergarten child. Champaign, IL, Research Press.

Mitchell, P., Parsons, S., & Leonard, A. (2007). Using virtual environments for teaching social understanding to 6 adolescents with autistic spectrum disorders. *Journal of Autism and Developmental Disorders, 37*(3), 589-600.

Minihan, A., Kinsella, W., & Honan, R. (2011). Social skills training for adolescents with Asperger's syndrome using a consultation model. *Journal of Research in Special Educational Needs, 11*(1), 55-69.

Nelson, C. M. (1988). Social skills training for handicapped students. *Teaching Exceptional Children, 20*(4), 19-23.

Palmer, S. & Dryden, W. (1994). *Counseling for stress problems.* Thousand Oaks, CA: Sage.

Rath, T. & Harter, J. K. (2010). *Well being: The five essential elements.* Gallup Press.

Ratto, A. B., Turner-Brown, L., Rupp, B. M., Mesibov, G. B., & Penn, D. L. (2011). Development of the contextual assessment of social skills (CASS): A role play measure of social skill for individuals with high-functioning autism. *Journal of Autism and Developmental Disorders, 41*(9), 1277-1286.

Riley, S. (2013). *Group process made visible: The use of art in group therapy.* New York: Routledge.

Ropars, K. (2013). Social skills training for children and adolescents with developmental disabilities. Accessed via website http://rtwiseowls.com/page/2/

Scattone, D., Tingstrom, D. H., & Wilczynski, S. M. (2006). Increasing appropriate social interactions of children with autism spectrum disorders using social stories. *Focus on Autism and Other Developmental Disabilities, 21*(4), 211-222.

Sheridan, B. A., MacDonald, D. A., Donlon, M., Kuhn, B., McGovern, K., & Friedman, H. (2011). Evaluation of a social skills program based on social learning theory, implemented in a school setting. *Psychological Reports, 108*(2), 420-436.

Special School District. (n.d.). Social skills index of skills. Accessed via website http://pbiscompendium.ssd.k12.mo.us/ResourcesSchools/SSD/SocialSkills/skillsin.htm.

Stanton-Chapman, T. L. & Snell, M. E. (2011). Promoting turn-taking skills in preschool children with disabilities: The effects of a peer-based social communication intervention. *Early Childhood Research Quarterly, 26*(3), 303-319.

Stephens, T. (1978). *Social skills in the classroom.* Columbus, OH: Cedars Press.

Strain, P. S., Odom, S. L., & McConnell, S. (1984). Promoting social reciprocity of exceptional children: Identification, target behavior selection, and intervention. *Remedial and Special Education, 5*(1), 21-28.

Stumbo, N. J. & Wardlaw, B. (2011). *Facilitation of therapeutic recreation services: An evidence-based and best practice approach to techniques and processes.* State College, PA: Venture Publishing.

Tetreault, A. & Lerman, D. C. (2010). Teaching social skills to children with autism using point-of-view video modeling. *Education & Treatment of Children (West Virginia University Press),* 395-419.

Tekinarslan, I. C. & Sucuoğlu, B. (2007). Effectiveness of cognitive process approached social skills training program for people with mental retardation. *International Journal of Special Education, 22*(7).

The Beck Institute, (2012). Cognitive Behavior Therapy. Retrieved from www.beckinstitute.org/what-is-cognitive-behavioral-therapy/

Tse, J., Strulovitch, J., Tagalakis, V., Meng, L., & Fombonne, E. (2007). Social skills training for adolescents with Asperger syndrome and high-functioning autism. *Journal of Autism and Developmental Disorders, 37*(10), 1960-1968.

Voorman, J. M., Dallmeijer, A. J., Van Eck, M., Schuengel, C., & Becher, J. G. (2010). Social functioning and communication in children with cerebral palsy: Association with disease characteristics and personal and environmental factors. *Developmental Medicine and Child Neurology, 52*(5), 441-447.

45. Stress Management and Coping

Heather R. Porter

The many aspects of what causes stress are discussed in the Therapy Basics chapter on Stress. People cope with stress in many different ways. Some people may go for a run to release excess energy, while others may comfort themselves with food or talk with friends. The techniques that people use may be conscious decisions (e.g., "I am under a lot of stress, so I am going to take a long hot shower to help myself unwind.") or unconscious decisions that are commonly engrained, learned behaviors (e.g., when under a lot of stress the person becomes very negative about everything).

The World Health Organization (1998) makes a clear distinction between coping and managing. Coping is defined as a capacity to respond and recover from something stressful. It implies that the individual has very little control over the situation, stressor, threat, or conflict. An example of coping would be eating less expensive food to handle stress about money or using substances such as alcohol or illicit drugs to handle relationship stress. Coping can help or make things worse. On the other hand, managing implies that a person has no need to cope because s/he has the knowledge and resources to control the situation, stressor, threat, or conflict. Examples of managing would be dipping into one's savings account or asserting one's needs in a healthy manner. Both coping and managing can also be viewed as a motivated and meaning-making process since it is a natural response for humans to try to make sense of things, as lack of meaning often results in distress (Aldwin, 2012).

The World Health Organization (1998) divides coping mechanisms into three categories. Although the categories were developed to describe coping mechanisms in the face of disaster (e.g., famine, village destruction, mass killings), they may be applicable to categorize the outcomes of the coping strategies employed by the individual.

Non-erosive: Non-erosive coping mechanisms result in little to no permanent damage (e.g., yoga, reducing meals, assertiveness).

Erosive: Erosive coping mechanisms result in harm or damage (e.g., illicit drug use, violence, anorexia nervosa).

Failed: Coping mechanisms employed fail and the person is overcome by the stressor. Damage and harm are irreversible. Dependence on external aid may be necessary. Examples include suicide, selling children, or prostitution.

Coping Styles and Responses

The Transactional Model of Stress and Coping (TMSC) provides a framework for evaluating the processes of coping with stressful events or situations (Glanz, Rimer, & Lewis, 2002). The word "transactional" is used to explain the interaction between the person and the environment, as stress results from an imbalance between demands and available resources to effectively cope with the stressor. When the stressor exceeds a person's available physical, financial, mental, or emotional resources, stress ensues. When a person experiences a stressor, the person evaluates the potential threat of the stressor in a primary appraisal. The primary appraisal is the person's opinion about the significance of the stressor including potential threats, challenges, loss, and possible harm. This is followed by a secondary appraisal of considering what the person can actually do about the situation including the amount of control the person has over the stressor and the resources the person has available to cope with the stressor.

Depending on the person's perceptions from the primary and secondary appraisals, the person implements a strategy called a coping effort to cope with the event. The coping can be problem-focused or emotion-focused. Problem-focused coping consists of strategies directed at changing the stressful event, such as defining the problem, identifying solutions, seeking out resources, learning skills to manage the stressor, and monitoring and reevaluating outcomes. Emotion-focused coping includes strategies aimed at changing the way the person thinks or feels about the stressful event, such as sharing feelings with other people, accepting the situation, distancing oneself from or avoiding the stressor, behaviorally acting out, turning to drugs or alcohol to forget about the problem. It is through problem-focused and emotion-focused coping that individuals move towards an outcome that brings about emotional homeostasis.

Although the TMSC only considers problem-focused and emotion-focused coping, Carver (2010) states that people often utilize a variety of coping styles, and that coping styles are not always clearly defined. For example, going out to a movie with a friend to engage in social conversation about things other than the stressor might be considered emotion-focused coping, as well as avoidance coping. Some examples of coping styles include:

Problem-focused coping: Involves taking steps to remove the stressor or impede its arrival to reduce its impact, such as sitting in a different seat on the bus to avoid a confrontation with another person.

Emotion-focused coping: Involves taking steps to reduce, minimize, or prevent the amount of emotional distress from a stressor, such as going out to lunch with a friend because you know she will make you laugh at a time when you need it most.

Approach coping or engagement coping: Involves taking steps to deal directly with the stressor or the emotions the stressor evokes, such as talking to a person with whom you are having a disagreement.

Avoidance coping or disengagement coping: Taking steps to avoid having to deal with the stressor, such as playing basketball to take your mind off of the stressor or turning to drugs or alcohol to escape from the stressor. Interestingly, smoking has been found to increase after adverse childhood experiences, negative life events, acute and chronic stressors, and perceived stress, as smokers commonly report that cigarette smoking reduces anxiety and alleviates negative moods. Alcohol use is associated with traumatic stress, unhappy marriages, and dissatisfaction with employment, well as a way to decrease

tension, anxiety, irritability, and depression for individuals with post-traumatic stress disorder. Opiates inhibit the stress cycle and produced feelings of euphoria (Grunberg, Berger, & Hamilton, 2010). There are many explanations as to why there is a strong relationship between stress and drug use, one of which is the self-medication hypothesis indicating that drugs might be self-administered to decrease CNS stimulation helping to combat feelings of stress, maintain one's performance while stressed, reduce distractions, and/or indirectly increase social support to alleviate and buffer stress (Grunberg et al., 2010).

Positive coping: Taking steps to engage in experiences that allow a person to experience positive emotions as a way of coping with the negative emotions associated with the stressor.

Meaning-focused coping: Taking steps to find meaning in the negative stressful event. This is also referred to a stress-related growth, post-traumatic growth, and finding benefits. It leads to comments like, "Having this injury is one of the best things that has ever happened to me because it made me turn my life completely around."

Spiritual coping: Engaging in spiritual activities to cope with a stressful event, often through prayer or relying on faith.

Indications

Interventions aimed at stress management and coping are warranted when a client expresses feelings of distress that are negatively impacting functioning, health, and/or quality of life. The ICF code d240 Handling Stress and Other Psychological Demands should be part of the diagnosis whenever the client expresses these feelings. The ICF code that describes the area where the client is feeling distress should also be part of the diagnosis. Almost any ICF code could be the cause of stress.

Not all clients will have the ability to identify and verbalize such feelings due to developmental ability, mental, cognitive, or communication impairment, or the conscious or unconscious choice to ignore rather than acknowledge the stressor. Consequently, if verbal or behavioral signs of stress are observed, the therapist should consider the use of these interventions.

Contraindications

There are no known contraindications to stress management and coping interventions. Therapists must be aware however, that interventions aimed at imagination, such as guided imagery and autogenics, could evoke hallucinations or illusions in populations with diagnoses that are prone to these experiences, such as schizophrenia.

Protocols and Processes

Upon exploration, some clients will be able to accurately identify the cause of stress. However, in other cases, clients may have difficulty identifying the cause or be unable to express feelings because of emotional or intellectual issues. It is also possible that the cause is not reality based. Projections and delusions can be stressors from within the client. Strategies employed to assist clients with stress management and coping will vary depending on the underlying causes of the stress and other variables such as developmental level and personal likes and dislikes.

Prior to exploring stress management and coping mechanisms and during the exploration process, the therapist needs to assess factors that are influencing the client's current stress response. Such factors include personality traits, individual perceptual styles, how information is perceived, situational determinants related to adapting coping techniques to the demands of the situation, cognitive approaches, social aspects of how the coping strategy meets the needs of others, and religious beliefs and practices, such as prayer, that influence coping responses (Aldwin, 2012). Other considerations include the person's developmental level, available resources, functional limitations that hinder utilization of specific stress management or coping strategies, and individual strengths or facilitators that have the probability of enhancing the stress management or coping response. In cases where individuals do not have the ability to communicate their thoughts and feelings, observation will be key in identifying triggers and responses.

Exploring stress management and coping strategies requires the therapist to evaluate variables that are unique to each client. A common approach to this process is to start out by briefly reviewing several types of stress management techniques that are initially thought to match the client's needs. This gives the therapist a general feel for what is appealing to or disliked by the client. Therapists must remember that although these techniques are labeled as stress management interventions, they do not have that effect on all people. Some people may find some of the techniques bothersome, frustrating, and annoying. We have found from experience that people who are highly stressed often have difficulty with relaxation training interventions that take a long time, such as guided imagery. They react better to simple techniques that offer an immediate physiological response, such as deep breathing. People who are highly stressed often seem to react better to interventions that challenge managerial skills such as problem solving, time management, and goal setting — techniques that reflect a sense of control, something that people who are highly stressed are often searching for.

Since therapists are aware that not all stress management and relaxation training strategies work with all people, provided below are guidelines to consider when identifying strategies:

Lifestyle: Interventions must easily fit into the client's lifestyle.

Interests: Techniques should align with the client's interests. Some clients do not like specific activities and will therefore balk at certain suggestions from a therapist.

Personality: The interventions must fit with the personality of the client.

Resources available: The activity must be available at a place and time that the client has access to.

Finances: Costs must be within the client's budget.

Level of support: Support from family and friends must be available, if it is required for the activity.

Health abilities and limitations: The client must be able to do the activities safely. Limitations include psychological issues, such as visualization being inappropriate for someone who has schizophrenia, and physical issues, such as having to walk at the mall in the winter because of weather.

Stress management and coping responses can be learned behaviors. Exploration of how the client responded to stressors in the past might provide insight into where and how behaviors were learned, as well as allow the therapist to assess for patterns of behavior and responses.

Interventions should be tailored based on the considerations described above. If the stressor is modifiable, then modifications are explored and addressed. If the stressor is not modifiable, such as death of a loved one or a history of abuse, healthy coping mechanisms can be explored and implemented to mediate the negative effects of the stressor on health and behavior.

Therapists who work with diverse populations, including recent immigrants, are aware that the client's coping mechanisms may be influenced by cultural beliefs and an upbringing that differs from Western culture. Therapists do not assume that unfamiliar coping mechanisms are unhealthy, but rather determine the healthiness of these coping mechanisms, as well as any other coping mechanisms, by asking two questions: (1) Is the mechanism employed causing harm to the client or others? and (2) Is it effective? The therapist is trying to figure out if the coping mechanism is resulting in better emotional, psychological, cognitive, physical, and social health. If the answer is no to either of these questions, alternative coping mechanisms should be taught through education and practical application.

Therapists who interact with clients on a regular basis have the responsibility to foster and strengthen healthy coping mechanisms and to ensure continuity of, and support for, access to healthy coping mechanisms. Therapists foster and strengthen healthy coping strategies through:

Education: Clients are educated directly or indirectly about the consequences of specific coping mechanisms.

Providing opportunities to engage in healthy coping mechanisms: Activities that encourage teamwork, relaxation, expression, and physical release of tension have inherent benefits to cope with stress. Therapists offer such programs, articulate their benefits to others, and ensure access to these activities.

Providing support and encouragement: When unhealthy signs of stress are observed or a client confides his/her conflict to a therapist, support and encouragement are provided to help the client implement healthy coping mechanisms, including referring the client to others as required.

Basic Clinical Approach

A basic clinical approach to stress management and coping typically includes five steps (Porter & burlingame, 2006): identify stressors and strengths, measure responses to stress, provide education, implement interventions, and reevaluate. Each is reviewed below.

Identify Stressors and Strengths

Therapists help clients identify their specific stressors and strengths. Knowing the source of stress and the resources (strengths) of the client is essential to building a stress treatment plan. An assessment tool developed by Eliot (1994) at the Institute of Stress Medicine is the *Quality of Life Index*. The tool (1) takes 10-15 minutes to administer, (2) takes 15 minutes to score, (3) indirectly educates the client to items that contribute to stress and the management of stress, (4) evaluates a wide spectrum of items related to stress including recreation and leisure and provides the therapist with several scores that are easy to see and integrate, and (5) looks at stress from the client's point of view. The last point is important because the most effective way to build a treatment plan for stress control "is to deal with the individual's perception of a stressful situation rather than with the actual situation or threat itself. We cannot control others; we can only control our reactions to them. There is much evidence that our unique perceptions and coping strategies are the primary catalyst for stress-linked disorders within our bodies" (Eliot, 1994, p. 87). Other assessment tools for consideration include the *Social Readjustment Rating Scale*, *Stress and Well-Being Inventory*, *Daily Hassles Scale*, *Perceived Stress Scale*, and *Profile of Mood States*.

In addition to assessment tools, therapists should conduct a clinical interview. Therapists should pose open-ended questions that encourage verbalizations of strengths and stressors (e.g., "What is different for you now?") and help the client to narrow down concerns about stressors and strengths so they can be turned into specific measurable objectives. The therapist also observes and evaluates indirect expressions of stress during activities by watching the client's defensive and coping mechanisms, behavioral responses to stressful situations, and physiological responses to stress.

Measure Responses to Stress

Once stressors have been identified, the therapist measures the client's response to stress. Measuring the client's physiological, cognitive, and behavioral response to stress will provide a baseline of functioning to show if the interventions are effective. If possible, measure the client's reactions to stress in a real-life setting, such as a community outing. If this is not possible, monitor responses in simulated environments or during designed challenges that allow for the observation of the client's response to stress. Designed challenges should be as close to the identified stressors as possible.

Physiological response: The easiest ways to measure a client's physiological response to stress is through blood pressure monitoring and observation of physiological changes. Eliot (1994) recommends that blood pressure should be taken every other day over the course of ten days with five days of monitoring in all. Blood pressure should be taken several times each day, especially when entering, during, or exiting a stressful situation and when the client is believed to be in a relaxed state. Each blood pressure reading is calculated to determine the mean arterial blood pressure. To calculate the mean subtract the diastolic blood pressure from the systolic blood pressure, divide the answer by three, and then add back the diastolic blood pressure (e.g., if the blood pressure is 120/80, 120-80 = 40, 40 divided by 3 equals 13, 13 plus 80 equals 93. 93 is the mean arterial blood pressure of 120/80). Eliot (1994) divides blood pressure means into categories to determine how a person reacts, as shown in Table 22. Therapists look for the highest mean over the course of the monitoring period. The highest peak is the best predictor of how the client will physiologically react to periods of high stress.

Table 22: Reactions to Stress

Each entry shows the reactor type, level assigned by Eliot, seriousness of the reaction, and mean arterial blood pressure

Hot Reactor, Level 4, Severe, 127 or greater

Hot Reactor, Level 3, Moderate, 117-126

Hot Reactor, Level 2, Mild, 107-125

Normal, Level 1, Normal, 97-106

Cool Reactor, N/A, N/A, 96 or below

Cognitive response: Therapists ask the client to focus on internal and external cognition as they relate to dealing with stress and then write their thoughts in a daily journal for a set period of time, usually one week. Therapists look for patterns in the thought processes of the client, especially defensive mechanisms and coping mechanisms, and develop a plan to change distorted thinking patterns into healthy thinking patterns.

Behavioral response: Therapists look for behavioral manifestations of stress when the client is experiencing a stressful situation. Behaviors are measured in terms of description and frequency. Stress is not always revealed in verbalizations and cognition is not always apparent. The therapist must often use behavioral observations to identify the existence of stress.

Provide Education

Clients are educated about the consequences of uncontrolled high levels of stress as it pertains to their specific situation. Many people do not fully understand the detrimental effects of stress on their lives. Gaining insight can help clients to take control of their lifestyle and implement positive lifestyle changes.

Implement Interventions

The step reflects the coming together of many key components. Clients identify triggers of stress, discover their signs and symptoms in response to stress, and learn to manage or cope with the stress so that stress does not become a barrier to health and therapeutic progress. Eliot (1994) comments on the relevance of managing stress through planned interventions and strategies. He says, "Life-threatening overreaction to stress is neither innate nor inevitable. We were not born with this trait. We have learned it. We can unlearn it" (p. 92). Therapists convey this message to clients to highlight the control that they have in making positive lifestyle changes.

Reevaluate

When the program is running, it is important to check periodically to be sure that it is effective. The stressors may have changed, the client may have learned to deal with some of the stress and need new goals, or the interventions may not feel comfortable any more. Depending on the particular situation, it may be appropriate to do a brief reevaluation daily at the start of a program. Later there can be weekly or monthly checkups.

Relaxation Training

There are many different ways to manage stress, but most of them require clear thinking and a positive emotional state. These are, of course, exactly the opposite of how people usually feel when they are stressed. Stress often leads to more stress. Relaxation training may be enough to deal with some stressful situations, but even if it isn't a complete answer, it will help the client to reach a state where other solutions to the stress seem possible.

Relaxation training focuses on specific techniques that induce a relaxation response when stress levels are high. Formal relaxation training interventions may be helpful, especially for clients who are experiencing non-modifiable stressors, are unable to identify the particular stressor, or are generally experiencing overall stress. Techniques include deep breathing, progressive relaxation, meditation, visualization or guided imagery, and autogenics.

Deep Breathing

When taking a breath, oxygen is taken into the lungs and then transported into the bloodstream to service organs and muscles. Oxygen is received by the cells and they release carbon dioxide, a waste product that the body does not need. The carbon dioxide is carried back to the heart and then to the lungs to be exhaled and the cycle repeats.

Shallow breathing (also known as chest or thoracic breathing) does not allow for a good exchange of oxygen and carbon dioxide. Inadequate amounts of oxygen are taken in and not enough carbon dioxide is exported out. When the body does not receive enough oxygenated blood and carbon dioxide builds up in the bloodstream, muscles tighten and the heart rate increases to try to increase the transport of oxygenated blood. Over time, inadequate oxygen intake and carbon dioxide buildup can contribute to headaches, fatigue, and irritability.

Clients who experience anxiety, anger, panic, depressive symptoms, or psychosomatic or physiologically based chronic pain will benefit from learning how to breathe deeply using their abdomen and diaphragm. People who lead sedentary or stressful lifestyles, are experiencing emotional events, or are wearing tight fitting clothes have also been found to breathe shallowly (Davis et al., 2000) and would

benefit from diaphragmatic breathing. Tight fitting clothes should be exchanged for more comfortable clothing.

Clients who have difficulty taking a deep breath, such as a client with tetraplegia or chronic obstructive pulmonary disease, should not be excluded from this technique. In fact, clients who are using oxygen through a nasal cannula or who do not have adequate upper body control to maintain the erect posture required to take in a full, deep breath can benefit greatly from learning how to breathe deeply. Although clients with chronic obstructive pulmonary disease may not be able to achieve the optimal level of deep breathing, breathing even a bit more deeply can be helpful in relieving some symptoms of thoracic breathing, as well as increasing the client's oxygen saturation level. Clients with complete tetraplegia should be positioned in an upright, seated position (a chest strap may be needed) to help achieve the most effective seated posture to improve breathing.

Clients are taught to breathe from the diaphragm by:

Teaching the difference between thoracic and diaphragmatic breathing: The client is instructed to place one hand centered on his/her chest and the other hand centered on his/her abdomen and to breathe normally. Which hand moves or moves more? If the hand on the chest moves more, then thoracic breathing is evident. If the hand on the abdomen moves more, then diaphragmatic breathing is evident.

Educating clients about the symptoms of thoracic breathing: Thoracic breathing may contribute to the current problems of the clients. For example, when a client with chronic back pain breathes shallowly, muscles do not receive a good amount of oxygen causing them to contract and tighten. Muscles are already tight due to pain. Muscles are now further tightened due to inadequate oxygen supply. When tightened muscles are stretched, pain results. The more pain, the less the client wants to move. The less the client moves, the tighter the muscles become and so the cycle continues affecting the client's ability to perform tasks, lead a quality life, and maintain independence. Deep breathing isn't a quick fix, but it does play a vital role in pain management.

Teaching technique of deep breathing: Lying on his/her back, the client places one hand centered on his/her chest and the other hand centered on his/her abdomen. If lying on the back is not appropriate, another position can be utilized. The client inhales slowly through the nose and pulls the breath down into the abdomen. The hand on the abdomen should rise comfortably. The client exhales slowly through the mouth. The client should make a whooshing sound when exhaling to bring more attention to the breath and free the client from constraining the natural sound of an exhalation. In some situations, however, the sound can be misinterpreted as a sigh of frustration or be inappropriate. The therapist explains this to the client and confirms that a quiet exhale is an appropriate adaptation to the technique for real-world application.

Benefits of diaphragmatic breathing can be experienced immediately. Muscles relax and blood pressure goes down. Learning how to breathe deeply only takes a matter of minutes, Davis et al. (2000) note, however, that "profound effects of the exercise may not be fully appreciated until after months of persistent practice" (p. 22).

Progressive Relaxation

Progressive relaxation reduces pulse rate, blood pressure, perspiration, and respiration rate and is commonly used in the treatment of muscular tension, anxiety, insomnia, depression, fatigue, irritable bowel, muscle spasms, neck and back pain, high blood pressure, mild phobias, and stuttering (Davis et al., 2000).

Clients are taught how to recognize muscle tension by progressively tightening and relaxing specific muscle groups. The client assumes a comfortable position, such as lying on the floor or sitting in a quiet and non-distracting environment. Relaxing music can be used but it is not necessary. The client is instructed to tighten a specific muscle group for about five seconds and then the client shifts focus to relaxation of that same muscle group. The client focuses on the relaxation of the muscle group for 20 to 30 seconds (Davis et al., 2000). Many people do not have an awareness of where they hold muscle tension when stressed, so every muscle group in the body is tightened and relaxed until the client increases his/her awareness of specific muscle groups that hold tension when s/he is under stress. The tightening and relaxing of muscles typically begins at the top or bottom of the body with the top of the body being the most common. Here is a list of muscle groups addressed in progressive relaxation in top to bottom order. A brief description of how to tighten the muscle group is provided for some of the groupings that are less commonly known.

- Forehead (wrinkle forehead)
- Eyes (shut eyes tightly)
- Jaw (clench teeth)
- Neck (pull in chin and squeeze muscles tight)
- Shoulders (shrug and tighten shoulder muscles)
- Arm (upper arm and forearm)
- Hands and wrists (make a fist and curl wrist in)
- Chest
- Upper back
- Stomach
- Lower back
- Buttocks
- Upper legs
- Calves
- Feet (curl toes)

This process usually takes about 20 to 30 minutes to complete and it is recommended that clients do it at least once, if not twice, a day for a period of one to two weeks. Following the two weeks, clients will begin to become aware of where they hold tension in their bodies when under stress and should then be able to relax the area without having to go through the entire progressive relaxation cycle. This is a very discreet relaxation training technique because once the client has a heightened awareness of muscle sensation, s/he can induce a relaxation response without other people noticing the intervention.

Progressive relaxation will not cause harm to a client, however, it is not appropriate to use with clients who have uncontrollable muscle dysfunction, such as tremors or spasms or who have extensive paralysis. If a client has paraplegia or mild to moderate muscle dysfunction, the therapist can adapt progressive relaxation to include only muscle groups that are not affected. It is also not an appropriate intervention for clients who have difficulty following simple directions or attending to a 20-minute task.

Meditation and Mind-Body Techniques

Meditation and other mind-body techniques train the mind to focus and, in a sense, open up the mind at the same time. They are excellent ways to promote relaxation when dealing with stressful situations. See the chapter on Mind-Body Interventions for more detailed information.

Davis et al. (2000) report that "meditation has been used successfully in the treatment and prevention of high blood pressure, heart disease, migraine headaches, and autoimmune diseases such as diabetes and arthritis. It has proved helpful in curtailing obsessive thinking, anxiety, depression, and hostility" (p. 37).

Being able to meditate for an extended period of time can be very difficult to start with. It should not be a stressful task, so the client should meditate only for as long as s/he feels comfortable. With practice, mediation time will increase and feelings of relaxation will deepen. The client may even become able to focus for a few minutes in his/her day-to-day environment to induce feelings of calm.

Meditation is not an appropriate intervention to use with clients who have hallucinations or distorted thought processes or clients who have difficulty attending to a task.

Visualization and Guided Imagery

Imagination is a powerful tool. Emotions are affected by what we imagine and our body is affected by what we feel. If we imagine sad things, feelings of sadness will arise and our body may respond with feelings of fatigue. If we imagine joyful things, our body may respond with more energy and a quickened heart and respiration rate. Emotions are tied to thoughts, thoughts affect our bodily functions, and thoughts are fueled by input whether real or imagined. Therefore it makes sense to harness that power and use it to our advantage to manage emotions and bodily processes and reduce stress.

When feelings and symptoms of stress surface, using imagination to take our thoughts to a happy, peaceful, and comfortable place will change our thought focus, thus affecting the response of our body. Clients are asked to sit in a comfortable position in a quiet and non-distracting environment.

In guided imagery the client is told to close his/her eyes and imagine himself/herself in a positive place or time that holds special meaning to the client. The therapist poses sensory questions to heighten the experience and induce positive feelings of "really being there." For example, what do you see, smell, hear, taste, and feel? Other questions may be more specific to the place chosen by the client and can be useful in one-on-one situations.

Visualization can be used to reduce symptoms of stress, including feelings of anxiety, panic, and depression. Although outcomes are mixed, visualization research has been conducted with clients who have cancer and clients who have chronic pain. In the cancer cases the client may visualize cancer cells as green balls and a "Pac-man" like critter going around the body gobbling up the cancer cells. For chronic pain the client may visualize special body chemicals flowing to pain sites to dissipate knots of pain.

Clients do not need to have an outside source, such as a therapist, to walk them through this process every time. Clients, once educated on how to stimulate their imaginary senses, will be able to apply this intervention independently. However, having another person lead the session may be a preferred method for the client. Guided imagery and visualization tapes and CDs can also be purchased at local music stores, bookstores, and self-help stores. For example, a CD may take the person on a trip through a nature trail by offering enhanced auditory input, such as a bubbling brook, birds, and leaves rustling in the wind. Therapists can even make personalized tapes for the client to meet his/her individual needs.

Visualization and guided imagery are not appropriate for clients experiencing hallucinations, clients who have difficulty attending to a task for a minimum of 20 minutes, clients who are paranoid, clients who have a strong tendency to dissociate from reality, or those who are unable to follow simple directions.

Autogenics

Autogenics is the process of obtaining a relaxed state by imagining the body as being warm and heavy. The client finds a comfortable position in a quiet and non-distracting environment. The source of instruction can be a tape, CD, therapist, or the internal dialogue of the client. The client is instructed to take a few deep breaths and then to imagine specific body areas as being warm and heavy. Only one body area is focused on at a time. Body areas typically include the face, right and left arm and hand, chest, stomach, back, front and back of both right and left legs, and the right and left feet. Visualization is a commonly used method to induce this type of imagination. For example:

"Imagine that you are on a raft in the water. Feel the water rise and fall under the raft. The sun is shining brightly and it is warm. The raft slowly floats to the right and your right arm is now in the sunlight.

Feel the warmth of the sun on your right arm. The arm feels warm. Take a deep breath. With every breath you sink deeper into the raft. You feel heavy. Your right arm feels warm and heavy." This continues with the various body parts entering the sunlight. Continue deep breathing, focusing on becoming heavier, sinking deeper into the raft, and the body becoming warmer in the intensity of the sun for each of the body parts.

Another example is for the client to imagine being on a raft in a pool and dipping his/her hand into the water. Instruct the client to imagine the water as a warm, orange liquid. "Imagine that your fingers are drawing the warm, orange liquid into your body as it gently swirls into each part of your body … up your arms … into your head … down into your chest …, and all the way down your legs until it reaches your toes. Your entire body feels warm and relaxed and heavy. Now imagine the warm, orange water draining out of each part of the body down through the toes and back into the pool. Feel the water rise and fall. With every breath your body sinks deeper into the raft. Your body feels warm and heavy."

Davis et al. (2000) report that autogenics "has been found to be effective in the treatment of muscle tension and various disorders of the respiratory tract (hyperventilation and bronchial asthma), the gastrointestinal tract (constipation, diarrhea, gastritis, ulcers, and spasms), the circulatory system (racing heart, irregular heartbeat, high blood pressure, cold extremities, and headaches), and the endocrine system (thyroid problems). Autogenics is also useful in reducing general anxiety, irritability, and fatigue. It can be employed to modify … reaction to pain, increase … resistance to stress, and reduce or eliminate sleeping disorders" (p. 84).

Autogenics is contraindicated for clients with high or low blood pressure, diabetes, or anyone with low blood sugar because of possible increases or sudden drops in blood pressure from this technique (Davis et al., 2000). It is also not appropriate for clients who experience hallucinations, illusions, or paranoia. As with any relaxation training exercise, if discomfort is experienced, the exercise should be stopped.

Some clients report immediate relief of stress-related symptoms following the first autogenics session and others will require extended practice of one to two times a day over a period of one or two months to experience symptom relief. Eventually, the client will be able to feel warm and heavy upon the initial thought.

Coping Skills Training

Unlike relaxation techniques, which solely focus on relaxing the mind and body, coping skills training focuses on addressing the underlying issues. This includes the use of Problem-Solving Therapy (PST), Cognitive Behavioral Therapy (CBT), Coping Effectiveness Therapy (CET), Mindfulness-Based Stress Reduction (MBSR), and Biofeedback.

Problem-Solving Therapy (PST)

PST is a cognitive-behavioral intervention that seeks to improve a person's problem-orientation to a stressor and develop rational problem-solving skills that eliminate becoming impulsive or avoidant and making the stress worse. This therapy helps the person change his/her attitudes and beliefs that hinder the ability to cope with stressors. It teaches the person how to set realistic goals, identify barriers, find alternative solutions, make effective decisions to maximize outcomes, monitor the outcomes from such decisions, and re-evaluate the situation (Nezu, Nezu, & Xanthopoulos, 2010). In a study of adults newly diagnosed with melanoma, participants received PST in combination with stress management interventions, group support, and psycho-education for six weeks (Fawzy, Fawzy, & Canada, 2001). At the end of six weeks, the group had significantly lower levels of anxiety, depression, and mood disturbance. There was an increase in granular lymphocytes and natural killer cells six months post treatment and longer overall survival at six years compared to the no-treatment control group.

Cognitive Behavioral Therapy (CBT)

CBT reasons that things, in general, do not cause stress. It is the person's perception of the event that causes stress. For example a person who experiences the death of a loved one may be distraught and inconsolable, yet another person who experiences a death of a loved one may view the passing as a beautiful experience that is part of life's journey. One person might lose his job and be enraged at the unjustness, yet another person might view it as an opportunity to explore something new. Consequently, CBT focuses on the connections between emotions, thoughts, and actions. It may be used to change specific cognitions that impact the stress response. CBT protocols look at identifying and expressing emotions appropriately, changing distorted thoughts, and using undistorted thoughts and healthy expression of emotion as bases for action. This has been found to be effective in coping with stress. For example, in women with breast cancer, CBT was found to reduce prevalence of moderate depression and significantly enhance benefit-finding (Antoni et al., 2001); decrease thought intrusion, anxiety, and emotional distress (Antoni et al., 2006); decrease serum cortisol levels (Cruess et al., 2000); and improve immune function (McGregor et al., 2004). Other stress reducing techniques, especially mindfulness strategies, are often used with CBT.

Coping Effectiveness Training (CET)

CET (Chesney et al., 2003) requires individuals to keep a daily dairy to log daily positive events and then share those entries with others in a group format. In the group, participants additionally engage in benefit finding and are encouraged to be humorous and light-hearted as a coping resource. Chesney et al. (2003) utilized this method with HIV-positive men and found decreased levels in perceived stress, burnout, and anxiety, as well as increased positive states of mind, compared to those in control groups.

Mindfulness-Based Stress Reduction (MBSR)

MBSR is rooted in Eastern meditation. It is the process of accepting that negative events and feelings are a natural part of life and are therefore viewed as more of a nuisance that doesn't deserve sustained focus. Instead, individuals are trained to focus on the positive aspects of life and positive emotions experienced during everyday, moment-to-moment activities. This, in turn, increases the experience of positive emotions and subsequent health benefits by providing a stress buffer and undoing effects of negative emotions (Hamilton, Kitzman, & Guyotte, 2006; Kabat-Zinn, 1990; Finan et al., 2010). MBSR has been found to reduce pain, anxiety symptoms, depression symptoms, and psoriasis symptoms, as well as increase positive mood (Finan et al., 2010).

Application of the Leisure and Well-Being Model in recreational therapy practice (Carruthers & Hood, 2007; Hood & Carruthers, 2007) also aligns well with this intervention, as the model focuses on cultivating positive emotions, building resources, and nurturing potential through various mechanisms including leisure experiences that teach and facilitate the ability to savor leisure by focusing attention on the positive aspects of the experience.

Biofeedback

Biofeedback uses a device that provides feedback to a client regarding his/her skin temperature, breathing rate, blood flow, muscle tension, and/or heart rate to help the client better understand how thoughts and emotions impact stress-related bodily responses. The goal is to learn how to control these responses by monitoring the feedback provided by the device. It is most often used in conjunction with relaxation training techniques such as deep breathing, progressive relaxation, guided imagery, positive self-talk, etc., as these mechanisms are used to assist in changing the bodily responses.

The biofeedback device provides the client with concrete feedback regarding the body's response to stress and relaxation, which enables the client to perfect his/her use of stress management interventions, with the ultimate goal of the client being able to successfully and effectively implement the relaxation training techniques without the biofeedback device (Nezu et al., 2010).

Other Interventions

There are a variety of other interventions, outside of formal relaxation training and coping skills training protocols, that can assist in achieving a relaxation response, as well as aid in the coping process.

Positive Emotions through Leisure

Recreational therapists are strongly rooted in utilizing a strengths-based and positive psychology approach in client treatment. Consequently, the cultivation of positive emotions is routinely woven into practice. A comprehensive review of the leisure literature found that positive emotion is an outcome of meaningful experiences and that people search for five overarching meanings in leisure activities: connection/belonging, identity, freedom/autonomy, control/power, and competence/mastery (Porter, 2009; Porter, Iwasaki, & Shank, 2011). It was also found that when people experience personal meaning in leisure activity, they reap the particular outcomes of positive emotions, hope, optimism, strength, creativity, and human growth and development.

Leisure as a context for meaning making has been validated in the literature (Iwasaki, 2008), and outcomes from meaning making through leisure have resulted in health benefits. For example, in a study of 101 adults with mental illness, leisure generated meanings significantly predicted the adjustment to and recovery from mental illness, increased leisure stress-coping and leisure satisfaction, more positive perceptions of active living, and lowered leisure boredom (Iwasaki et al., 2013). In another study of 26 adults with type 2 diabetes, individuals who experienced higher meaning during physical activity engaged in more minutes of physical activity. Regular engagement in physical activity, as shown in other research, is associated with better mental health outcomes (Porter, Shank, & Iwasaki, 2012).

It is also relevant to note that a person's ability to return a healthy psychophysiological state after stress depends on the person's resilience. This reserve capacity of psychophysiological systems to recover from challenging conditions is based on a sense of control, optimism, social support, early life experiences, learning, genetics, sleep, environment, and nutrition (Dhabhar, 2010, p. 57).

Too often, medical communities do not recognize the powerful benefits of positive emotions that arise from the experience of personal meaning in relation to health. However, "a growing body of evidence supports the notion that therapy need not focus principally on the reduction of cognitions and emotional states. Treatments that target the promotion of positive emotional resources are being viewed instead as excellent complementary, if not primary, treatment options. Clinically, the technique for maximizing a patient's general fund of positive emotion and emphasizing its importance as a resilience resource in times of elevated stress may not differ substantially from that employed for the reduction of negative emotion in cognitive therapy" (Finan et al., 2010, p. 216).

Social Relationships

Social relationships are not only a basic human need, but are vitally important in times of stress. Social support has been found to correlate with positive effects on an array of mental and physical health disorders, such as cardiovascular disease, depression, systemic lupus erythematosus, and progression of HIV infection (Taylor & Master, 2010). The quantity and quality of social relationships have also been reliably related to mortality (Taylor & Master, 2010). Social relationships act as a

stress buffer and decrease the negative effects of stress on both mental and physical health, as well as provide social network members with additional resources that can aid in avoidance or reduction of stressful life events (Uchino & Birmingham, 2010). Individuals who lack strong social networks have a higher rate of mortality and morbidity and are at a higher risk for infectious disease, cardiovascular disease and stroke, some forms of cancer, and dementia, as well as the onset and course of chronic illness, including illness adjustment, postsurgical recovery, disability transitions, and survival (Rook, August, & Sorkin, 2010).

While social support helps the individual return to emotional functioning at the pre-stressor baseline, a different kind of relationship called companionship has the potential to offer the individual much more. Receiving social support might cause someone to feel indebted, "less than," guilty, or obligated to help in return. In companionship the individuals are equals and share many other things outside of formal support. They may exchange jokes, engage in recreation and leisure activities together, share memories, and more. Consequently, there is some evidence that companionship may play a stronger role than social support in sustaining self-esteem among people experiencing stressors (Rook et al., 2010).

The experience of shared leisure activities, specifically, leads to the experience of positive affect, which in turn has been found to have health-protective effects associated with lower morbidity, fewer symptoms and less pain associated with health conditions, greater longevity among older adults, greater resilience and optimism, greater psychological resources that help people withstand life stress more effectively, and more ability to transcend current concerns and problems (Rook et al., 2010). On the other hand, "loneliness has been linked to persistently elevated negative emotions, more chronic stress, greater cardiovascular activation, reduced physical activity, and impaired sleep.... [B]oth loneliness and the threat of social exclusion also have been found to impair self-regulation, leading to poor control over emotions and health behaviors. All of these processes increase the risk of disease onset and progression" (Rook et al., 2010, p. 127-128).

Exercise

A review of the literature by Edenfield and Blumenthal (2010) found that engagement in both aerobic and anaerobic exercise reduces psychophysiological responses to stress. It has also been found that regular engagement in aerobic exercise affects brain chemistry, enhances self-esteem and self-confidence, decreases stress, contributes to both physical and mental well-being, and increases motivation and self-discipline (Pandey et al., 2010). Although the duration, frequency, and intensity of exercise required to achieve positive results is unclear, therapists should keep in mind that "in the relatively small number of sedentary samples studied in the exercise literature, mood enhancement seems most likely to have resulted when the prescribed exercise program was of mild-to-moderate intensity and performed on a voluntary basis. Exercise prescribed at a level that is of greater intensity than an individual's habitual exercise level may be less likely to positively impact mood" (Edenfield & Blumenthal, 2010, p. 310).

Additionally, exercises such as yoga have been found to reduce stress, relieve muscular tension and pain, improve oxygen consumption and respiration, decrease sympathetic nervous system activity, stimulate arterial blood flow, and enable individuals to acquire mental discipline and explore their mental potential (Pandey et al., 2010).

Individual Needs

Depending on the stressor and client's skills, knowledge, and resources, other interventions might be helpful in reducing stress and developing coping strategies. These include time management training, resource education and exploration, values clarification, goal setting, nutrition evaluation, assertiveness training, and/or anger management training. Consult the index of this text to learn more about these topics.

Outcomes and Documentation

If a client has been diagnosed with stress management and coping problems, the ICF code d240 Handling Stress and Other Psychological Demands should be part of the diagnosis. It will indicate the level of difficulty the client has with stress management. Other ICF codes in the diagnosis should indicate areas where not being able to handle stress and other psychological demands affects the health of the client. Changes in these codes can be used to demonstrate the efficacy of the treatment provided.

In addition to scoring the ICF codes, therapists should document the stressor, underlying causes of the stressor, coping mechanisms employed, healthiness of the coping mechanisms employed, assistance required to implement specific coping mechanisms, circumstances where the coping mechanisms are employed, effectiveness of coping mechanisms on specific symptoms, specific triggers that bring about a stress response, behavioral and cognitive reactions to stressors, and impact of stress level on particular health concerns.

References

Aldwin, C. M. (2012). *Stress, coping, and development: An integrative perspective* (2nd ed.). New York: Guilford Press.

American Psychiatric Association. (1994). *Diagnostic and statistical manual of mental disorders, IV edition.* Washington, DC: American Psychiatric Association.

Antoni, M. H., Lehman, J. M., Kilbourn, K. M., Boyers, A. E., Culver, J. L., Alferi, S. M., et al. (2001). Cognitive-behavioral stress management intervention decreases prevalence of depression and enhances benefit finding among women under treatment for early-stage breast cancer. *Health Psychology, 20*, 20-32.

Antoni, M. H., Wimberly, S. R., Lechner, S. C., Kazi, A., Sifre, T., Urcuyo, K. R., et al. (2006). Reduction of cancer specific thought intrusions and anxiety symptoms with a stress management intervention among women undergoing treatment for breast cancer. *American Journal of Psychiatry, 163*, 1791-1797.

Bernardi, L., Sleight, P., Bandinelli, G., Cencetti, S., Fattorini, L., Wdowczyc-Szulc, J., et al. (2001). Effect of rosary prayer and yoga mantras on autonomics cardiovascular rhythms: A comparative study. *British Medical Journal, 323*, 1446-1449.

Carruthers, C. & Hood, C. (2007). Building a life of meaning through therapeutic recreation: The Leisure and Well-Being Model, Part I. *Therapeutic Recreation Journal, 41*(4), 276-297.

Carver, C. (2010). Coping. In Contrada, R. & Baum, A. (2010). *The handbook of stress science: Biology, psychology, and health.* New York, NY: Springer Publishing Company.

Chesney, M. A., Chambers, D. B., Taylor, J. M., Johnson, L. S., & Folkman, S. (2003). Coping effectiveness training for men living with HIV: Results from a randomized clinical trial testing a group-based intervention. *Psychosomatic Medicine, 65*, 1038-1046.

Contrada, R. & Baum, A. (2010). *The handbook of stress science: Biology, psychology, and health.* New York, NY: Springer Publishing Company.

Cooper, C. L. (2013). *From stress to wellbeing: Volume 1: The theory and research on occupational stress and wellbeing.* New York, NY: Palgrave Macmillan.

Cousins Center. (2011). Research highlights 2007-2012. Accessed via website www.semel.ucla.edu/cousins/research.

Cruess, D. G., Antoni, M. H., McGregor, B. A., Kilbourn, K. M., Boyers, A., Alferi, S. M., et al. (2000). Cognitive-behavioral stress management reduces serum cortisol by enhancing benefit finding among women being treated for early stage breast cancer. *Psychosomatic Medicine, 62*, 304-308.

Davis, M., Eshelman, E. R., & McKay, M. (2000). *Relaxation & stress reduction workbook* (5th ed.). Oakland, CA: New Harbinger.

Dhabhar, F. S. (2010). Effects of stress on immune function: Implications for immunoprotection and immunopathology. In Contrada, R. & Baum, A. *The handbook of stress science: Biology, psychology, and health.* New York, NY: Springer Publishing Company.

Dhabhar, F. S. & McEwen, B. S. (1997). Acute stress enhances while chronic stress suppresses immune function in vivo: A potential role for leukocyte trafficking. *Brain, Behavior, & Immunity, 11*, 286-306.

Dziegielewski, S. F. (2013). *DMS-IV-TR in action: Includes DSM-5 update chapter*. John Wiley & Sons.

Edenfield, T. M. & Blumenthal, J. A. (2010). Exercise and stress reduction. In Contrada, R. & Baum, A. *The handbook of stress science: Biology, psychology, and health*. New York, NY: Springer Publishing Company.

Eliot, R. (1994). *From stress to strength*. New York, NY: Bantam Books.

Fawzy, F. I., Fawzy, N. W., & Canada, A. L. (2001). Psychoeducational intervention programs for patients with cancer. In A. Baum & B. L. Anderson (Eds.). *Psychosocial interventions for cancer* (pp. 235-267). Washington, DC: American Psychological Association.

Finan, P. H., Zautra, A. J., & Wershba, R. (2010). The dynamics of emotion in adaptation to stress. In Contrada, R. & Baum, A. *The handbook of stress science: Biology, psychology, and health*. New York, NY: Springer Publishing Company.

Fredrickson, B. L., Mancuso, R. A., Branigan, C., & Tugade, M. M. (2000). The undoing effect of positive emotions. *Motivation and Emotion, 24*, 237-258.

Garrido, M. M., Hash-Converse, J. M., Leventhal, H., & Leventhal, E. A. (2010). Stress and chronic disease management. In Contrada, R. & Baum, A. *The handbook of stress science: Biology, psychology, and health*. New York, NY: Springer Publishing Company.

Glanz, K., Rimer, B., & Lewis, F. (2002). *Health behavior and health education: Theory, research, and practice*. Indianapolis, IN: Jossey-Bass.

Gruenewald, T. L., Kemeny, M. E., Aziz, N., & Fahey, J. L. (2004). Acute threat to the social self: Shame, social self-esteem, and cortisol activity. *Psychosomatic Medicine, 66*, 915-924.

Grunberg, N. E., Berger, S. S., & Hamilton, K. R. (2010). Stress and drug use. In Contrada, R. & Baum, A. *The handbook of stress science: Biology, psychology, and health*. New York, NY: Springer Publishing Company.

Hamilton, N. A., Kitzman, H., & Guyotte, S. (2006). Enhancing health and emotion: Mindfulness as a missing link between cognitive therapy and positive psychology. *Journal of Cognitive Psychotherapy: An Internationally Quarterly, 20*, 123-134.

Hood, C. & Carruthers, C. (2007). Enhancing leisure experience and developing resources: The Leisure and Well-Being Model, Part II. *Therapeutic Recreation Journal, 41*(4), 298-325.

Iwasaki, Y. (2008). Pathways to meaning-making through leisure-like pursuits in global contexts. *Journal of Leisure Research, 40*(2), 231-249.

Iwasaki, Y., Coyle, C., Shank, J., Messina, E., & Porter, H. (2013). Leisure-generated meanings and active living for persons with mental illness. *Rehabilitation Counseling Bulletin, 57*, 46-56.

Julien, R. (2004). *A Primer of Drug Action, 10th edition*. New York: Worth Publishers.

Kabat-Zinn, J. (1990). *Full catastrophe living: Using the wisdom of your body and mind to face stress, pain, and illness*. New York: Delacorte.

Lazarus, R. S., Cohen, J. B., Folkman, S., Kanner, A., & Schaefer, C. (1980). Psychological stress and adaptation: Some

unresolved issues. In H. Seyle (Ed.). *Seyle's Guide to Stress Research*, pp 90-217. Academic Press: New York, NY

Mayo Clinic Staff. (2013). Chronic stress puts your health at risk. Accessed via website www.mayoclinic.org/healthy-living/stress-management/in-depth/stress/art-20046037.

McGregor, B. A., Antoni, M. H., Boyers, A., Alferi, S. M., Blomberg, B. B., & Carver, C. S. (2004). Cognitive-behavioral stress management increases benefit finding and immune functioning among women with early stage breast cancer. *Journal of Psychosomatic Research, 56*, 1-8.

Nezu, A. M., Nezu, C. M., & Xanthopoulos, M. S. (2010). Stress reduction in chronically ill patients. In Contrada, R. & Baum, A. *The handbook of stress science: Biology, psychology, and health*. New York, NY: Springer Publishing Company.

Pandey, A., Quick, J. C., Rossi, A. M., Nelson, D. L., & Martin, W. (2010). Stress and the workplace: 10 years of science, 1997-2007. In Contrada, R. & Baum, A. *The handbook of stress science: Biology, psychology, and health*. New York, NY: Springer Publishing Company.

Peters, M. L., Godaert, G. L. R., Baleiux. R. E., Brosschot, J. F., Sweep, F. C., & Swinkels, L. M. (1999). Immune responses to experimental stress: Effects of mental effort and uncontrollability. *Psychosomatic Medicine, 61*, 513-524.

Porter, H. (2009). Developing a Leisure Meanings Gained and Outcomes Scale (LMGOS) and exploring associations of leisure meanings to leisure time physical activity adherence among adults with type 2 diabetes. ProQuest #3359696.

Porter, H. & burlingame, j. (2006). Recreational therapy handbook of practice: ICF-based diagnoses and treatment. Enumclaw, WA: Idyll Arbor, Inc.

Porter, H., Iwasaki, Y., & Shank, J. (2011). Conceptualizing meaning-making through leisure experiences. *Society & Leisure, 33*(2), 167-194.

Porter, H., Shank, J., & Iwasaki, Y. (2012). Promoting a collaborative approach with recreational therapy to improve physical activity engagement in type 2 diabetes. *Therapeutic Recreation Journal, Special Issue Part I: Collaborative Practices and Physical Activity, XLVI*(3), 202-217.

Rook, K. S., August, K. J., & Sorkin, D. H. (2010). Social network functions and health. In Contrada, R. & Baum, A. *The handbook of stress science: Biology, psychology, and health*. New York, NY: Springer Publishing Company.

Sadock, J. & Sadock, V. (2003). *Kaplan & Sadock's synopsis of psychiatry* (9th ed.). Philadelphia, PA: Lippincott Williams & Wilkins.

Sadock, J. & Sadock, V. (2008). *Kaplan & Sadock's concise textbook of clinical psychiatry* (3rd ed.). Lippincott Williams & Wilkins.

Slavich, G. M., O'Donovan, A., Epel, E. S., & Kemeny, M. E. (2010). Black sheet gets the blues: A psychobiological model of social rejection and depression. *Neuroscience and Biobehavioral Reviews, 35*(1) 39-45.

Taylor, S. E. & Master, S. L. (2010). Social responses to stress: The tend-and-befriend model. In Contrada, R. & Baum, A. *The handbook of stress science: Biology, psychology, and health*. New York, NY: Springer Publishing Company.

Uchino, B. N. & Birmingham, W. (2010). Stress and support processes. In Contrada, R. & Baum, A. *The handbook of stress science: Biology, psychology, and health*. New York, NY: Springer Publishing Company.

World Health Organization. (1998). *Coping mechanisms*. Geneva, Switzerland: WHO.

46. Therapeutic Relationships

J. Randal Wyble

The nature of the relationship between the helper and client has long been identified as an important component in helping relationships. The term therapeutic relationship underlies the recognition that this relationship can have a positive impact on client outcomes, which are the focus of this relationship. Historically, this recognition first appeared in the field of psychotherapy with the focus on the impact of the therapeutic relationship that exists between therapist and client. In 1936, Rosenzweig (as cited in Weinberger, 2002) predicted that the various psychotherapeutic approaches that were being used at the time, despite varying in the techniques that they used, would produce similar outcomes. He predicted that the similarity in outcomes could be attributed in large part to common factors that existed across the various approaches. This would indicate that these common factors, separate from any specific techniques that were being used, had a significant impact on the outcomes associated with psychotherapy. This has since become known as the common factors approach.

Lambert (2005) defines common factors as "those dimensions of the treatment setting that are not specific to any particular technique" (p. 856). Highlighted among the common factors identified by Rosenzweig (as cited in Weinberger, 2002, p. 68) was the development of a therapeutic relationship. Since that time, research has supported many of the predications that Rosenzweig made, including the important contribution that therapeutic relationships have in outcomes resulting from psychotherapy. Fifty-four years after Rosenzweig's predication, in a review of related literature, Grencavage and Norcross (1990) found that the therapeutic relationship was the most frequently identified common factor and that clinicians and researchers were in agreement that it was an important factor that influenced outcomes in

psychotherapy. Additionally, research has repeatedly identified the presence of a therapeutic relationship as a predictor of positive outcomes in therapy (Kopta et al., 1999).

This idea, that the development of a therapeutic relationship between the therapist and a client can have a significant impact on outcomes, has expanded beyond the field of psychotherapy. It is now an integrated aspect of a variety of health fields, especially those that have a strong focus on the relationship between helper and client, as is the case in recreational therapy. An example of the strength of this integration in the field of recreational therapy is provided by Austin (2011) who states that "the therapeutic relationship is at the heart of recreational therapy" (p. 24), and furthermore, that such relationships provide the foundation by which people obtain therapeutic benefits.

Before continuing, it should be noted that, while the development of a therapeutic relationship is being discussed here as a recreational therapy technique, it is different in nature from many of the other techniques. Anger management and assertiveness training are examples of specific techniques that are typically used as recreational therapy interventions. The development of a therapeutic relationship, however, might best be described in terms of a contextual model or approach. In describing a contextual model, Wampold (2001) proposed that common factors in general, and specifically the development of a therapeutic relationship, play a crucial role in establishing a context in which positive change can occur. In other words, the presence of a therapeutic relationship provides a context which supports positive change and/or enhances the impact of other, more specific interventions. The following diagram (see Figure 2) was designed to provide a visual representation of the APIE (assessment, planning, implementation, evaluation) process in action. It illustrates the development of a therapeutic relationship during the assessment and planning portions of the process that then continues through the implementation and evaluation portions of the process as well. Additionally, this diagram captures the way a therapeutic relationship provides a context in which the intervention occurs. It should also be clear that the use of specific techniques and the presence of a therapeutic relationship do not occur independently of one another. Rather they are interwoven in that the use of specific techniques is often impacted by the presence of a therapeutic relationship and vice versa.

Indications

Developing a relationship with a client that is therapeutic is indicated at any time that it is felt that the relationship could impact the client outcomes. Indications of a need for a change in the therapeutic relationship may be indicated by deficits in ICF codes d5702 Maintaining One's Health, d740 Formal Relationships, or e340 Personal Care Providers and Personal Assistants. As discussed further in the next section, this does not indicate that the therapeutic relationship developed with Client A will have the same features as the therapeutic relationship developed with Client B. Granted, they will share general features but the extent and nature of these features will, at times, be different, as they need to be to make the relationship a therapeutic one.

Contraindications

While the idea of developing a therapeutic relationship is never contraindicated (in contrast to having a relationship that is not therapeutic), the nature of the relationship, especially as related to boundaries and self-disclosure, varies from client to client depending on client characteristics and issues of transference-countertransference. These concepts will be addressed further but, to clarify, the nature of the therapeutic relationship will, and should be, different based on the client. Additionally, in general there must be an awareness of boundaries that exist in therapeutic relationships that do not exist in other types of relationships. Maintenance of these boundaries is an essential aspect of developing and maintaining a therapeutic relationship. The development of other types of relationships, such as a friendship, in addition to a therapeutic relationship, is contraindicated for the period of time that the client is involved in active treatment.

Protocols

As stated earlier, the development of a therapeutic relationship differs in nature from typical

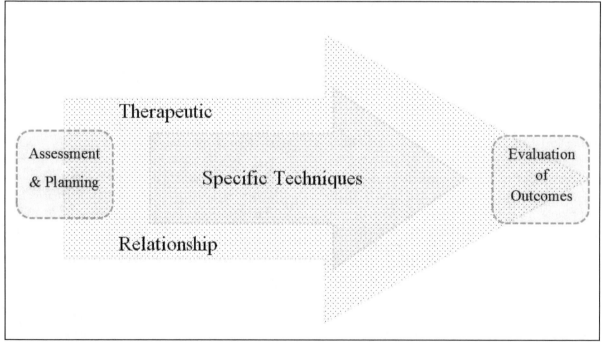

Figure 2: The Therapeutic Relationship

recreational therapy techniques and interventions. This protocol for its use is presented but it is critical to remember that it is an ongoing process that encompasses all interactions between a recreational therapist and a client and is not readily defined in terms of frequency or length of sessions.

Processes

While some variation exists as to the characteristics that are thought to make up a therapeutic relationship, there has recently been a great deal of focus on analyzing research in order to identify features that have been clearly linked to successful outcomes. This systematic review of research was conducted by the Task Force on Evidence-Based Therapy Relationships (Norcross & Wampold, 2011). This task force, commissioned by the American Psychological Association's Division of Psychotherapy and Division of Clinical Psychology, was created with the intended purpose of updating the research base associated with therapeutic relationships (Norcross, 2011). Due to the limited research on therapeutic relationships in the field of recreational ther-

apy, the information contained in this section reflects the information put forth by that task force. The information can be found in its entirety as a series of articles in a special issue of *Psychotherapy* (2011) and as part of the second edition of the book *Psychotherapy Relationships That Work* (Norcross, 2011). In addition, a summary of these findings has been published on a website sponsored by the Substance Abuse and Mental Health Services Administration which is listed in the resources section of this chapter. While this research comes from the field of psychotherapy, the focus of this chapter is on those specific features of relationships that have been generalized to related fields in which the helper-client relationship is identified as an essential component, as is the case with recreational therapy. Before looking at specific features that are supported by the literature, several general conclusions of the task force will be discussed.

As was expected, based on previous literature reviews, the task force concluded that therapeutic relationships contribute to outcomes independent of other, more specific types of interventions that are

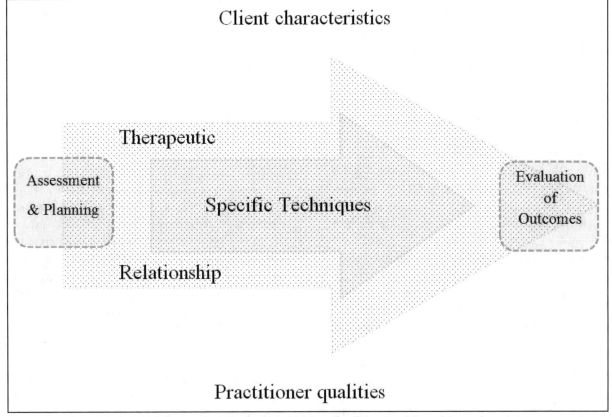

Figure 3: The Therapeutic Relationship Taking the Client and Practitioner into Account

being utilized (Norcross & Wampold, 2011). This means that at least a portion of the outcome can be attributed to the presence (or absence, in the case of negative outcomes) of a therapeutic relationship. Because of this, it was suggested that practice guidelines should focus on the features that make a relationship therapeutic. Additionally, it was concluded that, while the relationship contributes independently of more specific techniques, it also "acts in concert with treatment methods, patient characteristics, and practitioner qualities in determining effectiveness" (Norcross & Wampold, p. 98). To illustrate this, the diagram presented earlier, which presented the therapeutic relationship and specific recreational therapy techniques as separate yet interconnected entities, has been updated (see Figure 3). The factors of client characteristics and practitioner qualities have been added to the context in which the techniques (and in reality, all interactions with the client) takes place.

While acknowledging the impact of client characteristics and practitioner qualities, the focus will be now will be placed on the features of the relationship that have been supported by research as having a positive impact on treatment outcomes. Following that, there will be a presentation of specific techniques that can be used to promote these features.

The first features to be discussed are those that were first identified by Rogers (1957) in describing what he believed to be essential components of the therapeutic relationship in a client-centered therapy approach. These features have been identified with high frequency as necessary components for the development of therapeutic relationships since that time. He identified three features consisting of warmth, genuineness, and empathy. Of these three, as with the other components that will be discussed, the task force found evidence providing varying levels of support as to their effectiveness and designated them as having a large effect, medium effect, or small effect.

Warmth, also referred to as positive regard, was designated as having a medium effect on the basis of the meta-analysis of relevant research (Faber & Doolin, 2011). Warmth in a therapeutic relationship has been described in a variety of ways but generally implies that the therapist respects, accepts, and affirms the client. Rogers (1951), in a discussion on the concept of warmth and positive regard, indicated

that these are present when, through our attitudes and behavior, it is clear that we value, respect, and accept the client as a person. In their conclusions, Faber and Doolin (2011) suggested that when working with clients, it is the therapist's responsibility not only to generate feelings of warmth and positive regard towards the client, but also to clearly communicate these to the client.

Empathy, on the basis of the task force's meta-analysis, was designated as having a medium effect in contributing to positive outcomes as part of a therapeutic relationship (Elliott et al., 2011). Empathy is often described in layman's terms as putting yourself in another person's shoes. Rogers (1980) provides an expanded definition in defining empathy as the "sensitive ability and willingness to understand the client's thoughts, feelings and struggles from the client's point of view" (p. 85) and "It means entering the private perceptual world of the other" (p. 142). These definitions of empathy point out that there is both cognitive perception that is focused on the client's thoughts and perceptions and an emotional perception that is focused on the client's feelings. Conclusions drawn by Elliot et al. (2011) in their meta-analysis on research related to empathy include the need for therapists to understand what the person is discussing, in terms of thoughts and feelings, instead of focusing on what they are saying. Additionally, while accurate understanding may serve as a foundation for more open communication, so might inaccurate, yet well intentioned, attempts at understanding. In other words, a client may value the effort the therapist puts forth to be empathetic separate from the empathy itself, if the effort is felt to be genuine.

Genuineness, or congruence as it is sometimes referred to, is the last of the components originally identified and described by Rogers (1957). Based on the meta-analysis of research by the task force, this component was categorized as having a small effect on outcomes (Kolden et al., 2011). However, in the overall discussion of these components by members of the task force, as well as historically by Rogers (as cited by Kolden et al., 2011, p. 66), it is thought that genuineness may serve to enhance the overall impact by providing the foundation for the communication of warmth and empathy. Without a sense that the therapist is genuine, it is unlikely that the therapist's attempts to convey warmth/positive regard and/or empathy will elicit a favorable response from the client. Genuineness, as a component of a therapeutic relationship, implies a sense of being authentic, open, and honest in a relationship (Gelso & Hayes, 1998). However, it is recognized that communication of this, the therapist's experience in relation to the client, requires "careful reflection and considered judgment on the part of the therapist" (Kolden et al., 2011, p. 65). This last statement truly shows the interconnectedness of these three components in that genuineness is best conveyed through a warm, empathetic approach while at the same time, warmth and empathy are difficult to establish in a relationship without a sense of genuineness. Kolden et al. (2011) concluded that the therapist needs to take a mindful approach to genuineness with recognition of the complexity of conveying genuineness. Additionally, by being genuine in the relationship, the therapist could enhance the client's ability to reciprocate in a genuine way.

The next two features to be discussed, while not part of Roger's (1957) original focus, have been frequently identified as being components that contribute to the therapeutic nature of relationship. Additionally, the task force found support for both of these features during their meta-analysis of research. They are the features of goal consensus/collaboration and the management of countertransference.

Goal consensus and *collaboration* were found, when combined, to have a medium to large effect on outcomes when present in a helping relationship (Tyron & Winograd, 2011). Goal consensus involves the helper and client sharing a view of the goals of treatment and the processes that will be used to achieve these goals (Tyron & Winograd, 2011). The process of goal consensus rests, as do the other features discussed to this point, heavily on open and honest communication between the helper and the client. From goal consensus follows collaboration. Collaboration indicates active involvement by both the helper and the client to work together in the agreed upon manner to reach the treatment goals. Collaboration also indicates a willingness to revisit and revise agreed upon goals and processes as needed. However, collaboration, in and of itself, does not indicate the level of involvement on the part of the client. It only indicates that the client will take as active of a role as was agreed upon in the first place. For instance, if while reaching goal consensus it was

agreed upon by both the client and the recreational therapist that the recreational therapist make a majority of decisions in the initial phase of treatment, then successful collaboration would reflect that decision.

Countertransference in relationships between helpers and clients was first identified by Freud (Hayes, Gelso, & Hummel, 2011). At that time it was rather narrowly defined in terms specific to the process of psychoanalysis. Since that time it has evolved and has been defined in a variety of ways. The key element is that it causes a reaction on the part of the helper that results from the helper's unresolved conflicts when exposed to specific client characteristics (Gelso & Hayes, 2007). Such a reaction could be covert, such as the helper finding himself/herself bored listening to the client or feeling irritated by the client. Such covert or internal reactions often are manifested in overt ways such as the helper becoming distracted or cutting off the client abruptly. Another aspect of countertransference that is generally agreed upon at this time is that it is an expected part of the relationship and can provide information that will aid in development of a therapeutic relationship if managed properly. Through their meta-analysis of relevant research, Hayes, Gelso, and Hummel (2011) concluded that this proper management of countertransference had a variable impact on outcomes ranging from low to medium in magnitude. Proper management of countertransference means that the reaction is recognized and processed prior to it becoming expressed in the helper's behavior. For example, a recreational therapist who finds s/he is having a negative emotional reaction to a particular client recognizes this at the onset prior to having it impact interactions with the client. Baehr (as cited in Hayes, Gelso & Hummel, 2011, p. 93) found that therapists' level of empathy and engagement in self-care (resting, exercising, etc.) were positively related to lower levels of overt countertransference behaviors directed at clients.

Specific Techniques

Recommendations are provided on how to promote the features of therapeutic relationships that improve the impact the relationship can have on client outcomes. When considering these recommendations, remember that the development of therapeutic relationships is often seen as a mixture of art and science. While there are well defined, tangible steps that can be taken to develop the relationship, there are equally as many less defined, intangible factors at play that vary according with the situation and what the helper and the client, in terms of experiences and personal characteristics, bring to the relationship. The suggestions provided here are common techniques that can be found as part of various resources listed at the end of this chapter.

Warmth/Positive Regard

Develop attitudes of caring, support, and respect. One key step in this direction is being able to suspend value judgments. Value judgments occur when the recreational therapist judges the clients thoughts, feelings, and actions based on the recreational therapists own values or perspective.

Engage in active listening. Active listening involves the intentional use of verbal and non-verbal cues that communicate a purposeful intent to listen to what is being communicated. Active listening serves two purposes. First, it sends a message to the client that what they are communicating is valued. Second, it reinforces the client's continued communicating.

Convey the attitudes of caring, support and respect through words and actions.

Empathy

Employ the communication techniques of clarification. Clarification is an active listening technique that is used by the listener to check if s/he accurately understands the content of the communication. For instance, clarification often involves the recreational therapist stating back to the client what s/he believes the client is trying to communicate such as "and when you were at the mall you ran into people that hadn't seen you since the accident...that's what happened..."

In conjunction with clarification, use reflection. While clarification helps the recreational therapist gain an understanding of the content being communicated, reflection helps to provide an understanding of the experience focused on the emotions elicited by the content. For instance, a recreational therapist stating "and that made you feel so embarrassed" is an example of trying to understand the overall experience rather than just the content of what happened.

Genuineness

Use self-disclosure in a purposeful and planned manner. As recreational therapists, when considering any type of self-disclosure, two questions must be satisfactorily answered before self-disclosing. First, what is the purpose of my self-disclosure? When answering this, it is important to keep in mind that in a therapeutic relationship our focus is on the needs and goals of the client and so the answer should indicate that focus. Second, is what I am disclosing crossing the boundaries that separate professional from personal relationships? This question is sometimes difficult to answer and requires knowledge combined with experience. For this reason, new recreational therapists are often advised to err on the side of too little self-disclosure versus too much self-disclosure.

Keep your eyes on the prize. This refers back to the need of the recreational therapist to keep the purpose of the relationship first and foremost in his/her mind at all times. Consistently acting on behalf of the client reinforces the genuineness of the relationship.

Goal Consensus and Collaboration

Share relevant information with the client. This ensures the client feels that s/he is an active partner in the process of reaching a consensus. A key to this is to ensure that all of the relevant information is presented to the client. This might not be the same information that is relevant to the recreational therapist. In concert with this is the idea of providing opportunities for choice whenever available. Again, this reinforces the idea that the client is an active partner in the process of reaching a consensus.

Reinforce collaborative efforts. Once a plan has been made, reinforce the client in being collaborative. This often comes about naturally when progress is being made. However, in the face of disappointing results, it is essential for the recreational therapist to acknowledge and support the ongoing collaboration instead of abandoning the plan and falling into the "righting reflex" — a term used to indicate a helping professional's desire to take over and fix things.

Management of Countertransference

Develop and maintain self-awareness. This self-awareness indicates a monitoring of one's thoughts, attitudes and actions and the factors that are influencing those areas. Self-awareness provides the ability to pause and reflect when countertransference is first recognized. This action itself may serve to manage the countertransference before it causes any disruption in the relationship.

Take care of yourself. This is an outward expression of self-awareness in that engaging in self-care activities indicates recognition of the need to engage in self-care activities.

Outcomes and Documentation

Answering the question, what are the outcomes of a therapeutic relationship, is difficult because, as alluded to earlier, it is a general rather than specific approach. Additionally, therapeutic relationships are seen as providing a context in which positive change can occur and in which other, more specific techniques are employed. Due to this, outcomes are not specifically tied to the use of therapeutic relationships. Rather, outcomes are documented related to the specific techniques that are employed within the context of the therapeutic relationship. Three specific ICF codes that should be considered are d5702 Maintaining One's Health, d740 Formal Relationships, and e340 Personal Care Providers and Personal Assistants.

Resources

Evidence-Based Therapy Relationships

www.nrepp.samhsa.gov/Norcross.aspx

This site, published by the Substance Abuse and Mental Health Services Administration, summarizes the information that provided the foundation for a series of articles in a special issue of *Psychotherapy* (2011) and also appeared in the second edition of the book *Psychotherapy Relationships That Work* (Norcross, 2011).

Therapeutic Communication in Psychiatric Nursing

http://nursingplanet.com/pn/therapeutic_communication.html

This website provides an overview of specific therapeutic communication techniques. While written from a nursing perspective, the same techniques can be applied across disciplines to all professions that recognize the helper-client relationship as a potential change agent.

The Interview Phase

burlingame and Tostenrude (2010) provide a detailed description of many common techniques which can be utilized to enhance the helper-client relationship. Their discussion, as it relates to the assessment process, is on pages 96-99 of *Assessment Tools for Recreational Therapy and Related Fields*.

References

Austin, D. R. (2011). *Lessons learned: An open letter to recreational therapy students and practitioners.* Urbana, IL: Sagamore Publishing.

burlingame, j. & Tostenrude, D. (2010). The assessment process. In j. burlingame & T. Blaschko (Eds.), *Assessment tools for recreational therapy and related fields* (pp. 89-109). Enumclaw, WA: Idyll Arbor.

Elliott, R., Bohart, A. C., Watson, J. C., & Greenberg, L. S. (2011). Empathy. *Psychotherapy, 48*(1), 43-49.

Faber, B. A. & Doolin, E. M. (2011). Positive regard. *Psychotherapy, 48*(1), 58-64.

Gelso, C. J. & Hayes, J. A. (1998). *The psychotherapy relationship: Theory, research, and practice.* New York: Wiley.

Gels, C. J. & Hayes, J. A. (2007). *Countertransference and the inner world of the psychotherapist: Perils and possibilities.* Mahwah, NJ: Erlbaum.

Grencavage, L. M. & Norcross, J. C. (1990). Where are the commonalities among the therapeutic common factors? *Professional Psychology: Research and Practice, 21*(5), 372-378.

Hayes, J. A., Gelso, C. J., & Hummel, A. M. (2011). Managing countertransference. *Psychotherapy, 48*(1), 88-97.

Kolden, G. C., Klein, M. H., Wang, C., & Austin, S. B. (2011). Congruence/genuineness. *Psychotherapy, 48*(1), 65-71.

Kopta, S. M., Saunders, S. M., Lueger, R. L., & Howard, K. I. (1999). Individual psychotherapy outcome and process research: Challenges leading to greater turmoil or a positive transition? *Annual Review of Psychology, 50*, 441-469.

Lambert, M. J. (2005). Early response in psychotherapy: Further evidence for the importance of common factors rather than "placebo effects." *Journal of Clinical Psychology, 61*, 855-869.

Norcross, J. C. (2011). *Psychotherapy relationships that work: Evidence-Based Responsiveness* (2nd ed.). New York: Oxford University Press.

Norcross, J. C. & Wampold, B. E. (2011). Evidence-based therapy relationships: Research conclusions and clinical practices. *Psychotherapy, 48*(1), 98-102.

Rogers, C. R. (1951). *Client-centered therapy.* Boston: Houghton Mifflin.

Rogers, C. R. (1957). The necessary and sufficient conditions of therapeutic personality change. *Journal of Consulting Psychology, 21*, 95-103.

Rogers, C. R. (1980). *A way of being.* Boston: Houghton Mifflin.

Tyron, G. S. & Winograd, G. (2011). Goal consensus and collaboration. *Psychotherapy, 48*(1), 50-57.

Wampold, B. E. (2001). *The great psychotherapy debate: Models, methods, and findings.* Mahwah, NJ: Erlbaum.

Weinberger, J. (2002). Short paper, large impact: Rosenzweig's influence on the common factors movement. *Journal of Psychotherapy Integration, 12*(1), 67-76.

47. Therapeutic Thematic Arts Programming (TTAP Method®)

Linda Levine-Madori

The prevalence of mild cognitive impairment (MCI) in the general population is reported to be as high as 25% for adults 65 years of age and older, and the progression from MCI to Alzheimer's disease (AD) is reported to be approximately 12-14% per year (Reisberg et al., 1988; Yu et al., 2009). In a national review of all research on AD conducted over the past decade through the National Institute on Aging's (NIA) (2005) Progress Report on Alzheimer's Disease, multimodal interventions (defined as experiences stimulating all regions of the brain in the areas of affect, behavior, sensation, imagery, and interpersonal and intrapersonal relationships) were proven to be the most successful in early stages and moderate stages of AD for decreasing deficits in speech, language recall, and short-term memory. Such interventions provide a wide variety of stimuli, positively affecting and increasing neuronal activity responses and plasticity of the cells deep within the brain.

One such multimodal intervention is the Therapeutic Thematic Arts Programming Method (TTAP Method) (Levine-Madori, 2007, 2009, 2012). TTAP Method is a multimodal, structured, art/recreation psychotherapeutic approach that uses a nine-step process with common recreational therapy modalities. The method acts as a catalyst for enhancing social interactions and cognitive stimulation of the participants. (See Table 23.)

Table 23: The TTAP Method Nine-Steps

Step 1: Individual thought to group ideas
Stimulation: linguistic
Brain region: Broca's area

Step 2: Group ideas to music/guided imagery
Stimulation: musical/visual

Brain region: visual/auditory cortex

Step 3: Music/guided imagery to 2D image
Stimulation: visual
Brain region: temporal lobe

Step 4: Image into 3D image/sculpture
Stimulation: spatial
Brain region: parietal/occipital lobe

Step 5: Sculpture into movement
Stimulation: kinesthetic
Brain region: motor cortex

Step 6: Movement into words/poetry/stories
Stimulation: linguistic
Brain region: frontal lobe

Step 7: Words into food for thought
Stimulation: spatial
Brain region: sensory cortex

Step 8: Food for thought into photography
Stimulation: intrapersonal
Brain region: reticular formation

Step 9: Photography into themed event
Stimulation: interpersonal
Brain region: Broca/Wernicke's area

Multiple regions of the brain are stimulated at any given time through multimodal interventions. However, the brain region listed is the focus of the corresponding step (Madori, 2007).

The method was developed out of neuroscience research, which demonstrates that personally meaningful life experiences and activities that challenge the mind result in continued positive changes in the human brain (Cappeliez, O'Rourke, & Chaudhury, 2005). Activities that combine reminiscing and sharing of life stories are most meaningful and have been proven to provide therapeutic stimulation to all areas of the brain, thus directly affecting the neuroplasticity of the brain, specifically the hippocampus region (Buckwalter, Burgener, & Buettner, 2009; Alzheimer's Association, 2006). Blooms' Taxonomy of Learning is also incorporated into the TTAP Method approach in that each of the nine steps is designed to stimulate the visual, musical, linguistic, interpersonal, intrapersonal, kinesthetic, and spatial learner to reach participants with different learning styles. Enhancing social interaction by stimulating all types of learners ensures a higher likelihood of full participation from each participant in the group and has a protective effect on the hippocampus. Additionally, research suggests that higher levels of social interaction possibly decrease the likelihood that individuals with AD will decline in language abilities and short-term memory (Snowdon, 2001; Alders & Levine-Madori, 2010).

Each of the steps in the nine-step process utilizes creative therapeutic activities including self-expression; music with guided meditation; drawing and painting (2D images); sculpture (3D images); movement; words, poetry, and stories; food for thought; photography; and themed events. Other activities can be utilized or some activities deleted depending on the needs of the individual or group. The activities maximize interaction among participants, stimulate all aspects of brain functioning, address social and emotional needs, and integrate opportunities for life review (Levine-Madori, 2007, 2009, 2012). Through the use of themes within the steps the individual and the group are able to share themselves and learn through others, which provides dynamic person-centered approaches. Themes can include environmental themes, such as weather, holidays, and vacations or personal themes, such as family, love, friendships, and relationships. Sharing rich and intimate stories about their life, allows individuals to bond deeply with each other on cognitive, social, emotional, physical, and spiritual levels. The TTAP Method also works to enable a "flow" effect, a term coined by psychologist Mihály Csíkszentmihályi (1990) to describe a state of complete immersion in an activity.

The TTAP Method identifies specific regions of the brain stimulated during an expressive arts recreational therapy activity and identifies which learning processes are being employed during each activity. The replicable identification of learning processes

and brain functions provides a structured approach to research in recreational therapy and the arts. It also offers many benefits to the therapist including: (1) the ability to assess, plan, implement, develop, and evaluate programming to meet the individual's needs at that moment, (2) a systematic structure that decreases anxiety and burnout on the part of the therapist, and (3) better documentation of intervention because it is based on a known protocol.

Previous research on brain plasticity, neural regeneration, and the phenomena of cognitive reserve demonstrates that positive changes in neural activity can be activated by visual, auditory, and sensory stimulation (Rentz, 2002). During the TTAP Method program, participants are provided with visual, auditory, and sensory stimulation as well as stimulation to three distinct brain systems: the affective system, the strategic system, and the recognition system. Brain research indicates that the brain can change in mass and density through increased stimulation in these three areas, even in the last stages of life.

Since 2000, when Harvard University developed the use of CAT and PET scans, scientists have studied how the living brain is activated and responsive when engaged in meaningful and emotional interactions (Stern, 2003). Research from the National Institute on Health (National Institute on Aging, 2005) found that different regions of the brain are activated during activity, which increases the effects of neuroplasticity, thus correlating the use of the creative arts to "brain exercise, brain habilitation, and brain rehabilitation" that aren't being stimulated throughout the individual's daily activities. The TTAP Method systematically identifies the specific areas of the brain that are being utilized when involved in creative arts activities. The structured approach found in the TTAP Method activity assessments and protocols captures how recreational therapy and the creative arts can be utilized to enhance brain functioning. It documents brain rehabilitation, thus providing a measure of efficacy in art and recreational therapy research. Additionally, the person-centered approach in the TTAP Method has been found to increase socialization as participants naturally and effectively use long-term memory to share and reminisce during therapeutic activity. The TTAP Method makes every activity a past, present, and future opportunity for the residents.

Transcending Dementia: A New Psychology of Art, Brain, and Cognition (Levine-Madori, 2012) gives an in-depth analysis of how the TTAP Method is successfully utilized with all three stages (mild, moderate, and advanced) of AD and is recognized as a Best Practice Approach through the Office on Aging and the New York State Therapeutic Recreation Association.

The integration of various artistic activities elicits an integration of higher cortical thinking such as planning, attentiveness, problem solving, and emotional investment, in both the topic of discussion and in goal accomplishment. This promotes faster cognitive and emotional processing and facilitates learning and memory (Burgener, Gilbert, & Mathy, 2007). Guided imagery, synchronized with music, allows the individual to access positive long-term memory (Levine-Madori, 2007). Guided imagery has also been shown to significantly decrease cortisol levels, thereby enhancing mood and subsequent cognitive performance, even for those with moderate AD in skilled nursing facilities (Levine-Madori, 2009).

In the area of recreational therapy and social research on activities and their effect on aging individuals, specifically those diagnosed with AD, findings have increasingly shown that activities and social involvement play a significant role in cognition, socialization, and overall well-being, and have been proven to have an impact on longevity (Buettner, 2006; Buettner & Fitzsimmons, 2009). This is specifically cited in a study of Cohen-Mansfield (1994). The researcher surveyed 369,000 clients across five countries and found that activity involvement is highest among individuals with adequate cognition. Similarly, many studies focused on those diagnosed with AD have concluded that social engagement and social support is currently the only proven intervention that is sustained through time and goes beyond any current pharmaceutical intervention (Khachaturian et al., 2008).

Research on recreational therapy for residents diagnosed with severe AD has also supported the importance of activities on behavior (Cohen-Mansfield, 1992; Buettner, 1999, 2006; Buettner & Ferrario, 1998). Findings included reduced levels of agitation, increased social interactions, a marked decrease in overall neediness, and a strong correlation between increased activity participation and higher levels of cognitive functioning. The studies also found that the daily lives of residents could be positively affected through increasing the length of time spent in recreational therapy programming.

Thus, we now recognize that those who have no social stimulation have a more rapid decline into the disease (Buettner, 1999, 2006). Further, Levine-Madori (2005) studied 110 individuals diagnosed with mild to moderate Alzheimer's disease admitted into five different nursing homes in the New York area. This two-point data study compared a yearlong participation in therapeutic activities and time involved in programming from the initial point of entry into the skilled nursing facility and one year later. This study found significant correlations between the frequency of participation and length of time in therapeutic programming and higher levels of cognitive levels and psychosocial well-being after the one-year period. What were not followed were those that had no activity and the correlation to decline in cognition and socialization, which was studied in the Alders and Levine-Madori study in 2010. This study investigated the role of various activities on cognitive performance in a community sample of Hispanic elderly subjects. The aim of the study was to determine whether differences in cognitive performance could be accounted for by activity (using the TTAP Method), particularly when the influence of other variables, such as gender, country of origin, acculturation, education, and frequency of self-initiated tasks, were taken into account. A total of 24 subjects were interviewed in a Hispanic community center by bilingual interviewers, allowing for culturally sensitive interaction. Cognitive functioning was measured with the neurological *Clock Drawing Test* (CDT). The CDTs were blindly scored by three raters, using the clock drawing interpretation/scoring system described by Sunderland (1989). Participants were also given a pre and post self-report known as the *Cognitive Failures Questionnaire* (CFQ), pertaining to the frequency of everyday deficits in attention, perception, memory, and motor coordination. Additionally, personal and demographic information was collected at the onset of the investigation, including education, age, gender, country of origin, date of immigration to U.S., and level of social support. The TTAP sessions consisted of a weekly two-hour session for 12 weeks. Participants who attended the TTAP Method sessions had an average increase of 2.2 points in the CDT and an average increase of 3.5

points in the CFQ. Those who did not attend the TTAP Method sessions had an average increase of 0.1 point in the CDT score and an average decrease of 7.5 points in the CFQ. These findings indicated that the TTAP Method sessions contributed positively and significantly to self-perceived cognitive functioning and cognitive performance.

Another research study by Levine-Madori and Bendel-Jones (2011) found that more time in therapeutic programming correlated with less agitation and boredom among participants in a long-term care facility and geriatric psychiatric unit. This decrease in agitation and aggressive behaviors has been documented in the research in 2011 by Edward Hospital geri-psychiatric unit in Naperville, IL, to save over $160,000 yearly in nursing staff costs (Levine-Madori, 2012).

Communication, in all forms, is a crucial aspect of social support as it serves in maintaining or retaining feelings of connectedness to oneself and to the larger community of peers, friends, and family. The TTAP Method employs dynamic interaction by incorporating avenues for both non-verbal and verbal communication in a group context. As a result of the nine-step structure, the TTAP Method increases the total time a participant spends in programming, exposing the participant to longer levels of increased stimulation.

Recent research suggests that when social and emotional needs are addressed, feelings of self-worth, self-esteem, mood, and overall quality of life are enhanced. The TTAP Method, in its thematic orientation, structures sessions in order to meet the specific needs of persons with AD, These include the exploration of feelings of hope, love, grief, and sorrow, as well as fortitude. The TTAP Method was created and designed to address a range of emotional and social needs by increasing opportunities to engage participants in positive individualized and person-centered social involvements (Levine-Madori, 2007; Levine-Madori, 2012).

Cognitive difficulties, specifically short-term memory loss, are a defining feature of AD and are one of the central problems experienced on a daily basis. For a person with early stage AD, memory losses can have a major impact on daily living skills, which impedes self-confidence and can lead to anxiety, depression, and withdrawal from activities and other social involvements (Snowdon, 2001).

Social withdrawal can result in a general increase in symptoms including enhanced memory loss. This increase in symptoms beyond those attributable to the disease process is an example of excess disability. The TTAP Method, through its person-centered approach, enhances feelings of self-worth, which has a direct correlation to creating enhanced social support systems, thus decreasing the likelihood of withdrawal among participants.

Depression coupled with feelings of hopelessness can have a detrimental impact on cognitive functioning. Emotions directly affect cognition and, therefore, subsequent motor coordination, memory, self-esteem, and the perception of health. Cognitive evaluation tests show that cognitive performance is significantly impaired during depressive states and 15-30% of individuals with AD have clinically significant levels of depression symptoms (Gilley et al., 2004). Successful depression treatment, through the use of multi-modal interventions such as the TTAP Method, has been correlated to significant alleviation of cognitive impairments and overall improvement in independent functioning.

The TTAP Method utilizes, during the group recreational therapy sessions, a continual process of life review at each of the nine steps. The process is part of the method in which the individual looks back on his/her life, reflects on the past, and revisits positive events and unresolved difficulties and conflicts. The continual reminiscence and life review allows individuals to revisit profound life events, thus serving as a useful intervention for depression and as a promising intervention among older adults with dementia.

The TTAP Method provides a structured and systematic approach to life review which has shown to help the older adult adjust to the many life changes and challenges, positively affecting well-being. Moreover, the TTAP Method incorporates life review in successive steps which has been shown to promote memory retention, perceived social values of self, decreased disorientation, reduced fear and anxiety, and improved self-esteem and social interaction (Levine-Madori, 2009, 2012; Levine-Madori & Bendel-Jones, 2011).

Indications

The therapist can adapt any or all of the expressive arts aspects of the TTAP Method to meet the specific needs of clients, although it has been primarily used as an early intervention to assist older adults in retaining cognitive and psychosocial abilities, especially those with mild cognitive impairment and Alzheimer's disease (Rentz, 2002; Levine-Madori, 2009; Alders & Levine-Madori, 2010; Levine-Madori, 2012). The TTAP Method has also been used with individuals who have autism and children and adolescents with emotional, cognitive, and social problems.

The primary ICF codes that the TTAP method will improve are in b1 Mental Functions. These include b114 Orientation Functions, b117 Intellectual Functions, b122 Global Psychosocial Functions, b126 Temperament and Personality Functions, b130 Energy and Drive Functions, b140 Attention Functions, b144 Memory Functions, b147 Psychomotor Functions, b152 Emotional Functions, b160 Thought Functions, b164 Higher-Level Cognitive Functions, b167 Mental Functions of Language, b180 Experience of Self and Time Functions, d163 Thinking. Other areas the TTAP Method covers are found in Activities and Participation codes d2 General Tasks and Demands, d3 Communication, d7 Interpersonal Interactions and Relationships, and d910 Community Life. If these are seen in the diagnosis of the client, the therapist should consider using the TTAP method.

In rehabilitation, residential, community, and long-term care facilities more and more groups are held with multi-functional participants. The TTAP Method allows all participants, residents, and consumers to interact on their individual level. In a group of mixed cognitive functioning individuals, one individual might talk about a memory in great detail, whereas another individual might give fewer details. The TTAP Method allows all participants to be heard, share, and get positive feedback from peers, thus creating deeper bonds. When it comes to the actual art process, individuals can be designated tasks, such as cutting and gluing, while others can simply point to an image or photo that reminds them of the specific theme or discussion.

The method is currently being studied with emotionally disturbed adolescents, psychiatric populations, hospice care, community day programs, cognitively challenged individuals living in community residential facilities, individuals who have continued from the initial Cornell study, assisted living programs, individuals diagnosed with mild and moderate stage Alzheimer's disease, and the geri-psychiatric populations. Contact Dr. Linda Levine Madori at linda@levinemadoriphd.com for assistance in grant writing and research design.

Contraindications

The first two steps of the TTAP Method approach are conversation and music and meditation. The therapist must be aware that meditation can reach deep into the sub-conscious and bring up negative feelings, emotions, or events (Levine-Madori, 2007, 2009). Individuals can also react negatively to a certain piece of music, which could remind them of a person, place, or time. This risk has been proven over the years to be small, but the therapist must be ready to comfort and support the individual in whatever need is uncovered.

The use of certain art materials and supplies may also be contraindicated or require close supervision. Glue, clay, scissors, paints, pastels, and string, for example, may be inappropriate for some clients because of object misuse, suicide precautions, or respiratory precautions. The therapist may need to change or modify the activity or supplies to ensure safety. Supplies and equipment might also require modifications or adaptations to accommodate impairments. To ensure safety and maximize outcomes, the therapist will need to determine the appropriate number of group participants.

Protocols and Processes

The primary objectives of the TTAP Method are to: (1) enhance and increase cognitive, social, emotional, physical, and spiritual domains through specifically designed assessment, program protocols and documentation; (2) define the specific regions of the brain used during each therapeutic intervention including the affective system, strategic system, and recognition system, (3) depict through charts, each area of the brain that is stimulated through each of the nine steps; (4) provide multiple opportunities for the individual to integrate personal life experiences into group programming, thus enhancing the creative process; (5) provide a nine-step structure in which the individual can reintegrate in a supportive social environment that fosters feelings of safety and support to increase social participation and self-worth; (6) engage participants in a multitude of creative arts experiences while emphasizing each person's learning styles in the group; and (7) naturally increase time in programming.

Given that the TTAP Method can be used with various populations and has the ability to target a variety of needs, specific protocols can be designed based on individual or group needs. Specific protocols used in a 14-week study at the Cornell Memory and Evaluation Clinic in 2010 for individuals diagnosed with MCI and early-onset AD can be found in Levine-Madori (2012). In this particular study, the participants met as a group once a week for 60 to 90 minutes. Cornell protocols are included in the publication *The TTAP Method for Cognitive Rehabilitation* (Levine-Madori, 2012).

Sample Protocol

Steps utilized: Step #1 Conversation, Step #2 Meditation, and Step #3 Drawing/Painting

Materials: Music, DVD player, 18"x24" white paper, tempera paints, brushes, paper towels, water bowls, colored markers, colored pencils, pastels, and tissues

Rationale: Guided imagery is a way to calm the mind. While playing music, the therapist speaks slowly to the participants, first relaxing the body and then the mind. This program allows all participants to freely access their long-term memory to be utilized in the conversation and graphic element of this session. All participants create a personal mental image of a garden as a special summer place. Free association of these summer memories will enhance recall of quality times to share in detailed language, thus providing the opportunity for individual life review. The life review provides positive and significant effects for each individual. The group experience instills a sense of overall positive well-being and increases social and verbal interactions.

Structure of session: If conducting for research purposes, time the duration of each session. Session structure is shown in Table 24.

Table 24: Structure of Session

Time: Approximately 5 minutes
Introductions of group
Goals of the group are explained as follows:
1. Explain to group members the importance of mental stimulation through body relaxation and guided imagery.
2. Listen to music that aids in the formulation of mental images.
3. Reminisce about past, present, and future experiences.
4. Share with the group reminiscing and life events that might come to mind during the meditation.

Time: Approximately 10 minutes
Participants are invited to sit and listen to soothing music (e.g., classical, nature sounds, meditative).
The therapist guides the meditation to visualize a garden and promotes awareness in the meditation of sensory experiences, such as the sound of the birds, feel of the breeze, and smell of the flowers.

Time: Approximately 5-10 minutes (until conversation subsides)
Participants are asked: When you were listening to the music and meditation, what were you thinking about? Did you "see" a garden, what did it look like, what were the details? What season were you in? Were you concentrating on the sounds? What sounds could be heard? What did those sounds remind you of? Did any memories come to you while you were listening to the music?
Hand out items that symbolize the garden, such as real flowers, tree branches, dirt, a small water fountain, etc., to provide help facilitating the garden discussion and sensory stimulation.

Time: Approximately 20-35 minutes
Participants will have the option of creating an image evoked from the music and meditation using paints, pastels, or colored pencils and markers.
As closure, participants are invited to share their artwork with others in the group.

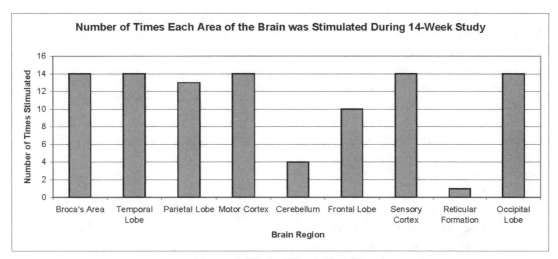

Figure 4: Brain Stimulation Counts

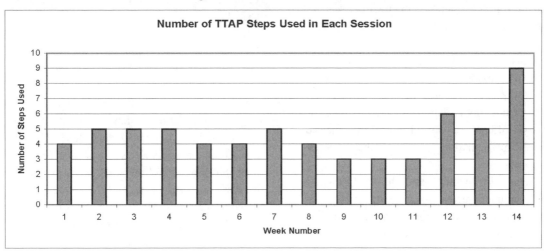

Figure 5: TTAP Steps per Session

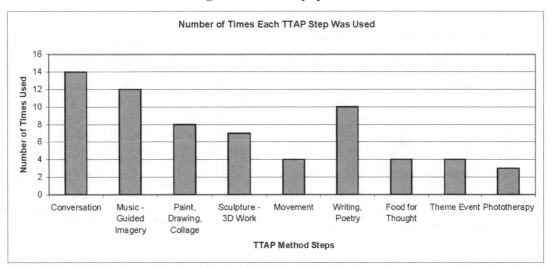

Figure 6: TTAP Step Use

Outcomes and Documentation

The TTAP Method is a structured recreational therapy program that identifies the therapeutic activity with a specific region of the brain. This structured approach aides in the therapist's ability to better document exactly what has been done in each treatment session. As illustrated, therapists can identify the number of times brain regions were utilized (Figure 4), explain and expand on the number of steps utilized in the program (Figure 5), and track the number of steps used in programming (Figure 6). This offers an effective and valid way in which to enhance documentation, which can clearly represent habilitation or rehabilitation progress, enhancing documentation in notes, reports, or research. Assessment forms can be found in Levine-Madori (2007, 2012).

Charts in the TTAP Method book (Levine-Madori, 2007) provide a means of documenting with specific details the variables of time in activity, frequency of the actual brain regions stimulated, learning style offered, steps used in each therapeutic program, and participation, as well as the scope of treatment provided.

The Centers for Medicare and Medicaid Services MDS 3.0 includes recreation and art therapy as treatment services. Information pertaining to frequency, duration, and scope of treatment is required for recreational therapy and the therapeutic service rendered must follow proven procedures to restore, remediate, or rehabilitate functional abilities. The TTAP Method gives order to therapy sessions and assimilates the MDS 3.0 requirements needed to achieve funding.

Additionally, therapy session protocols outlined in the appendix of the TTAP Method manual were designed according to the American Therapeutic Recreation Association practice guidelines (Buettner & Kolanowski, 2003). Concepts from the Need-Driven Dementia-Compromised Behavior Model (NDB) (Penrod et al., 2007) and Buettner's (1988) Neurodevelopmental Sequencing Program (NDSP) were incorporated into the theoretical foundations of the nine steps.

By providing therapy interventions that facilitate various cognitive processing styles, the TTAP Method aims to identify and meet a wide and varied scope of care. In this way, it structures a desired outcome process, such as that described in the NDB. Detailed treatment notes, such as those facilitated through the TTAP Method, track changes in the identified problems, symptoms, beliefs, or behaviors in order to assess the effectiveness of treatment on an ongoing basis. Changes in the ICF codes discussed in the Indications section can also be used to document the effectiveness of the treatment.

Note

TTAP Method is a registered trademark of Linda Levine-Madori.

Resources

Linda Levine-Madori, Ph.D., CTRS, ATR-BC, LCAT

www.ttapmethod.com

Linda@Levinemadoriphd.com

Dr. Levine-Madori's website is a comprehensive site for TTAP Method resources. Recreational therapists can purchase the TTAP Method manual for more detailed information on how to utilize and apply the TTAP Method (Levine-Madori, 2007). A variety of other books and resources, such as videos, are also available that compliment the manual. Dr. Levine-Madori also offers a TTAP certification course. Anyone interested in utilizing the TTAP Method in research is required to take the TTAP Method Certification Course, which has been approved for continuing educational credits across all healthcare professions.

References

Alders, A. & Levine-Madori, L. (2010). The effect of art therapy on cognitive performance of Hispanic/Latino older adults. *Art Therapy, 27*(3), 127-135.

Alzheimer's Association. (2006). *Warning signs you should know.* Chicago, IL: Author.

Buckwalter, K., Burgener, S., & Buettner, L. (2009). Review of exemplar programs for persons in early stage Alzheimer's disease. *Research in Gerontological Nursing, 1*(4), 295-304.

Buettner, L. (1988). Utilizing developmental theory and adapted equipment with regressed geriatric patients in therapeutic recreation. *Therapeutic Recreation Journal, 22,* 72-79.

Buettner, L. (1999). Simple Pleasures: A multilevel, sensorimotor intervention for nursing home residents with dementia. *American Journal of Alzheimer's Disease, 14,* 41-52.

Buettner, L. (2006). Peace of Mind: A pilot community based program for older adults with memory loss. *American Journal of Recreation Therapy, 5*(1), 42-48.

Buettner, L. & Ferrario, C. (1998). Therapeutic recreation as an intervention for nursing home residents with dementia and agitation: An efficacy study. *Annuals of Therapeutic Recreation, 7*(1), 15-26.

Buettner, L. & Fitzsimmons, S. (2009). *N.E.S.T. approach: Dementia practice guidelines for disturbing behaviors.* State College, PA: Venture Publishing.

Buettner, L. & Kolanowski, A. (2003). Practice guidelines for recreation therapy in the care of people with dementia. *Geriatric Nursing, 24*(1), 18-23.

Burgener, S., Gilbert, R., & Mathy, R. (2007). The effects of a multi-modal intervention on cognitive, physical, and affective outcomes of persons with early stage dementia. *Journal of Alzheimer's Disease and Related Disorders, 12,* 143-156.

Cappeliez, P., O'Rourke, N., & Chaudhury, H. (2005). Functions of reminiscence and mental health in later life. *Aging & Mental Health, 9*(4), 295-301.

Cohen-Mansfield, J. (1992). Agitation in elderly person: An integrative report of findings in a nursing home. *International Psychogeriatrics, 4*(4), 221-240.

Cohen-Mansfield, J. (1994). Reflections on the assessment of behavior in nursing home residents. *Alzheimer's Disease and Associated Disorders, 8*(10), S217-S222.

Csíkszentmihályi, M. (1990). *Flow: The Psychology of optimal experience.* New York: Harper and Row.

Khachaturian, Z. S., Petersen, R. C., Gauthier, S., Buckholtz, N., Corey-Bloom, J. P., Evans, B., … Bain, L. R. (2008). A roadmap for the prevention of dementia: The inaugural Leon Thal Symposium. *Alzheimer's & Dementia, 4*(3), 156-163.

Gilley, W., Wilson, L., Bienias, L., Bennett, A., & Evans, A. (2004). Predictors of depression symptoms in persons with Alzheimer's disease. *Journal of Gerontology: Psychological Sciences, 59*(2), 75-83.

Levine-Madori, L. (2005). Therapeutic recreation participation of Alzheimer's disease patients living in skilled nursing homes (unpublished doctoral dissertation). New York University, NY.

Levine-Madori, L. (2007). *Therapeutic Thematic Arts Programming for Older Adults (TTAP),* Baltimore, Maryland: Health Professionals Press.

Levine-Madori, L. (2009). Using the therapeutic thematic arts programming, TTAP Method®, for enhanced cognitive and psychosocial functioning in the geriatric population. *American Journal of Therapeutic Recreation, 8*(1), 25-31.

Levine-Madori, L. (2012). *Transcending dementia through the TTAP Method: The new psychology of art, brain, and cognition.* Baltimore, Maryland: Health Professionals Press.

Levine-Madori, L. & Bendel-Jones, T. (2011). The use of thematic creative arts in mental health: Changing social systems through TTAP Method. *American Society of Aging 44th National Conference,* March, California.

National Institute on Aging. (2005). Progress report on Alzheimer's disease. NIH Publication No. 05-5724. Bethesda, MD: Author. Retrieved from www.alzheimers.org/pr04-05/index.asp.

Penrod, J., Yu, F., Kolanowski, A., Fick, D., Loeb, S., & Hupcey, J. (2007). Reframing person-centered nursing care for persons with dementia. *Res Theory Nurs Pract, 21*(1), 57-72.

Reisberg, B., Ferris, H., de Leon, J., Sinaiko, E., Franssen, H., Kluger, A., et al. (1988). Stage-specific behavioral, cognitive, and in vivo changes in community residing subjects with age-associated memory impairment (AAMI) and primary degenerative dementia of the Alzheimer type. *Drug Development Research, 15,* 101-114.

Rentz, C. (2002). Memories in the Making©: Outcome-based evaluation of an art based program for individuals with dementing illnesses. *American Journal of Alzheimer's Disease and other Dementias, 17*(3), 175-181.

Snowdon, D. (2001). *Aging with grace: What the nun study teaches us about leading longer, healthier, and more meaningful lives.* New York: Bantam Books.

Stern, Y. (2003). The concept of cognitive reserve: A catalyst for research. *Journal of Clinical and Experimental Neuropsychology, 25*(5), 589-593.

Sunderland, T. (1989). Clock drawing in Alzheimer's disease: A novel measure of dementia severity. *Journal of the American Geriatric Society, 37,* 725-729.

Yu, F., Rose, K., Burgener, S., Cunningham, C., Buettner, L., Beattie, E. Bossen, A., Buckwalter, K., & McKenzie, S. (2009). Cognitive training for early-stage Alzheimer's disease and dementia. *J Gerontol Nurs., 35*(3), 23-29.

48. Transfers

Heather R. Porter

Performing transfers (moving from one surface to another) is a basic mobility skill. The most common transfers taught to clients in hospital settings are bed, chair, toilet, and wheelchair transfers. Recreational therapists assist client in performing these transfers. They also teach transfer techniques for uncommon surfaces related to recreation, leisure, play, and community activities not typically reviewed in a hospitalized setting. These might include riding lawn mowers, boats, movie seats, and horses, depending on the interests of the client.

Typically, recreational therapists perform transfers that require moderate assistance or less. If the client requires more than moderate assistance, the therapist seeks out the appropriate staff (PT, OT, or nurse) to determine the best technique.

Some of the common techniques employed to enhance learning transfers include repetition of task, physically guiding the client in a move, verbal cues, demonstration of desired skill, verbal review of steps in a transfer, positive feedback, physical assistance, and a gait or transfer belt. A gait or transfer belt is a common piece of safety equipment used when clients are ambulating and transferring. There are various styles of belts. In general, it is a piece of strong fabric that typically has belt loops sewn along the outside of the belt and is wrapped and secured snugly around the client's waist, but not too tight, so the therapist can comfortably fit fingers underneath the belt (Acello, 2006). The therapist grasps either the belt itself using an underhand grasp or the belt loops to have a secure hold on the client while s/he is ambulating or transferring. Gait/transfer belts are particularly helpful when clients are wearing loose-fitting clothing that does not provide the therapist with a secure hold, such as sweat pants or a dress. Clients may experience pain, discomfort, or harm from someone holding onto or grabbing body parts. The belt provides a safe method of providing assistance. The belt can also be helpful in controlling the speed and direction of a fall.

Transfer training is not a cookie cutter approach. The technique and instructions vary according to the client's abilities and limitations. A few considerations follow (Hegner, Acello, & Caldwell, 2009; Nelson, 2005; Lockette, 2011).

Prior to performing the transfer

Type of transfer: There are a variety of transfer techniques that can be used. Choosing the best one depends on the client's abilities and limitations. Clients may have specific cueing, assistance, and technique requirements identified by members of the treatment team. The recreational therapist explores the client's specific needs by asking the client; checking in the medical chart; or asking the client's primary nurse, physical therapist, or occupational therapist.

Secondary conditions that impact transfer technique: It is not uncommon for clients to have a secondary condition that requires a modification of the transfer technique. For example, a client who has left upper extremity paralysis needs to learn how to transfer using the support of only one arm or hand. Other medical conditions that may affect the client's transfer performance include orthostatic hypotension, amputation, fragile skin, pressure ulcers, pain, or spasms.

Client's strength and endurance: Therapists must consider whether the client has enough strength and endurance to complete the transfer safely. For example, a client who is deconditioned may have great difficulty in performing a floor transfer because it requires too much strength.

Client's available range of motion: Therapists consider the available range of motion of the client and its impact on performing transfers. If range of motion is restricted, modifications of transfer techniques may be required. For example, a client who has recently had a total knee replacement will have limited knee flexion, resulting in the need to extend the affected leg when going from a standing to a sitting position rather than placing the foot on the floor and flexing the knee.

Client's cognitive and perceptual skills: Therapists evaluate and problem solve for cognitive and perceptual problems that may interfere with a client's ability to perform a transfer, such as difficulty remembering the steps or poor awareness of body position.

Assistance is available: To ensure safety, the therapist must be able to provide the level of support needed by the client. If the therapist is unable to provide the level of assistance needed, the therapist seeks out available assistance, which might require a second person or a Hoyer lift. It is also important to consider the abilities, limitations, and reliability of people who will assist the client with transfers after discharge. For example, if a client requires moderate assistance to perform a car transfer but his fishing buddy has a bad back, he might not be able to help him with a stand-pivot transfer thus impacting the client's ability to go fishing. Consequently, the therapist would need to explore other transfer techniques (e.g., may be able to transfer with a transfer board with minimal assistance) or problem solve for other available resources (e.g., use of paratransit to get to the fishing dock). Every attempt is made to ensure that assistance is available, safe, and appropriate.

Proper support: Therapists must be sure that the client is provided with the appropriate supports to ensure safe transfers. For example, if a client requires the support of armrests to transfer, it is important to make sure that armrests are available or alternative techniques are taught, as in transferring onto or off of a sofa that only has one armrest.

Stability of transfer destination: Check the stability of the items to be used during the transfer to make sure that they provide a safe transfer opportunity. For example, check chairs to make sure they will not slide or move because of a slippery tile floor or because the chair has wheels.

Proper equipment: Therapists make sure that transfer equipment is available and appropriate for the specific transfer. For example, a client may be able to independently transfer from a wheelchair to a bed using a transfer board, but the transfer board will not work to transfer from a boat dock onto a boat. Also, make sure the client has the appropriate equipment needed to perform the transfer, such as a walker, braces, or splints.

Condition of equipment: Inspect the wheelchair and transfer devices to make sure they are safe and secure.

Proper height: Transfers must be within the specific height precautions or parameters of the client. For example, if a client has total hip precautions, the client is not allowed to flex the hip past 90°. This means that floor transfers and transfers to low surfaces, such as car seats that flex the hip more than 90°, are contraindicated. The therapist should also adjust the height of the transfer surfaces whenever possible to ensure proper body mechanics, such as adjusting the height of bed so it is even with the therapist's waist. The therapist may also adjust his/her height to accommodate the transfer. For example, if the therapist is tall and the client is short, the therapist might sit on a stool in front of the client to assist the client with the transfer.

Proper shoes and clothing: Both the caregiver and the client should wear non-slip, rubber-soled flat shoes. Avoid wearing long clothing that can drag on the floor or big, flowing clothing that makes it difficult to see body parts.

Space: Make sure there is enough space to perform the transfer safely. Move items out of the way, as appropriate. Too tight of an area can hinder movement, thus impairing performance and safety. Make sure the floor isn't slippery.

During the transfer

Transfer to stronger side: Whenever possible place the transfer destination on the client's stronger side.

Position of caster wheels: When transferring to or from a wheelchair, make sure the caster wheels are facing forward as it adds more stability to the wheelchair. To do this, roll the wheelchair backwards so the caster wheels move into the forward position.

Wheels are locked: Make sure wheels on a bed and wheelchair are locked to prevent movement during the transfers.

Tubing: Make sure all tubes including oxygen tubing, feeding tubes, and IV lines, are carefully repositioned as needed so they do not interfere with the transfer.

Communication: Explain the steps that will be taken to transfer the client and explain to the client how s/he can help. Give specific, clear, and short instructions.

Hand placement: Never allow a client to place his/her hands on the therapist's body during a transfer (e.g., wrap hands around neck). Therapists should never place their hands under a client's arms or shoulders because it can cause injury.

Body mechanics: Use good body mechanics. Lifting 10 pounds away from the body exerts a force of 100 pounds on the lumbar spine. Consequently, proper body mechanics are a must. Maintain a sturdy, broad base of support with feet shoulder-width apart. Keep the client close to your body to avoid stress on the back. Lift with the legs not with the back by tightening the stomach, bending your knees, and using large leg muscles to lift. Push instead of pull, whenever possible, because pushing makes it easier to maintain a normal lumbar curve.

Indications

If lack of transfer skills are limiting the client's ability to perform activities being addressed by recreational therapy, then transfer goals should be established. The ICF notes mobility issues with subcodes in d4 Mobility. Transfer training should be considered when deficits are noted in d410 Changing Basic Body Position and d420 Transferring Oneself.

Contraindications

It is rare that transferring a client is contraindicated. However, contraindications do exist for certain transfer techniques. Some examples include:

If a client is obese and requires maximum assistance, a stand-pivot transfer would be contraindicated due to safety concerns. A Hoyer lift might be required.

If a client is non-weight bearing on bilateral lower extremities or has bilateral lower extremity amputations without prosthetics, a stand-pivot transfer would be contraindicated. A transfer board might be required.

If a client has right upper extremity paralysis, the client would not be able to push up with bilateral upper extremities on the armrests to move into a standing position, thus possibly requiring more physical assistance from the therapist.

It is impossible to list all of the potential contraindications for transfer techniques in this chapter. The therapist must fully understand the task analysis of the transfer and compare it to the client's abilities, limitations, precautions, and parameters to determine appropriateness.

The use of a gait (transfer) belt is contraindicated if the client has a colostomy, a gastrostomy tube, recent abdominal surgery or a fresh incision, severe cardiac or respiratory disease, fractured ribs, pregnancy, an abdominal pacemaker, implanted medication pump, or abdominal aneurysm (Acello, 2006).

Protocols and Processes

There are over 20 types of transfers and types of transfer lifts (Nelson, 2005). In an effort to impart basic transfer techniques, step-by-step directions for common transfer techniques are provided below.

Stand-Pivot Transfer (SPT)

In brief, the client stands upright, pivots on his/her lower extremities towards the destination, and sits down. The client should perform the following actions with assistance from the helper, as required.

1. Position the wheelchair so that the wheelchair and the destination site are at a 90° angle from each other ("L" form). This will minimize the amount of stepping and pivoting required to reach the transfer destination. Whenever possible, the client should position himself/herself to transfer toward his/her stronger side.

2. Lock the brakes on the wheelchair and swing the leg rests out of the way.

3. Scoot forward to the end of the seat. This may be done by walking the buttocks forward one cheek at a time, placing the hands on the armrests and lifting the buttocks to the end of seat, or leaning against wheelchair back and pushing the buttocks forward. If the client is unable to scoot to the edge of the seat, the therapist may assist the client by squatting in front of client, placing his/her hands around the client's buttocks, and pulling the buttocks forward.

4. Place feet flat on the floor and tuck the feet behind the knees.

5. Place both hands on the armrests of the wheelchair.

6. On the count of three, stand up by leaning forward, keeping the nose over the toes, straightening the knees and trunk, looking straight ahead, straightening the shoulders, tucking in the buttocks. If the client requires assistance with standing, the therapist stands on the affected side of the client. The therapist holds onto the client at the trunk in the back by grabbing the waistband of the pants or the belt to assist with standing. The therapist places the other hand on client's chest to provide support so that the client does not go too far forward. The therapist provides cueing and further assistance as needed.

7. Pivot the feet so that the buttocks are now in line with the transfer destination.

8. Back up to the transfer destination until the legs touch the transfer destination.

9. Reach back and place both hands on the transfer destination and slowly lower himself/herself onto the destination site. No plopping.

Sit-Pivot Transfer

A sit-pivot transfer has the same abbreviation as a stand-pivot transfer (SPT). Since the stand-pivot transfer is more commonly used, the abbreviation SPT is typically reserved for the stand-pivot transfer and the words "sit-pivot transfer" are written out. The sit-pivot transfer is performed exactly the same as the SPT with the exception that the client does not reach a full upright position in standing, but rather a half standing position.

Transfer Board Transfer (TB)

In brief, in a sitting position, place one end of the board underneath the client's buttocks and the rest the other end on the transfer destination. Perform small buttocks lifts using support of the arms and legs to move to the destination.

There are short boards and long boards. Short boards are used for short-distance transfers, such as wheelchair to mat or wheelchair to bed. Long boards are used for traversing longer distances, such as car transfers. A typical transfer board is made out of wood and is tapered at each end. There is a hole on one end of the board that allows the client to grasp and manipulate the board. The client should perform the following actions with assistance from the helper, as required.

1. Position the wheelchair so that the wheelchair and the destination site are at a 90° angle from each other ("L" form) or position the wheelchair next to the destination, each other facing in the same direction. The placement of the large power wheels on the wheelchair will determine which position to use. If the power wheels are set forward and there is not a lot of room at the side of the seat to place the transfer board, use the 90° angle position. If the power wheels are set back and there is plenty of room at the side of the seat to place the transfer board, use the parallel position.

2. Lock the wheelchair brakes and remove the armrest that is next to the destination site.

3. Scoot forward to the end of the seat. This may be done by walking the buttocks forward one cheek at a time, placing the hands on the armrests and lifting the buttocks to the end of seat, or leaning against wheelchair back and pushing the buttocks forward. If the client is unable to scoot to the edge of the seat, the therapist may assist the client by squatting in front of client, placing his/her hands around the client's buttocks, and pulling the buttocks forward.

4. Lean to the side with one buttock cheek raised. Place the board carefully under the buttock being careful to not shear the skin. Make sure the other end of the board is resting securely on the destination and then lower the buttock onto the board.

5. Perform small hops (buttocks lifts) across the board using arm and leg support until the destination is reached. Do not slide across the board because it can shear the skin.

6. Lean to the side and remove the board from under the buttocks when the destination is reached.

Hoyer Lift Transfer

A Hoyer lift is a large piece of equipment used to transfer a client from one surface to another. It is used with clients who require maximum assistance or who are totally dependent to transfer. Body weight is a primary barrier to being able to transfer the person manually. For example, a child who weighs 30 pounds, despite being dependent for transfers, can easily be transferred manually. A client who weighs 250 pounds and is dependent for transfers can't be transferred manually and will require the use of a Hoyer lift. The therapist will need specialized training on how to operate a Hoyer lift. Only a general outline is provided of how to perform a bed to wheelchair Hoyer lift transfer:

In brief, the client is hoisted from one place to another using a piece of equipment called a Hoyer lift. The seat of the Hoyer lift is made out of a strong material that is placed around the client and buckled into place. The final outcome is the construction of a seat resembling a child's swing with a back. The swing is attached to a metal frame with wheels so that the client can be lifted up in the swing and then rolled to the next destination. The swing is then lowered onto the transfer surface and the buckles are undone.

1. With the bed flat, position the sling underneath the client. To do this, fold the sling in half the long way. Roll the client away from you and lay the folded sling underneath the client against his/her back. Roll the client back onto his/her back. Roll the client to the other side to grab the end of the folded sling, and flatten the sling on the bed. The sling is now totally open and flat underneath the client.

2. Raise the head of the bed and connect the sling straps and hooks.

3. Position the Hoyer lift under the client's bed with the Hoyer legs fully open and locked.

4. Lower the cradle of the Hoyer lift over the bed and attach the sling.

5. Raise the Hoyer lift until the client is clear of the bed surface.

6. Unlock the brakes, gently swing the Hoyer lift to the wheelchair, and then re-lock the brakes.

7. Lower the client down onto the wheelchair.

8. Unhook the sling from the Hoyer lift and then remove the sling from underneath the client.

Dependent Lift of Two

1. Client is in a seated position.

2. One person approaches the person from behind, places his/her arms underneath the armpits of the client and grasps the client's opposite wrist or forearm, so the therapists right hand grasps the client's left wrist or forearm and the therapist's left hand grasps the client's right. The therapist pulls the client's arms under the client's chest for support when lifting.

3. The second person approaches the client from the front. The second person places both his/her hands underneath the client's knees.

4. On the count of three, both therapists lift the client up and over to the transfer destination.

Floor Transfers (Between Floor and Wheelchair)

From the Wheelchair to a Kneeling Position on the Floor

1. Position the wheelchair so that it is ready for the transfer. Brakes are locked, casters are rotated in the most forward position, and the cushion is removed if necessary to decrease the height of the transfer.

2. Client scoots to the edge of the wheelchair.

3. Client places his/her feet on the floor and tucks them underneath knees as tolerated based on knee flexion.

4. Client places one hand on the seat of the wheelchair and flexes forward at the trunk slowly reaching with the other hand for the floor.

5. Client slowly lowers himself/herself toward the floor until s/he reaches the floor in a hands-and-knees position.

From a Kneeling Position on the Floor to the Wheelchair

This technique can be difficult with a wheelchair that does not have swing away leg rests.

1. Position the wheelchair so that it is ready for the transfer. Brakes are locked, casters are rotated in the most forward position, and the cushion is removed if necessary to decrease the height of the transfer. It is replaced once the client is seated on the wheelchair seat.

2. With both knees bent to one side and buttocks on the floor, client places his/her hands on either side of the seat or armrest.

3. Client lifts himself/herself into a tall kneeling position.

4. Client continues to lift the torso until the hips clear the edge of the seat.

5. Client rotates his/her hips to one side and moves one hand to the other armrest so that the buttocks are fully on the wheelchair seat.

From the Wheelchair to a Long Sitting Position on the Floor

1. Position the wheelchair so that it is ready for the transfer. Brakes are locked, casters are rotated in the most forward position, and the cushion is removed if necessary to decrease the height of the transfer.

2. Client scoots to edge of wheelchair seat and straightens his/her legs out to one side so that s/he is sitting at an angle in the wheelchair.

3. Client places one hand on the wheelchair seat or armrest and reaches towards the floor with the other hand.

4. Client slowly lowers himself/herself to the floor into a long sitting position.

From a Long Sitting Position on the Floor to the Wheelchair

1. Position the wheelchair so that it is ready for the transfer. Brakes are locked, casters are rotated in most forward position, and the cushion is removed if necessary to decrease the height of the transfer. It is replaced once the client is seated on the wheelchair seat.

2. Client positions himself/herself with his/her back to the wheelchair seat and legs straightened out in front of him/her on a diagonal away from his/her body.

3. Client reaches behind and finds two stable areas for his/her hands to lift himself/herself back into the wheelchair. This could be one hand on the wheelchair seat and another on the lower part of the wheelchair frame.

4. Client pushes flexed elbows into extension and slides buttocks onto the wheelchair seat.

5. Client readjusts position on the wheelchair.

Back Approach for Transfer from the Wheelchair to Long Leg Sitting on the Floor

1. Position the wheelchair so that it is ready for the transfer. Brakes are locked, casters are rotated in most forward position, and the cushion is removed if necessary to decrease the height of the transfer.

2. Client scoots forward on the wheelchair seat and extends his/her legs directly out in front.

3. Client places both hands on the wheelchair seat and slowly lowers his/her buttocks onto the floor.

4. As the client begins to lower himself/herself to the floor his/her knees will bend up towards the chest.

Back Approach for Transfer from Long Leg Sitting on the Floor to the Wheelchair

1. Position the wheelchair so that it is ready for the transfer. Brakes are locked, casters are rotated in most forward position, and the cushion is removed if necessary to decrease the height of the transfer. It is replaced once the client is seated on the wheelchair seat.

2. Client sits with his/her back to the wheelchair seat.

3. Knees are bent up towards chest.

4. Client positions both hands on the wheelchair seat and lifts his/her buttocks onto the wheelchair seat.

Outcomes and Documentation

Therapists commonly document the type of transfer performed, equipment utilized, environment in which the transfer was performed, and type and amount of physical assistance and cueing provided. For example, "At local health club, client required moderate assistance and minimal verbal cues to look up and straighten knees when performing stand-pivot transfers between wheelchair and locker room bench." ICF codes d410 Changing Basic Body Position and d420 Transferring Oneself can be used to track changes in the client's ability.

References

Acello, B. (2006). *Competency exam prep and review for nursing assistants* (4th ed.). Boston, MA: Cengage Learning.

Hegner, B. R., Acello, B., & Caldwell, E. (2009). *Nursing assistant: A nursing process approach — Basics*. Boston, MA: Cengage Learning.

Nelson, A. L. (2005). *Safe patient handling and movement: A guide for nurses and other health care providers*. New York, NY: Springer Publishing Company.

Lockette, K. (2011). *Caregiver's complete guide for safe mobility and independence in the home*. Minneapolis, MN: Two Harbors Press.

49. Values Clarification

Alexis McKenney

Every day, every person confronts decisions that require a response based on personal beliefs, attitudes, and values (McKenney & Dattilo, 2011). This is not always easy because individuals may not be sure about what it is they believe or value (Simon, Howe, & Kirschenbaum, 1995). Values are "those aspects of our lives that are so important and pervasive that they include feelings, thoughts, and behaviors" (Simon et al., 1995, p. 10), and center on the standards individuals and societies set for themselves (Lee, Whitehead, & Balchin, 2000).

Recreational therapists might use values clarification strategies when assisting individuals in clarifying values specific to making healthy lifestyle choices and exploring barriers to participation. These strategies are based on the concept of values relativity, meaning that participants adopt their own values rather than those that have been prescribed (Brady, 2010). Ultimately, these strategies are used to help people better understand themselves and the larger society through the process of clarification (Pinch, 2003).

The theory of values clarification is grounded in the argument that, when confronted by complicated decisions, some people struggle with feelings of confusion, apathy, or inconsistency (Raths et al., 1978). Consequently, they struggle with finding clarity in their values and finding life patterns that are purposeful and satisfying. According to McKenney and Dattilo (2011), "The theory of values clarification focuses on the belief that people can be helped to clarify their values, which in turn will result in a behavior change" (p. 16). For example, if an individual finds clarity in his or her leisure values, then that person is apt to seek more purposeful and meaningful leisure experiences. Similarly, if a person is, for example, struggling with committing to exercising regularly, values clarification could result in that person making healthier life decisions and committing to acting upon them on a more consistent basis.

This chapter provides a summary of how values clarification can serve as a recreational therapy protocol.

Indications

Research specific to values clarification has focused primarily on its effects on participants' self-esteem and self-concept. Participants have included students enrolled in general education classes ranging from middle school to high school. Consequently, the research does not demonstrate effectiveness specific to individuals with disabilities. Nevertheless, low self-esteem and problems with self-concept are symptoms associated with selected diagnoses as outlined in the *Diagnostic and Statistical Manual of Mental Disorders* (American Psychiatric Association, 2013). For example, low self-esteem is one of six criteria used to diagnose persistent depressive disorder (dysthymia).

ICF codes that might indicate a need for values clarification include b126 Temperament and Personality Functions, and b130 Energy and Drive Functions. Self-esteem and self-concept are not addressed directly in the ICF because they are not considered traits that are found in all cultures, but the codes listed above cover aspects of self-esteem and self-concept and can be used to document deficits in those areas. The need for values clarification might also be present if there are deficits in life activities and interpersonal codes, such as d230 Carrying Out Daily Routine, d240 Handling Stress and Other Psychological Demands, d570 Looking After One's Health, and d710 Basic Interpersonal Interactions. If the therapist determines that one of the reasons for deficits in these codes is an issue with values, a values clarification intervention may be appropriate.

Contraindications

Values clarification as a protocol requires that recreational therapists remain neutral as they assist individuals in exploring and choosing values (McKenney & Dattilo, 2011). For years, educators have questioned whether it is possible for facilitators to remain neutral when they disagree with values that are expressed (Lockwood, 1978). For example, Lockwood questioned what one should do if a person believes racism is acceptable. Lickona (1991) provided the following example of what can happen when values clarification was used with a group of adolescents with behavioral problems:

> When we shared our lists, the four most popular activities listed by students were sex, drugs, drinking, and skipping school. I asked why these were the most popular, and these are the things my students said: *I don't need this class to graduate, so why come?*; *School isn't important; Everyone drinks and smokes dope; Pot doesn't harm you; All my friends do it, so why can't I?*; *Sex is the best part of life; and Sex, drugs, and rock and roll rule* (p. 237).

Recreational therapists working with children or adolescents who are diagnosed with behavior disorders or who exhibit behavioral problems might consider using an alternative protocol, such as a cognitive developmental approach to facilitating moral development discussions (McKenney & Dattilo, 2011).

Protocols

To better understand values clarification as an RT protocol, it is important to first differentiate between values, the valuing process, value indicators, and values clarification. Values guide a person's behavior when confronted with different life situations (Lee, Whitehead, & Balchin, 2000). They provide standards for behavior, as well as a basis for goal setting (Mosconi & Emmett, 2003).

The valuing process involves the steps an individual takes in clarifying his or her values (Raths, Harmin, & Simon, 1978). These steps, which include choosing, prizing, and acting, must all be taken for an individual's choices to be considered values. Choosing involves having individuals freely explore alternative possibilities for their beliefs and behaviors, consider possible consequences that may result, and choose from the alternatives. Prizing involves encouraging individuals to feel content with their choices, as well as being willing to proudly share their choices with other people. When acting upon their values, individuals are deciding what they would be willing to do with their choices and committing to regularly act on them.

If the aforementioned criteria of choosing, prizing, and acting are not all met, then the beliefs an individual expresses are referred to as value indicators (Raths et al., 1978). Examples of value indicators include goals, interests, beliefs, and worries. A person, for example, may express an interest in swimming, but not actually engage in any swimming activities.

Finally, values clarification is a protocol used to help individuals explore what is important to them and build their own value system (Simon et al., 1995). Participants introspectively ask questions that help them consider what they believe and who they are as human beings (Leeds, 2010). This approach then helps participants to apply the valuing process to beliefs and behavior patterns, with emphasis being placed on how decisions affect their lives (Leeds, 2010; Mosconi & Emmett, 2003).

Evidence-Based Practice

Limited research exists that examines the effects of values clarification and, overall, it lacks adequate rigor. Nevertheless, effects of school-based values clarification activities on self-concept, self-esteem, and value awareness have been found. For example, Covault (1975), Guziak (1975), and Fitzpatrick (1977) all implemented values clarification programs lasting one hour per week, one time a week from eight to 16 weeks. Covault found that, compared to a control group, the treatment group demonstrated significant improvement in self-concept, initiation in classroom activities, and attitudes toward learning. Participants in the Guziak study were found to improve in self-concept and initiation in classroom activities, show less apathetic, flighty, uncertain, inconsistent, drifting, over-conforming, and over-dissenting behaviors. Participants in the Fitzpatrick study showed increases in self-concept, personal adjustment, sense of personal feeling, feelings of belonging, reading comprehension, reading efficiency, and total reading achievement.

After implementing a 40-hour, semester long values clarification program with 60 senior high school students, DePetro (1975) found small but significant gains in self-esteem scores. However, gains on participants' value priorities were not found. This suggests that the study's values clarification strategies were designed to help individuals simply clarify values rather than impact self-esteem. In a similar study, Tinsley, Benton, and Rollins (1984) examined the effects on values clarification on 103 participants enrolled in middle school. Participants experienced a significantly greater degree of confusion after participating in the intervention. The researchers concluded that, although values clarification may help participants begin the process of self-examination, confusion may be experienced as well. Consequently, the researchers suggested that values clarification techniques might be better used as part of a program, rather than as an entire program.

Processes

Values clarification centers upon helping people to develop their own value systems. The values clarification approach typically uses one or a combination of three methods, which include the individual clarifying response, group discussions, and value sheets. Values clarification programs are usually about 12 weeks in length, one hour long, and one time a week. The following includes a brief description of each of these methods as they might be used in implementing values clarification.

Individual Clarifying Response

The individual clarifying response is used to encourage participants to think about something they said or did while interacting with other people. An effective response is one that encourages participants to think more about their thoughts and beliefs than they might otherwise. Furthermore, the response should emerge from dialogue, not be planned in advance. The following includes guidelines for individual clarifying responses, including that they: (1) are not moralizing or criticizing, (2) place responsibility on participants to decide what *they* want, (3) are stimulating, but not insistent (4) help participants understand their ideas, (5) do not result in an extended discussion, (6) are individually tailored, (7) are not made in response to everything said, (8) do

not provoke "right" answers; and, (9) are used creatively (Raths et al., 1978).

Group Discussions

To avoid having private discussions emerge or cause participants to lose interest, group discussions should be carefully planned. Raths et al. (1978) suggested that four steps should be used to help in facilitating discussions that result in personal reflection.

Step 1: First, recreational therapists should select a topic carefully. Topics should be value-rich, such as friendship, justice, or leisure. To initiate a discussion, a recreational therapist might use quotations, websites, pictures, scenes from movies, or other sources (McKenney & Dattilo, 2011).

Step 2: Next, it is important that recreational therapists encourage participants to think before speaking. This might be accomplished by asking participants to sit silently and ponder a question or issue for a few minutes before the discussion begins. The recreational therapist might ask participants to write down thoughts as they start to experience reactions.

Step 3: The third step involves structuring discussions in a manner that promotes sharing. This can be done by dividing participants into small groups, allowing opportunities for discussion, or by asking each person to share one by one.

Step 4: Finally, recreational therapists want to encourage participants to learn by asking them to sit alone and reflect for a period of time before providing lead statements, such as, "I learned that…" or by providing worksheets with similarly open-ended statements.

Values Sheet

A values sheet provides participants with another way to take time to think prior to making decisions. A values sheet should include a provocative statement along with corresponding questions, fill-in the blank statements, or a set of open-ended questions (Raths et al., 1978). Regardless of how the values sheet is structured, the purpose of the sheet is to raise an issue that stimulates thinking among participants. Examples of suggestions that Raths et al. (1978) offered for developing value sheets include: (1) avoid "yes-no," "either-or," or "why" questions, (2) include "you" on the sheets, (3) offer choices; and, (4) create small rather than large groups for discussions.

Other strategies might include a SWOT analysis, values shields, Likert scales, or unfinished sentences (Leeds, 2010). A SWOT analysis is a process that includes participants identifying Strengths, Weaknesses, Opportunities, and Threats as they relate to situations or issues they are confronting. Values shields involve participants identifying and drawing what is important to them with the use of symbols, such as a family crest. Likert scales include a series of difficult and/or contentious statements that allow participants to identify the degree to which they agree or disagree with the statements. Unfinished sentences include a list of incomplete sentences written by the recreational therapist and designed to elicit feelings and opinions.

Outcomes and Documentation

If the intervention was based on ICF codes in the client's assessment, changes in the codes caused by the intervention should be documented. The most likely codes were provided in the Indications section.

Self-esteem can be measured and documented through the use of self-concept and self-esteem scales (Covault, 1973; DePetro, 1975; Fitzpatrick, 1977; Guziak, 1975). Examples of self-esteem tools include: the *Self-Esteem Scale* (Rosenberg, 1965, 1979), the *Tennessee Self-Concept Scale* (Fitts, 1964), and the *Feelings of Inadequacy Scale* (Coopersmith, 1967). Additional scales include career decision-making, occupations, and leisure activities scales (Tinsley, Benton, and Rollins, 1984). An example of a career decision-making scale is the *Career Decision Scale* (Osipow, 1987). Numerous examples of leisure-related scales can be found in burlingame and Blaschko's (2009) book, *Assessment Tools for Recreational Therapy and Related Fields*.

Resources

Therapeutic Recreation Directory

www.recreationtherapy.com/tx/txvalue.htm

Books

The following books provide information on values clarification and resources for activities used in teaching clients.

burlingame, j. & Blaschko, T. (2009). *Assessment tools for recreational therapy and related fields*. Enumclaw, WA: Idyll Arbor.

Coopersmith, S. (1967). *The antecedents of self-esteem*. New York: W. H. Freeman.

Edginton, S. R. & Edginton, C. R. (1994). *Youth programs: Promoting quality services*. Champaign, IL: Sagamore.

Fitts, W. (1964). *Manual: Tennessee concept scale*. Nashville, TN: Counselor Recording and Tests.

Osipow, S. H. (1987). *Manual for Career Decision Scale*. Lutz, FL: Psychological Assessment Resources, Inc.

Rosenberg, M. (1965). *Society and the adolescent self image*. Princeton, NJ: Princeton University Press.

Rosenberg, M. (1979). *Conceiving the self*. New York: Basic Books.

Stumbo, N. J. (1992). *Leisure education II: More activities and resources*. State College, PA: Venture.

Stumbo, N. J. & Thompson, S. R. (1986). *Leisure education: A manual of activities and resources*. State College, PA: Venture.

Stumbo, N. J., (1997). *Leisure education III: More goal-oriented activities*. State College: PA: Venture.

Stumbo, N. J., (1998). *Leisure education IV: Activities for individuals with substance addictions*. State College: PA: Venture Publishing, Inc.

References

American Psychiatric Association. (2013). *Diagnostic and statistical manual of mental disorders* (5th ed.). Washington, DC: Author.

Brady, L. (2010). Classroom-based practice in values education. In T. Lovat et al. (Eds.). *International handbook on values education and student wellbeing* (pp. 211-224). New York: Springer.

Caldwell, L. L. (2001). The role of theory in therapeutic recreation: A practical approach. In N. J. Stumbo (Ed.), *Professional issues in therapeutic recreation: On competence and outcomes* (pp. 349-364). Champaign, IL: Sagamore.

Coopersmith, S. (1967). *The antecedents of self-esteem*. New York: W. H. Freeman.

Covault, T. (1973). The application of value clarification teaching strategies with fifth grade students to investigate their influence on students' self-concept and related classroom coping and interacting behaviors. Unpublished doctoral dissertation, Ohio State University, Columbus, OH.

Creswell, J. W. (2009). *Research design: Qualitative, quantitative, and mixed methods approaches* (3rd ed.). Thousand Oaks, CA: Sage.

DePetro, H. (1975). Effects of utilizing values clarification strategies on self-esteem of secondary school students. Unpublished doctoral dissertation, University of Northern Colorado, Greeley, CO.

Fitts, W. (1964). *Manual: Tennessee Concept Scale*. Nashville, TN: Counselor Recording and Tests.

Fitzpatrick, K. (1977). Effects of values clarification on self-concept and reading achievement. *Reading Improvement, 14*, 233-238.

Guziak, S. (1975). The use of values clarification strategies with fifth grade students to investigate influence on self-concept and values. Unpublished doctoral dissertation, Ohio State University, Columbus, OH.

Lee, M. J., Whitehead, J., & Balchin, N. (2000). The measurement of values in youth sport: Development of the youth sport values questionnaire, *Journal of Exercise and Sport Psychology, 22*, 307-326.

Leeds, J. (2010). Transitioning values education into values action. In T. Lovat et al. (Eds.), *International handbook on values education and student wellbeing* (pp. 795-809). New York: Springer.

Lickona, T. (1991). *Educating for character. How our schools can teach respect and responsibility*. New York: Bantam Books.

Lockwood, A. L. (1978). The effects of values clarification and moral development curricula on school-age subjects: A critical review of recent research. *Review of Educational Research, 48,* 325-364.

McKenney, A. & Dattilo, J. (2011). Values clarification. In J. Dattilo & A. McKenney, *Facilitation techniques in therapeutic recreation* (2nd ed.) (pp. 593-614). State College, PA: Venture.

Mosconi, J. & Emmett, J. (2003). Effects of a values clarification curriculum on high school students' definitions of success. *Professional School Counseling, 7,* 68-78.

Osipow, S. H. (1987). *Manual for career decision scale.* Lutz, FL: Psychological Assessment Resources, Inc.

Pinch, K. (2003). Surely you don't mean me? Leisure education and the park and recreation professional. *California Parks and Recreation Magazine, 59,* 36-39.

Raths, L. E., Harmin, M., & Simon, S. B. (1978). *Values and teaching: Working with values in the classroom* (2nd ed.). Columbus, OH: Charles E. Merrill.

Rogers, C. R. (1961). *On becoming a person.* Boston, MA: Houghton Mifflin.

Rosenberg, M. (1965). *Society and the adolescent self image.* Princeton, NJ: Princeton University Press.

Rosenberg, M. (1979). *Conceiving the self.* New York: Basic Books.

Simon, S. B., Howe, L. W., & Kirschenbaum, H. (1995). *Values clarification: A handbook of practical strategies.* Chesterfield, MA: Values Press.

Tinsley, H. E. A., Benton, B. L., & Rollins, J. A. (1984). The effects of values clarification exercises on the value structure of junior high school students. *The Vocational Guidance Quarterly, 32, 160-167.*

50. Walking and Gait Training

Heather R. Porter

Gait refers to the body mechanics used to walk. It includes the elements of rhythm, cadence, and speed. It also includes walking using a device, such as crutches, canes, or walkers, but does not include moving around in a wheelchair.

Moving our bodies from point A to point B is a complex task that involves many different body functions and structures. For example, most of us rely on our vision to make sure we don't run into anything. Our bones help us remain upright against the pull of gravity and our muscles help us stay balanced while allowing movement. We use visual cues, vestibular information about balance, and proprioceptor nerves to let us know where our body parts are. Coordinating all of these is required for safe walking. By looking at a client's gait we can assess many aspects of a client's overall abilities.

Gait Cycle

A gait cycle is the time and actions required for one foot to touch the ground twice. This cycle typically takes about one second and has both a stance phase and a swing phase. The stance phase is the time that the foot is in contact with the ground and the swing phase is the time that the foot is in the air. Typically 60% of the cycle is spent in the stance phase and 40% is spent in the swing phase. Both feet are on the ground at the same time for approximately 20% of the cycle. The term used to describe the time that both feet are on the ground is *double-support time*.

During each cycle there are three functional tasks that the body must accomplish: (1) weight acceptance, (2) single-limb support, and (3) limb advancement. Weight acceptance is the most challenging because it requires the integration of many tasks including establishing an initial contact with the ground in a smooth manner, anticipating the required knee flexion to absorb the shock of the body's weight (around 15° on level surfaces), coordinating muscle actions to accept the weight of the body and provide stability, and proprioceptor feedback to help keep the body's center of gravity moving forward to accomplish the next step. The primary muscles used in the weight acceptance are hip extensors, quadriceps, and dorsiflexors. Hip extensors provide limb stability. Quadriceps control knee flexion during weight acceptance. Dorsiflexors control the heel strike, place the foot on the ground, and prepare it for accepting the body's weight.

During the single-limb support phase, the two primary tasks are to support the body's total weight and simultaneously get ready to advance the leg. The primary muscles used in the single-limb support phase are hip abductors, trunk muscles, quadriceps, and plantar flexors. Hip abductors stabilize the hip during the weight-bearing phase. Trunk muscles help maintain an upright position. Quadriceps help prepare for the forward motion of the body's center of gravity. Plantar flexors control the tibia, which controls the forward movement during the weight-bearing phase.

The last phase of the cycle is the limb advancement phase where the body prepares for the swing of the leg and then executes the action. To facilitate the swing action the knee must be bent to around 35° (on level ground) in the pre-swing phase advancing to a 60° bend to keep the toes above the ground during the swing phase. The primary muscles used during this phase are the dorsiflexors, hamstrings, hip flexors, knee flexors, and quadriceps. Dorsiflexors keep the toes from touching the ground. Hamstrings cause the bend at the knee. Hip flexors move the leg forward. Knee flexors also control the position of the knee. Quadriceps extends the leg at the end of the advancement phase.

Normal Gait

A normal gait is called a heel-toe gait. In the heel-toe gait the heel strikes the ground first with the rest of the foot rolling down to the ground after the heel strike during the weight acceptance phase. Rose (2003) lists four attributes associated with normal gaits: "1. an adequate range of joint mobility; 2. appropriate timing of muscle activation across the gait cycle; 3. sufficient muscle strength to meet the demands involved in each phase of the gait cycle; and 4. unimpaired sensory input from the visual, somatosensory [skin and deep tissue sensations], and vestibular [sense of balance] systems" (p. 179).

While mobility is the general category associated with the process of movement from point A to point B, moving by using the legs (perhaps with the help of devices) requires functional skills that are found under b7 Neuromusculoskeletal and Movement-Related Functions and b1 Mental Functions. To better understand what constitutes a normal gait the therapist should be familiar with the concepts of stride length, cadence, central pattern generators, avoidance strategies, and accommodation strategies.

There are two characteristics, *stride length* and *cadence*, that influence how fast the client walks. Stride length is the distance covered between the time one heel touches the ground (heel strike) and the next time that same heel touches the ground. Cadence is the number of steps a client takes in a specified length of time, often measured over a distance of 50'. Not only do stride length and cadence help the therapist determine if a client is able to move through the community at a reasonable speed, but it can also indicate if the client is at an increased risk of falling. A slow cadence and short stride length are signs of an increased risk of falling (Rose, 2003). One way to measure stride and cadence is described in the *Fifty-Foot Walk Test* (see Appendix A in this chapter).

The spinal cord has groupings of nerves, often referred to as *central pattern generators*, that allow us to maintain a rhythm during movement. Central pattern generators are nerves that produce patterns of actions that are independent of sensory input. For individuals to be functionally independent in the community they must be able to use mental functions to neurologically override or modify the rhythm of movement created by their central pattern generators. For example, if a client is walking through a shopping mall and comes to a set of steps leading to the next level of the mall, he must be able to adjust his walking pattern by stepping higher to place his feet on the step. Clients with global mental function impairments, such as Alzheimer's, have difficulty with this process.

Patla (1997) describes two critical strategies for community mobility that are frequently impaired by disease, trauma, or old age. The first is *avoidance strategy* — the ability to momentarily modify one's movement patterns to avoid a barrier. The ability to change direction to walk around a mud puddle is an example of avoidance strategy. Clients with Parkinson's disease have difficulty stopping the gait cycle and are therefore at a greater risk of falling or otherwise hurting themselves. Clients with damage to the cerebellum area of the brain also have difficulty using avoidance strategies.

The second critical strategy for safe mobility is *accommodation strategy*. Clients accommodate the rhythm pattern associated with movement to adjust to a change in the environment. Slowing down, picking the foot up, and stepping over the dog's bone left in the center of the living room floor is an example of using an accommodation strategy. Clients with peripheral neuropathies (damage to the nerves in the arms and legs) will have more difficulty adjusting to changes in the walking surface because they will not be able to perceive them. Clients with visual impairments will have significantly more problems avoiding obstacles.

Abnormal Gaits

There are impairments (diseases and disorders) that affect the gait cycle and clients' abilities to function in their community. The list below contains some of the more common gait patterns (burlingame, 2001).

Antalgic gait: A gait that has a shortened limb support phase because the client is avoiding putting weight on a leg that hurts. A limp.

Arthogenic gait: Also referred to as hip-hiking. A gait noted by the elevation of one hip and the swinging out of the leg (instead of a straight through swing). This gait is often caused by a deformity or stiffness of the hip or the knee.

Ataxic gait: A gait characterized by an unsteady, wide gait that has two different forms: spinal ataxia and cerebellar ataxia. Spinal ataxia is caused by a disruption of sensory pathways in the central nervous system. This gait is frequently seen in clients with tabes dorsalis (slow wasting away of the nerve roots in the spine due to syphilis), multiple sclerosis, or other disease processes that affect the central nervous system. The ataxic gait tends to become worse when the client closes his/her eyes. In addition to the broad-based gait, spinal ataxia is also identified by "double tapping" when the heel comes down first followed by the toes, making a double slapping sound. Cerebellar ataxia is caused by lesions in the cerebellum of the brain. Cerebellar ataxia is characterized by an inability to walk in a straight line but does not worsen when the client's eyes are closed.

Dystrophic gait: Movement is achieved by rolling the hips from side to side producing a pronounced waddling or penguin gait. Because of the nature of this gait, the client's ability to run, climb stairs, or hike up inclines is impaired. The most common reason for this gait is muscular dystrophy, but it is also seen in a variety of myopathies (diseases of the muscles that cause weakness or wasting that is not the result of nerve dysfunction). This gait is also referred to as a myopathic gait.

Festinating gait: A gait in which the individual takes small steps while leaning forward. It is common for the client to strike the ground with only the toes and ball of the foot (tiptoeing) during the limb support phase. Due to the forward position of the client's center of gravity, the gait becomes steadily faster as the client tries not to fall forward. Other abnormal characteristics of this gait include a loss of reciprocal arm swing and difficulty initiating movement during the limb advancement stage of the gait cycle. This gait is frequently seen in individuals with Parkinson's disease.

Footdrop gait: A gait where the client slaps the foot to the ground after lifting the knee high on the affected side only (the client is unable to pull the toes up to get a heel strike, therefore the toes hit first or the whole foot slaps down flat). This gait causes increased jarring to the body. It limits, to some degree, the client's ability to achieve a high skill level in physical activities requiring highly coordinated foot and leg movements. The footdrop gait is frequently due to weak or paralyzed dorsiflexor muscles.

Gastrocnemius-soleus gait: An abnormal gait where the affected side is dragged along due to the lack of heel lift on push off (limb advancement phase). Activities that involve going up inclines are affected most. Since this gait is usually due to weakened gastrocnemius and/or soleus muscles, a strengthening program involving activities that mildly stress those muscles may lead to increased function.

Hemiplegic gait: also known as a *flaccid gait* This gait has two primary elements: a swinging (circumduction) or pushing of the affected leg forward combined with a forefoot strike with a missing heel strike on the affected leg (also referred to as "footdrop").

Other problems with gait include dorsal (posterior) column deficits. The dorsal columns are responsible for mediating proprioceptive input from muscles and joint receptors. Proprioceptive input includes both position sense (awareness of the position of a joint at rest) and kinesthetic sense (awareness of movement). Problems observed may include a wide-based and swaying gait pattern, uneven step lengths, excessive lateral displacement, advancing leg lifted too high and then dropped abruptly, and dysmetria. Visual feedback helps compensate for proprioceptive deficits, therefore the client will perform better in well-lit areas compared to poorly lit areas.

Indications

Recreational therapists assist with walking and gait training skills when functional ambulation is identified as a realistic goal. ICF codes that indicate a need to consider walking and gait training are part of d4 Mobility, usually d450 Walking, d455 Moving Around, d460 Moving Around in Different Locations, and d465 Moving Around Using Equipment.

Functional ambulation is defined as requiring minimal assistance or less to walk, with or without mobility aids and devices. If the client is not a primary ambulator (e.g., utilizes a wheelchair as the primary mode of mobility); has undergone medical treatment or surgery that could impair ambulation ability, such as endurance, strength, or balance; or has a medical condition, such as stroke or amputation, that could impact ability to ambulate, the recreational therapist must receive medical clearance from the treating physician, along with any related precautions and parameters, including weight-bearing restrictions, fall precautions, and vital-sign parameters. If other members of the treatment team are working on ambulation with the client, the recreational therapist should additionally reach out to the other treatment team members to ascertain more detailed information about the client's abilities and needs related to ambulation, such as the need for specific movement cueing to facilitate proper gait patterns.

Contraindications

If functional ambulation is not a realistic client goal or the physician does not clear the client for ambulation in recreational therapy, gait training and walking skills are not incorporated into the recreational therapy treatment plan. In a rehabilitation setting, involvement of recreational therapy in walking and gait training might not be appropriate while the client is in the early stages of gait training. In this situation, it might be more appropriate for one discipline (e.g., physical therapy) to work with the client until basic skills are learned to minimize client confusion that might be caused by different disciplines teaching different techniques.

Recreational therapists, especially those who work in long-term residential care where staff-to-client ratios are low, might find that walking is contraindicated, despite the client's abilities, due to safety issues regarding the lack of staff that can provide the level of assistance needed for ambulation due to fall precautions. Consequently, despite having the ability to ambulate, many do not. This results in loss of key physical abilities, such as strength and endurance. It can also foster dependency on others, increase risks associated with sedentary behavior, such as depression, blood clots, or muscle atrophy, and lead to other negative behaviors including increased isolation and agitation. This is a current healthcare challenge that deserves considerable attention. Recreational therapists are positioned to play a major role.

Protocols and Processes

Guarding Techniques

One of the tasks of the therapist is to help the client improve his/her ability to use the walking and moving skills learned on the unit in real-world situations. While the unit or the therapy gym offers a few challenges, normal environments offer greater challenges, such as uneven terrain, ramps, curbs, elevators, escalators, doors and doorways, curb cuts, and stairs.

The physical therapist assesses and addresses gait training. Once the client develops a gait pattern, the physical therapist consults with the recreational therapist about helping the client use these walking and moving techniques in a community environment. The physical therapist will review the techniques employed, the amount of assistance needed, the type of equipment used, the client's endurance level, walking and moving distance, cueing techniques, and other concerns. Once the physical therapist clears the client for walking and moving outside physical therapy sessions, the recreational therapist can begin his/her work. Walking on uneven surfaces is much different than walking on smooth, level indoor flooring and requires practice, patience, and the problem-solving support and education offered by the recreational therapist.

Walking and moving outdoors (and in different environments) offers greater physical and cognitive demands due to uneven surfaces, weather, obstacles, and tasks, as these examples show: Outdoor walking and moving requires more cardiopulmonary and muscular endurance. Barriers challenge problem-solving skills. Incorporation of a task (e.g., picking flowers) requires integration of many learned skills and the need to develop new skills that were not developed in a clinical setting.

Every client will present with different needs for walking and moving. Some may require only close supervision, while others may require a more hands-on approach, such as blocking the knee from buckling while walking or supporting the client who has a strong lean to the right to stand upright. The recreational therapist must be aware of the client's individual needs. The best way to do this is to talk with the physical therapist. If the recreational therapist is not familiar with the specific techniques employed by the physical therapist, the recreational therapist should ask for instruction.

The general procedure has the therapist position himself/herself in the optimal position for assisting the client. One of the most common guarding techniques is described here. Since a client is more prone to fall to his/her weaker side, the therapist stands on the client's weaker side slightly behind the client. If the front of client is 12 o'clock, the therapist stands on client's right side at 4 o'clock or left side at 8 o'clock. The therapist holds the client's transfer belt or waistband with one hand (on side of client's waist) and places the other hand in front of the client's shoulder. For example, if the therapist is standing on the client's right side, the therapist reaches around with his/her left hand and grasps the left side of the client's transfer belt or waistband and places his/her right hand in front of the client's right shoulder.

Even if the client is documented as being independent or requiring only supervision for walking, the recreational therapist should assume the guarding position described above when walking with the client (whether on level indoor surfaces or uneven outdoor surfaces) until the therapist is confident in the client's skills. It is normal for a client to be rated at a particular level of assistance in the clinic and then require a greater amount of assistance in a different environment. If the client begins to lose his/her balance while walking, the therapist in the guarding position can react as follows:

If the client begins to fall backwards: the therapist can stop the momentum of the fall, supporting the back of the client with the arm that is extended along the back of the client to allow the client to move back into an upright position. The therapist additionally takes a lateral step with the leg that is closest to the client to gain a strong base of support. If the client requires physical assistance to get back into an upright position, the therapist can push the client forward with the hand that is on the transfer belt or waistband. Pushing is ergonomically preferred to pulling and the dynamic between the therapist's base of support and strength help reduce the client's impaired line of gravity and balance. If the therapist is unable to support the client enough to regain an upright position, the therapist, because s/he is slightly behind the client and has taken a lateral step, can bend his/her knee so that the therapist's thigh becomes a resting seat for the client. The therapist needs to make sure that his/her foot is firmly on the ground for this technique and it is best if the foot is pointed toward the client. Placement of the foot on the ground and lowering the client onto the knee or thigh allows the therapist to use gravity, alignment, and base of support to work in his/her favor.

If the client begins to fall to his/her stronger side: This is unlikely because people tend to fall to the weaker side, but if it happens, the therapist takes a lateral step with the leg that is closest to the client to attain a strong base of support. At the same time, the therapist raises his/her elbow while still holding

the client's waistband or gait belt. Raising the elbow allows the therapist's forearm to provide support. Raising the elbow, along with the lateral step, also allows for the creation of an arm "cradle" to help support the client. This stops the momentum of the fall and allows the client to move back into an upright position with the therapist's assistance, as needed.

If the client begins to fall forward: the therapist's hand that is in front of the client's shoulder provides support. The arm can be extended across the chest, if needed, to provide extra support. The therapist also takes a forward step with the leg that is furthest away from the client to attain a strong base of support. This stops the forward momentum of the client to allow the client to move back into an upright position with the therapist's assistance, as needed. The therapist can additionally use his/her hand that is holding the client's waistband or gait belt to guide the client back into an upright position.

If the client begins to fall to his/her weaker side: the therapist provides support with the hand that is in front of the shoulder by moving it to the outside of the shoulder to stop the momentum of the fall. This allows the client to move back into an upright position with the therapist's assistance, as needed. The therapist can also block the fall using the entire side of his/her body by taking a forward step with the foot that is furthest away from the client.

New therapists should practice these techniques until they are comfortable. Supervising therapists should imitate various clients and have the new therapist guard them for walking and moving. As part of the practice, the supervising therapists should imitate common types of loss of balance and falls, allowing the new therapist to learn how to support and "catch" the client.

Walking on Uneven Surfaces

Walking on uneven surfaces presents challenges for clients who have deficits in their walking skills. This section looks at general guidelines and ways to handle specific circumstances.

General Guidelines

Go slow: Walking on uneven surfaces challenges balance more than even indoor surfaces. Clients can compensate for increased challenges by decreasing speed. Guide the client to walk at his/her own pace and not be pressured to move at a faster pace than s/he can safely move. For example, if a car is stopped and waiting for the client to cross the parking lot, the client should walk at a comfortable pace and not give in to the pressure of hurrying-up.

Make sure that the device and footing are secure: Attention to outdoor surfaces is imperative for safety. Clients are to look at least five feet ahead of them at all times. Clients are not to look down at their feet. Because of divided attention challenges, such as looking at store windows and walking at the same time, the clients may not anticipate uneven surfaces ahead. For example, if the client does not recognize ahead of time that s/he is going to have to step over a section of buckled sidewalk, loss of balance may occur. Encourage clients to stay aware of outdoor surfaces when walking. The client can minimize loss of balance if constant attention is given to things in the environment that challenge the stability of the mobility device or make footing less than optimal. This is especially true for clients with impaired gait and gait accommodation strategies.

If the client feels that s/he is losing balance, STOP: Clients may have a tendency to step forward when they are losing their balance in the hope of regaining balance. However when walking outdoors the next step forward could challenge the client's balance even more and increase the chances of falling. Encourage clients to be aware of their balance at all times and, if they feel that they are losing their balance, they should stop immediately, regain balance, and then proceed. For more information on strategies for regaining balance, see the Balance Training chapter.

Grass, Cobblestone, Broken Sidewalk, Uneven Ground

Educate the client about the common guidelines for walking and moving on uneven surfaces (described previously). When advancing the assistive device, make sure that all points of the assistive device are stable. For example, if one walker leg is in a ditch, the walker becomes unstable and increases the client's risk of falling. If the client is advancing a foot, ensure that footing is secure. If a prosthetic leg is advanced, be sure that the client knows how to compensate visually for lack of sensation. If the assistive device or footing is not secure, the client repositions the assistive device and footing until stability is achieved. Once the assistive device is secure, the client can carefully take a step forward,

making sure that footing is secure. The client should adjust footing as needed.

Hills and Inclines

The client's gait pattern may need to be altered so that each sequenced step is halted rather than maintaining a smooth movement. This is done to control speed and balance. One example would be roll walker forward, STOP, advance one foot, STOP, advance other foot, STOP, advance walker, STOP. Practicing the correct methods should improve the client's skill level.

Curbs

Curbs can be major barriers for clients with impaired mobility. A common sequence of stepping up and down a curb is described below, but the recreational therapist needs to know the technique the physical therapist is using with the client, as techniques vary and clients need to have consistent techniques. See Device Specific Mobility below for information on specific techniques for going up and down curbs using a specific device.

Going up curbs: Walk close to the curb and place the assistive device on the sidewalk on top of the curb. Step up on the curb with the unaffected or stronger leg and then follow with the weaker leg. Clients with new impairments concentrate so much on walking that they often forget which leg goes first. A few mnemonics to help remember which leg goes up first are "Up with the good," "The good go to heaven," and "Up with the good things in life."

Going down curbs: Walk to the edge of the curb and place the assistive device in the street. Step down with affected or weaker leg and then follow with the stronger leg. Mnemonics to help remember which leg goes down first are "Down with the bad," "The bad go to hell," and "Down with the bad things in life."

Escalators

Discourage using escalators with clients who have balance problems or who use an assistive device. Encourage the use of elevators instead. Escalators require the client to have good reaction time. Trying to open or close devices on an escalator can be very difficult. If the client does lose his/her balance and fall, the injury could be severe. Escalator rails usually do not move at exactly the same pace as the footplates. This difference in speed may cause some clients to lose their balance.

Device Specific Mobility

Refer to the Wheelchair Mobility chapter for information on wheelchair mobility skills. Other mobility devices are described below.

Canes

Canes as walking sticks are the most commonly used mobility device (School of Public Health, 2004). While canes increase independence, they also can make fashion statements offering clients the opportunity to express personal flair. Canes are offered in a variety of woods, metals, and modern materials. Some are made of multiple elements. For example, the handle may be made of brass, while the shaft is made of plastic designed to look like a plaid fabric. Wooden canes can easily be painted and shellacked to meet the individual's style. (Sand off the original shellac first so that new paint sticks.)

Cane Components

Canes have four common components.

Cane Handles

There are many options for cane handles. The handle is the interface between the client and the walking aid so it needs to meet the needs of the client based on his/her abilities and impairments and the activities selected. To increase comfort, cane handles may be covered with foam or other materials that pad the handle. All handles should be evaluated for ease of cleaning. The primary types of handles are

Ball-topped handle: a sphere located on top of the shaft of the cane. This type of cane places too much pressure on the palm of the hand and forces the wrist into a dorsiflexion position. This cane is not a good choice to use when the client must support a lot of weight on the cane or use the cane for extended periods.

Crooked handle: A semicircular top formation of the cane. This type of cane is the one that is typically pictured in older movies and books. Because of the shape of the curved handle, the little finger and index finger must help grasp the cane in a partially flexed position while the two center fingers are flexed more. This is an unnatural position for the hand and can increase fine motor fatigue.

Pistol handle: A pistol handle is a cane grip that extends from the cane shaft at approximately a 90° angle. This type of handle is especially good for clients with weak grasps. Research has found that 85% of cane users find pistol handles to be more comfortable than crook-handles (Wylde, 2004). Pistol handles are also called "T" handles. Ergonomically this type of handle puts most of the pressure on the centerline of the palm, increasing pain, callusing, and nerve compression.

Cane Shaft

A number of materials are used for the shaft of a cane. In most cases, the material used in the shaft decides the weight of the cane. (The exception is with quad bases.) Aluminum shafts are usually the lightest with wood shafts being heavier. One of the added benefits of aluminum shafts is that many of them have height adjustment buttons to raise and lower the height of the cane. This not only allows a cane purchased at a local drug store to be fitted to a client, but it also allows the length of the cane to be adjusted based on the type of activity or the height of shoe heels.

Some cane shafts are foldable. Folding canes are made of many different materials, including wood.

There are two common accessories applied to cane shafts: wrist straps and cane holders. Wrist straps are straps clipped onto the shaft just below the handle. With the wrist strap around the wrist a person may "drop" the cane to use two hands for an activity and always have the cane close by. A cane holder is not actually a holder but a short 90° extension on the shaft (located below the handle) that can be used to lean the cane against a table or wall without the cane falling over.

Cane Bases

Canes have one-point or four-point bases of support that are located at the bottom of the cane shaft. Four-point bases provide more stability than single base canes. Some clients may use single point bases for many activities and choose to use quad bases for activities that challenge the client's balance. Standard aluminum canes with adjustable buttons allow the client to interchange a one-point base with a quad (four-point) base.

Single bases: Single base canes are also referred to as single point canes (SPC). Single point canes are effective in resolving minor instability and balance difficulties, as well as preventing falls. Minor instability and balance difficulties are common in the aging process.

Four-point bases: Four-point bases are referred to as quad canes. They provide increased stability compared to a single base cane. There are two types of quad canes, small-base quad canes (SBQC), also called narrow-base quad canes (NBQC), and wide-base quad canes (WBQC), also called large-base quad canes (LBQC). A SBQC has a smaller base, thus challenging the client's balance more than a LBQC. The shaft of the cane is to the side of the base, not centered on the base. Therefore, the bases on the quad cane are right and left sensitive. The base must jut out away from the client. The base of a quad cane is adjustable. It can rotate to the left or the right so that it can be properly adjusted for the client.

Cane Tips

Cane tips are the unit that makes contact with the ground. They are selected based on the type of traction needed. There are many choices and the selection is made by considering the client's abilities and the activity.

Most cane tips are removable, allowing replacement of worn tips or the placement of specialized tips. An easy way to remove an old cane tip is to place it in a lightly closed door and twist and pull the cane.

Icy conditions often cause clients to be homebound. Canes with rubber tips do not provide a good base of support on icy or snow-covered surfaces. Specialized ice attachments are available, most having retractable spikes so that the cane may be used in an icy parking lot and (with the spikes retracted) inside also.

A tripod base is available that fits most canes. A tripod tip is a rubber tip with three "toes" extending two inches from the bottom of the tip with rubber "webs" between the toes. The toes are usually located at four, eight and twelve o'clock (if placed on a clock face). Tripod tips are helpful for walking on soft surfaces, such as dirt trails or lawns. Canes with a tripod base can stand upright without being held or propped against something.

Clients should have extra tips available, especially while traveling, as smaller towns may not have places to purchase new tips.

Cane tips must be replaced when they are worn because they will not grip the surface well, thus increasing the risk of falling. Worn cane tips will also make the cane shorter, therefore being a less effective support.

Weight

The rule of thumb is to ensure that the cane selected for use is light enough that the client will not have difficulty lifting the device even when s/he is experiencing mild fatigue and that it is strong enough to support the weight of the client. Therapists also consider the weight of the cane in relation to its use. For example, a client who was living in a tough neighborhood feared being attacked by local gangs. He was a young, strong client who had a below-knee amputation. The physical therapist prescribed a heavy-duty black metal cane with a 500-pound weight capacity weighing approximately two pounds. That was above the weight normally prescribed since a standard aluminum cane has a 250-350 pound weight capacity and weighs approximately one pound. The client possessed the strength to easily tolerate and manipulate the increased weight of the cane. The cane was specifically chosen to function as a supportive ambulation device, as well as double as a self-defense device should such a situation arise. Part of recreational therapy treatment involved teaching the client self-defense techniques using the cane to decrease anxiety and increase confidence related to participating in community activities.

Fitting the Device

Unless the client uses the cane for a limited time during recovery, the expectation should be that the client will have two or more canes or multiple interchangeable parts for use during different types of activities.

The handle of the cane should be level with the client's hip joint. Some prescribing guidelines suggest that having the top of the cane reach the client's wrist when the arm is at his/her side is a better measurement. To know where to cut a wooden cane for proper length, turn it upside down so that the rounded cane handle rests on the floor and make a mark on the cane where it reaches the client's wrist and then cut it at that mark. Depending on the type of activity, the cane may need to be longer. For instance, if the client is hiking over hilly ground, the height of the cane handle may need to be six inches above the client's elbow to provide support going downhill. Canes that are adjustable for length may be good choices in this situation. If the client hikes above the tree line, aluminum canes (usually the type of cane that is adjustable) may not be the safest choice, as the cane may become a lightning rod during a thunderstorm.

Canes that are too long increase stress on the shoulder and arm causing pain and decreasing endurance. Canes that are too short increase strain on the wrist and the back. Properly fitted canes for basic walking place the client's elbow at a 15-20° angle. When selecting the handle type, it is important that the handle fits the contour of the client's hand. A larger handle grip may be more comfortable for clients with arthritis.

Authorization

A prescription is not required for canes, but clients are encouraged to get assistance from a therapist or physician when selecting canes.

Use

The cane is usually placed on the opposite side of an injury or weakened side. One exception is when the client has a muscular or nerve problem whereby the muscles just stop working properly in mid step or without warning. Then a cane on the same side as the problem limb becomes a tool to catch the step or stop the client from falling over.

Benefits

Canes increase a client's options and independence by augmenting balance. Because canes are relatively inexpensive and interchangeable, using a cane provides a client with the ability to custom fit the cane to the activity.

Design Challenges

Almost all canes used today lack design components based on solid ergonomic principles (Diez, 1997). Cane handles using ergonomic principles would meet the following requirements: They would allow the wrist to remain in a near neutral position (straight wrist with minimal flexion, extension, or deviation). There are two benefits to using a cane with the wrist in a near neutral position: grip strength is greater in a neutral position versus a flexed position and risk of developing carpal tunnel syndrome is reduced. They are cylindrical in shape and large enough in size to allow the surface pressure exerted on the hand and fingers to be more widely distributed.

Two other ergonomic challenges posed by most of the canes available today are related to repetition and vibration. Repetitive damage may occur as the wrist and fingers repetitively bend to move the cane forward during walking. Vibration and jarring occur each time the client places the tip on the ground during the gait cycle. With instruction, clients can minimize these actions to reduce long-term damage to tissue and joints.

Treatment Direction

The recreational therapist participates in several aspects of treatment:

- Teach clients how to use a cane when walking over different surfaces (e.g., uneven outdoor surfaces).
- Contribute to the selection of an appropriate cane length based on activity or heel size.
- Assist clients in identifying appropriate cane tips to maximize safety in specific tasks.
- Help clients problem solve for proper cane placement when it is not in use. For example, where and how to place a cane when sitting at a table at a restaurant or on a city bus.

Walking

During the gait cycle the client places full weight on the "good" leg. During the weight acceptance and limb support phase of the gait cycle on the weaker side the client distributes his/her weight between the weaker leg and the cane. To simplify this description, tell the seated client to place the cane in the hand that is on his/her stronger side (If the client has weakness in his left leg, he is to hold the cane in his right hand). Push up from the chair to get into a standing position. Advance the cane 12-18" in front of the current position of the stronger leg. Step forward with the leg opposite the cane until the foot is directly across from the cane. The cane and the opposite foot are now the same distance in front of the back foot. Now advance the leg on the cane side. The leg should step forward past the cane and the opposite leg. Repeat the stepping process.

Steps or Curbs

Use a handrail if it is available. To help remember which foot to lead with when going up and down stairs you can remember the following saying, "Up with the good, down with the bad."

To go up steps or up a curb: Client holds the cane in the hand that correlates with his/her stronger side. Step up with the strong leg onto the first step. Then bring the cane up onto the first step. Now step up with the weaker leg onto the first step. Both legs and the cane are all on the first step. This is called a "step to step" pattern, rather than a "step over step" pattern. Repeat the pattern for the rest of the steps.

To go down steps or down a curb: Client holds the cane in the hand that correlates with his/her stronger side. Lower the cane down onto the first step. Lower the weaker leg down onto the first step. Lower the stronger leg down onto the first step. Repeat the pattern for the rest of the steps.

Crutches

There are three types of crutches: axillary crutches, forearm crutches, and platform crutches. Axillary crutches are the most common crutch. People who have a minimal injury, such as a cast on one leg or a sprained ankle, and are required to maintain weight-bearing precautions are typically prescribed axillary crutches. The crutches tuck underneath the arms and there is a bar for each hand to hold. The overall height and the hand bar height are both adjustable. Forearm crutches (also called Lofstrand crutches) have a cuff that slips onto the top of the forearm and horizontal handles for the client to hold. Forearm crutches are best for clients who have moderate problems with stability and generalized weakness throughout the lower extremities. Platform crutches (also known as triceps crutches) are similar to forearm crutches while providing more support because they have an additional upper cuff.

Weight

Axillary crutches weigh about three pounds a pair. Forearm crutches weigh about five pounds a pair. Platform crutches weigh about six pounds.

Fitting

Axillary crutches: Ask the client to stand normally (feet shoulder width apart) and lift his/her arms out to the side. Adjust the crutch so that it sits about two inches below the client's armpit (axilla) when the base of the crutch is six to eight inches out from the client's foot. The hand bar is then adjusted so that the elbow is bent 30° when the crutches are in line with the client's feet. An easy way to set this angle is to adjust the hand bar so that it is at the height of the client's wrist.

Forearm crutches: This crutch should allow the client to flex his/her elbow 15-30°. The increased flexion allows the arm to bear greater weight. Ask the client to stand in a normal position (feet shoulder-width apart). Place the base of the crutch two to four inches outside the foot and six inches forward of the foot. Adjust the cuff so that it sits 1-1½ inches below the back of the elbow.

Platform crutches: Ask the client to stand normally (feet shoulder-width apart). Place the base of the crutch two to four inches outside the foot and six inches forward of the foot. Adjust the upper cuff so that it sits about two inches below the skin fold of the armpit. Adjust the lower cuff so that it sits 1-1½ inches below the back of the elbow.

Authorization

Simple axillary crutches may be purchased from local stores. A prescription is needed for forearm or platform crutches.

Use

There are various ways to walk with crutches (crutch gaits). There are also specific techniques for standing and sitting with crutches and going up and down steps and curbs. See the discussions below.

Benefits

Crutches provide support for movement.

Treatment Direction

Recreational therapists assess the client's ability to use crutches in a community setting and in functional tasks. They provide necessary training and recommendations (e.g., in a crowded community environment the crutches may not offer the client enough support to maintain balance, so a walker is recommended). Recreational therapists also make recommendations for crutch accessories, such as a crutch bag.

Crutch Gaits

There are six different crutch gaits. They are sorted in this discussion from lowest to highest energy requirements. A repertoire of crutch gaits is helpful because the client can use a slow or fast gait to meet the demands of a situation. Also, each crutch gait uses different muscles so it allows the client to rest or exercise muscles as needed.

Drag-to gait: This gait is used when the client has very limited control or weight-bearing ability in the lower extremity and good to strong strength in the upper extremity. The client begins by placing both crutches in front of the body. The crutches are slightly wider than shoulder width and placed between one and two feet in front of the client. The client leans into the crutches, placing most of his/her body weight on the crutches. The client then drags his/her feet forward until they are between the crutches.

Four-point alternate gait: This is a low and stable gait that is used when a client is able to move each leg separately and bear considerable weight on each leg. Advance the right crutch forward to a comfortable reach (approximately 12"). Advance the left foot forward so that it is even with the right crutch. Advance the left crutch forward past the right crutch (about 12"). Advance the right foot so that it is even with the left crutch.

Two-point alternate gait: This gait is a little faster than the four-point gait and requires a bit more balance. Simultaneously advance the right crutch and the left leg a comfortable distance (about 12"). Simultaneously advance the left crutch and the right leg a comfortable distance.

Three-point alternate gait: This is a fairly quick gait that requires significant upper arm and body strength because the arms bear the majority of the weight. It also requires a moderate amount of balance. Simultaneously advance both crutches and the weaker leg a comfortable distance. The crutches and the weaker leg should be at the same distance in front of the back leg when landing. Next, advance the strong leg so that it is even with the crutches and the weaker leg. To do this, most of the weight is born through the arms

Swing-to-gait: This gait is faster than the three-point gait and it requires even more upper arm and body strength to support the entire body weight. This is a common crutch gait for axillary crutches. Weight bear on the good leg(s). Simultaneously advance both crutches forward a comfortable distance (about 12"). Place all of the body weight through the crutches by leaning forward and then swinging both legs simultaneously forward to meet the crutches.

Swing-through-gait: This is the fastest crutch gait and is commonly used by runners. Weight bear on the good leg(s). Simultaneously advance both crutches forward a comfortable distance. (Runners typically extend this reach as far as possible.) Place all of the body weight through the crutches by leaning forward

and then swinging both legs simultaneously past the crutches. Quickly advance the crutches past the landing area of the feet.

Sit to Stand

Scoot to the edge of the seat. Place both crutches in the hand that correlates with the stronger leg. Use the chair armrests to push up to a standing position. Move crutches to both hands.

Stand to Sit

Back up until the chair touches the back of the legs. Transfer crutches into the hand the correlates with the stronger leg. Stretch injured leg forward so that the knee is straightened and the heel rests on the floor. Reach back for the chair armrests for support to sit back into the chair.

Stairs and Curbs

Going up and down stairs and curbs with crutches demands a lot of strength and balance. There are several possible techniques besides the ones described here. The recreational therapist, like all health professionals, consults the other members of the treatment team to identify which technique is currently recommended for the client.

Non-weight bearing on one leg: If a client is non-weight bearing on one leg, it is dangerous to go up and down steps. It is recommended that alternatives be identified (e.g., elevator, bumping up the stairs on the buttocks). To go up curbs, push up on the crutches to hop up onto the curb on the strong leg and then bring up the crutches. To go down a curb, lower the crutches down the curb and then hop down the curb on the strong leg.

To go up stairs or a curb, weight bearing on both legs: Step onto the first step with the strongest leg. Then, step onto the step with the weaker leg and both crutches simultaneously. Repeat this pattern to the top of the stairs. If there is a handrail, tuck both crutches underneath one arm and use the handrail like it is the other crutch.

To go down the stairs or a curb without a handrail, weight bearing on both legs: Simultaneously lower the weaker leg and both crutches down onto the first step. Then lower the stronger leg onto the first step. Repeat this pattern to the bottom of the stairs.

Walkers

There are two types of walkers: standard walkers and rolling walkers. There are some variations that may be used in special cases, as discussed below. Walkers also have several attachments that make them easier for the client to use.

Standard Walkers

Standard walkers have four legs and feet. On the bottom of each foot is a rubber tip that keeps the walker from slipping when the client puts weight on it. Most standard walkers fold but some do not (each side folds into the center so that the walker becomes flat). There are handgrips on each side of the walker to help the client grip the walker. They are usually made out of foam, rubber, or plastic. Standard walkers are used when a client needs bilateral upper extremity support to advance a lower extremity. Some examples: a client who has weight-bearing parameters, a client who has had a lower extremity amputation using the walker to hop on one leg, or a client learning to walk with a lower extremity prosthesis where there is difficulty bearing weight through the prosthetic limb.

The hemi-walker is a variant on a standard walker. It is a small, four-legged device that is held with one hand to the side of the body. It is different from a quad cane because all four legs originate from the top of the device rather than just four small feet on a bottom platform. It provides more support than a quad cane and less support than a standard walker. Hemi-walkers are commonly used by clients who have paralysis of one upper extremity and require an assistive device that provides more support than a cane to walk.

Rolling Walkers

Rolling walkers are different from standard walkers because they have small wheels on the front or the front and back of the walker. Rolling walkers are used with clients who do not have weight-bearing precautions or impairments. They are commonly used with clients who have endurance and strength issues, such as cardiopulmonary issues, because they do not require the client to lift the walker to advance it like a standard walker.

Reverse Walkers

Reverse walkers are used for pediatrics. It looks like the child is using the walker backwards (it goes around the child's back). They typically have upright handles and automatic brakes that engage when the child puts pressure on the handgrips. The weight of the device is to the back of the child. Therefore it encourages the child to stand upright.

Eva walkers

Eva walkers provide maximum walking support. They are much larger than a typical walker and they are used only in a rehabilitation setting as a device for gait training. They are not sent home with the client. They have a large pad that wraps around the front and sides of the walker for the client to rest his/her forearms. There are also two upright handles for the client to grasp. The Eva walker has a wider and stronger base than a traditional walker.

Seated Walkers

There is a type of rolling walker that is geared towards the active adult. It is modern and sleek and comes in various colors. The usual features include a basket on the front, swivel wheels for increased agility, larger wheels than a typical walker with pneumatic or solid rubber tires to help traverse uneven community surfaces, hand brakes, and a built-in seat that flips down when the client needs to take a rest. It is commonly prescribed for clients who are able to walk consecutive short community distances (walk 150', rest for 10 minutes, walk another 150', and so on), need the security of having an immediate place to sit and rest, have the cognitive ability to operate and manipulate the device safely (put brakes on before sitting), and engage in community tasks requiring longer distances.

Walker Attachments

Glides: Glides are small ski-like attachments that hook onto the bottom of the back feet of a rolling walker, only when the back feet do not have wheels. It keeps the back feet from catching on the floor (rubber feet on tile floors sometimes stick and catch) and keeps the walker from squeaking when the back feet rub against the floor. If the walker does not have glides and it is squeaking and catching, get two small Dixie cups from the water fountain and set each back walker foot inside a cup. It will stop squeaking and glide across a tiled floor. This is not a substitute for glides, but it works in a pinch. Another idea is to put a slit into a standard tennis ball and set each of the back feet of the walker inside a ball.

Platform: A platform attachment is a metal rod that attaches to the side of a walker. On top of the rod is a forearm rest with an upright handle to the front of it for the client to hold. A Velcro strap wraps around the forearm to hold it on the forearm rest. These are commonly used for gait training with rolling walkers. They are also used for clients who have enough lower extremity strength to walk, have limited mobility or strength in one or both upper extremities, and require bilateral upper extremity support for balance.

Swing seat or foldaway seat: Plastic or canvas seats are available for walkers. They hook to the four legs so that the client can sit "inside" the walker. Therapists must be careful when making this recommendation because the seat is not very stable (especially on rolling walkers) and it can be a tight squeeze to get into and out of the seat, possibly putting the client at an increased risk of falling. It is a good thing to have one in the equipment closet and to evaluate the client's ability to safely use this product before recommending it. If a client is fearful about not being able to find a place to sit and rest, consider the seated rolling walker or teach the client how to plan for and recognize resting areas in the community (see the Energy Conservation Training chapter).

Baskets and pouches: There are a variety of baskets and pouches that can be attached to the front or side of a walker. These are very important attachments so that the client does not attempt to carry items while also trying to hold the walker. They are not covered by insurance companies because they are not seen as medically necessary. Many clients are on a tight budget and find it difficult to spend $25.00 for a basket. Some hospitals have volunteers who make pouches out of cotton fabric and give them to the clients for free. Clients can also use a wicker bike basket and tie it to the front of the walker with heavy string. Clients who are going to use baskets or pouches must be warned that putting too much weight in the pouches or basket will affect the client's safety and performance. Too much weight in the front basket can cause the walker to tip forward and, if it is a standard walker, advancing the walker can become difficult because of the extra weight. Transporting extra weight using a standard walker increases energy demands. This could result in decreased walking distance, such as the client who was able to walk 150' without a basket but is able to walk only 100' with five pounds of items in pouches. If clients need to carry bulky items, such as transporting laundry from one room to another or carrying several grocery items

from the car into the house, the therapist may consider the use of a backpack. Like the swing seat, the client's ability to use a backpack and to determine an appropriate weight limit must be assessed. Other ideas for transporting items include the use of a fanny pack (instead of a pocket book) and an apron with pockets.

Weight

A standard or rolling walker weighs approximately six pounds. A hemi-walker weighs about four pounds. An Eva walker weighs about 40 pounds. A seated rolling walker weighs about 17 pounds.

Fitting

Most walkers are height adjustable in one-inch increments. The height of the walker, just like the cane, should allow a 15-30° elbow flexion. A simple way to achieve this it to have the client place his/her hands down by his/her side and then adjust the walker height so that the walker handle comes up to the client's wrist. The width of the walker varies depending on the size of the person. A common width for an adult walker is 20" and a youth walker is 16". With hands down by the side, each walker handle should meet the client's hands. It should not adduct or abduct the shoulder.

Authorization

Walkers can be purchased from local stores. A letter of medical necessity is needed for insurance reimbursement.

Use

There are different techniques for walking with a standard walker, a hemi-walker, and a rolling walker. There are also specific techniques for going up and down curbs and stairs.

Benefits

Walkers offer bilateral upper extremity support for people who have trouble with their balance. The variety of walkers offers the therapist flexibility in choosing an appropriate device to best suit the client's needs in real-life tasks.

Design Challenges

Walkers are pretty basic pieces of equipment and there aren't many fancy components to confuse the client. Simple is sometimes a good thing, especially for people who have cognitive impairments. The equipment companies have answered the call to develop walkers that are more functional in life activities by providing additions like folding seats, baskets, pouches, and brakes. They are lightweight and relatively inexpensive.

Treatment Direction

Recreational therapists evaluate a client's ability to use a walker in a community setting, on uneven outdoor and indoor surfaces, and while doing functional tasks, such as carrying items and transferring. They make recommendations for types of walkers, walker accessories, changes in technique, and ways to overcome physical barriers. For example, if a client lives alone on the second floor of a duplex and lacks the ability to carry the walker up and down the steps, how is he going to be able to take it out with him to go shopping? Is it possible for the client to get two walkers, one for inside the apartment and one to keep by the front door? Is it safe to keep it at the front door? Just because a device is functional in a clinic does not mean that it fully meets the needs of the client in real life.

If the recreational therapist is working with a client who was very active in the community, has a long-term or progressive disability, and is now anxious that a basic rolling walker may potentially limit community participation because he may not be able to find a seat or transport items, the recreational therapist should consult with the physical therapist and explore the possibility of prescribing a seated rolling walker.

Walking

Using a standard walker: Advance the walker a comfortable arm's length and then step forward with the weaker leg first and then the stronger leg following. Advance the walker forward, and then step again. Do not step into the walker. The client's feet should be next to the back feet of the walker after the step is complete. Stepping too far into the walker will cause the client to lose balance. Advancing the walker too far ahead and taking small steps will cause the client to lean forward and not stand upright.

Using a hemi-walker: The hemi-walker is in the hand on the stronger side. During the gait cycle the client places full weight on the "good" leg. During the weight acceptance and limb support phase of the gait cycle on the weaker side the client distributes his/her weight between the weaker leg and the hemi-walker.

Using a rolling walker: There are two ways to use a rolling walker.

Continual pushing technique: The client continually pushes the walker forward while stepping (a smooth walk). The client should maintain an upright position. The client should not step too far into the walker. (See standard walker use above.) Clients who use this technique need to be very aware of their surroundings so they can note changes in surfaces and lift the walker appropriately to transition from one surface to another. For example, small walker wheels tend to get stuck easily on raised sidewalk blocks, pebbles, etc.

Halting technique: Clients who do not have the awareness discussed above (whether from a cognitive impairment or general anxiety with the task) should be instructed to push the walker forward until the back legs of the walker are just past the client's feet. Halt the walker and then step forward. Push the walker forward again, step again, and so on. This decreases the chances of the walker becoming stuck on an object and the client stepping before the walker has fully advanced, causing the client to step too far into the walker and risk loss of balance and a fall. This is also a good technique for clients to use when they are walking outside on uneven surfaces. For example, a rolling walker does not roll easily on grassy surfaces. So if a client wants to walk across a patch of grass, s/he will need to roll the walker slowly forward in halting motions as previously described. In some instances, the client may need to pick up the walker and advance it like a standard walker. The therapist should be aware of the added stress that lifting the walker puts on the client and assess whether or not this is an appropriate technique. Things to watch for include shortness of breath, loss of balance, and increased blood pressure or heart rate. The halting technique is also good for going up and down inclines because, when s/he is going down a hill, the client sometimes feels that the walker is starting to get away from him/her and, when going up the hill, the client often begins to push the walker too far forward and begins to lean forward as if pushing the walker up the hill. A halting technique will minimize these occurrences and increase the client's safety.

Curbs

To go up a curb: Move up as close as possible to the curb. Lift the walker up onto the sidewalk. While holding onto the walker handgrips, step up with the stronger leg onto the sidewalk and then lift the weaker leg onto the sidewalk.

To go down a curb: Move to the edge of the curb. Lower the walker down into the street. While holding onto the walker handgrips, step down to the street with the weaker leg and then lower the stronger leg.

Stairs

It is not recommended for a client to go up and down stairs with a walker, but it is not impossible. Clients can be taught to use the folded walker like a crutch for going up and down stairs. This requires a moderate amount of skill, strength, and balance and is not a general recommendation. Therefore, if the client desires to learn this skill or if it is foreseen that this skill will be needed to access the client's real-life environment, the recreational therapist should consult with the physical therapist to decide who will instruct the client in this skill after determining the best technique to use.

Outcomes and Documentation

Mobility related to walking and gait training improves physical processes, such as strength, balance, and coordination, as well as functional ambulation. Walking better can improve activity engagement, life participation, and independence, as well as decrease risks for conditions associated with sedentary behavior. Increased walking ability, as well as ability to overcome architectural obstacles, including curbs, stairs, and uneven surfaces, can also minimize access issues.

In the ICF, walking skills are part of d4 Mobility (e.g., d450 Walking, d455 Moving Around, d460 Moving Around in Different Locations, d465 Moving Around Using Equipment). Recreational therapists might additionally use other ICF codes related to walking and conditioning (e.g., b4 Functions of the Cardiovascular, Hematological, Immunological, and Respiratory Systems, b7 Neuromusculoskeletal and Movement-Related Functions).

Common criteria used in mobility charting include distance, time, equipment utilized, amount of assistance needed, cueing, type and frequency of cueing, type of surface (smooth, uneven, paved, gravel, grassy), description of environment (e.g., crowded, noisy), and abnormal gait patterns observed. Recreational therapists also document the location of mobility and the situation or task in which

functional mobility is challenged, as different locations and activities challenge different mobility skill sets and introduce new challenges. For example, a leisurely walk at the park doesn't challenge reactive movements as much as a game of laser tag.

Challenging mobility application skills in various environments and tasks (as appropriate) is necessary for skill development, as well as building mobility confidence and problem-solving skills. Recreational therapists also document mobility related skills, such as the client's ability to don and doff mobility devices like an ankle foot orthosis, utilize mobility equipment appropriately, employ learned mobility techniques, and problem solve for new mobility challenges, such as slippery surfaces or a curb that is higher in the community than the practice curb in the therapy gym.

References

burlingame, j. (2001). *Idyll Arbor's therapy dictionary*, (2nd ed.). Ravensdale, WA: Idyll Arbor, Inc.

Diez, M. (1997). Ergonomic projects. http://ergo.human.cornell,edu/ErogPROJECTS/97/diez.htm.

Patla, A. E. (1997). Understanding the roles of vision in the control of human locomotion. *Gait and Posture, 5*:54-69.

Rose, D. (2003). *Fallproof! A comprehensive balance and mobility training program*. Champaign, IL: Human Kinetics.

School of Public Health. (2004). *Take a step towards independence: Canes*. University of Buffalo, New York. http://cat.buffalo.edu/newsletters/canes.php.

Wylde, M. (2004). Referenced in product catalog. *The house of canes and walking sticks*. www.houseofcanes.com.

Appendix A: Fifty-Foot Walk Test

The *Fifty-Foot Walk Test* is a fairly simple test that can be used in the hospital or in the community. The test takes three measurements: (1) the speed the client walks normally (called the "preferred speed"), (2) the speed that the client walks when asked to walk fast, and (3) the number of steps the client uses to walk 50'. The therapist needs three supplies: (1) a stopwatch, (2) something to mark the floor or sidewalk with, and (3) a measuring tape that is at least 100' long.

The therapist measures the amount of time it takes the client to walk 50'. To measure the client's actual speed and not include the length of time it takes the client to start and stop, the therapist needs to have a seventy-foot long, straight, and flat surface. If the therapist is using chalk to mark the sidewalk four marks are made:

- One at zero (the starting point)
- One at 10' (the point to start timing the client and counting the number of steps taken by the client)
- One at 60' (the point to stop timing the client and stop counting the number of steps taken by the client)
- One at 70' (the finishing point)

Standing near the zero mark, the therapist lets the client know that s/he wants to watch the client walk from the starting line to the finish line (the mark at 70'). This will be done twice, once at the walking speed that is comfortable for the client and once at a fast walk. The therapist makes sure that the client knows where the "start" and "finish" lines are located. The marks at 10' and 60' are not mentioned.

As the client is walking, the therapist walks just slightly behind the client (at about four o'clock or eight o'clock). This ensures that the client is choosing his/her own pace and not attempting to match the pace of the therapist. It is also provides a better vantage point for the therapist to count the number of steps the client takes between the 10' and 60' markers.

Dividing 50' by the number of steps the client took determines the client's stride length. To time the client's speed (both the preferred and fast) the therapist starts the stopwatch when the client passes the 10' mark and stops the stopwatch when the client passes the 60' mark. The client's score is reported in feet per second and the average number of feet (and inches) per stride. The norms reported by Bohannon (1997) were taken from a relatively small sample and were obtained in a clinical setting and not in the community. These norms are found in Table 25.

Table 25: Reference Values for the Fifty-Foot Walk Test

Ages 60-69
Preferred Speed
Men 4.46 feet per second
Women 4.25 feet per second

Maximum (Fast) Speed
Men 6.34 feet per second
Women 5.82 feet per second

Ages 70-79
Preferred Speed
Men 4.36 feet per second
Women 4.17 feet per second

Maximum (Fast) Speed
Men 6.82 feet per second
Women 5.74 feet per second

From Rose (2003), p. 80.

These norms provide the therapist with a benchmark, but further study is needed by recreational therapists to establish norms when using an outdoor course with a broader range of ages. An unexpected finding of these numbers is that men in their seventies generally moved faster than men in their sixties. This anomaly is probably due to the relatively small sample size.

In the standard testing situation the therapist does not talk to the client during the time the client is walking and being timed. A modification to the *Fifty-Foot Walk Test* is called the *Walkie-Talkie Test*. This test measures whether the client can walk and talk at the same time. The functional ability to walk and talk at the same time is a mental function called "dividing attention" (b1402 Dividing Attention). As the therapist walks with the client along the 70-foot-long course the therapist asks the client an open-ended question that cannot be answered with either a "yes" or "no." If the client stops to answer the question, the client receives a "positive" score on this test. A positive score means that the client needs assistance and may not be ready to enter groups or activities that require the client to perform multiple tasks. If the client is able to both walk and answer the question at the same time, the client has a "negative" score. This means that the client is likely to function appropriately in tasks that require divided attention.

As a side note, the speed that a client walks may or may not be an issue affecting recreation, leisure, and community activities. Additionally, walking speed may be slowed purposely for safety. For example, a client who uses a walking device and/or has poor balance desires to water her flowers in the backyard. In this scenario, the client may be instructed to purposely slow down her walking speed to decrease her risk of falls and to increase attention to the placement of the walking device with each step to make sure it is stable. In another example, a client who walks at a slow speed and needs to cross a busy road with a fast traffic light may need to work on increasing walking speed to ensure a timely street crossing. Consequently, therapists are not only aware of the distance, device, and level of assistance for walking, but also the speed of walking as it pertains to a client's safety and optimal task participation.

References

Bohannon, R. W. (1997). Comfortable and maximum walking speed of adults aged 20-79 years: reference values and determinants. *Age and Aging, 26*:15-19.

Rose, D. (2003). *Fallproof! A comprehensive balance and mobility training program*. Champaign, IL: Human Kinetics.

51. Wheelchair Mobility

Heather R. Porter

It is estimated that 1.6 million people living outside of institutions in the United States use a wheelchair for mobility; with 1.5 million using manual wheelchairs (majority are older adults — 57.5%) and the remaining using power wheelchairs (majority are children, adolescents, and adults — 69.7%) (Kaye, Taewoon, & LaPlante, 2002). The leading conditions associated with wheelchair and scooter use include stroke, arthritis, multiple sclerosis, lower extremity amputation, paraplegia, other orthopedic impairment of the lower extremities, heart disease, cerebral palsy, rheumatoid arthritis, and diabetes (Kaye et al., 2002). A significant number (93%) of individuals who use a wheelchair report some form of activity limitation, of which 66.1% report that the limitation is severe enough to render them unable to perform major life activities (Kaye et al., 2002). Although there are many factors that limit activity, wheelchair skills training has been identified as one of the major factors that make "the difference between dependence and independence in daily life [and] is therefore a vital part of the rehabilitation process" (Kilkens et al., 2004).

Moving from point A to point B in a wheelchair is more than the ability to roll forward or backward. Examples of wheelchair mobility skills required to move around in various environments include:

Basic maneuvering: Stopping; turning; ascending and descending ramps, curbs, and curb cuts; moving over uneven terrain; moving through elevators, doors, and doorways.

Advanced skills for maneuvering: Stairs, escalators, slopes that exceed 1:12 grade. ADA accessibility guidelines limit ramps to a one-inch rise for every 12 inches of length. Many ramps are steeper than that and require advanced skills for going up and down.

Weather-related challenges: Heavy rain, snow, ice, extreme wind.

Accessing pubic mobility devices: Community scooters, such as the ones found at grocery stores for clients using mobility devices, and public transportation (bus, train, taxi).

Transfers into public transportation: Using low pivot transfers, stand-pivot transfers, one-man vs. two-man transfers. This may include using a step-up block or a transfer board and knowing how to accommodate for low car ceilings and door handles that are in the way.

Changing the wheelchair configuration: Opening and closing the wheelchair, removing or folding footrests, removing armrests, and removing support braces.

Special precautions: Head-in-first vs. buttocks-in-first car transfers with trunk flexion precautions, such as after hip replacement surgery, modifying the height of the vehicle seat to meet total hip replacement or other precautions.

Strapping and tie down: Procedures for securing the wheelchair in a vehicle with the client still in the wheelchair or securing the client into one of the seats of the vehicle without the wheelchair.

Indications

Wheelchair mobility skills training is appropriate for clients who will be using a wheelchair or scooter. ICF codes in d4 Mobility indicate a need for using a wheelchair. If there is a deficit in d465 Moving Around Using Equipment, teaching wheelchair mobility skills is indicated. Other ICF codes that might trigger this training include d175 Solving Problems, d177 Making Decisions, d410 Changing Basic Body Position, d420 Transferring Oneself, d470 Using Transportation, and d660 Assisting Others.

Contraindications

The techniques described below, although common, are not universal. Be sure to modify techniques as needed according to client or caregiver needs and abilities, to eliminate or reduce the risk of injury or harm. If the recreational therapist is teaching wheelchair mobility skills to a caregiver, ask the caregiver if s/he has any physical limitations that would be a contraindication for assisting the client with wheelchair mobility, such as lifting restrictions, cardiac restrictions, feeling uncomfortable about helping, etc. If the caregiver has limitations, the therapist should not, under any circumstances, allow the caregiver to perform wheelchair mobility skills that are contraindicated due to a limitation.

The therapist must decide if s/he should train the caregiver on how to instruct another and transfer the training task to the caregiver or schedule another training session with the newly identified caregiver. This decision is based on availability of the other caregiver and time constraints, as well as other factors, such as the caregiver's ability to clearly communicate and teach the required skills.

A little preliminary work helps avoid this type of situation. Contact the caregiver ahead of time to discuss availability and limitations. Document conversations with caregivers and statements of health for the rest of the treatment team to consider. A sample chart note might be "Mary Smith, the client's daughter, notified via phone about the wheelchair mobility skills training session scheduled for 6/28 at 4 P.M. Daughter states no restrictions or limitations to perform skills, and stated plan to attend the session." or "Mary Smith, client's daughter, attended 4/12 RT treatment session for wheelchair skills training. Upon questioning, daughter reported a history of lower back pain but reported no limitations or restrictions. Daughter was asked to get clearance from primary physician to perform physical tasks without restrictions, otherwise another caregiver will need to be identified to assist client with wheelchair skills. Daughter's availability for training is minimal; therefore daughter instructed on techniques but not allowed to perform the task. Daughter scheduled to attend 4/18 session for community integration training with client. If daughter receives clearance further training will occur at that time."

Protocols and Processes

Prior to initiating wheelchair mobility skills training, the recreational therapist collaborates with the other primary therapists (PT, OT) to provide a consistent message, technique, and approach. At evaluation, the therapist establishes the client and/or caregiver's baseline of skills and knowledge regarding wheelchair mobility and evaluates, through a discussion, the specific mobility obstacles and challenges faced in the client's real-life environment and activities. This usually involves gathering performance information and then meeting with the client to ask questions and evaluate skills.

When conducting the assessment, it is important to evaluate the appropriateness of the wheelchair that the client is currently using (see Appendix A). It is not uncommon for clients in a rehabilitation hospital to receive a standard inpatient wheelchair for moving from therapy to therapy. The type of wheelchair being used in the facility may not be the type of wheelchair that the client will be issued when going home. For example, the client may use a standard cross-brace wheelchair in the hospital while a rigid wheelchair is on order for use after discharge. It is also not uncommon for hospital wheelchairs to have "problems" that hinder wheelchair skills training. For instance, some facilities bolt the anti-tipper bars onto the wheelchairs so that they do not fall off or get misplaced. This might work well for the hospital setting, but it is not appropriate for community and home life. A client will not bolt his/her anti-tipper bars at home. In fact, the client and caregiver will need to flip up or remove the anti-tipper bars to perform some of the wheelchair skills, such as bumping the wheelchair up a curb.

Another common problem with standard hospital wheelchairs is that they are often a heavy-duty style (about 40-50 pounds) so that they last while clients are often prescribed a lightweight wheelchair for discharge (about 28-36 pounds). The added weight of a heavy-duty wheelchair can be especially difficult for older caregivers. For example, lifting a 50-pound wheelchair into a car trunk is more difficult than lifting a 28-pound wheelchair. There are also problems if the leg rests and armrests are part of the wheelchair frame (can't be removed or are bolted onto the wheelchair), rigid backrests are bolted to the frame preventing the wheelchair from folding, and old, heavy-duty wheelchairs have not been folded in years so that they seem to be almost rusted in a fixed position.

Consequently, it can be very frustrating, when the therapist is ready to evaluate or teach a client or caregiver how to perform a specific wheelchair skill, to discover that the wheelchair the client is currently using is not appropriate. Prior to conducting a wheelchair mobility session, be sure to first evaluate the appropriateness of the wheelchair. Make sure it is similar to the type of wheelchair that the client is going to use after discharge and that all of the parts of the wheelchair are working. If it is not appropriate, identify another wheelchair to use for the session. This can typically be accomplished by talking to the physical therapist or wheelchair room mechanic to borrow a wheelchair that is appropriate for the training session.

In the wheelchair mobility training sessions, the recreational therapist focuses on:

- Wheelchair mobility techniques.
- Maximizing independence and overall mental, emotional, physical, and social health related to wheelchair mobility.
- Awareness of, and problem solving for, social and physical barriers that can facilitate or hinder mobility.
- Safety precautions to reduce risk of harm or injury from impaired performance of mobility skills.
- Improving mobility task performance to increase self-esteem, confidence, and likelihood of activity and community participation.

When teaching wheelchair mobility skills, the following techniques can be helpful:

Clearance and preparation for the caregiver: The caregiver must wear rubber-soled shoes for good traction, limit accessories that can get in the way, and be medically cleared, as appropriate, prior to performing any training in wheelchair skills.

Real-life environment: Wheelchair mobility skills should be evaluated in the client's real-life setting (home, neighborhood, activities). Although performance in the client's real-life environment is ideal, this is sometimes not possible due to time constraints or distance. If this is the case, the area neighboring the hospital or the immediate area around the hospital, residential facility, or community center typically offers enough different challenges to allow the

evaluation to be done without having to use public or private transportation. If going out into the community is not possible and it is a bad weather day that makes it unsafe or impractical for practicing wheelchair mobility skills outside, use available indoor equipment, such as the practice curb in the clinic, the ramp in the hallway, the public bathroom in the hospital, and hospital elevators. It is also possible to lay a piece of carpet on the gym floor and position chairs or cones for obstacles.

Teach skills one at a time: Most clients and caregivers learn new skills best when the therapist works on just one new skill at a time. If the client is unable to attend the session (e.g., not feeling well), but the caregiver is available, the therapist may want to consider training the caregiver without the client being present, especially if the caregiver's availability for training is limited. Utilize "errorless learning techniques" to minimize learning errors as described in the chapter on Errorless Learning.

Emphasize proper body mechanics and techniques: Teach and emphasize the use of proper body mechanics to minimize harm or injury, such as bending the knees and holding items close to the body when lifting. See the Body Mechanics and Ergonomics chapter for more information.

Use a long mirror: A long mirror can be positioned so that the client can see what the therapist is doing as s/he helps maneuver the wheelchair. For example the long mirror can be positioned next to the curb so that the client can see what the therapist or caregiver is doing to bump the wheelchair up the curb. This offers the client a visual demonstration of the skill and acts as a teaching tool for the client. For clients who will be needing assistance with the skill, seeing the skill performed helps the client to better understand the steps involved, thus improving his/her ability to instruct another person on how to provide assistance. For the client who is learning how to perform the skill independently, a long mirror provides visual feedback of performance (e.g., is the client leaning far enough forward prior to backing down a two-inch curb independently). Seeing his/her actions in conjunction with feeling the correct position is ideal for learning physical skills.

Demonstrate before practice: If the therapist is teaching a caregiver to perform a skill, demonstrate the skill several times and then ask the caregiver (and client as appropriate) to verbally repeat the steps involved. Once they are able to repeat the steps verbally, ask the caregiver to try the skill and ask the client to practice verbally instructing the caregiver to perform the specific steps involved in the skill. The therapist stands close to the client and caregiver offering cueing and physical assistance as needed. The therapist may need to provide step-by-step instructions at first. The goal is to maximize the caregiver's and client's ability to perform the skill without the therapist's help. Once one skill is accomplished, the therapist moves on to the next skill until all of the skills have been addressed.

Provide references: Provide the client and caregiver with materials to help recall information taught, including handouts and videos. If providing handouts, make sure they are easy to read, preferably at a fifth-grade reading level or lower. If the therapist is providing a digital video, such as recording the technique on an iPhone, record the actual client or caregiver performing the skill. Therapists could then provide the client and caregiver with a library of short video clips that can be referenced at a later date, as needed.

Explore "what if" scenarios: Once skills are learned, explore "what if" situations associated with each skill to foster problem solving. Therapists must be careful, however, not to overload the client or caregiver with "what ifs" that could induce feelings of fear and anxiety. For example, after the client or caregiver feels comfortable going down a four-inch curb, start working on "what ifs" such as "What if the curb is higher than four inches?"

If the client does not have a caregiver who is able to provide assistance, or the client is unable to instruct another on wheelchair mobility skills because of limitations, the therapist will need to identify alternatives. These may include:

- Identifying specific places in the client's real-life environment that are totally wheelchair accessible.
- Identifying services and other outside sources that provide assistance, such as a door-to-door transportation service that includes physical assistance overcoming barriers — such as curbs — that occur between each "door-to-door."
- Exploring the possibility of hiring a caregiver for mobility-related activities.
- Exploring assistance available in a facility or program, such as availability of program staff to

assist with wheelchair mobility during the program.
- Bringing identified problems that significantly impact the client's lifestyle to the attention of the treatment team for problem solving, such as asking the team to consider a power wheelchair instead of a manual wheelchair if the client lacks endurance to self-propel the wheelchair at school.

Specific wheelchair mobility techniques for manual wheelchairs are provided below. They are written in simple English so they can be easily converted into a handout (if needed), for caregiver or client reference.

Manual Wheelchair Mobility with Assistance

Pushing the Wheelchair

When pushing a wheelchair, hold both handgrips and stand up straight. Look at least five to ten feet in front of the wheelchair to avoid obstacles.

Keep the wheelchair a safe distance from the curb edge and other obstacles.

Stopping the Wheelchair

To stop the wheelchair, hold the handgrips tightly and stop walking.

Turning

To turn the wheelchair to the right, pull back on the right handgrip and push forward on the left handgrip.

To turn the wheelchair to the left, pull back on the left handgrip and push forward on the right handgrip.

Uneven Surfaces

Going over rough ground can be hard. It is better to pull the wheelchair backward rather than pushing it forward.

Lead with the large back wheels so the small front wheels don't get stuck on small obstacles like cracks or bumps or gravel.

If you push the wheelchair forward over rough ground, raise the front end and roll on the back wheels. Stay on the balance point as described next. If the small wheels in front get stuck, the wheelchair may stop abruptly. This is very dangerous. The client may be thrown from the wheelchair if s/he is not wearing a seatbelt.

Balance Point

This is a basic wheelchair mobility skill. It is the process of tipping the wheelchair back onto the large wheels with the front wheels in the air. Find the balance point where all the weight is centered directly over the back wheels. It will feel as if there is no pull forward or backward. This skill will get you over many obstacles including curbs and raised sidewalk squares. This is how the helper gets to the balance point.

- Tell the client that you are going to tip the wheelchair backwards.
- If the anti-tipper bars are turned down, turn them up or remove them completely. This will allow the wheelchair to be tipped backwards.
- Place one foot on a tipper bar.
- Hold on tightly to both handgrips.
- Push down on the tipper bar with your foot and pull back on the handgrips at the same time. Pull your hands back to your hips. Do not push down.
- Push with your foot and pull with your arms until the wheelchair is in balance.

Curbs

To go up a curb:

- Stop the wheelchair about six inches away from the curb.
- Find the balance point, as described above.
- Roll the wheelchair forward until the back wheels hit the curb.
- Put your foot back on one of the tipper bars and slowly lower the caster wheels onto the sidewalk.
- Turn sideways, bend your knees, and place your hip against the back of the wheelchair.
- Using your hip and taking small side steps, bump the back wheels up over the curb. Use your hip instead of your arms to put less stress on your back.

To go down a curb:

- Back the wheelchair up to the edge of the curb.
- Stand sideways in the street with your hip facing the wheelchair.
- Roll the wheelchair backwards so that it rests against your hip.
- Bend your knees and take small steps away from the curb, as needed, to lower the back wheels onto the street.

- After the back wheels are on the street, face the wheelchair, push down on one of the tipper bars, and find the balance point.
- In the balance point, roll the wheelchair backwards until the caster wheels and the leg rests are clear of the curb.
- Place your foot back on the tipper bar and lower the caster wheels onto the ground.

Ramps

To go up a ramp: Approach the ramp. If the ramp does not smoothly meet the sidewalk (e.g., there is a lip), assume the balance point to get the caster wheels over the lip. Once the caster wheels are on the ramp you can use one of two techniques:

If it is a slight incline, you can push the wheelchair up the ramp facing forward. Be sure to keep a relatively straight back and use your legs to push the wheelchair up the ramp. *Do not use your back!*

If it is a steep ramp, turn sideways and place your hip against the back of the wheelchair. Take small side steps. *Do not put your feet together!* Each time you step, be sure to leave a space between your two feet. This will give you a good base of support.

To go down a ramp use one of these two techniques:

If it is a slight incline and the person does not have any problems with trunk control, go down the ramp facing forward. Hold the curve of the handgrips near the back of the wheelchair seat for a better grip.

If it is a steep ramp or the person does not have good trunk control, take the wheelchair down the ramp backwards. Turn sideways and place your hip against the back of the wheelchair and do side steps down the ramp. *Do not put your feet together!* Each time you step, be sure to leave a space between your two feet. This will give you a good base of support. By standing sideways, you will be able to turn your head to the side to see where you are going.

Escalators

Most escalators say no strollers and wheelchairs. Elevators should always be your first choice. Sometimes there is an emergency. Then you may need to know how to go up and down an escalator. Only consider this option:

- If there are no elevators available. Be sure to check for private elevators, such as a service elevator. Wait for the elevators to be fixed if you can.

- If the stairs aren't safe, maybe because of a fire. Usually stairs are safer than escalators.
- If there are no emergency personnel to help. They can bump the wheelchair down the stairs. They can also move the client with a blanket carry and bring the down wheelchair empty and folded.

Going up an escalator: Make sure the escalator is wide enough to handle the wheelchair. Remove the anti-tipper bars. The person in the wheelchair leans forward. Roll the wheelchair onto the escalator. The first two steps start together and flat. As the steps separate, the front wheels will be on the top step and the back wheels will be on the lower step.

The helper supports the back of the wheelchair to keep it from rolling backwards. Do not put the brakes on. The helper may find it best to place both hands flat against the back of the wheelchair rather than holding the handgrips.

The person in the wheelchair can hold the escalator hand rims if the hand rims are going at the same speed as the escalator footplates. If they are not, the person should just lean forward with his/her hands on the lap.

At the top, the helper pushes the wheelchair off the escalator.

Going down an escalator: Make sure the escalator is wide enough to handle the wheelchair. Remove the anti-tipper bars. The person in the wheelchair leans forward.

The helper steps backwards and pulls the wheelchair backwards onto the escalator. The helper supports the back of the wheelchair to stop it from rolling backwards. As the steps separate, the front wheels will be on the top step and the back wheels will be on the lower step. Do not put the brakes on. The helper may find it best to place both hands flat against the back of the wheelchair rather than holding the handgrips.

The person in the wheelchair can hold the escalator hand rims if the hand rims are going at the same speed as the escalator footplates. If the are not, the person should just lean forward with his/her hands on the lap.

At the bottom, the helper steps off the escalator and pulls the wheelchair off.

Elevators

It is best to pull the wheelchair into an elevator backwards. Align the wheelchair with the door opening. This allows you and the client to easily see where you are when the doors open. You can view the floor numbers and easily exit the elevator.

Stairs

Going up and down stairs is hard and always takes two people working together. One person should never try this alone. For going up or down stairs, the strongest person should be in the back of the wheelchair.

To go up steps: Remove the leg rests. Back the wheelchair up until the large wheels rest against the bottom step.

The person in back must be at least one step ahead of the wheelchair at all times. The back person holds the curve of the handgrips closest to the back seat of the wheelchair. The front person holds the front wheelchair frame.

Slightly tip the wheelchair into a wheelie position. The greater the tilt, the harder it is to control the wheelchair on the steps. By tipping the wheelchair backwards, the person's legs will swing under the seat so that they will not be in the way of the front person.

The back person is the counter. On the count of three, the back person rolls the wheelchair up onto the first step as the second person pushes the wheelchair toward the step.

The back person readjusts his foot location. The front person holds the wheelchair in place by pushing it into the step.

Again, on the count of three they roll the wheelchair up another step and so on to the top of the stairs. When you reach the top landing, lower the front caster wheels onto the landing and replace the leg rests.

To go down steps: Use the reverse of going up steps. There are only a few differences: Instead of rolling up the step you roll down the step. The person in back should have one foot on the same step as the wheelchair and one foot above it.

Narrow Doorways

If a doorway is too narrow, place a chair on the other side of the doorway and transfer through the door onto the chair. Fold up the wheelchair. Roll it through the doorway. Open it and then transfer back onto the wheelchair.

If the narrow door is in the client's home, s/he should consider enlarging the door. This can be done by removing the woodwork around the door or installing swing away hinges that allow the door to swing completely open so that the width of the door is not an issue. This provides an extra inch or so in width.

Manual Doors

Forward facing method (the person in the wheelchair is able to help): Approach the door normally. The person in the wheelchair pushes or pulls the door open with the arm closest to the door hinge. The helper holds the door open and pushes the wheelchair through the door.

Forward facing method (the person in the wheelchair is unable or limited in ability to assist): Approach the door normally. Helper opens the door and uses his/her back and feet to hold the door open. Helper grabs the side of the wheelchair and pulls the wheelchair through the doorway.

Backward facing method: This is a good choice if there is a raised doorsill.

If the door opens away from you, back up to the door. The helper pushes the door open with his/her back and legs. Using a foot to keep the door open, s/he pulls the wheelchair through the doorway.

If the door opens towards you, the helper pulls the door open. S/he maintains the opening with his/her foot. There are two choices: (1) Push the wheelchair backwards through the doorways by holding the side or front of wheelchair. (2) Walk backwards through the door while pulling the wheelchair through the doorway backwards. The person's arms are held inside the wheelchair so that the door rubbing along the wheelchair does not hurt the person's hands and arms.

Car Transfers

The stand-pivot transfer (SPT) and transfer board transfer (TBT) are the most common ways to get into and out of an automobile.

Stand-Pivot Transfer

A stand-pivot transfer needs to have the car on a level surface. It can be in a driveway or parking lot but not up against a curb.

Open the car door. Push the wheelchair up to the open car door and position it at a slight angle. The wheelchair should not be side by side with the seat of the car because the large back wheels and the armrest will be in the way of the person transferring.

Remove the leg rests. You may need to reposition the wheelchair to remove the leg rests since they have to swing out to the side and the car would be in the way.

Lock the brakes on the wheelchair. Remove the armrest that is closest to the car. The client scoots forward in the wheelchair and places his/her feet flat on the ground slightly behind the knees.

The client leans forward and stands up. If the client needs help to stand, place the wheelchair farther from the seat of the car. This gives the caregiver room to stand in front of the client and assist with the transfer. Sometimes the caregiver can assist the client from behind by reaching over the back of the wheelchair seat. The client pivots on his/her feet and turns his/her body so that his/her back lines up with the seat of the car.

The client can hold the car dashboard or back of the seat for support. Do not hold the car door because it moves and gives a false sense of security. Slowly lower buttocks onto the seat of the car. Swing legs into car. Buckle seatbelt.

Transfer Board

Follow the steps listed in the stand-pivot transfer to the point the client scoots forward in the wheelchair.

One end of the transfer board is placed under the client's buttocks and other end rests on the seat of the car. A long board is often better than a short board because the transfer distance is long.

The client does a series of small lifts across the board until his/her buttocks are on the seat of the car. Lift legs into the car.

The client then leans towards the middle of the car so that pressure is taken off the buttocks and the board is pulled out from underneath.

Public Bathrooms

Getting a wheelchair into a public bathroom can be difficult, especially if it is not fully accessible. The height of the toilet, availability of bathroom bars, width of the stall, height of the sink, and placement of the soap and towel dispensers may not meet the client's needs. This means the client may need more assistance in a public bathroom than at home.

There are several transfers. Some wheelchairs have a zipper back. With those, the client can back into the bathroom stall, unzip the back of the wheelchair, and slide back onto the toilet. Clients can transfer onto the toilet using a stand-pivot transfer or a transfer board. If the client chooses one of these transfers, it is important to practice it in a tight space. Several options should be practiced because public bathrooms can vary. Clients should learn their bowel routine to reduce the need to transfer onto a toilet.

Folding a Manual Wheelchair

There are different procedures for reducing the bulk of a wheelchair. They depend on its design. The basic procedures for the most common types of wheelchairs are described below.

Cross-brace wheelchair: Remove the leg rests. Remove the seat cushion. Remove any backpacks or bags on the back of wheelchair. Remove the back of the wheelchair (if hardback). The helper approaches the wheelchair at an angle, bends at the knees, and grabs the front and back of the wheelchair seat. Pulling up on the wheelchair seat will cause the wheelchair to fold.

Rigid wheelchair: Remove leg rests (if applicable), armrests, seat cushions, and any pouches or backpack from the wheelchair. Grab the string that runs along the back of the wheelchair. Pull the string away from the wheelchair and push the back of the wheelchair forward so that it collapses onto the wheelchair seat. Tilt the wheelchair on its side so that one wheel is off the ground. Stabilize the wheelchair with one hand. With the other hand push the wheel lock button found in the middle of the wheel. This will release the wheel and it can be pulled off the wheelchair frame. Use the same process to remove the other wheel. Remove or flip up the anti-tipper bars, if applicable.

Transporting a Wheelchair in a Car

Place a sofa-sized throw blanket over the open trunk. Half should be inside the trunk and half outside the trunk. This will help keep the car paint from getting scratched. It will also help when getting the wheelchair out of the trunk. When sliding the wheelchair into the trunk, the blanket may get wadded up under the wheelchair. Try to arrange the blanket so that it does not slide into the trunk with the wheel-

chair. Instead of leaning far into the car trunk to pull the wheelchair out (which can hurt your back), grab the blanket and pull on it. The blanket will help guide the wheelchair up and out of the trunk so that you don't have to lean in so far.

In and out of the trunk (one-person lift)

Fold the wheelchair according to previous directions. It is best to fold the wheelchair next to the trunk as everything taken off can be placed in the trunk. If the trunk is small, place the wheelchair parts in the trunk after the wheelchair is placed in the trunk. That way the wheelchair can easily slide into the trunk without getting caught on the wheelchair parts.

Lock the brakes on the wheelchair. Stand to the side of the wheelchair. Spread your feet apart for better balance and proper body mechanics. Your stance should be the width of the wheelchair. Bend your knees and tilt the wheelchair towards your body so that it rests against you. Lean over the top of the wheelchair so that your arms hang over the other side of the wheelchair. Grab the wheelchair frame wherever you are most comfortable. Do not hold the wheels as they could become unlocked and move. Pull the wheelchair into your chest. Using your legs, lift the wheelchair up so that it juts out in front of you. Place the wheelchair in the trunk. Put all of the accessories that are not already in the trunk into the trunk.

In and out of the trunk (two-person lift)

Follow the steps in the one-person lift to position the wheelchair and set the brakes.

Stand on opposite sides of the wheelchair. One person holds the handgrips and the tipper bars. The other person holds the front frame of the wheelchair. On the count of three, both people bend their knees and lift the wheelchair into the car trunk.

Alternatives

Wheelchairs can also be placed into the back of pick-up trucks and sport utility vehicles. They can also go on the floor of the back seat of a large two-door car. Run a seatbelt through the frame. Buckle it to keep the wheelchair from flying around in an accident.

An overhead wheelchair carrier or a car trailer may also be used. Car Transfers and Wheelchair

Loading in the Independent Wheelchair Skills talks about carriers. Transporting Wheelchairs in the Power Wheelchair and Scooter section talks about trailers.

Manual Wheelchair Mobility without Assistance

Propelling the Wheelchair

There are two common ways to propel a wheelchair that use the least energy and keep good posture. In general, using both arms at the same time is the most energy efficient.

Push and glide: Grip the hand rims slightly behind the trunk. Push the rims forward with both arms in a long stroke. Release the hand rims while maintaining proper posture and allow the wheels to glide freely.

Circular push: Grip the hand rims a little behind the top of the hand rim. Push to full extension of the arms and as far forward and down as body balance allows. At full extension release the hand rims. The hands circle back to the initial grip. Re-grasp the hand rims and push forward and down again. The arms should look like they are moving in a circle around the wheel.

Stopping the Wheelchair

To stop the wheelchair grip the hand rims tightly, stopping the motion of the wheels. When going down an incline, hold the hand rims loosely and let them slide through the hands. Tighten and loosen the grip as necessary to decrease or increase speed.

Turning

To turn the wheelchair to the right pull backwards on the right hand rim while pushing forward with the left hand rim.

To turn the wheelchair to the left pull backwards on the left hand rim while pushing forward with the right hand rim.

Rough Terrain

When going over uneven surfaces, you can go forwards or backwards. Choose the method based on the type of front tires and your upper body strength. If the surface is not too uneven or bumpy and the wheelchair has large front tires, you may be able to move the wheelchair forward. Small, hard-plastic casters will not go over rough surfaces as easily. They can get stuck in small cracks and divots. If this is the case, it's better to pull the wheelchair over the surface

backwards. Large power wheels go over the surface more easily and the front casters should follow.

Either way, if the front casters get stuck, try turning the wheelchair side to side. This should work the casters out of the rut. In addition to avoiding getting stuck, the correct technique will also reduce the chance of tipping over or falling out of the wheelchair. If the wheelchair stops quickly while moving forward, you can be thrown from the wheelchair. This is a reason to wear a seatbelt.

Wheelies

This is a basic skill for community mobility. Many techniques require a wheelie to complete. The client should wear head protection while learning how to do a wheelie. A bicycle helmet works well for this.

To teach the wheelie position, the therapist flips up or removes the anti-tipper bars. Then the therapist uses the handgrips and the lever bars to tip the wheelchair back to the balance point. The client holds the balance point by moving the wheelchair and his/her body. Learning on a soft surface, such as a mat, will make it less scary. Therapists tell clients not to practice wheelie skills alone until the therapist says it is all right.

Once you can maintain the balance point, work on starting a wheelie as follows: Place your hands on the wheel rims slightly in front of the trunk. Grip the rims tightly. Push forward. Lean back in the wheelchair to get the front wheels off the ground. Hold the wheelie position as practiced above. To put the front wheels down lean forward and use body position and handgrips. Check to make sure feet are properly placed on the footrests.

Work on movement wheelies. These are wheelies where you move forward, backward, to the left or right, and in a full circle while in a wheelie position. You will need these skills for community mobility, such as rolling down a curb in the wheelie position.

Curbs

To go up a curb from a static position: Roll the wheelchair a few inches from the curb. Pop a wheelie and move forward until the casters are on the curb. To get the back wheels onto the curb, begin with the casters as close to the edge of the curb as possible. You may need to back the wheelchair up a bit depending on the height of the curb. This will help to give the back wheels some room to gain momentum.

Lean forward in the wheelchair and push forward on the tires or hand rims to roll the back wheels up onto the curb. Some people find it helpful to rock the back wheels up onto the curb (e.g., one… give a push… two… give a harder push… three… push with all your strength). Rocking also helps build momentum to get the back wheels up onto the curb.

To go up a curb in a dynamic position: This method requires much less strength but very good timing and skill. Roll towards the curb with all four wheels on the ground. Just before reaching the curb, pop into a wheelie position. Lower the caster wheels onto the curb BEFORE the back wheels hit the curb. Lean forward in the wheelchair and push hard on the hand rims to bring the back wheels up onto the curb in one smooth motion.

To go down a curb from a static position: Back the wheelchair to the curb edge. Lean forward in wheelchair and place your hands on tires or hand rims. Slowly lower the back wheels onto the street in a controlled roll. To lower the caster wheels, place one hand forward on the tire or hand rim and the other hand slightly behind the torso on the tire or hand rim. Pull back with the forward hand and push forward with the back hand. This will cause the wheelchair to spin to one side. Spinning the caster wheels off of the curb to the side prevents the roller bar or footplates from becoming stuck on the curb.

To go down a curb in a dynamic position: This method is much quicker; however it does require good timing and skill. As you approach the curb in a forward direction, pop into a wheelie. While in the wheelie position, bump down the curb on the back wheels and then lower the caster wheels to the street.

Ramps

To go up a ramp: Pop a small wheelie if there is an edge or lip to the ramp. Not all ramps flow smoothly from one surface to the other. Lean forward in the wheelchair. Place both hands on the tires or hand rims of the wheelchair and push simultaneously. If the ramp is really steep (greater than a 1:12 ratio) and it has a decent width, try pushing up the ramp in a zigzag fashion. This will cut the grade of the ramp.

To go down a ramp forwards: If the ramp does not have any obstacles that could pose a danger, such as holes or debris, and it is not too steep to handle, go down the ramp forwards. Place both hands on the tires or hand rims and lean back in the wheelchair. Control the roll down the ramp by opening and closing your hands to loosen and tighten the grip as needed.

To go down a ramp backwards: If the ramp is too steep to handle or there are obstacles like pebbles and sticks that could pose a danger, go down the ramp backwards. Place both hands on the tires or hand rims and lean forward in the wheelchair. Slowly loosen and tighten your grasp to control the roll of the wheelchair down the ramp.

Stairs

Going up and down stairs with a wheelchair is very hard. You will need a lot of upper body strength and determination. Young people with low paraplegia are most likely to be able to perform these skills.

Going up stairs on your buttocks: Transfer from the wheelchair to the second step. Tilt the wheelchair back onto the step (unfolded). Bump up one more step. Reposition the legs on next step. Pull wheelchair up one step and stabilize the wheelchair on the step while bumping up another step. If the wheelchair is difficult to stabilize while bumping up to the next step, try to hold the wheelchair with one hand and use the other hand to assist in raising the buttocks to the next step.

Going up stairs in a wheelchair: Buckle seatbelt. Tilt the wheelchair backwards so that the back of the wheelchair rests on the steps. Grab the rail with the closest hand (e.g., hold the right rail with the right hand). The other hand grabs the wheelchair tire or hand rim. Use the hand on the rail to pull the wheelchair up one step while the hand on the tire or hand rim also helps to roll the wheelchair up one step by pulling backwards on the tire or hand rim. Reposition the hands and continue.

Going down stairs in wheelchair backwards: Buckle seatbelt. Back the wheelchair up to the top step. Hold one rail with BOTH hands, one hand above the other. Slowly lower the wheelchair down the stairs one step at a time, repositioning hands as needed.

Going down stairs in wheelchair forwards: Buckle seatbelt. Initiate a wheelie position at the edge of the top step. Lower down the stairs in a wheelie position. Use the tires or hand rims to control the descent. To assist in stabilizing the wheelchair, pull back on the tires or hand rims.

Doorways

It is important to know the width of the wheelchair. This is especially true if the wheelchair has wider than normal width or a camber. Measure the width from outer hand rim to outer hand rim. A standard doorway is 32" wide. A standard-width wheelchair should fit through most household and community doors. However, there will be times, even with a standard wheelchair, that it won't. Here are several ways to work around this: Remove molding around the door. Install swing-away hinges. Remove the door. Use alternatives for doors, such as curtains or pocket doors. Expand the doorway by remodeling.

To transfer through a narrow door: Place a chair on the other side of the doorway. It would be side by side for a transfer board transfer or at an angle for a stand-pivot transfer. Transfer from the wheelchair to the other chair through the doorway. Collapse the wheelchair enough to roll it through the doorway. Open the wheelchair and transfer from the chair to the wheelchair.

Manual Doors

Door opens away from you, forward method: Approach the door. Push the door open as much as possible with one hand. While pushing the door open with the one hand, place the other hand on the tire or hand rim and push the wheelchair through the door. It is usually hard to get all the way through. The leg rests will often be all that gets through the door. They will help hold the door open while you give the door another push and propel yourself the rest of the way through. If the door is light enough, you may be able to give the door one more big push and then quickly push the wheelchair through the door with both hands on the tires or hand rims. It's a good idea to place your hands on top of the tires when pushing. This way, if the door swings back when you are pushing the wheelchair through the door, it will hit the outside of the hand rim and not your hands. You may also push with just one hand when going through the door while using the other hand to keep the door open.

Door opens away from you, backwards method: Back up to the door. Pull back on both tires or hand rims and push through the door. Using the tires instead of the hand rims may save you a scrape from the door.

Door opens towards you: Approach the door in a forward position. Stay to the side of the door. For example, if the door handle is on the right side, align the wheelchair on the right side of the door so that the left hand can easily pull the door open. This also positions the wheelchair farther away from the door hinge, which will make it easier when going through the doorway. When pulling the door open with the left hand, pull back on the right tire or hand rim to assist in opening the door. Push forward on the right tire or hand rim to spin the wheelchair forwards and to the left. This will help block the door open with the leg rests.

If the door is very heavy and you cannot hold the door open to spin the leg rests into the door, this method might be helpful: When approaching the door, leave about two feet between the door and the wheelchair. Put on the wheelchair brakes. Reach forward with the left hand and pull the door open. Since the brakes are on, the wheelchair will not move. Reposition the left hand to the inside of the door. Release the right brake and spin the leg rests into the doorway. Release the left brake. Now you have blocked the door open. Once the door is blocked open, push the door open further with the left hand and push the wheelchair through the door with the right tire or hand rim. If it is difficult to hold the door open with one hand and push with the other, give the door one big push and propel through the door using both hands. You can also plow through the door at an angle with power from both hands, using the force of the wheelchair to open the door. Place your hands on top of the tires when pushing through a door. If the door swings closed, it will hit the hand rim and not your hand.

Escalators

To go up or down an escalator in a wheelie position: Approach the step of the escalator. Get in a wheelie position. Hold the rails of the escalator while in a wheelie position for the descent or ascent. Use hands on the rails to keep the wheelie. At the end of the escalator, get ready to let go of the rails.

There is usually a lip at the end of the escalator. You have to maintain the wheelie position long enough to clear the lip. Then let go of the rails. Quickly place both hands on the tires and hand rims. Lower the front wheels to the ground and push the back wheels off the last escalator step.

To go up or down an escalator in a non-wheelie position: Use the methods described in the Wheelchair Mobility with Assistance. Adjust for having no assistant.

Elevators

Pull the wheelchair into an elevator backwards. Align the wheelchair with the door opening. Then you can see where you are when the doors open, view the floor numbers, and easily exit the elevator.

Folding a Manual Wheelchair

See Folding a Manual Wheelchair in the Dependent Wheelchair Skills section. The steps are the same.

Car Transfers

The stand-pivot transfer (SPT) and transfer board transfer (TBT) are the most common ways to get into or out of a car. Refer to Car Transfers in the Wheelchair Mobility with Assistance. The techniques are the same without the assistant. Clients who have leg involvement with no or little arm involvement may not be able to stand upright for the stand-pivot transfer. They may also have problems with the position of the legs for transfer board transfers. They may find one of these techniques easier:

Place one or both legs in the car before the transfer or during the transfer. For example, place both legs on the floor in the front seat. Use a sit-pivot to transfer to the seat of the car.

Place one leg on the front seat floor and the other foot flat on the ground outside the car. Complete two lifts across the transfer board. Lift the other leg onto front seat floor. Then complete the final lifts across the transfer board onto the seat of the car.

If you want to drive, ask your therapist for a referral to an adaptive driving program. They are best suited to evaluate driving ability. Adaptive equipment might be suggested. These include an elbow switch for turn signals, a knob on the steering wheel, and push/pull levers for the gas and brake.

Wheelchair Loading

There are many ways to load a manual wheelchair into the car:

Rigid Wheelchair into Passenger Seat

Transfer into the driver seat. Fold the wheelchair outside of the vehicle. As you take off each component, place it on the floor of the opposite side of the car. For example, if you are sitting in the driver seat, place the items on the floor of the front passenger seat. Slide the seat all the way back. If the steering wheel tilts, move it into the best position for bringing the wheelchair into the vehicle. You may also need to recline the driver seat for extra room. Grab the wheelchair and lift it. Bring it across your body and place it on the passenger seat. Strap the wheelchair in with the seatbelt by running it through the frame of the wheelchair.

Cross-Brace Wheelchair into Back Seat

This requires a large two-door car. Transfer into the driver seat. Fold the wheelchair outside of the vehicle. Place wheelchair parts on the floor of the passenger side. Place both feet on the ground outside of the vehicle. Slide the driver seat all the way forward. Roll the wheelchair behind the front seat. Slide the driver side seat back into the correct position. The wheelchair will be stabilized by being "crushed" between the front and back seat.

Rigid or Cross-Brace Wheelchair Pulled across a Bench Seat

You must have a large two-door car with a bench seat. Transfer to the passenger side of the vehicle. Fold the wheelchair outside of the vehicle and place the wheelchair components on the floor of the back seat. Grab the wheelchair. Pull the wheelchair in as you scoot across to the driver side of the vehicle. Strap the wheelchair in with the seatbelt by running it through the wheelchair frame.

Cross-brace Wheelchair into Overhead Wheelchair Carrier

This technique cannot be used with a rigid wheelchair. A special overhead wheelchair carrier can be bought and placed on a car roof. (It looks like a luggage box.)

Transfer into the driver seat. Fold the wheelchair. (See Folding a Cross-brace Wheelchair in Dependent Wheelchair Skills.) Place the wheelchair parts on the floor of the passenger side. Place both legs back into the car. Push the special button installed inside the car that automatically lowers a strap from the carrier down by the side of the car. Hook the wheelchair frame to the straps. Push the button inside the car again. The straps automatically lift the wheelchair up, turn it sideways, and slide it into the overhead car carrier.

Power Wheelchairs or Scooters

Power wheelchairs are typically very heavy and pose some difficulty when the client is trying to overcome obstacles in the community. This section provides a general outline of community mobility skills for someone using a power wheelchair in the community. Although power wheelchairs or scooters are battery operated and do not require the physical assistance of another person, there may be occasional times when the power wheelchair or scooter will need to be placed into manual mode and require the physical assistance of another person. One of the most common reasons for needing help is when the battery runs out of power. This section addresses how to operate a power wheelchair in power mode and manual mode. This information is also helpful if the client is considering using a community scooter, such as using an electric scooter provided by a grocery store.

Accessibility Issues

The weight of the wheelchair, the battery, and the positioning and type of wheels prevent power wheelchairs from being tipped backwards onto back wheels to a balance-point position with the front wheels in the air. Since power wheelchairs are unable to be tipped backwards, they can't be bumped up or down curbs and stairs, nor should one ever consider taking a power wheelchair or scooter up or down an escalator. Therefore, it is very important to make sure that the client's real-life living situation and the places the client goes in the community are free of such obstacles. It is also recommended that the therapist educate the client about community accessibility issues and the Americans with Disabilities Act (ADA).

Pushing the Wheelchair

Manual mode: Power wheelchairs can be placed into manual mode, allowing the caregiver to manually push the wheelchair. Typically, the wheelchair is turned from power to manual by releasing the wheel locks that are located in the center of the back wheels. Because of the weight of the wheelchair, plus the weight of the individual in the wheelchair, pushing a power wheelchair is not an easy task, especially on uneven outdoor surfaces. When pushing a wheelchair, hold both handgrips, stand up straight, and look at least five to ten feet in front of the wheelchair to avoid obstacles. Keep the wheelchair a safe distance from the curb edge and obstacles. If the wheelchair is too heavy to push in this manner, try turning sideways. Take side steps and use your hip (the whole side of your body if needed) to push the wheelchair a short distance at a time. The power wheelchair is usually only placed in manual mode if there is a problem, such as a dead battery or a client who isn't feeling well enough to operate the wheelchair. This should not be an everyday occurrence.

Power mode: Power wheelchairs can be operated by the individual in the wheelchair through a variety of modalities including a joystick, sip and puff, or head control. The right modality will be determined primarily by the physical and occupational therapists or through a referral to a power wheelchair clinic. Recreational therapists contribute to this process by providing feedback about the client's ability to utilize the modality in a functional setting. For example, if the client's hand continually slips off the joystick control on bumpy outdoor surfaces and the client requires assistance to reposition the hand, this suggests a different type of control may be needed — one that stabilizes the client's hand. A square control that the client's hand slips into rather than a U-shaped control that the client's hand rests on may work better.

Stopping the Wheelchair

Manual mode: To stop the wheelchair, hold the handgrips tightly and stop walking.

Power mode: To stop the wheelchair, a specific function will need to be performed. It may be to lift the hand off of joystick or make one long blow on sip and puff.

Turning

Manual mode: To turn the wheelchair to the right, pull back on the right handgrip and push forward on the left handgrip. To turn the wheelchair to the left, pull back on the left handgrip and push forward on the right handgrip.

Power mode: To turn the wheelchair to the right or left a specific function will need to be performed, such as turning the head in the direction desired or pushing the joystick in the direction desired.

Uneven Surfaces

Manual mode: In the Dependent Community Wheelchair Skills section, recommendations are made to pull the wheelchair backwards on uneven surface. Unfortunately, pulling a power wheelchair in manual mode is almost impossible due to the weight. Sometimes, the front wheels and the back wheels on a power wheelchair are the same size, thus allowing the caregiver to push the wheelchair forward over the uneven surface with the same ease (or difficulty) as going over the uneven surface backwards.

Power mode: Power wheelchairs typically go over uneven surfaces such as grass, hills, and broken sidewalk with ease in forward motion. However, depending on the wheel size, alternative methods may need to be used.

Elevators

It is best to go onto an elevator backwards, aligning the front of the wheelchair with the door opening. This allows the client to easily see where s/he is when the doors open, view the floor numbers, and easily exit the elevator. Usually the hallways outside of the elevators allow more room for turning around than the inside of the elevator does, especially if there are other people inside the elevator.

Ramps

Manual mode: Ramps can be very difficult in manual mode due to the weight of the wheelchair. This can quickly turn into a very dangerous situation if the caregiver loses control. If it is necessary to push a power wheelchair up or down a ramp in manual mode, have a minimum of two people holding the back of the wheelchair for safety/ One way is for each person to have one hand on the handgrip and one hand clutching the top of the wheelchair back. The wheelchair should be pushed up a ramp forwards and guided down a ramp backwards. When you are going down a ramp, the caregivers are to stand sideways using their hips or sides of the body to control the roll of the wheelchair.

Power mode: Power wheelchairs should go up and down ramps easily. However, the client must use common sense when evaluating a ramp. If the ramp is full of debris, such as sticks, rocks, or trash, or the surface does not seem secure and stable (e.g., loose gravel), the client should consider another route.

Manual Doors

Manual mode: Due to the weight of a power wheelchair it will be difficult for one person to push a power wheelchair through a manual door. The person assisting will need two hands to push the wheelchair and another person to hold the door open. Ask for assistance from a passerby to hold the door open and push the wheelchair forwards through the door.

Power mode: An individual using a power wheelchair typically has poor arm strength and function, therefore will need assistance to open manual doors. Look for automatic doors or doors with a handicap button that opens the door automatically when pressed. If the client is unfamiliar with the door and it has a handicap button, press the button and watch to see how much time is allowed to get through the door. If the door opens and closes rather quickly, the client may still need to request assistance to hold the door open when s/he is going through.

Car Transfers

Stand-pivot transfers and transfer board transfers are typical ways to get in and out of a car. However, individuals who use a power wheelchair may require much more assistance with transfers, sometimes needing maximum assistance from two people. It may be advantageous to explore vehicles that do not require the individual to transfer in and out of the wheelchair, such as a mini-van with a ramp and tie downs to stabilize the wheelchair inside the vehicle. This is especially true if the caregiver is unable to provide the level of assistance needed.

Another thing to consider is how the wheelchair will be transported. Some power wheelchairs fold or disassemble and others do not. Some power wheelchairs, although they are collapsible, do not fold easily despite their marketing promises. Therefore, it may not matter if the client can transfer in and out of the car if the car is unable to transport the wheelchair. The client who has a power wheelchair that does not fold (or does not fold easily) or whose caregiver is unable to disassemble the wheelchair should consider other alternatives for transporting the wheelchair. Examples of alternatives include vans with a lift or ramp, a car trailer for the wheelchair, or a trunk lift. Another option is using alternative transportation that provides van service with a lift, such as paratransit services.

Driving

If the client is interested in driving, his/her physician may refer him/her to an adaptive driving program. These programs evaluate the client's ability to drive and make recommendations for vehicle adaptations, such as a knob on steering wheel and push/pull lever for gas and brake. Because the client is likely to be unable to load the power wheelchair or scooter by himself/herself, s/he may need to consider a van. There are many different types of vans to choose from and the professionals in the adaptive driving program will be able to provide the dimensions and specifications to meet the client's needs and recommend a particular style of vehicle.

Public Bathrooms

In addition to the comments on public bathrooms in the Manual Wheelchair Mobility with Assistance section there are additional concerns for clients using power wheelchairs or scooters. Whether in power or manual mode, it can very difficult to maneuver a power wheelchair in a bathroom stall due to the wheelchair's size and poor turning radius. If the bathroom stall is wide enough to accommodate the power wheelchair or scooter, it may still be difficult to close the stall door. An additional concern is the level of assistance that the client will need to use the bathroom. Many clients who have a power wheelchair require maximum assistance for transfers, therefore requiring the client to explore alternatives for bowel and bladder care, such as a Texas catheter or incontinence pad. Individuals who use a scooter and are able to walk a short distance may opt to park the scooter outside of the stall and walk into the stall.

Wheelchair Breakdown in the Community

If at any time there is a problem with the power wheelchair, call the technical assistance center. If the client is out in the community and a problem with the wheelchair can't be fixed quickly, put the wheelchair in manual mode and request the assistance of others to move to a safe location. Most times, a client who is using a power wheelchair is with or around other people who could offer assistance. If the client is by himself/herself or if the people with the client are not able to provide the assistance needed, call someone who can help. It is a good idea for the client to keep a cell phone with him/her at all times for such an emergency. Even if the client is unable to operate a cell phone, s/he can instruct another person to turn on the phone and dial the number. The worst-case scenario is that the client will be unable call someone and the assistance available is not sufficient. In that case, the client can call or request another person to call the local emergency number (e.g., police or fire) and report a concern for safety. Request that the emergency operator remain on the line until help arrives. Although emergency personnel are trained professionals, the client cannot assume that they will know how to handle the specific situation. Teach the client how to be prepared to offer needed instruction.

The client should at least be able to describe how to dismantle the wheelchair so the emergency personnel can transport the client and the wheelchair home and how the personnel can assist the client in transferring into and out of their vehicle.

Treatment

Traditionally, in the rehabilitation setting, the physical and occupational therapists, along with the wheelchair vendor identify and choose appropriate wheelchair options to present to the client. Recreational therapists are increasingly becoming more involved in the wheelchair selection process. The recreational therapist offers a view of the client's lifestyle that other therapists do not have. By having a holistic understanding of the client's current and desired recreational and community activities, along with the knowledge of the application of wheelchair components, recreational therapists can offer quality input.

Recreational therapists assist clients in test-driving wheelchairs by scheduling community integration sessions that allow the client to test one or more wheelchairs in a real-life environment.

Recreational therapists teach clients how to manipulate mobility devices and overcome obstacles in a community environment.

Recreational therapists teach clients how to problem solve for barriers that may occur with their wheelchair/scooter in a community setting (e.g., battery dies, flat tire).

Recreational therapists are part of the wheelchair prescription team to voice concerns and ideas about wheelchair and scooter prescriptions.

Outcomes and Documentation

Several criteria are used in wheelchair mobility skills training. The criteria with sample chart notes include:

Percentage: "Client able to verbally sequence the steps involved in bumping a wheelchair up a curb with 75% accuracy."

Assistance: "Mary Smith, client's daughter, able to bump wheelchair up and down a four-inch curb with minimal assistance from therapist."

Cueing: "Client able to instruct caregiver on how to propel wheelchair up a steep ramp with minimal verbal cues from therapist."

Ability: "Client able to independently bump wheelchair up a four-inch curb."

Performance time and distance: "Client able to negotiate a six-foot ADA-compliant ramp in 30 seconds."

Physical strain: "Client exhibits signs of fatigue — shortness of breath, degraded technique — when propelling the wheelchair over uneven outdoor surfaces."

Technique: "Client able to successfully demonstrate push and glide wheelchair propulsion technique."

Sample ICF codes related to wheelchair mobility skills training might include: d175 Solving Problems, d177 Making Decisions, and d4 Mobility, especially d410 Changing Basic Body Position, d420 Transferring Oneself, d465 Moving Around Using Equipment, d470 Using Transportation, and d660 Assisting Others.

Appendix A: Wheelchairs, Scooters, and Accessories

There are three main types of seated mobility devices: manual wheelchairs, power wheelchairs, and scooters. The type of seated mobility chosen reflects the needs of the client. If a client is going to need the wheelchair for only a short period of time (e.g., total joint replacement), the client will probably rent a standard manual wheelchair, rather than purchase one. For a client who is ordering a custom wheelchair for long-term use, choosing a wheelchair can be difficult because it must match the client's physical needs, cognitive abilities, living environment, and activity patterns. Clients are presented with many different options and at times it can become a very confusing and frustrating process for the client, especially when the wheelchair chosen will not be replaced by the insurance company for several years.

Some therapists prefer to order a custom wheelchair while the client is in inpatient rehab because it takes six to eight weeks for the wheelchair to be made. This may not always be ideal because it doesn't let the client test-drive the wheelchair. What sounds good and looks good may not always feel right to the client. A developing trend is to send the client home with a trial wheelchair that is closely related to the wheelchair in consideration. This gives the client an opportunity to try out several different wheelchairs over a short period of time in his/her real-life environment in order to make a more informed choice.

Manual Wheelchairs

Advantages: Manual wheelchairs are lightweight. They do not require a battery and they have fewer parts than a power wheelchair, thus requiring less maintenance. When compared to power wheelchairs and scooters, manual wheelchairs are less expensive to repair (no electric components), quieter (no motor), and more discreet (you see more of the person and less of the wheelchair). Manual wheelchairs are easily transportable and foldable and provide more flexibility than power wheelchairs or scooters for overcoming obstacles. They are able to pop a wheelie and negotiate curbs and steps. Manual wheelchairs also help to maintain and improve muscle and cardiopulmonary strength and endurance and provide secondary health benefits related to the physical activity of pushing.

Disadvantages: Manual wheelchairs require upper body strength and endurance. Years of wheelchair propulsion can cause shoulder problems. A high degree of strength is required to overcome community barriers, such as hills, and the speed of the wheelchair varies depending on the client's physical ability, as well as endurance level, which can fluctuate throughout the day.

Types

There are two types of manual wheelchair frames, rigid and cross-brace.

Rigid frame: The rigid frame is one tubular piece. It has a modern or sport-like appearance and is lighter than a cross-brace wheelchair. A rigid frame is stronger and more energy efficient than a cross-brace wheelchair because it does not have a jointed frame piece, which is an advantage for an active person. A solid frame, however, is more sensitive to body movement and can be a challenge to manipulate on uneven surfaces. Rigid wheelchairs have a tighter turning radius and offer a variety of options that cannot be ordered on a cross-brace wheelchair. These include seat bucket options and special sport designs for tennis, rugby, basketball, and racing. To fold a rigid frame wheelchair the wheels pop off and the back folds down making it look like a box. A folded rigid wheelchair does not fit easily into a standard car trunk. The client will need a van, pickup truck, or sport utility vehicle with a hatchback. In a standard car the client can sit in the driver seat, fold the wheelchair, and then pull it across his/her body and place it on the passenger seat. This is the most common situation because most clients who purchase a rigid frame wheelchair have paraplegia and are unable to load a wheelchair into a trunk independently. Rigid frame wheelchairs are custom ordered. They are not a standard rental wheelchair.

Cross-brace frame: The cross-brace frame wheelchair has a cross-frame. The frame looks like an "X" under the wheelchair seat. This design allows the wheelchair to fold flat by taking off the leg rests and armrests, removing the seat cushion, grabbing the front and the back of the wheelchair seat, and pulling up. The wheelchair will then collapse flat. When folded, the wheelchair can be placed flat in a trunk or put into a rooftop carrier. A button in the car opens the rooftop carrier and lowers a metal contraption down next to the driver-side door, the driver loads the wheelchair onto the contraption and then pushes the button to raise it up and slide it into the rooftop carrier. Roof top carriers are not available for rigid frame wheelchairs. The roof top carrier is an excellent choice for a client who does not have the strength to pull in or load the wheelchair without assistance. The cross-brace wheelchair has a traditional appearance and is stable on uneven surfaces. However, active clients often complain that the wheelchair shakes too much because the center joint in the cross-brace can become loose with active use. It also requires more energy to push than a rigid frame wheelchair. Cross-brace wheelchairs do not have as many options as rigid frame wheelchairs. Clients who have a short-term need for a wheelchair, such as a client who has a total hip replacement and requires the use of a wheelchair for a month or two for long-distance mobility, are typically given a standard cross-brace rental wheelchair. A client who has a long-term need for a manual wheelchair can opt for a cross-brace wheelchair and it will be custom tailored (like the rigid frame wheelchair) to meet the specific needs of the client related to width, height, and other options. Clients who opt for a cross-brace wheelchair are usually those with progressive muscular disabilities, such as multiple sclerosis, who would benefit from a wheelchair with greater stability.

Power Wheelchairs

Advantages: Powered wheelchairs conserve cardiopulmonary and muscular energy. When compared to a manual wheelchair, they provide greater ease overcoming uneven terrain like grass and ramps and require the use of only one body part to control the wheelchair. The other limbs are available for other tasks. Power wheelchairs are custom fitted and designed for the client with the goal of independent operation. Assistance from others may be required to change or charge the battery and perform routine maintenance. Power wheelchairs can also be designed with power tilt and recline to aid in pressure relief and comfort.

Disadvantages: Power wheelchairs can be difficult to transport. Some power wheelchairs can be dismantled and placed into a car trunk (the typical pieces weighing about 30 pounds). However, the client would need to be able to transfer into a car and have another person who could dismantle and reassemble the wheelchair as well as provide assistance to transfer into the car. Another option is a wheelchair trailer that hooks onto a tow ball on the back of a car. The client transfers into the car and another person drives the wheelchair around to the back of the car and loads it on the trailer. Most clients who purchase a power wheelchair have significant motor loss making car transfers almost impossible. Therefore, most clients choose to purchase a custom van with a ramp or lift. Clients who desire to drive and have the ability to drive using adaptive equipment can also have a van tailored so that the power wheelchair locks down as the driver seat. When compared to the manual wheelchair, power wheelchairs require higher maintenance because there are more parts. They are more expensive. They do not provide cardiovascular or muscular exercise (possibly promoting further deterioration). They are also bigger pieces of equipment that lets others see more of the wheelchair than the person. Some power wheelchairs can go up small curbs of two to four inches. They do not have the flexibility of a manual wheelchair, which can be folded and carried up a flight of steps and can bump up high curbs.

Types

Power wheelchairs are described as being front wheel drive, rear wheel drive, or mid-wheel drive.

Front wheel drive: The front wheel drive wheelchair gives the person the sensation that s/he is pulling the wheelchair behind him/her. They are very agile, making a full rotation in a tight space. They take skill to operate and may be difficult for those with cognitive deficits. The wheels in the front are larger and help to overcome small obstacles. A tilt option may make the wheelchair unstable because weight transferred to the back may raise the front wheels making it difficult to operate.

Rear wheel drive: The rear wheel drive gives the person the sensation that s/he is being pushed forward. The larger wheels are in the back. There is a greater sense of control at the sacrifice of agility since the wheelchair needs more room to make a full rotation. Anti-tippers may be needed because the wheelchair may have a tendency to tip with acceleration and inclines.

Mid-wheel drive: The mid-wheel drive has a tight turning radius and requires good upper body balance to operate. It doesn't perform well on rough terrain and is best on hard, flat surfaces.

Scooters

Advantages: Scooters are less expensive than power wheelchairs and some believe that they are more socially acceptable than a power wheelchair in the American culture. Like the power wheelchair, they conserve cardiovascular and muscular energy. However, when compared to the power wheelchair, the scooter is not able to meet complex positioning needs including tilt or recline and custom headrests and backrests. It is a good option for older adults who would not otherwise be able to engage in community tasks due to limited mobility and those who may be in the early stages of a disease such as multiple sclerosis. Scooters can be dismantled and put into a car trunk, but they are heavy. There is a chain hoist that can be attached to the inside of a car trunk to lift, swing, and lower the scooter into the trunk. The scooter does have some unique extras that the manual wheelchair and power wheelchair do not have such as a basket on the front or back to transport items and the ability to place items on the running board.

Disadvantages: In contrast with the power wheelchair, the client requires good arm strength and adequate hand use to steer the scooter and operate buttons. The client also has to have good trunk control due to limited seat support. Although different seating options are available, they are not as extensive or adaptable to meet complex trunk and upper extremity needs. Scooters don't work well at tables and desks because the front steering system gets in the way. Like the power wheelchair, the scooter requires the use of a battery and does not provide cardiopulmonary or muscular exercise, possibly leading to deconditioning. Scooters cannot be tipped backwards to climb curbs and other physical obstacles, therefore the environment must be fully accessible.

Components of the Seat

Cushions

The primary function of a cushion is to prevent pressure ulcers and maintain postural stability. There are four main types of cushions:

Foam: Foam cushions are inexpensive. The therapist can easily carve out areas in the cushion to decrease pressure on sensitive areas that are at a high risk for skin breakdown or that currently have skin breakdown. Foam cushions, however, wear out quickly (become flat). When the cushion becomes flat, it will not meet the comfort needs of the client and can result in secondary problems, such as skin breakdowns. Foam cushions come in a range of densities.

Gel: Gel cushions have gel fluids placed in pouches inside the cushion. They easily adapt to pressure distribution needs and clients say they are comfortable. Gel cushions are heavier than foam cushions and they do not absorb impact well resulting in bouncing up and down. Some gel cushions can bottom out, so look for cushions that have separate compartments in the cushion if weight makes this an issue. Gel cushions can leak.

Air/dry floatation: Support is maintained by air. One example is the Roho cushion with small, interconnected rubber balloons arranged in rows. They are waterproof, but they are less stable than other cushions. Air leaks can occur so air pressure should be checked frequently. They are lightweight.

Honeycomb: Honeycomb cushions have individual beehive like cells. The skin is kept cooler. The cushions are lightweight, shock absorbent, and washable. There is no risk of leakage, and they provide good support. They have a low profile appearance. They are relatively new, and no weaknesses have been noted so far.

Seat Width (also referred to as chair width)

This is the width of the wheelchair seat. If it is too wide, it can be difficult to manipulate the hand rims (wheels) on a manual wheelchair. It also promotes poor posture and adds more weight to the wheelchair.

Seat Depth

This is the length of the seat (front to back). If it is too shallow (short) it places increased pressure on the buttocks and lessens stability. If it is too deep, the client will not be able to rest effectively against the back of the seat. It will also add more weight to the wheelchair.

Seat Height

This is how high the seat is off the ground. The correct seat height depends on the length of the client's legs, clearance needed for footrests or running board, the integration of the seat height in standard environment to match things like desk and table heights, personal preferences of the client, and any restrictions due to the build of the wheelchair.

Seat Angle (manual wheelchairs)

The seat does not have to be parallel to the floor; it can be angled forward ("seat dump") or backward ("squeeze"). Clients with higher-level spinal cord injuries who lack good trunk and upper body control may benefit from a seat that is angled back because it keeps them back in the wheelchair for added safety. However it can also make transferring in and out of the wheelchair more difficult, as well as possibly promote secondary problems with the back or skin breakdowns.

Back Support

There are many types of wheelchair backs including rigid, cloth, and vinyl. Cloth and vinyl backs fold down on a rigid wheelchair or fold in half vertically on a cross-brace wheelchair. Rigid backs are removable and come in a variety of heights, widths, lateral supports, and curves to meet the needs of the client. Scooters do not have separate back supports because the seat is a one-piece unit.

Back Angle

Some seat backs are adjustable. Although upright is usually desirable, the person's disability and positioning needs may make an angled back or tilt/recline back optimal.

Components of Propulsion

Push Handles (wheelchairs only)

Push handles are small handles that protrude from the top back of a manual or power wheelchair. If the back of the wheelchair is low so that it only comes up to the middle of the client's back (a common feature of manual rigid wheelchairs) push handles interfere when the client propels the wheelchair because they are hit by the back of the upper arm. Hence the wheelchair may not have push handles. Push handles are helpful in case the client needs assistance. Push handles can also provide support for the client who has poor trunk control and needs to lean forward. S/he can hook one arm around a push handle and lean forward with the other arm to retrieve an item.

Tires

Tires that are air-filled are called pneumatic tires. They provide a comfortable ride. However, they puncture easily and often need to be replaced. Clients with pneumatic tires must be able to independently fix a flat tire and need to keep a patch kit, inner tube, and tools on the wheelchair in case of an emergency. Solid rubber tires have a rougher ride but they never go flat. They are heavier than pneumatic tires. Rubber or foam filled inserts are available for tires instead of having a solid rubber tire. These tires won't go flat since no air is required and they have a softer ride than a solid rubber tire.

Power Wheels (manual wheelchair)

Power wheels, the back wheels on a manual wheelchair, come in different diameters. They must be ergonomically correct in relation to the seat height because too high a wheel can overstrain arms and be difficult to start propulsion. Too low a wheel can result in decreased force to propel the wheelchair. Spoked wheels are heavier than molded wheels and require adjustment for wheel balance. Molded wheels take more of an impact than spoked wheels and do not require adjustments.

Wheel placement: Power wheels can be moved more forward or backwards with an axle adjustment. The more forward the back wheels, the tippier the wheelchair. The more backward the wheels, the more stable the wheelchair. For the client to learn how to do wheelies and/or slight caster tips, the wheels will need to be placed slightly forward. Start out with wheels in a more stable position and move them forward to the optimal position. You don't want the wheelchair to be too tippy for safety reasons. The weight and height of the person also determine how to position the wheels to achieve optimal stability and tip. In addition, the therapist considers the placement of the wheels in relation to the stress on the upper body to propel the wheelchair. If they are too far back it will be difficult for the client to push the wheels.

Camber: Camber is the angle of the wheels. The wheels tilt in at the top and out at the bottom. The more camber a wheel has, the wider the total width of the wheelchair, which can make it difficult to maneuver through doorways and tight spaces. Camber provides the wheelchair with a greater wheelbase and therefore gives the wheelchair greater turning and lateral stability, for example when the client is leaning over the side. Some wheelchairs have a fixed camber while others are adjustable. Sport wheelchairs can have extreme camber so that the person does not fall out of the wheelchair easily. Everyday wheelchairs may have a slight camber to accommodate normal living movements. Camber adjustments can also cause the wheels to toe-in or toe-out making the wheelchair more difficult to steer and propel.

Hand rims (manual wheelchair)

Like power wheels, hand rims come in different diameters. Hand rims are usually made out of metal and are attached to the outside of the power wheel. The client uses the hand rims to propel the wheelchair. The smaller the diameter, the more force the client needs to apply to propel the wheelchair. Most people who use wheelchairs push the wheelchair using the palms and heels of the hand on both the hand rim and the tire. This technique requires less force to propel the wheelchair and puts less stress on the hands. The problem with this technique is that clients can injure their hands because tires can pick up glass and other debris that could cut the skin. Clients who find this technique helpful must wear fingerless gloves (see Push Gloves later in this section) to protect their hands. For clients who have hand limitations, knobs can be placed on the hand rims. These are short nubs that stick out from the hand rim that allows the client to use the hand to push the wheelchair without the use of fingers. Therapists can also wrap hand rims in TheraBands, which make the hand rim easier to grip. There are also devices that allow the user to push with only one hand.

Casters

Casters are the small wheels on the front of manual wheelchairs. They come in a variety of sizes and materials. Smaller casters are usually made of solid plastic. They have good agility and turn easily, but they have a bumpy ride and don't roll over obstacles easily, which means that the client will have to do a mini-wheelie to get over door thresholds and small cracks and may get stuck on sidewalk cracks or street grates. Sudden and unexpected stops from a caster that gets stuck can cause injury if the person is thrown from the wheelchair. Pneumatic casters are air filled. They give a soft ride, overcome small obstacles easily, and are not as hard on the wheelchair frame, therefore adding extra years to the life of the wheelchair. However, they can puncture easily. Solid rubber casters are another option. They come in a variety of sizes. They are a softer ride than the small plastic casters and will not go flat like pneumatic casters.

Control Systems (power wheelchair and scooter)

Power wheelchairs can be controlled by a joystick, sip and puff (breath controlled), chin control, or head control. Scooters are controlled by a two handed front steering system.

Batteries (power wheelchair and scooter)

There are two types of wheelchair and scooter batteries (gel cell and wet cell). How long and far the wheelchair will go depends on battery size and many other factors: weight of the wheelchair, wheel size, surfaces negotiated, amount of equipment on the wheelchair, extra weight carried on wheelchair (e.g., heavy school backpack), and driving style (stop and go really fast, slow and steady pace). Both types of batteries must be charged and well maintained at all times.

Gel cell: Gel cell batteries require less maintenance than wet cell batteries, but they don't last as long as a wet cell battery and they are slightly less powerful.

Lead cell/wet cell: Wet cell batteries can be charged more times than a gel cell battery so they have a longer life span. They are popular among active users who would otherwise have to replace expensive batteries more often. They generally have about 10% more power (amp hours) than gel cell batteries.

Components for Safety

Wheel Locks (manual and power wheelchair, scooter)

Wheel locks or brakes are used to keep the wheelchair from moving. They are especially important when getting in or out of the wheelchair and when parked on an incline. There are a variety of wheelchair brakes. The most typical are mounted to the front of the wheel. However, for the person using a manual wheelchair, they can get in the way when propelling the wheelchair and hurt the thumb. Wheelchair brake extensions are also available. This is a long tube that slips over the top of the brake, requiring less strength to engage and disengage the brake. The client may want to consider scissor brakes that disappear under the wheelchair when disengaged so they do not get in the way when propelling the wheelchair. This type of brake, however, can be challenging for clients who have difficulty with trunk control and balance as it requires the client to lean farther down compared to a standard front-locking brake. Brakes can also be mounted to the back of the wheel.

Brakes will need adjustment from time to time because they can become loose or misaligned. If the wheelchair has pneumatic tires, brakes should be adjusted when the tires are at their correct tire pressure. If brakes become less effective, tires may need to be filled. The client can also request two different types of brakes and remove one or the other as needed, for example removing standard front locking brakes and using the scissor brakes when playing a sport. Some power wheelchair locks come on automatically when there is no weight on the seat of the wheelchair. This feature prevents clients from falling when they transfer into or out of a wheelchair without setting the brakes. It is especially useful for clients with cognitive deficits.

Power wheelchairs have a locking mechanism that is usually found in the middle of the back wheels. A small round metal plate sits inside the wheel and, when turned in a certain direction, will put the wheelchair in manual or power mode. Manual mode allows the wheelchair to be pushed by another person. Power wheelchairs and scooters do not have manual locks. The wheels lock when the wheelchair or scooter is turned off. The seat can be locked on a scooter. For example, the client can swivel the scooter seat to the right and then lock it in place so that it does not move when standing or transferring.

Anti-Tippers (manual and power wheelchairs)

Anti-tippers are downward-sloped attachments that click into the lever bars. The lever bars are the two bars that extend out the back of the wheelchair between the two wheels. The anti-tippers are easily removable or can be flipped up out of the way. Depending on the person's agility and skill, some clients can do this themselves while others require the assistance of another to remove or flip the anti-tippers. They resemble the shape of a half moon, round part down towards the ground. They prevent the wheelchair from tipping backwards. This is a good safety precaution for clients who have a tendency to tip backwards. They can also be an obstacle and annoyance for the independent person who needs to tip the wheelchair back to overcome obstacles, such as bumping up a curb. If the client typically has a helper with him/her and would require the assistance of another to overcome such obstacles, it is better to err on the side of safety and opt for the anti-tipper bars. Anti-tippers can be designed to be one inch or more from the ground so different clearances can be achieved. This way a client who feels safer with anti-tippers but needs to tip the wheelchair back a maximum of three inches to overcome obstacles in his/her community can have anti-tippers with a four-inch clearance.

Grade Aids (manual wheelchair)

A device that resembles the shape of a half moon that attaches below the wheel lock. They are easily locked and unlocked in the same manner as wheel locks. When locked, it prevents the wheel from rolling backwards. This is especially helpful for clients who lack the strength or hand function to overcome inclines (e.g., multiple sclerosis, high-level spinal cord injury with minimum hand and arm involvement).

Seatbelt (manual and power wheelchairs)

Although every wheelchair should have a seatbelt, some of them do not. The client may also choose not to wear it or remove it from the wheelchair. Seatbelts are a vital component of the wheelchair. Should the wheelchair come to an abrupt stop, the client can be thrown from the wheelchair resulting in serious injury. The seatbelt also provides additional trunk support.

Components for Arms and Legs

Armrests (manual and power wheelchairs, scooter)

Armrests are helpful for many reasons. They help hold the seat cushion in place, offer support and stability, help with changing position in the wheelchair and performing weight shifts, and provide an extra handle to maintain balance when reaching for an item with one arm. Armrests can also get in the way. If they are too long, the client may have difficulty propelling the wheelchair or using a desk or table because the armrests bump up against the table edge preventing the client from getting close enough to the table. There are many different types of armrests: standard upholstered armrests in various lengths, flip-up armrests that swing up and behind the wheelchair so there is no need to manually remove the armrests when transferring or using a table, tubular armrests that look sleek and modern (although they aren't as comfortable as standard armrests), and molded or sculpted armrests that are specially designed to provide arm support for clients who lack full upper body function, as in a high level spinal cord injury. Armrests should not be too high or too low. Too high can cause pain in the neck and shoulders and too low can encourage a slumping posture resulting in back problems.

Footrests (manual and power wheelchairs; scooter has a running board)

There are two different kinds of footrests.

Fixed leg rests: Fixed leg rests (also referred to as roll bars) are part of the wheelchair frame and do not swing out of the way. They can be found on some pediatric power wheelchairs, but are most common on manual rigid frame wheelchairs. Fixed leg rests are sleek and modern. They tuck the feet right below or slightly behind the knees, thus shortening the length of the wheelchair. They also act as a roller bar that aids in keeping the wheelchair from tipping forward. Transferring can be a bit cumbersome at first due to the added obstacle, but problems can be overcome. Feet and legs are kept from sliding off the roller bar with a calf strap that wraps behind and in front of the legs (usually with a Velcro closure). Roller bars, like swing away leg rests, can be angled to help keep the feet from sliding off.

Swing away leg rests: Swing away leg rests are two single footrests (one for each foot) and swing out to the side of the wheelchair. They are used on manual and power wheelchairs. They are removable. Swing away leg rests can be moved out of the client's way. Therefore, they can be advantageous for transferring because the client can place his/her feet flat on the floor unobstructed. Removing the leg rests also lowers the client's knees so s/he can fit under a table by placing the feet flat on the floor instead of on the leg rests. Swing away leg rests lengthen the wheelchair due to the space needed for the footplates.

Both leg rests can also be narrowed, depending on the style of the wheelchair, thus keeping the legs closer together and giving the client a tighter turning radius. Footrests must be high enough to accommodate uneven surfaces and small obstacles, such as a raised sidewalk block, but not so high that they create inappropriate knee and hip flexion.

Miscellaneous Components and Accessories

Suspensions (manual wheelchair)

Some rigid and cross-brace manual wheelchairs have suspension systems (springs) that allow better wheel contact with the ground when going over uneven surfaces, as well as a more comfortable, softer ride.

Clothing Guards (manual and power wheelchairs)

Clothing guards are typically a flat plastic piece that partially covers the side of the armrest. This prevents clothing from coming into contact with the wheels.

Cup Holders

There are various types of cup holders that attach onto the wheelchair armrest or frame. A bottle of water could also be easily kept in a backpack on the back of the wheelchair. Water is important for hydration and taking medication.

Pouches

Backpack-like pouches for the back, side, or underside of a wheelchair or scooter.

Crutch Holders (manual wheelchair, but could be put on a power wheelchair or scooter)

This is a small metal tray that attaches to one of the tipper bars and a Velcro strap that wraps around the push handle. The crutches sit on the tray and the Velcro strap goes through the crutch handles to hold them in place.

Toolkits (manual and power wheelchair, scooter)

Small toolkits have the tools and equipment needed to perform light repairs on a wheelchair or scooter. Clients can also ask the wheelchair vender for a list of recommended tools and supplies to be purchased independently.

Push Gloves or Cuffs (manual wheelchair)

These are gloves that the client wears when pushing a wheelchair. They are often fingerless. Some have a thumb protector. The palm of the glove usually has a patch of leather, suede, or rubber that gives extra friction for pushing the wheelchair. Weight training gloves from a local sporting goods store are commonly preferred.

Backpacks

Backpacks can be purchased at a local store. The arm straps on the backpack can be hooked around the push handles of the wheelchair so that the backpack hangs on the back of the wheelchair. Choose a backpack that is waterproof, won't show a lot of dirt (a dark color), and one that has zippers and pockets that match the client's needs and abilities. For example, if a client has limited hand function, choose a backpack with large pockets and zippers. Small pockets may be difficult for this client to get his/her hand inside and a backpack with a drawstring may be difficult to operate. Look at the number of pockets in the backpack. How many pockets does the client need (e.g., one for cathing supplies, one for change of clothes, one for a cell phone)? Consider the weight of the backpack and the fashion statement that it makes.

Weight

The weight of a wheelchair varies greatly depending on the type and extent of materials used, the weight of the cushion, and the type of wheels chosen. Spoked wheels are heavier than molded wheels. Solid rubber tires are heavier than pneumatic tires.

Power wheelchair: 100-180 pounds (250-500 pound capacity). This excludes the batteries, which typically weigh about 75 pounds.

Scooter: approximately 150 pounds (300-pound capacity).

Standard cross-brace aluminum wheelchair: approximately 41-50 pounds (250-pound capacity) and 46 pounds (350-pound capacity).

Standard cross-brace lightweight wheelchair: 28-36 pounds (250-pound capacity).

Standard rigid frame wheelchair: 19-27 pounds (250-pound capacity).

Titanium rigid frame wheelchair: approximately 18 pounds (250-pound capacity).

Sport wheelchair: 15-27 pounds (250-pound capacity).

General Maintenance

Manual Wheelchair

Chair: At least once a week clean the wheelchair with a mild detergent and soft cloth.

Cushion: If washable, wash the cushion or cushion cover at least once a week. Wash more frequently if required due to soiling.

Frame: Look for any cracks, scratches, sharp edges, loosened bolts, or thin material on the cloth seat or back, foam tubing on handgrips, etc.

Tires: Are they worn? Do they need to be replaced? If pneumatic, check the tire pressure.

Casters and wheels: Remove any debris that may be caught around casters or power wheels.

Axles and joints: Do they need lubricating?

Wheels: Do they spin freely? Do bearings need to be replaced?

Spoke tension: Check at least monthly.

Casters and forks: Should not shake with propulsion.

Alignment: Do all four wheels touch the ground? Does the wheelchair need to be aligned?

Wheel locks: Do they lock tightly? Do they need adjustment?

Power Wheelchairs and Scooters

Become familiar with the sound of the wheelchair. Should anything sound "off," a full inspection of the wheelchair should be performed. This includes checking all the components listed for the manual wheelchair, as well as additional components special to the power wheelchair and scooter including electrical connections, belts, batteries, and tilt/recline mechanisms.

Fitting

Clients are fitted for a wheelchair or scooter by the vendor and the physical therapist.

Authorization

A physician's order, a certificate of medical necessity (CMN), and supporting documentation that justify prescription of a wheelchair are required.

Benefits

Using a wheelchair or scooter provides an opportunity for mobility. Mobility enables people to engage in life tasks for health. However, inappropriate use of a wheelchair or scooter can cause physical health deterioration. Clients should avoid using a wheelchair more than recommended or using a scooter or wheelchair that provides more assistance than the client needs.

Design Challenges

The wheelchair and scooter have many parts and every part has many different kinds of designs. It is impossible to discuss all of the design challenges of the wheelchair and scooter, however the primary challenges revolve around material, weight, strength, and durability; usability; cost; reliability; power and speed; and flexibility and adjustability of parts and accessories to meet the individual needs of the client.

References

Kaye, S., Taewoon, K., & LaPlante, M. P. (2002). Wheelchair use in the United States. Disability Statistics Center. Accessed via website http://dsc.ucsf.edu/publication.php?pub_id=1&section_id=1.

Kilkens, O. J., Dallmeijer, A. J., de Witte, L. P., van der Woude, L. H., & Post, M. W. (2004). The wheelchair circuit: Construct validity and responsiveness of a test to assess manual wheelchair mobility in persons with spinal cord injury. *Archives of Physical Medicine and Rehabilitation, 85,* 424-431.

Appendix A. Common Clinical Symbols and Abbreviations

Symbols and abbreviations are commonly used in clinical documentation. The following is a list of common symbols and abbreviations as they are used in many healthcare facilities. Prior to using any of the symbols and abbreviations below consult with your employer, as every agency should have a list of approved symbols and abbreviations that limits the symbols and abbreviations allowed for use in agency documentation. An approved symbol and abbreviation list ensures that everyone in the agency is using the same symbols and abbreviations to decrease confusion and increase consistency.

Functional Assessment Scale (FAS)

No Helper

Level of Assistance 7
Complete Independence: Ⓘ
 Client: 100%, timely, safely
 Therapist: 0%

Level of Assistance 6
Modified Independence: Mod Ⓘ
 Client: 100% Requires increased time or device
 Therapist: 0%

Helper

Level of Assistance 5
Supervision: Ⓢ
 Client: 100%
 Therapist: No hands on assistance. Requires auditory, gestural, or demonstrative cues (no tactile cues — tactile cues are min assist).

Level of Assistance 5
Close Supervision: cl Ⓢ
 Client: 100%
 Therapist: Within a few feet of the client

Level of Assistance 5
Distant Supervision: d Ⓢ
 Client: 100%
 Therapist: Within a few yards of the client

Level of Assistance 4
Minimal Assistance: Min Ⓐ
 Client: 75-99% of the work
 Therapist: 1-25% of the work

Level of Assistance 3
Moderate Assistance: Mod Ⓐ
 Client: 50-74% of the work
 Therapist: 26-50% of the work

Level of Assistance 2
Maximal Assistance: Max Ⓐ
 Client: 25-49% of the work
 Therapist: 51-75% of the work

Level of Assistance 1
Total Assist or Dependent Ⓓ
 Client: 0-24% of the work
 Therapist: 76-100% of the work

Symbols

~	approximately
@	at
δ	change
↓	decrease
↓'d	decreased
↓'ing	decreasing
♀	female
√	flexion
>	greater than
≥	greater than or equal to
↑	increase
↑'d	increased
↑'ing	increasing
<	less than

$\leq$	less than or equal to
♂	male
'	minutes or feet
−	negative
⊖	negative
#	number
‖	parallel bars
%	percent
1°	primary
?	question
?'s	questions
2°	secondary to (due to)
"	seconds or inches

Weight Bearing Status (WBS)

FWB	Full Weight Bearing (100%)
NWB	Non-Weight Bearing (0%)
PWB	Partial Weight Bearing (~ 50%)
TDWB	Touch Down Weight Bearing (~ 25%)
TTWB	Touch Toe Weight Bearing (~ 25%)
UWB	Usual Weight Bearing
WBAT	Weight Bearing As Tolerated

Abbreviations

ā	before
Ⓐ	assistance
AAC	augmentative/alternative communication
AAD	appropriate assistive device
abs	abdominals
ac	before meals
ACD	augmentative communication device
ADL	activities of daily living
adm	admission
AEA	above elbow amputation
AFO	ankle foot orthosis
AIDS	acquired immune deficiency syndrome
AKA	above knee amputation
AMA	against medical advice
amb	ambulation
amt	amount
ant	anterior
A&O	alert and oriented
approx.	approximately
AROM	active range of motion
AS	air splint
ASAP	as soon as possible
as tol	as tolerated
attn	attention
ax cxs	axillary crutches

Ⓑ	bilateral
B&B	bowel and bladder/bed and bath
BEA	below elbow amputation
BKA	below knee amputation
BI	brain injury
bid	twice a day
B/L	bilateral
BLE	bilateral lower extremities
BM	bowel movement
BP	blood pressure
BPM	beats per minute
BUE	bilateral upper extremities
bx	biopsy

c̄	with
CA	cancer
CAD	coronary artery disease
CAT	computerized axial tomography
cath	catheter
cc	chief complaint
CG	contact guard
CHF	congestive heart failure
CHI	closed head injury
chol	cholesterol
CI	community integration
c/o	complains of
cont	continue
COPD	chronic obstructive pulmonary disease
CPM	continuous passive motion
CPR	cardiopulmonary resuscitation
CVA	cerebrovascular accident
cx	cancel

D&A	drug and alcohol
dbp	diastolic blood pressure
dc	demonstrative cue
d/c	discharge
DJD	degenerative joint disease
DM	diabetes mellitus
DNR	do not resuscitate
DOA	dead on arrival
DRG	drug
drsg	dressing
DVT	deep vein thrombosis
dx	diagnosis

EC	energy conservation
ECF	extended care facility

EEG	electroencephalogram		IBW	ideal body weight
e.g.	example		Ience	independence
EKG	electrocardiogram		IEP	individualized education plan
ELOS	estimated length of stay		I'ly	independently
EOB	edge of bed		I&O	intake and output
EOM	edge of mat		Ind.	individual
ER	emergency room		Indiv.	individual
ESL	English as second language		IP	inpatient
ETOH	alcohol		ITP	individual treatment plan
eval	evaluation		IV	intravenous
ex	exercise			
ext	extension		JC	joint commission
F	female		KAFO	knee ankle foot orthosis
FF	full flight (of stairs)			
flex	flexion		Ⓛ	left
freq	frequency		Lb	pound
FT	full time		LBQC	large base quad cane
f/u	follow up		LD	learning disability
fx	fracture		LE	lower extremity
			LLE	left lower extremity
gc	gestural cue		LLQ	left lower quadrant (usually of the eye)
grp	group		lg	large
GSW	gunshot wound		LOB	loss of balance
			LOC	locus of control; loss/level of consciousness
HA	headaches		LOS	length of stay
Hb	hemoglobin		LPT	low pivot transfer
Hbg	hemoglobin		LRE	least restrictive environment
hemi	one side (e.g., hemiplegia, hemianopsia)		LTC	long-term care
HEP	home exercise program		LTG	long-term goal
HHA	household activities		LTM	long-term memory
HHC	home healthcare		LUE	left upper extremity
HHD	household distance (ambulation)		LUQ	left upper quadrant
HHM	household mobility			
HIV	human immunodeficiency virus		m	male
HNP	herniated nucleus pulposus (herniated disc)		MAFO	modified or molded ankle foot orthosis
h/o	history of		max	maximum
HOH	hard of hearing		MDS	minimum data set
H&P	history and physical		MET	metabolic equivalent
HPI	history of present illness		MH	mental health
hr	hour		MI	myocardial infarction or mental illness
HR	heart rate		min	minimal
hs	bedtime; hour of sleep (hora somni)		mins	minutes
HS	high school		mod	moderate
ht	height		MR	mental retardation (term no longer used)
HTN	hypertension		MR/DD	mental retardation/developmentally disabled
HW	hemi-walker		MVA	motor vehicle accident
hx	history			
			n/a	not applicable

NBQC	narrow base quad cane
neg	negative
NH	nursing home
NKA	no known allergies
NKDA	no known drug allergies
NL	normal limits
NOK	next of kin
NOS	not otherwise specified
NPO	nothing by mouth (nil per os)
NR	do not repeat
nsg	nursing
NT	not tested, not tender
N&V	nausea and vomiting
OOB	out of bed
op	outpatient
Ox3	oriented to person, place, and time
$\bar{p}$	after
P	pulse
pc	after meals
p.c.	after meals
PH	past history
PMH	past medical history
PM&R	physical medicine and rehabilitation
po	by mouth/orally
p.o.	by mouth/orally
post	after
post op	postoperative
PROM	passive range of motion
prn	as needed or as necessary
pt	patient
PTA	prior to admission
PW	platform walker
Px	prognosis
q	every
qa	quality assessment
qd	every day
qh	every hour
q2h	every two hours (number can vary)
qhs	every night at bedtime
qid	four times a day
qn	every night
qod	every other day
qoh	every other hour
qpm	every night
Ⓡ	right

re:	regarding
RLE	right lower extremity
RLQ	right lower quadrant
R/O	rule out
ROM	range of motion
RR	respiratory rate
RUE	right upper extremity
RUQ	right upper quadrant
RW	rolling walker
Rx	prescription
Ⓢ	supervision
$\bar{s}$	without
SBP	systolic blood pressure
SBQC	small base quad cane
SH	social history
SIB	self-injurious behavior
SNF	skilled nursing facility
SOB	shortness of breath
S/P	status post
SPC	single point cane
SPT	stand-pivot transfer
SROM	self range of motion
SSDI	social security disability income
SSI	supplemental security income
stat	right away; immediately
STG	short-term goal
STM	short-term memory
SW	standard walker
Sx	surgery
Sxs	symptoms
sz	seizure
TBA	to be assessed
TBD	to be determined
TBT	transfer board transfer
TC	tactile cue
temp	temperature
TENS	transcutaneous electrical nerve stimulation
Ther/Ex	therapeutic exercise
Thpy	therapy
TID	three times a day
TLSO	thoracic lumbar sacral orthosis
TO	telephone order
TTY	teletypewriter
Tx	treatment
Txfer	transfer
UE	upper extremity

URI	upper respiratory infection
UTI	urinary tract infection
VC	verbal cue or visual cue
VH	visual hallucination
via	by way of
VO	verbal order
VS	vital signs
VTO	verbal telephone order
WBQC	wide base quad cane
w/c	wheelchair
WFL	within functional limits
WNL	within normal limits
w/o	without
WS	weight shift

wt	weight
x	times (e.g., 3x means three times)
y/n	yes/no
y/o	year old (e.g., 3 y/o means three year old)
yr	year

References

burlingame, j and Skalko, T. (2001). *Idyll Arbor's Therapy Dictionary* (2nd ed.). Ravensdale: WA: Idyll Arbor.

burlingame, j. & Blaschko, T. (2009). *Assessment Tools for Recreation Therapy and Related Fields* (4th ed.). Ravensdale: WA: Idyll Arbor.

Free Dictionary (2015). *Acronyms and abbreviations*. Retrieved from http://acronyms.thefreedictionary.com.

United Spinal Cord Resource Center (n.d.). Alphabetical listing of medical abbreviations. Retrieved from www.spinalcord.org/resource-center/askus/index.php?pg=kb.page&id=1413.

Appendix B. Anatomical Orientation and Positioning

In anatomy, certain terms are used to denote orientation. For example, a structure may be horizontal, as opposed to vertical. Anatomical positioning is defined by looking at a subject facing you with arms down by his/her side and palms facing forward. Some of the terms of anatomic orientation are as follows:

Abduction: The process of moving a body part away from midline.

Adduction: The process of moving a body part toward the midline.

Anterior: The front, as opposed to the posterior.

Anteroposterior: From front to back, as opposed to posteroanterior.

Caudal: Toward the feet (or tail in embryology), as opposed to cranial.

Cranial: Toward the head, as opposed to caudal.

Deep: Away from the exterior surface or further into the body, as opposed to superficial.

Distal: Further from the beginning, as opposed to proximal; further from the torso.

Dorsal: The back, as opposed to ventral.

Extension: Straightening or unbending a flexed limb. Moving two ends of a jointed part away from each other.

Flexion: Moving two ends of a joint closer together.

Horizontal: Parallel to the ground, as opposed to vertical.

Inferior: Below, as opposed to superior; toward the feet.

Lateral: Toward the left or right side of the body, as opposed to medial; away from the middle (medial).

Medial: In the middle or inside, as opposed to lateral; towards the midline that divides left and right.

Posterior: The back or behind, as opposed to the anterior.

Posteroanterior: From back to front, as opposed to anteroposterior

Pronation: Rotation of the forearm and hand so that the palm is down (and the corresponding movement of the foot and leg with the sole down), as opposed to supination.

Prone: With the front or ventral surface downward (lying face down), as opposed to supine.

Proximal: Toward the beginning, as opposed to distal; closer to the torso.

Sagittal: A vertical plane passing through the standing body from front to back. The mid-sagittal, or median plane, splits the body into left and right halves.

Superficial: On the surface or shallow, as opposed to deep.

Superior: Above, as opposed to inferior; toward the head.

Supination: Rotation of the forearm and hand so that the palm is upward (and the corresponding movement of the foot and leg), as opposed to pronation.

Supine: With the back or dorsal surface downward (lying face up), as opposed to prone.

Transverse: A horizontal plane passing through the standing body parallel to the ground.

Ventral: Pertaining to the abdomen, as opposed to dorsal.

Vertical: Upright, as opposed to horizontal.

Index

S

About the Editor

Heather Porter, Ph.D., CTRS, is a faculty member in the Rehabilitation Sciences Department at Temple University in Philadelphia, PA. She has a dual BS in Recreational Therapy and Sport/Recreation Management, an MS in Counseling Psychology with a Certificate in Marriage and Family Counseling, and a Ph.D. in Health Studies (Recreational Therapy and Public Health). She has a strong clinical background in inpatient and outpatient physical rehabilitation and has been teaching recreational therapy in higher education for over 18 years. She is committed to strengthening recreational therapy research and disseminating research information to practitioners, consumers, payers, legislators, and the general public. Most notably, she coordinates an annual Recreational Therapy Evidence-Based Practice Conference and maintains an open-access database for recreational therapy research and resources that has been utilized by over 60 countries (www.rtwiseowls.com). Dr. Porter also provides consultations to recreational therapy academic programs on how to integrate evidence-based research into academic coursework, and is recognized as a leader in the community seeking to integrate the World Health Organization's *International Classification of Functioning, Disability, and Health* into healthcare practice.